Veterinary Clinical Pathology

Veterinary Clinical Pathology

Edited by Georgiana Baldwin

AMERICAN
MEDICAL PUBLISHERS
www.americanmedicalpublishers.com

American Medical Publishers,
41 Flatbush Avenue,
1st Floor, New York,
NY 11217, USA

Visit us on the World Wide Web at:
www.americanmedicalpublishers.com

ISBN: 978-1-63927-524-3

Cataloging-in-Publication Data

Veterinary clinical pathology / edited by Georgiana Baldwin.
p. cm.
Includes bibliographical references and index.
ISBN 978-1-63927-524-3
1. Veterinary clinical pathology. 2. Veterinary medicine--Diagnosis.
3. Veterinary pathology. I. Baldwin, Georgiana.
SF772.6 .V48 2022
636.089 607--dc23

Table of Contents

Preface

Veterinary pathology is a field of medicine which focuses on the diagnosis of diseases in animals by examining tissues and body fluids. It deals with the diagnosis of diseases in all kinds of animals such as food-producing animals, zoo animals and companion animals. It also plays an important role in drug discovery and safety. Veterinary pathology is divided into two branches, namely, clinical pathology and anatomical pathology. Veterinary clinical pathology focuses on laboratory analysis to diagnose diseases. It makes use of tools from several disciplines such as molecular pathology, microbiology, chemistry and hematology. This book outlines the processes and applications of veterinary clinical pathology in detail. It will provide a fair idea about this discipline and help in developing a better understanding of the latest discoveries and studies in this field. The book is meant for students who are looking for an elaborate reference text on veterinary clinical pathology.

After months of intensive research and writing, this book is the end result of all who devoted their time and efforts in the initiation and progress of this book. It will surely be a source of reference in enhancing the required knowledge of the new developments in the area. During the course of developing this book, certain measures such as accuracy, authenticity and research focused analytical studies were given preference in order to produce a comprehensive book in the area of study.

This book would not have been possible without the efforts of the authors and the publisher. I extend my sincere thanks to them. Secondly, I express my gratitude to my family and well-wishers. And most importantly, I thank my students for constantly expressing their willingness and curiosity in enhancing their knowledge in the field, which encourages me to take up further research projects for the advancement of the area.

Editor

Laboratory investigations into the origin of *Mycoplasma synoviae* isolated from a lesser flamingo (*Phoeniconaias minor*)

Salvatore Catania[1*], Federica Gobbo[1,2], Ana S. Ramirez[3], Davide Guadagnini[4], Elisa Baldasso[1], Maria Luisa Moronato[1,2] and Robin A. J. Nicholas[5]

Abstract

Background: The role of wild birds in the transmission and spread of mycoplasmas is not clear. Up to now different *Mycoplasma* species have been isolated from wild birds many of which are not considered pathogens sensu stricto for domestic flocks. This report describes the first isolation of *Mycoplasma synoviae* in a captive lesser flamingo (*Phoeniconaias minor*) held in a zoo in Italy and the laboratory investigations performed to elucidate its origin. Results showed that the strain was similar to the MS-H vaccine strain using the *vlh*A methods although no vaccination with this product was used in the zoo.

Case presentation: This paper describes investigations into a case in which 10 of 12 adult lesser flamingos (*Phoeniconaias minor*) died after having recently been moved from the Netherlands to a new zoo in Northern Italy. While most of the birds appeared to have died from the stress of movement and poor adaptation to their new environment, *Mycoplasma synoviae*, an important poultry pathogen in the layer and meat industry, was isolated for the first time from the trachea of one animal presenting catarrhal tracheitis and fibrinous airsacculitis. Genetic analysis of the conserved region of the *vlhA* was not able to differentiate the flamingo strain from the MS-H vaccine strain. However differences in the sequences of the *obg* gene of the flamingo and vaccine strain were detected. A test for temperature-sensitivity (*ts*) gave a ts^{-} phenotype for the flamingo strain, in contrast to the ts^{+} status of the MS-H strain. Based on this information and knowing that the flamingos were not vaccinated against *M. synoviae*, it is highly likely that the flamingo was infected with a genetically similar wild strain by contact with infected birds.

Conclusions: This case provides evidence for the potential role of international trade of ornamental birds as a possible route of introduction of new mycoplasma strains between countries, and moreover highlight that *vlh*A gene sequencing was not sufficient to discriminate the wild strain isolated from the flamingo from the MS-H vaccine strain.

Keywords: *Mycoplasma synoviae*, *Vlh*A, Lesser flamingo, *Phoeniconaias minor*, Aereosacculitis

Background

Mycoplasma synoviae, an important pathogen of poultry, can cause respiratory and articular disease, loss of production in the layer and meat industry [1]. In the poultry sector, control of mycoplasmosis is mainly based on the production and maintenance of mycoplasma-free breeders, with high levels of biosecurity measures applied to the flocks.

The role of wild birds in the transmission and spread of mycoplasmas is still unknown, despite the isolation of different *Mycoplasma* species from several avian species [2–8]. These include *M. gallinaceum, M. iners, M. pullorum, M. columbinum, M. anatis, M. sturni, M. buteonis, M. falconis, M. gypis, M. corogypsi* and *M. neophronis*; however none of these are considered pathogens sensu stricto for domestic flocks [9]. In contrast, some reports described infections of wild birds with

* Correspondence: scatania@izsvenezie.it
[1]Istituto Zooprofilattico Sperimentale delle Venezie, viale dell'Universita' 10, Legnaro, 35020 Padova, Italy
Full list of author information is available at the end of the article

pathogenic mycoplasmas of poultry, the most important of which is the infection of house finches (*Carpodacus mexicanus*) with *M. gallisepticum* in North America, causing a severe outbreak of conjunctivitis [10, 11]. However, the strain involved in these outbreaks was genetically different from vaccine, reference or field strains of *M. gallisepticum* isolated from commercial poultry [12].

In an epizootiological study of over 560 wild birds in Spain, *M. synoviae* was isolated from the tracheal and oropharynx samples of one red-legged partridge and three house sparrows [2]. Furthermore, *M. meleagridis* was isolated from captive falcons in the Middle East [13] and from free-ranging birds of prey in Europe [14]. In the latter case, infection could have arisen from a contaminated waste disposal site. Recently some authors have reported for the first time the isolation of *M. iowae* from the Eurasian stone-curlew (*Burhinus oedicnemus*) found in Gran Canaria [15]. More research is needed to understand the role of wild species in the maintenance and spreading of different strains of poultry pathogens species.

The lesser flamingo (*Phoeniconaias minor*) is a gregarious and social bird, very much appreciated by most ornithologists for its elegance. It is mainly distributed in Africa particularly in Tanzania, Kenya, Namibia, Botswana and South Africa, but there are also some breeding sites in south western and southern Asia. Several groups of this species are kept in captivity in the collection of some zoos worldwide [16]. Because of the particular reproductive behaviour of flamingos, breeding in captivity is difficult. In this report we describe the first isolation of *M. synoviae* from a captive lesser flamingo and investigate the variability of strains involved in the infection.

Case presentation

At the end of April 2010 a group of 12 adult lesser flamingos was moved from the Netherlands to a new zoo in northern Italy. These birds were kept in a large zoological garden enriched with a pond. The pond water was changed completely every week and the concrete surfaces were cleaned to avoid any growth of algae. The feeding program applied was considered appropriate for this species and birds received the same diet prescribed by the previous owner with the addition of a specific dietary supplement to supply birds during the critical and stressful phases.

The aviary in which the new birds were introduced already contained other flamingos but no aggressive behaviour or dominance interactions were seen. No other birds were present in the aviary. A few days after introduction, all new birds became sick, showing wet and ruffled feathers, hypomotility, lethargy, apathy, weakness, hypothermia and poor adaptation to the new environment. After 5 days some of the new birds started to die despite the administration of antibiotic treatment with enrofloxacin (100 mg/1 kg of moist food for 14 days) and mortality continued for some days. In total 10 out of 12 flamingos died showing similar clinical signs before death. These clinical signs and mortality are frequent findings in the acclimatizing phase of wild birds to captivity when this was considered common practice.

Materials and methods

Four carcasses of lesser flamingos were submitted to the Diagnostic Unit of Istituto Zooprofilattico Sperimentale delle Venezie, Legnaro (PD, Italy) for necropsy examination and other diagnostic procedures. Several tissues (liver, intestine, lung, air sac and brain) were collected and submitted for bacteriological test; liver, intestine and foot pad lesion were collected for virological investigations and finally air sac was submitted for histopathological and mycological examinations.

The specimens were cultured for routine microbiological procedure both aerobically and anaerobically at 37 ° C. Tracheal swabs were collected from all carcasses and submitted for mycoplasma isolation using a selective broth medium for avian mycoplasmas (Mycoplasma Experience [ME], Reigate, UK) and incubated at 37 ° C under CO_2 conditions for at least 15 days. During this time the cultures were checked daily and when a colour change or turbidity was seen, the broth was inoculated onto ME semi-solid medium, if no change was seen after 15 days, an aliquot of the broth was inoculated onto ME semi-solid medium (ME, Reigate, UK). The inoculated agar plates were checked for mycoplasmas daily for 15 days, after this period samples were considered negative. In order to identify the *Mycoplasma* species, DNAs were extracted from broths of suspect samples, and a 16S-rDNA PCR and denaturing gradient gel electrophoresis (DGGE) method was performed [17]. The results were also confirmed with a specific PCR for *M. synoviae* [18]. Moreover in order to confirm the purity of MS we performed the 16S rDNA identification. Briefly PCR products were cleaned-up using the Performa DTR Ultra 96-well kit (Edge BioSystems, Gaithersburg, MD). Treated PCR products were sequenced using BigDye Terminator v3.1 cycle sequencing kit (Applied Biosystems, Foster City, CA) in a 16-capillary ABI PRISM 3130xl Genetic Analyzer (Applied Biosystems, Foster City, CA). Sequence data were assembled and edited with SeqScape software v2.5 (Applied Biosystems).

In addition, the analysis of the variable lipoprotein haemagglutinin-A (*vlh*A) [19] and the *sp0B*-associated GTP binding (*obg*) [20] genes were applied to the *M. synoviae* isolates in order to detect intraspecific differences.

The following oligonucleotide primers were used in the study: obg-F (5'-GTT GAT AAA GGT GGA CCA G -3'), obg-R (5'-TTA GTG CAG ATA TCT CAA TG-3') [21] and vlhaF (5'-ATT AGC AGC TAG TGC AGT GGC C-3') and vlhaR2 (5'-AGT AAC CGA TCC GCT TAA TGC-3') [19]. The positive amplified PCR products, obtained from both techniques, were then sequenced at the IZS (Venezie) where PCR products were purified with ExoSAP-IT (USB Corporation, Cleveland, OH) and sequenced in both directions using the Big Dye Terminator v3.1 cycle sequencing kit (Applied Biosystems, Foster City, CA). The products of the sequencing reactions were cleaned-up using the Performa DTR Ultra 96-well kit (Edge BioSystems, Gaithers- burg, MD) and analyzed on a 16-capillary ABI PRISM 3130xl Genetic Analyzer (Applied Biosystems, Foster City, CA, USA). Sequence data were assembled and edited with SeqScape software v2.5 (Applied Biosystems). Sequences obtained were submitted to GenBank®(NIH genetic sequence database) resulting respectively in HG4[21]742.1 (*vlhA* gene) and KJ802785 (*obg* gene) accession numbers.

In order to compare the sequences with other Italian *M. synoviae* strains the MEGA 5.05 [22], Bioedit 7.0.0 [23] and BLAST search (http://www.ncbi.nlm.nih.gov/BLAST/) were used.

Once the strain of *M. synoviae* was identified, a differential growth at two different temperature (33°, and 39.5 °C) was performed in order to elucidate its temperature-sensitive phenotype (ts^- or ts^+). The capacity of the strain to replicate at different temperature was established using the *colours changing unit* (CCU) method on a 96-well plate, as described by others [24, 25]. The temperature-sensitive phenotype was attributed when a difference $\geq 10^3$ CCU/ml occurs in the strain cultivated at the two different temperatures.

Moreover we decided to apply an additional test using three different temperatures (30°, 37° and 42 °C) in order to create larger differences between the lower and higher temperature of cultivation. The same test was performed with the MS-H vaccine strain in order to have a control sample.

Finally the *vlhA* and *obg* PCRs were applied also to the isolates grown at the three selected incubation temperatures (30°, 37° and 42 °C). All temperature-sensitive results were summarized in the Table 1.

Discussion

Gross-pathology findings of the four birds included poor state of nutrition, absence of feed in the gastrointestinal tract and severe enteritis with some haemorrhagic intestinal areas. Only one bird (#2) showed catarrhal tracheitis and fibrinous airsacculitis (Fig. 1). All birds showed the same lesions such as chronic and septic lesions of the foot pads with joint enlargement, which were probably related to the bad conditions of the transport cage floor. Bacteriology results revealed pure cultures of *Staphylococcus spp.* (coagulase positive) from the air sac lesion as well as in the affected foot pad and *Escherichia coli* and *Clostridium perfringens* in the gut sample.

Mycological examination of the air sac revealed the presence of *Candida spp.* and *Rhodotorula spp.*. Moreover histopathology of the air sac showed several chronic inflammatory reactions with a necrotic centre surrounded by multinucleated giant cells (Fig. 2).

After only 24 h of incubation, the ME broth culture originating from the tracheal swab of bird #2 showed a colour change and 24 h later typical mycoplasma colonies were observed on the ME agar surface. *M. synoviae* was identified by three techniques: a specific *M. synoviae* PCR [18], a specific *Mycoplasma* DGGE [17] and by sequencing of the16S gene that confirmed only the presence of *Mycoplasma synoviae.* Figure 3 shows the same DGGE profile for the flamingo isolate as other *M. synoviae* field strains, as well as the positive controls including *M. synoviae.*

After applying the PCR for *vlhA* gene to the isolate, a single amplicon was produced. This product was submitted for sequencing and the sequence obtained was compared with *M. synoviae* strains isolated in the previous year in the Italian geographical areas. The strain isolated from the flamingo did not match any Italian *M. synoviae* strains detected previously in our laboratory.

Based on the genotype classification of Bencina et al. [26] the strain was designated as genotype C subtype 3, whereas, according to the recent classification of Hammond et al., [19], the *M. synoviae* isolated from the flamingo represented a new group.

The BLAST search showed a similarity of 100 % with four *M. synoviae* strains, all isolated in Australia (GenBank® Accession n°: DQ661614, AY913827, AY913822, AY913823) (Additional file 1).

Table 1 Temperature-sensitive results. In the table are reported the growth results at different temperature expressed in UCC/ml

	Temperature –sensitive test		Additional temperature test		
	33 °C	39.5 °C	30 °C	37 °C	42 °C
IZSVe/2010/5711	1.8×10^4	3.36×10^5	1.155×10^2	1.155×10^6	1.15×10^2
MS-H	1.8×10^8	1.27×10^2	1.15×10^6	2.255×10^6	0

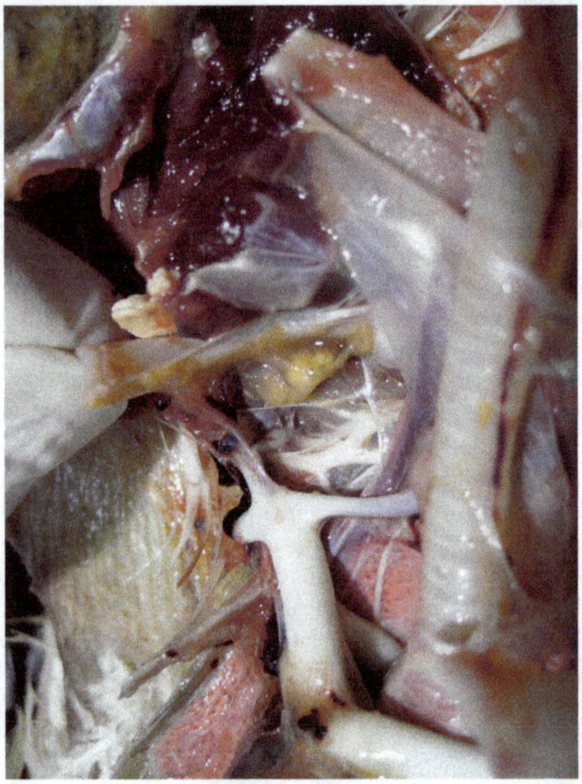

Fig. 1 Gross pathology findings. Fibrinous airsacculitis in bird #2

Moreover the sequence obtained from the strain isolated from the lesser flamingo (IZSVe/2010/5711 GenBank® Accession n°. HG421742.1) had a 100 % of similarity in the *vlhA* gene sequence with MS-H vaccine strain (AB501271) (Fig. 4, Additional file 1).

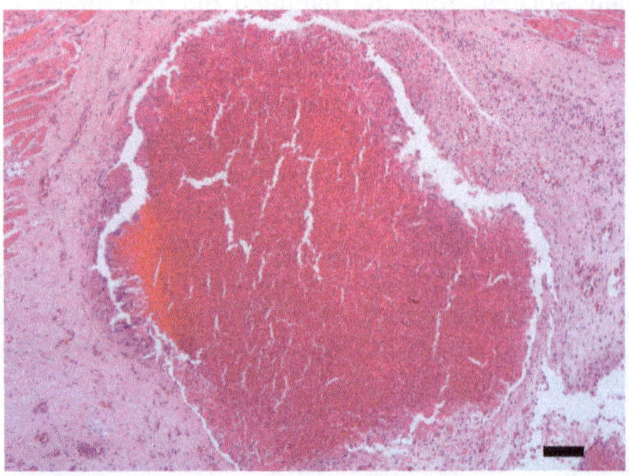

Fig. 2 Histopathology findings. The cervical air sac is severely expanded by a focal nodular lesion composed of abundant heterophils partially surrounded by a single to double layer of macrophages and occasional multinucleated giant cells (heterophilic granuloma), the remaining tissue is diffusely enlarged by strong fibroplasia and moderate lymphoplasmacytic infiltration

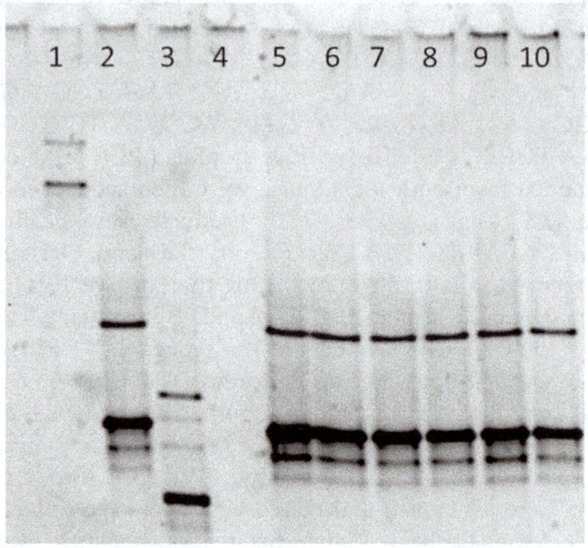

Fig. 3 DGGE gel. In the lanes 1, 2 and 3 there are *Mycoplasma gallisepticum*, *Mycoplasma synoviae* and *Mycoplasma meleagridis* controls respectively. From lane 5 to 10 there are diagnostic samples positive for *Mycoplasma synoviae*: in lane 5 *Mycoplasma synoviae* NCTC (reference strain) and in lane 6 the strain isolated from flamingo (HG421742.1 IZSVE/2010/5711)

The temperature did not affect the variability in both *vlhA* and *obg* sequences (data not shown).

The BLAST analysis of the *obg* gene showed similarity of 99 % with *M. synoviae* strains isolated in Australia (GenBank® Accession n°. KF875993.1, KF875997.1, KF875995, KF875994.19, [21]). Then nucleotide sequence was also compared to those investigated by Shahid et al. 2014 [21] (Additional file 2)

The *obg* gene of flamingo strain (IZSVe/2010/5711 GenBank® Accession n°. KJ802785) differed from others in some nucleotide positions resulting in a different sequence from the MS-H and re-isolates (ts^-, ts^+) and parental strain [21]. Moreover in position 367 the flamingo obg sequence presented a G.

The temperature-sensitive test demonstrated a ts^- phenotype because at 33 °C the titre was 1.8×10^4 CCU/ml, whereas at 39.5 °C the titre was 3.36×10^5 CCU/ml for the flamingo strain. In contrast the same test applied to the MS-H strain resulted in a titre of 1.8×10^8 CCU/ml for the lower temperature, while at 39.5 °C the titre was 1.27×10^2 CCU/ml. The additional test performed with a different range of temperature demonstrated a titre of 1.155×10^2 CCU/ml; 1.15×10^6 CCU/ml; 1.155×10^2 CCU/ml at 30, 37 and 42 °C respectively. Moreover the same test applied at MS-H vaccine strain showed a titre of 1.15×10^6 CCU/ml; 2.255×10^6 CCU/ml at 30 °C, 37 °C respectively, whereas there was no evidence of growth at 42 °C.

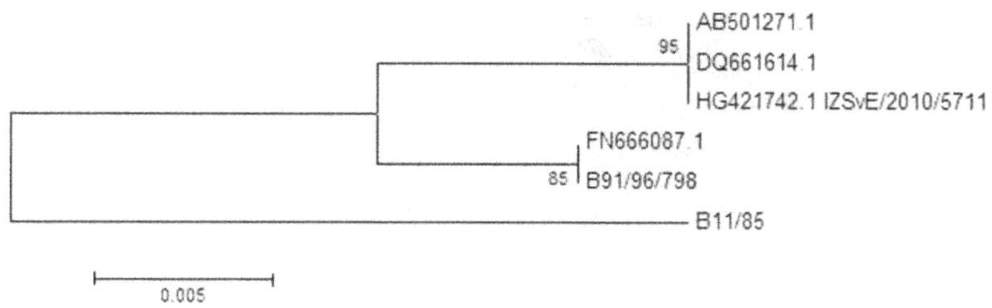

Fig. 4 Phylogenetic analysis of the *vlhA* gene. Basing on the *vlhA* gene, the flamingo isolate (HG421742.1 IZSVE/2010/5711) clusters with the MS-H vaccine strain (AB501271) and the Australian isolate DQ661614. They are all classified as type C - subtype three by Bencina et al. [26] and group 13 by Hammond et al. [19]. The strains FN666087.1 and B91/96/798 are classified as type C3 - group 5; the strain B11/85 is a C1 – group 4. The strains FN666087.1, B91/96/798 and B11/85 have been introduced as examples of different genotypes to build the phylogenetic tree

Conclusions

On the basis of gross pathology and histopathology findings it was concluded that the death of the birds was due to stress caused by movement and poor adaptation to their new captive conditions. The role of *M. synoviae* in this case, however, was not clear; indeed the air sac showed other opportunistic pathogens including fungi and bacteria such as *Staphylococcus spp.*. From the four tracheal samples, only one was positive for *M. synoviae* whereas the other three tracheal swabs were negative for *Mycoplasma spp.*. It is interesting to highlight that the positive sample were isolated from the trachea of the bird with fibrinous airsacculitis. Similar findings have been reported in birds of prey where bacteria and/or fungi were isolated simultaneously with *M. meleagridis* [14]. It is also interesting to point out that this strain of *M. synoviae* grew quickly (within 24 h in vitro) unlike most strains which take many days.

The significance of the flamingo strain depends on what genetic classification system is used for *M. synoviae*. Based on Bencina's *vlhA* scheme [26] the strain was classified as the type C3, a strain which has never been detected in Italy before as far as we are aware. However, based on Hammond's classification [19] this would represent the first isolation of a new genotype in the EU.

Regarding the identical *vlhA* gene sequence, we examined the possibility that the flamingo strain may have derived from the temperature-sensitive (ts^+) *M. synoviae* vaccine strain MS-H by differential growth at different temperatures. This showed that the flamingo strain grew poorly at low temperature which strongly suggested that it is a wild strain. However there remains the possibility that a ts^+ strain could occasionally revert to a ts^- MS-H strain [20, 27, 28]. This is highly unlikely given that there was no evidence that the flamingos had been vaccinated with the MS-H vaccine. Indeed during the period of isolation the use of MS-H within Europe, in particular, Italy, was not authorised. Finally the possibility of laboratory contamination can be excluded because strict quality control tests are performed daily.

Based on our data, the diagnostic application of the *vlh*A gene analysis is of limited value for the differentiation of field and vaccine strains (Fig. 4) as was previously proposed by Ogino et al. for Japanese strains [29], and has recently suggested for European strains by Dijkman et al. (2014) [30]. Shahid et al. [25] proposed a microtitration system coupled with real time PCR to distinguish the *ts* phenotype of *M. synoviae* because in Australia the *vlhA* sequencing is often inconclusive.

Moreover, investigating the *obg* sequence variability in the flamingo, different single nucleotide polymorphisms (SNPs) were detected, allowing to better distinguishing it from related MS-H strains. Analysis showed that the flamingo strain had a G in position 367, which based on previous results [21] classified it as a field strain and not related to the MS-H strain.

The majority of *M. synoviae* strains circulating in Italy which are non-vaccine wild type field strains can be identified by the *vlhA* method (unpublished data), while the microtitration system or the analysis of *obg* gene [21] could be used to distinguish the C-type strains which in Italy account for about 10 % of the rest.

Finally this clinical case provides good evidence for possible opportunistic transmission and spread of avian pathogens, which is compounded by the international trade in ornamental or zoo birds and may represent possible vectors of avian pathogens. These types of bird live in the open-air where strict biosecurity measures are not applied, thus enabling the direct and indirect contact with autochthonous fauna, increasing the risk of spreading infections if exotic microorganisms have contact with free populations. Hence these ornamental species could play an important epidemiological role in spreading infectious disease to the industrial poultry.

Additional files

Additional file 1: Alignment of partial *vlhA* sequences. *Mycoplasma synoviae* strains' *vlhA* sequences showed a similarity with the lesser flamingo isolates (HG421742.1 IZSVE/2010/5711). In this figure we insert only one of the strains that showed a 100 % of similarity for the

Australian isolate; its accession number is DQ661614 because the other one reported in the results showed the same sequence. The AB501271 is the *vlhA* sequence of MS-H vaccine strain. Finally, the accession number FN666087 is one of the two EU strains that showed the higher similarity.

Additional file 2: Alignment of partial *obg* sequences. The *obg* gene sequences of *Mycoplasma synoviae* isolated from flamingo (KJ802785 IZSVE/2010/5711) was aligned with MS-H (KC990837.1), re-isolate *ts*$^-$ (KC990838.1) and *ts* + (KC990839.1) and parental strain *ts*$^-$ (KC990840.1). Nucleotide differences are specified by the nucleotide, while dot represented no nucleotide changing.

Abbreviations

DGGE: Denaturing Gradient Gel Electrophoresis; DNA: Deoxyribonucleic acid; EU: European Union; ME: Mycoplasma experience; MS: Mycoplasma synoviae; obg: spOB-associated GTP binding protein; PCR: polymerase chain reaction; SNPs: single nucleotide polimorphisms; ts: temperature sensitive; vlhA: variable lipoprotein hemagglutinin A.

Competing interests

The authors declare that they have no competing interests.

Authors' contributions

S-C carried out the necroscopies and diagnosis, management of the additional test perfomed; F-G carried out the necroscopies, the diagnosis, the isolation of *Mycoplasma synoviae* and the thermosusceptibility test; AS-R performed sequencing analysis; D-G managed the birds in the zoo and reported the anamnestic informations and the follow-up; E-B performed biomolecular tests and sequencing analysis, ML-M contributed to cultivation, biomolecular tests and sequencing analysis. RAJ-N supervised the activities and contributed to the draft. All authors read and approved the final manuscript.

Acknowledgments

We gratefully acknowledge the "Histopathological Laboratory" of the Istituto Zooprofilattico delle Venezie (Legnaro - Padova) who provided invaluable technical support.

This work was supported by the Italian Ministry of Health with the Project RC IZSVE 15/10 "Le micoplasmosi nel settore avicolo industriale: studio e messa a punto di nuove metodiche e protocolli diagnostici al fine di valutare e studiare il differente ruolo dei ceppi circolanti tra le differenti tipologie di produzioni avicole"

Author details

[1]Istituto Zooprofilattico Sperimentale delle Venezie, viale dell'Universita' 10, Legnaro, 35020 Padova, Italy. [2]Università degli Studi di Padova, Dipartimento di Medicina Animale, Produzioni e Salute (MAPS), Legnaro, Padova, Italy. [3]Unidad de Epidemiología y Medicina Preventiva, Facultad de Veterinaria, Universidad de Las Palmas de Gran Canaria, C/Trasmontala s/n, Arucas 35413Islas Canarias, Spain. [4]Parco Faunistico LE CORNELLE, Valbrembo, Bergamo, Italy. [5]Nutshell Lane, Farnham, Surrey GU9 0HG, UK.

References

1. Bradbury JM. Recovery of Mycoplasmas from Birds. In: Miles R, Nicholas R, editors. Mycoplasma Protocols. Totowa: Humana Press; 1998. p. 45–51.
2. Poveda JB, Carranza J, Miranda A, Garrido A, Hermoso M, Fernandez A, Domenech J. An epizootiological study of avian mycoplasmas in southern Spain. Avian Pathology. 1990;19:627–33.
3. Poveda JB, Giebel J, Flossdorf J, Meier J, Kirchhoff H. Mycoplasma buteonis sp. nov., Mycoplasma falconis sp. nov., and Mycoplasma gypis sp. nov., Three Species from Birds of Prey. Int J Syst Bacteriol. 1994;44:94–8. doi:10.1099/00207713-44-1-94.
4. Pennycott TW, Dare CM, Yavari CA, Bradbury JM. Mycoplasma sturni and Mycoplasma gallisepticum in wild birds in Scotland. Vet Rec. 2005;156:513–5.
5. Loria GR, Ferrantelli E, Giardina G, Li Vecchi L, Sparacino L, Oliveri F, McAuliffe L, Nicholas RA. Isolation and characterization of unusual Mycoplasma spp. from captive Eurasian Griffon (Gyps fulvus) in Sicily. J Wildl Dis. 2008;44:159–63.
6. Lierz M, Hagen N, Hernadez-Divers SJ, Hafez HM. Occurrence of mycoplasmas in free-ranging birds of prey in Germany. J Wildl Dis. 2008;44:845–50.
7. Stipkovits L, Szathmary S. Mycoplasma infection of ducks and geese. Poult Sci. 2012;91:2812–9.
8. Suárez-Pérez A, Ramírez AS, Rosales RS, Calabuig P, Poveda C, Rosselló-Móra R, Nicholas RA, Poveda JB. Mycoplasma neophronis sp. nov., isolated from upper respiratory tract of Canarian Egyptian Vulture (Neophron percnopterus majorensis). Int J Syst Evol Microbiol. 2012;62:1321–5.
9. Brown R.B. Phylum XVI. Tenericutes Murray 1984a, 356^{VP} (Effective publication: Murray 1984b, 33). In: Bergey's Manual of Systematic Bacteriology. 2nd Ed. Volume 4. New York Dordrecht Heidelberg London: Springer. p. 567–613.
10. Ley DH, Berkhoff JE, McLaren JM. Mycoplasma gallisepticum isolated from house finches (Carpodacus mexicanus) with conjunctivitis. Avian Dis. 1996;40:480–3.
11. Fischer JR, Stallknecht DE, Luttrell P, Dhondt AA, Converse KA. Mycoplasmal conjunctivitis in wild songbirds: the spread of a new contagious disease in a mobile host population. Emerg Infect Dis. 1997;3:69–72.
12. Ley DH, Berkhoff JE, Levisohn S. Molecular epidemiologic investigations of Mycoplasma gallisepticum conjunctivitis in songbirds by random amplified polymorphic DNA analyses. Emerg Infect Dis. 1997;3:375–80.
13. Lierz M, Schmidt R, Runge M. Mycoplasma species isolated from falcons in the Middle East. Vet Rec. 2002;151:92–3.
14. Lierz M, Schmidt R, Brunnberg L, Runge M. Isolation of Mycoplasma meleagridis from free-ranging birds of prey in Germany. J Vet Med B Infect Dis Vet Public Health. 2000;47:63–7.
15. Suarez-Perez A, Ramirez AS, Rosales RS, Calabuig P, Poveda CG, Vega-Orellana OM, Mederos LE, Nicholas RAJ, Poveda JB. Isolation of Mycoplasma spp., from Eurasian Stone Curlew (Burhinus oedicnemus insularum) in Canary Island. Italy, Chianciano. In: Proceedings of the 18th International Congress of the International Organization for Mycoplasmology IOM. 2010. p. 107.
16. ISIS. International Species Information System. 2009. http://www2.isis.org/Pages/Home.aspx
17. McAuliffe L, Ellis RJ, Lawes JR, Ayling RD, Nicholas RA. 16S rDNA PCR and denaturing gradient gel electrophoresis; a single generic test for detecting and differentiating Mycoplasma species. J Med Microbiol. 2005;54:731–9.
18. Lauerman LH, Hoerr FJ, Sharpton AR, Shah SM, Van Santen VL. Development and application of a polymerase chain reaction assay for Mycoplasma synoviae. Avian Dis. 1993;37:829–34.
19. Hammond PP, Ramírez AS, Morrow CJ, Bradbury JM. Development and evaluation of an improved diagnostic PCR for Mycoplasma synoviae using primers located in the haemagglutinin encoding gene vlhA and its value for strain typing. Vet Microbiol. 2009;136:61–8.
20. Shahid MA, Markham PF, Markham JF, Marenda MS, Noormohammadi AH. Mutations in GTP binding protein Obg of Mycoplasma synoviae vaccine strain MS-H: implications in temperature-sensitivity phenotype. PLoS One. 2013;8(9):e73954.
21. Shahid MA, Markham PF, Marenda MS, Agnew-Crumpton R, Noormohammadi AH. High-Resolution Melting-Curve Analysis of obg Gene to Differentiate the Temperature-Sensitive Mycoplasma synoviae Vaccine Strain MS-H from Non-Temperature-Sensitive Strains. PLoS One. 2014;9(3), e92215.
22. Tamura K, Peterson D, Peterson N, Stecher G, Nei M, Kumar S. MEGA5: molecular evolutionary genetics analysis using maximum likelihood, evolutionary distance, and maximum parsimony methods. Mol Biol Evol. 2011;28:2731–9.
23. Hall TA. BioEdit: a user-friendly biological sequence alignment editor and analysis program for Windows 95/98/NT. Nucleic Acids Symp Ser. 1999;41:95–8. 1999 London University Press.
24. Morrow CJ, Markham JF, Whithear KG. Production of temperature-sensitive clones of Mycoplasma synoviae for evaluation as live vaccines. Avian Dis. 1998;42:667–70.
25. Shahid MA, Ghorashi SA, Agnew-Crumpton R, Markham PF, Marenda MS, Noormohammadi AH. Combination of differential growth at two different temperatures with a quantitative real-time polymerase chain reaction to determine temperature-sensitive phenotype of Mycoplasma synoviae. Avian Pathology. 2013;42:185–91.
26. Bencina D, Drobnic-Valic M, Horvat S, Narat M, Kleven SH, Dovc P. Molecular basis of the length variation in the N-terminal part of Mycoplasma synoviae hemagglutinin. FEMS Microbiol Lett. 2001;203:115–23.

27. Markham JF, Scott PC, Whithear KG. Field evaluation of the safety and efficacy of a temperature-sensitive Mycoplasma synoviae live vaccine. Avian Dis. 1998;42:682–9.
28. Noormohammadi AH, Jones JF, Harrigan KE, Whithear KG. Evaluation of the non-temperature-sensitive field clonal isolates of the Mycoplasma synoviae vaccine strain MS-H. Avian Dis. 2003;47:355–60.
29. Ogino S, Munakata Y, Ohashi S, Fukui M, Sakamoto H, Sekiya Y, Noormohammadi AH, Morrow CJ. Genotyping of Japanese field isolates of Mycoplasma synoviae and rapid molecular differentiation from the MS-H vaccine strain. Avian Dis. 2011;55:187–94.
30. Dijkman R, Feberwee A, Landman WJM. Variable lipoprotein haemagglutinin A (vlhA) gene sequence typing of mainly Dutch Mycoplasmma synoviae isolates: comparison with vlhA sequences from Genbank and with amplified fragment length polymorphism analysis. Avian Pathol. 2014;43(5):465–72.

An Exploratory Descriptive Study of Antimicrobial Resistance Patterns of *Staphylococcus* Spp. Isolated from Horses Presented at a Veterinary Teaching Hospital

James Wabwire Oguttu[1], Daniel Nenene Qekwana[2] and Agricola Odoi[1,3*]

Abstract

Background: Antimicrobial resistant *Staphylococcus* are becoming increasingly important in horses because of the zoonotic nature of the pathogens and the associated risks to caregivers and owners. Knowledge of the burden and their antimicrobial resistance patterns are important to inform control strategies. This study is an exploratory descriptive investigation of the burden and antimicrobial drug resistance patterns of *Staphylococcus* isolates from horses presented at a veterinary teaching hospital in South Africa.

Methods: Retrospective laboratory clinical records of 1027 horses presented at the University of Pretoria veterinary teaching hospital between 2007 and 2012 were included in the study. Crude and factor-specific percentages of *Staphylococcus* positive samples, antimicrobial resistant (AMR) and multidrug resistant (MDR) isolates were computed and compared across *Staphylococcus* spp., geographic locations, seasons, years, breed and sex using Chi-square and Fisher's exact tests.

Results: Of the 1027 processed clinical samples, 12.0% were *Staphylococcus* positive. The majority of the isolates were *S. aureus* (41.5%) followed by *S. pseudintermedius* (14.6%). Fifty-two percent of the *Staphylococcus* positive isolates were AMR while 28.5% were MDR. Significant ($p < 0.05$) differences in the percentage of samples with isolates that were AMR or MDR was observed across seasons, horse breeds and *Staphylococcus* spp. Summer season had the highest (64.3%) and autumn the lowest (29.6%) percentages of AMR isolates. Highest percentage of AMR samples were observed among the Boerperds (85.7%) followed by the American saddler (75%) and the European warm blood (73.9%). Significantly ($p < 0.001$) more *S. aureus* isolates (72.5%) were AMR than *S. pseudintermedius* isolates (38.9%). Similarly, significantly ($p < 0.001$) more *S. aureus* (52.9%) exhibited MDR than *S. pseudintermedius* (16.7%). The highest levels of AMR were towards β-lactams (84.5%) followed by trimethoprim/sulfamethoxazole (folate pathway inhibitors) (60.9%) while the lowest levels of resistance were towards amikacin (14.%).

Conclusions: This exploratory study provides useful information to guide future studies that will be critical for guiding treatment decisions and control efforts. There is a need to implement appropriate infection control, and judicious use of antimicrobials to arrest development of antimicrobial resistance. A better understanding of the status of the problem is a first step towards that goal.

Keywords: Horse, *Staphylococcus aureus*, *Staphylococcus pseudintemedius*, *Staphylococcus epidermidis*, *Staphylococcus chromogens*, Antimicrobial resistance, Multi-drug resistance, MDR, Gauteng, South Africa

* Correspondence: aodoi@utk.edu
[1]Department of Agriculture and Animal Health, College of Agriculture and Environmental Sciences, University of South Africa, Florida Science Campus, Johannesburg, South Africa
[3]Biomedical and Diagnostic Sciences, College of Veterinary Medicine, University of Tennessee, Knoxville, USA
Full list of author information is available at the end of the article

Background

Staphylococcus are Gram-positive cocci that comprise of over 50 species and subspecies, some of which are common commensals of various body sites of different animals [1, 2]. Although many *Staphylococcus* spp., are of no clinical significance, some are important opportunistic pathogens [1, 3, 4]. In equine medicine *S. aureus*, *S. intermedius* and *S. hyicus*, have been associated with clinical infections [2]. From a public health point of view, there are increasing reports of highly virulent staphylococcal infections that can be transmitted between horses and humans [5–7]. For example, a Canadian study reported that 96% of the *Staphylococcus* samples from horses and 93% from humans displayed similar genetic profiles [8]. Another study done in the Netherlands reported that *S. aureus* isolated from a 16 year old girl was genetically similar to that isolated from a horse [5]. Busscher et al. [3] also reported identical Methicillin Resistant *Staphylococcus aureus* (MRSA) from horses and their caregivers.

Infections with antimicrobial drug resistant *Staphylococcus* spp. in both equine and human medicine has been associated with high morbidity, mortality and treatment costs. In animals, infections with antimicrobial drug resistant *Staphylococcus* spp. has also been associated with significant animal welfare implications due to animals staying sick for long periods in event of treatment failures [9–12]. Although coagulase-positive staphylococci (CoPS) are the most important groups associated with severe infections, coagulase-negative staphylococci (CoNS) have emerged as important pathogens as well. Moreover, all *Staphylococcus* spp., regardless of their coagulase activity, have potential to develop resistance to different classes of antimicrobials used for human and animal treatment [13]. Just like CoPS, resistance to antimicrobials such as gentamycin, macrolides, tetracycline, streptomycin, trimethoprim, sulfamethoxazole and fluoroquinolones is commonly observed among CoNS isolates from pets and horses [13, 14].

Excessive use of broad spectrum antimicrobials has been hypothesized as the main driver of antimicrobial drug resistance in *Staphylococcus* spp. [15]. For example, Bagcigil et al. [16] reported high levels of resistance to multiple antimicrobial agents including β-lactams in horses with previous history of treatment with β-lactams. Failure to complete the course of antimicrobial treatment has also been identified as a risk factor for development of resistance among staphylococcal isolates from horses [17]. Recent studies show that colonization with *Staphylococcus* spp. carrying antimicrobial resistance genes increases the risk of infection with resistant *Staphylococcus* [2, 17]. Transfer of resistance genes between pathogenic organisms and commensal flora has also been hypothesized as a risk factor for infection with resistant isolates [18]. Morton et al. [19] were able to demonstrate horizontal transfer of one conjugate mupirocin plasmid by finding the same plasmid in different staphylococcal isolates from patients in different areas of the hospital, which suggested that isolates had acquired new genes. Moreover, conjugative plasmids can move between CoPS and CoNS [19]. Furthermore, molecular epidemiological analyses by pulsed-field gel electrophoresis has shown that horizontal transfer of plasmid borne genes within and between different equine staphylococcal species is possible [20].

Despite the existence of evidence suggesting that horses play a significant role as sources of staphylococcal infections for humans [5, 6], it is surprising that studies of staphylococcal infections in Africa in general, and South Africa in particular, have mainly focussed on humans [12, 21, 22]. Available studies in human medicine suggest a high prevalence of resistant staphylococcal infections, especially MRSA, associated with both hospital and community acquired infections [9]. Therefore, studies of horses are critically needed to fill this knowledge gap. Given the paucity of data on both the burden of staphylococcal infections and the antibiotic resistance profiles among *Staphylococcus* isolates from horses in Africa, the present study is an exploratory descriptive investigation of the burden of staphylococcal infections and their antimicrobial drug resistance patterns among horses presented at the University of Pretoria veterinary teaching hospital from 2007 to 2012. This exploratory investigation is expected to provide useful information to guide future hypothesis driven studies in this region of the world.

Methods

Study area

This study was conducted using retrospective laboratory data collected from Gauteng province in South Africa. Gauteng province is approximately 18,178 km^2 in size, and has an estimated population of 13.2 million people (24% of the South African population). During the time period covered by this study, the province had a total of five metropolitan municipalities: Ekurhuleni, Sedibeng, Johannesburg, Tshwane and West Rand. The province has a subtropical climate, and is cooler in Johannesburg and slightly warmer in Pretoria. Gauteng is located in the Highveld region of South Africa, and has an annual summer rainfall of approximately 700 mm. It has four seasons: summer (November–March), autumn (April–May), winter (June–August) and spring (September–October). Winter is the driest season, while December and January are the wettest months. The province experiences annual maximum temperatures of about 22 °C in the south and 25 °C in the north [23, 24].

Data source

Laboratory records of all 1027 clinical samples from horses, from Gauteng Province, presented at the University of Pretoria bacteriology diagnostic laboratory for isolation and susceptibility testing of *Staphylococcus* spp. from January 2007 to December 2012 were included in the study. The data were received as paper records, reviewed and entered into an electronic database. The following fields were extracted for each record: horse breed, sex, age (in months), date sample was submitted as well as culture and antimicrobial susceptibility test results. The data were assessed for duplicate entries and if any horses had been sampled multiple times during the study period. No duplicates were identified. The dataset did not contain multiple tests from the same horse, neither were there mixed infections in the samples analysed. The breeds of horses were re-classified to identify the top 10 breeds. All other breeds that had small numbers were grouped into one category and called other breeds.

Isolation of *Staphylococcus* spp. and testing for antimicrobial susceptibility

The Bacteriology Laboratory at the University of Pretoria veterinary teaching hospital, from where the study data were obtained, follows standardized protocols for isolation of *Staphylococcus* spp. based on the methods described in Quinn et al. [25]. Susceptibility testing of samples was conducted using the Kirby Bauer disc diffusion technique following the guidelines described in the Clinical and Laboratory Standards Institute (CLSI) document [26]. The isolates were subjected to antimicrobial susceptibility testing against a panel of 9 drugs using the disc diffusion method. Antimicrobial resistance (AMR) was defined as resistance to at least one antimicrobial while multidrug resistance (MDR) was defined as resistance to 3 or more classes of antimicrobials [27]. Thus, some of the isolates classified as AMR were also included in the MDR group if they exhibited resistance to 3 or more classes of antimicrobials.

Statistical analysis

Shapiro-Wilks test [28] was used to test normality of continuous variables. Non-normally distributed continuous variables were summarized using medians and interquartile ranges. Age was categorized into four categories: foals (<1 year old), yearlings (1–2 years old), fillies and colts (2–4 years old) and adults (>4 years old). Crude and factor-specific percentages of *Staphylococcus* positive samples, AMR and MDR isolates as well as their 95% confidence intervals were computed. The factors (categorical variables) considered were: species of *Staphylococcus*, geographic location, season, year, breed, age group and sex. Associations between these categorical variables and percentages of *Staphylococcus* positive samples, AMR and MDR isolates were assessed using Chi-square and, in cases of small expected cell sizes, Fishers Exact test. Significance was assessed at $p \leq 0.05$. Due to the small sample sizes involved in this exploratory descriptive investigation, adjusted associations using multiple regression models could not be assessed. All statistical analyses were performed in STATA [29].

Results

A total of 1027 clinical samples from horses in Gauteng Province were submitted to the University of Pretoria bacteriology diagnostic laboratory from 2007 to 2012 and were included in this study. Of the 1027 processed samples, 12.0% (123/1027) were positive for staphylococci, the majority of which were *S. aureus* (41.5%) followed by *S. pseudintermedius* (14.6%), *S. epidermidis* (4.9%), *S. equinus* (0.8%), and *S. chromogens* (0.8%). The remaining 37.4% of the samples did not have species information. Of the *Staphylococcus* positive samples, a total of 52.0% (64/123) had isolates that exhibited antimicrobial resistance to at least one antimicrobial (AMR), while 28.5% (35/123) had isolates that exhibited multidrug resistance (MDR). Significantly ($p = 0.002$) more samples had isolates that exhibited AMR (52.0%; 95% CI: 42.8–61.1) than those that had MDR (28.5%; 95% CI: 20.7–37.3%).

Distribution by animal characteristics

The samples that were submitted and processed, came from 29 different breeds of horses. The five most common breeds contributing samples were: Thoroughbreds (26.8%), European warm blood (12.6%), Arab (11.6%), South African warm blood (6.4%) and Friesian (6.0%) (Table 1). A significant ($p = 0.001$) association was observed between breed and the percentage of *Staphylococcus* positive samples, with the highest percentage of *Staphylococcus* positive samples observed among crossbreeds (20.5%), followed by Boerperds (18.9%) and European breeds (17.8%). There was also a significant ($p = 0.015$) association between breed of the horse and the percentage of samples carrying resistant isolates, with the highest percentage of samples with resistant isolates being observed among the Boerperds (85.7%) followed closely by the American saddler (75%) and the European warm blood (73.9%). Similarly, there was a significant ($p = 0.006$) association between the percentage of samples carrying MDR isolates and horse breed, with the American Saddler having the highest percentage (75%) of MDR followed by European warm blood (56.5%), Thoroughbreds (33.3%) and the Boerperds (28.6%).

The median age of the horses was 4.3 years, but ranged from 0 to 25.7 years (interquartile range: 0.7–9 years). The majority of the samples were from adults (50.6%), followed by foals (27.1%). Yearlings contributed

Table 1 Host factor distribution of equine samples from Gauteng Province (South Africa) tested for *Staphylococcus*, 2007–2012

	All Samples Processed (*n* = 1027)			Staphylococcus Positive Samples (*n* = 123)		
Breed	n[a]	%[b]	95% CI[c]	n[a]	%[b]	95% CI[c]
American Saddler	39	3.8	2.8, 5.2	4	10.3	3.8, 24.6
Arab	119	11.6	9.8, 13.7	8	6.7	3.4, 12.9
Boerperd	37	3.6	2.6, 4.9	7	18.9	9.2, 35.0
Crossbreed	39	3.8	2.8, 5.2	8	20.5	10.5, 36.2
European warm blood	129	12.6	10.7, 14.7	23	17.8	12.1, 25.4
Friesian	62	6.0	4.7, 7.7	2	3.2	0.8, 12.1
Nooitgedachtpony	43	4.2	3.1, 5.6	5	11.6	4.9, 25.3
South African warm blood	66	6.4	5.1, 8.1	1	1.5	0.2, 10.1
Thoroughbred	275	26.8	24.2, 29.6	21	7.6	5.0, 11.4
Welshpony	25	2.4	1.6, 3.6	3	12.0	3.8, 31.9
Percheron	13	1.3	0.7, 2.2	0	0	-
All other breeds	73	7.1	5.6, 8.9	6	8.2	3.1, 17.1
Unspecified or missing	107	10.4	8.7, 12.4	35	32.7	24.0, 42.5
Age Group						
Foal (< 1 year)	278	27.1	24.4, 29.9	58	20.9	16.2, 26.1
Yearling (1–2 years)	83	8.1	6.5, 9.9	9	10.8	5.1, 19.6
Filly or Colt (2–4 years)	146	14.2	12.1, 16.5	13	8.9	4.8, 14.7
Adult (> 4 years)	520	50.6	47.5, 53.7	43	8.3	6.0, 11.0
Sex						
Males	499	48.6	45.5, 51.7	48	9.6	7.2, 12.6
Females	434	42.2	39.2, 45.3	44	10.1	7.6, 13.4
Unspecified or missing	94	9.2	7.5, 11.1	31	33.0	23.6, 43.4

[a]number of samples
[b]percentage of samples
[c]95% confidence interval

the lowest percentage of samples (8.1%) (Table 1). A significant ($p = 0.001$) association was observed between age group and percentage of *Staphylococcus* positive samples. Foals had the highest percentage (20.9%; 95% CI: 16.2, 26.1%) of *Staphylococcus* positive samples followed by yearlings (10.8%; 95% CI: 5.1, 19.6), fillies/colts (8.9%; 95% CI: 4.8, 14.7%) and adults (8.3%; 95% CI: 6.0, 11.0%). However, there was no significant difference ($p = 0.360$) in the levels of antimicrobial resistance across age groups. On the contrary, a significant ($p = 0.012$) association in the levels of samples that had MDR isolates was observed across age groups, with fillies/colts having the highest levels (46.2%; 95% CI: 19.2, 74.9%) followed by adults (42.0%; 95% CI: 27.0, 57.9%), foals (17.2%; 95% CI: 8.6, 29.4%) and yearlings had the lowest (11.1%; 95% CI: 0.2, 48.2%).

Significantly ($p = 0.001$) more samples from males (48.6%) than from females (42.2%) were processed. However, there were no significant ($p = 0.438$) differences in the percentages of *Staphylococcus* positive samples obtained from males (9.6%) and females (10.1%) (Table 1). Similarly, no significant ($p = 0.231$) differences in the percentage of samples with resistant isolates were observed between males (64.6%); 95% CI: 49.5, 77.8%) and females (52.3%; 95% CI: 36.7, 67.5%). Interestingly, there was a significantly ($p = 0.024$) higher percentage of MDR isolates among samples from male (41.7%; 95% CI: 27.6, 56.8) than female horses (20.5%; 95% CI: 9.8, 35.3%).

Temporal patterns

The largest percentage of samples were submitted during summer (40.8%) while the lowest (15.6%) were submitted during the spring (Table 2). Although spring (14.4%) and autumn (14.1%) tended to have higher percentages of *Staphylococcus* positive samples than the other two seasons, there was no significant ($p = 0.357$) association between season and percentage of *Staphylococcus* positive samples (Table 2). However, a significant ($p = 0.002$) association between

Table 2 Temporal and Geographic distribution of equine samples from Gauteng Province assessed for antimicrobial susceptibility, 2007–2012

	All Samples Processed (*n* = 1027)		*Staphylococcus* positive samples (*n* = 123)		AMR[c] Isolates (*n* = 64)		MDR[d] *Isolates* (*n* = 35)	
	%[b]	95% CI[a]	%	95% CI[a]	%	95% CI[a]	%	95% CI[a]
Season								
Summer	40.8	37.8, 43.8	10.0	7.4, 13.3	64.3	48.6, 77.4	38.1	24.6, 53.8
Autumn	18.6	16.3, 21.1	14.1	9.9, 19.9	29.6	15.2, 49.6	14.8	5.5, 34.2
Winter	25.0	22.5, 27.8	12.1	8.6, 16.7	58.1	40.0, 74.2	41.9	25.8, 60.0
Spring	15.6	13.5, 17.9	14.4	9.7, 20.7	47.8	28.3, 68.1	8.7	2.1, 29.9
Year								
2007	34.1	31.2, 37.0	7.7	5.3, 11.0	55.6	36.4, 73.2	14.8	5.5, 34.2
2008	15.5	13.4, 17.8	8.2	4.8, 13.6	53.8	27.0, 78.6	15.4	3.6, 47.0
2009	16.1	13.9, 18.4	12.1	7.9, 18.1	55.0	32.9, 75.3	35.0	17.2, 58.3
2010	8.8	7.2, 10.7	13.3	7.7., 22.1	33.3	12.4, 63.9	8.3	1.0, 44.1
2011	7.1	5.7, 8.9	6.8	2.9, 15.5	60.0	16.6, 91.9	20.0	2.1, 74.8
2012	18.5	16.2, 21.0	24.2	18.6, 30.8	52.2	37.7, 66.3	43.5	29.8, 58.2
Municipality								
Johannesburg	20.0	17.6, 22.5	11.7	7.6, 16.9	54.2	34.0, 73.0	33.3	17.2, 54.5
Tshwane	61.2	58.2, 64.2	11.6	9.2, 14.4	49.3	37.9, 60.8	26.0	16.5, 37.6
Ekurhuleni	10.1	8.4, 12.1	10.6	5.4, 18.1	63.6	32.3, 86.5	36.4	13.5, 67.7
Sedibeng	2.4	1.6, 3.6	20.0	6.8, 40.7	40.0	5.3, 85.3	20.0	0.5, 71.6
West Rand	6.2	4.9, 7.9	10.0	7.8, 26.9	60.0	26.3,87.8	30.0	6.7, 65.2

[a]95% confidence interval
[b]Percent
[c]AMR: Antimicrobial resistant (defined as resistance to at least one antimicrobial)
[d]MDR: Multidrug resistant (defined as resistance to at least three classes of antimicrobials; includes a subset of AMR isolates)

season and percentage of isolates resistant to at least one antimicrobial was observed. Summer had the highest (64.3%; 95% CI: 48.6, 77.4%) and autumn the lowest (29.6%; 95% CI: 15.2, 49.6%) percentage of antimicrobial resistant isolates (Table 2). On the contrary, there was no significant ($p = 0.137$) association between the percentage of MDR isolates and season.

A comparison of the percentage of samples submitted and processed each year revealed that significantly more samples were processed in 2007; and the lowest percentage of samples were received and processed in 2011. Moreover, there was a significant ($p < 0.001$) association between year and the percentage of *Staphylococcus* positive samples, with the largest percentage of positive samples occurring in 2012 (24.2%) (Table 2). Thus, except for the anomaly observed in 2011, there was an increasing trend in the percentage of *Staphylococcus* positive samples during the study period (Table 2). By contrast, there were no significant ($p = 0.707$) differences in the percentage of AMR isolates across the years, neither were there significant differences ($p = 0.304$) in the percentage of MDR isolates across the years.

Geographic patterns

The geographic distribution of sample submissions was a reflection of the distribution of horse populations across the different municipalities with Tshwane submitting most (61.2%) of the samples followed by Johannesburg (20%) (Table 2). Although the percentage of *Staphylococcus* positive samples varied from 10% in Ekurhuleni municipality to 20% in Sedibeng municipality (Table 2), these differences were not statistically significant ($p = 0.563$). The percentage of isolates that were resistant to at least one antimicrobial varied from 40% in Sedibeng to 63.6% in Ekurhuleni (Table 2). Again, there were no significant ($p = 0.857$) differences in the percentage of isolates that were resistant to at least one antimicrobial. Similarly, the percentage of MDR isolates varied from 20% in Sedibeng to 36.4% in Ekurhuleni municipality (Table 2). As was the case with AMR isolates, there were no significant ($p = 0.891$) differences in the percentage of MDR isolates across the municipalities.

Antimicrobial susceptibility profiles

There was a significant ($p < 0.001$) difference in the percentages of samples with resistant isolates across the

Staphylococcus spp., with *S. aureus* (72.5%) showing much higher levels of resistance than *S. pseudintermedius* (38.9%) (Table 3). Similarly, there was a significant (p = 0.0001) difference in the percentages of samples with MDR isolates across species, and again *S. aureus* (52.9%) exhibited higher levels of MDR compared to *S. pseudintermedius* (16.7%) (Table 3).

Significant ($p < 0.05$) differences in the levels of resistance to each antimicrobial was also observed, with resistance to β-lactams being the highest (ampicillin: 84.5%; penicillin: 74.1%) followed by Trimethoprim/sulfamethoxazole (folate pathway inhibitors) (60.9%), while the lowest level of resistance was towards amikacin (14.1%) (Table 3). Most MDR isolates tended to exhibit resistance to trimethoprim/sulfamethoxazole (53.1%), followed by gentamicin (48.9%) (Table 3). Only 9.1% of these isolates exhibited resistance towards amikacin and only 18.8% displayed resistance towards enrofloxacin. The distribution of the number of classes of antimicrobials to which isolates were resistant is shown in Table 4.

The majority of MDR combinations observed involved *S. aureus* (Table 5). Multidrug resistance involving combinations of four antimicrobials tended to occur more frequently in young foals as compared to combinations that involved more antimicrobials. Most samples with MDR isolates came from Tshwane municipality (Table 5) and involved mainly European warm blood (31.1%) and Thoroughbreds (20.0%). It is interesting to note that a high percentage (35.6%) of MDR isolates were from horses less than 1 month old (Table 5).

Table 3 Distribution of antimicrobial resistance by species of *Staphylococcus* and antimicrobial agent

	Resistant Isolates		MDR Isolates	
	%	95% CI	%	95% CI
Species		n = 123		n = 35
S. aureus	72.5	58.3, 83.3[a]	52.9	38.5, 67.1[a]
S. pseudintermedius	38.9	19.2, 63.0[b]	16.7	3.6, 41.4[b]
S. spp[1]	30.4	18.7, 45.4[b]	2.2	0.1, 11.5[c]
All other species[2]	75.0	34.9, 96.8[a]	50.0	15.7, 84.3[a]
Antimicrobial & Antimicrobial Class		n = 64		n = 35
Aminoglycosides[3]				
Gentamycin	54.6	42.1, 66.7[a]	48.9	38.1, 59.8
Amikacin	14.1	7.3, 25.2[e]	9.1	4.0, 17.1
B-lactams[4]				
Ampicillin	84.5	72.3, 91.9[b]	37.5	27.4, 48.5
Penicillin	74.1	61.0, 84.0[b]	37.5	27.4, 48.5
Ceftriaxone	44.8	32.3, 58.1[c]	30.0	20.3, 41.3
Fluoroquinolones[5]				
Enrofloxacin	23.4	14.5, 35.7[c]	18.8	10.1, 30.5[b]
Folate Pathway Inhibitors[6]				
Trimotherim-sulfamethoxazole	60.9	48.2, 72.3[a]	53.1	40.2, 65.7[a]
Tetracyclines[7]				
Doxycyline	46.9	34.8, 59.4[a,d]	35.9	24.3, 48.9[c]
Phenicols				
Chloramphenicol	44.1	31.7, 57.2[d]	31.3	20.2, 44.1[c]

[1]Samples that were not identified to species level and were thus reported as *Staphylococcus spp.*
[2]Other species included *S. equinus*, *S. chromogens* and *S. epidermidis*
[3]Gentamycin and amikacin
[4]Penicillin, ampicillin, ceftriaxone
[5]Enrofloxacin
[6]Sulphamethoxazole
[7]Chloramphenicol
[a-d]Estimates with different superscripts are significantly different at 5% significance level

Discussion

The current study is an exploratory descriptive analysis of antimicrobial resistance patterns of *Staphylococcus* spp. isolated from horses presented at a veterinary teaching hospital in South Africa. Since very little is known regarding the epidemiology of antimicrobial resistance in horses in Africa and many other developing economies, this study is intended to provide preliminary information to guide future more detailed hypothesis driven epidemiological studies of antimicrobial drug resistance among *Staphylococcus* spp. not only in horses, but other domestic species as well.

Contrary to findings by Leekha et al. [30] the present study did not find significant seasonal differences in the percentage of *Staphylococcus* positive samples. This could be due to aggregation of cases by pre-defined seasons, as was done in the present study. Other authors have argued that this aggregation leads to loss of information if infection occurrences are not seasonal but follow other cyclical patterns such as biannual patterns [30]. Some authors have suggested use of time-series analytical approaches in such situations [31]. Unfortunately, due to the exploratory nature and the small samples sizes of the current study, time-series analysis could not be performed. The significant association observed between season and percentage of antimicrobial resistance could be attributed to weather

Table 4 Distribution of number of antimicrobial classes to which equine samples exhibited resistance (n = 64)

Number of antimicrobial classes to which isolates exhibited resistance	Number of isolates	Percent	95% CI[a]
1	17	26.6	16.3, 39.1
2	12	18.8	10.1, 30.4
3	7	10.9	4.5, 21.2
4	12	18.8	10.1, 30.4
5	8	12.5	5.6, 23.2
6	8	12.5	5.6, 23.2

[a]95% confidence interval

Table 5 Antimicrobial resistance patterns of staphylococcal isolates from equine samples from Gauteng Province (South Africa), 2007–2012

Horse Age (months)	Breed of Horse	Municipality	Year	Staphylococcus Species	Antimicrobial Resistance Patterns [a]
0	Thoroughbred	Tshwane	2008	*S. aureus*	AMP-DOX-PEN
0	Europeanwarmblood	Mogale City	2011	*Staph. spp.*	AMP-PEN-SUL
132	Crossbreed	Tshwane	2007	*S. aureus*	AMI-AMP-PEN
0	Boerperd	Tshwane	2007	*S.pseudintermedius*	AMP-DOX-PEN
0	Boerperd	Tshwane	2007	*S.aureus*	AMP-DOX-PEN
0	Unpecified or Missing	Tshwane	2007	*Staph. spp.*	AMP-CEF-PEN
131	Europeanwarmblood	Johannesburg	2008	*S. aureus*	AMP-PEN-SUL
48	Europeanwarmblood	Tshwane	2012	*S.aureus*	AMP-GEN-PEN-SUL
182	Boerperd	Tshwane	2012	*S.aureus*	AMP-GEN-PEN-SUL
1	Arab	Tshwane	2007	*S. equinus*	AMP-CEF-PEN-SUL
96	All other breeds	Tshwane	2012	*S. epidermidis*	DOX-ENR-GEN-SUL
40	All other breeds	Tshwane	2007	*S. aureus*	AMP-CEF-GEN-PEN-SUL
96	Europeanwarmblood	Tshwane	2012	*S. epidermidis*	DOX-ENR-GEN-PEN-SUL
0	Unpecified or Missing	Tshwane	2012	*S. aureus*	AMP-CEF-CHL-PEN-SUL
83	Europeanwarmblood	Johannesburg	2012	*S. aureus*	AMP-CHL-GEN-PEN-SUL
48	Europeanwarmblood	Tshwane	2012	*S. aureus*	AMP-DOX-GEN-PEN-SUL
84	Thoroughbred	Tshwane	2012	*S. aureus*	AMP-CEF-GEN-PEN-SUL
0	Europeanwarmblood	Johannesburg	2008	*S. aureus*	AMP-CEF-GEN-PEN-SUL
0	Unpecified or Missing	Tshwane	2012	*S. aureus*	AMP-CEF-CHL-GEN-PEN-SUL
0	Unpecified or Missing	Emfuleni	2012	*S. aureus*	AMP-CEF-CHL-GEN-PEN-SUL
0	Unpecified or Missing	Tshwane	2012	*S. aureus*	AMP-CEF-DOX-GEN-PEN-SUL
84	Thoroughbred	Ekurhuleni	2007	*S. aureus*	AMP-CEF-DOX-GEN-PEN-SUL
168	Europeanwarmblood	Ekurhuleni	2012	*S. aureus*	AMP-CEF-CHL-GEN-PEN-SUL
0	American Saddler	Ekurhuleni	2007	*S. aureus*	AMP-CEF-DOX-GEN-PEN-SUL
81	Thoroughbred	Tshwane	2009	*S. aureus*	AMP-CEF-DOX-GEN-PEN-SUL
0	American Saddler	Ekurhuleni	2007	*Staph. spp.*	AMP-CEF-DOX-GEN-PEN-SUL
48	Europeanwarmblood	Westonaria	2012	*S. aureus*	AMP-CHL-DOX-GEN-PEN-SUL
19	Europeanwarmblood	Westonaria	2012	*S. aureus*	AMP-CHL-DOX-ENR-GEN-PEN-SUL
108	Thoroughbred	Tshwane	2009	*S. aureus*	AMP-CEF-CHL-DOX-GEN-PEN-SUL
0	Arab	Johannesburg	2012	*S. aureus*	AMI-AMP-CHL-DOX-GEN-PEN-SUL
168	Europeanwarmblood	Johannesburg	2012	*S. aureus*	AMP-CEF-CHL-DOX-GEN-PEN-SUL
36	Europeanwarmblood	Westonaria	2010	*S.pseudintermedius*	AMP-CEF-CHL-DOX-ENR-GEN-SUL
111	All other breeds	Tshwane	2009	*S.pseudintermedius*	AMP-CEF-CHL-DOX-GEN-PEN-SUL
96	American Saddler	Tshwane	2012	*S.aureus*	AMI-AMP-CEF-CHL-GEN-PEN-SUL
0	Nooitgedachtpony	Tshwane	2009	*S. aureus*	AMI-AMP-CEF-CHL-DOX-ENR-GEN-PEN
120	Europeanwarmblood	Johannesburg	2009	*S.epidermidis*	AMI-AMP-CEF-DOX-ENR-GEN-PEN-SUL
182	Boerperd	Tshwane	2012	*S.aureus*	AMP-CEF-CHL-DOX-ENR-GEN-PEN-SUL
48	Europeanwarmblood	Tshwane	2012	*S.epidermidis*	AMP-CEF-CHL-DOX-ENR-GEN-PEN-SUL
155	Thoroughbred	Johannesburg	2012	*S.aureus*	AMI-AMP-CHL-DOX-ENR-GEN-PEN-SUL
83	Thoroughbred	Johannesburg	2011	*S.pseudintermedius*	AMI-AMP-CEF-CHL-DOX-ENR-GEN-PEN-SUL
0	Unpecified or Missing	Tshwane	2009	*S.aureus*	AMI-AMP-CEF-CHL-DOX-ENR-GEN-PEN-SUL
72	Thoroughbred	Tshwane	2009	*S.aureus*	AMI-AMP-CEF-CHL-DOX-ENR-GEN-PEN-SUL

[a]AMI = Amikacin; AMP = Ampicillin; CEF = Ceftriaxone; CHL = Chloramphenicol; DOX = Doxycycline; ENR = Enrofloxacin; GEN = Gentamicin; PEN = Penicillin; SUL = Sulphametho

conditions such as temperature and humidity. However, it may also be due to seasonal differences in staffing levels (i.e., fewer regular staff during vacation months) and seasonal differences in antimicrobial drug use due to differences in infection rates from other bacteria resulting in differences in selection pressure [30].

Although the percentages of *Staphylococcus* positive samples increased over time, there were no similar increases in the number of samples submitted for processing. Therefore, the observed increases in percentage of *Staphylococcus* positive samples may be a reflection of a true increase in the number of staphylococcal infections over the years. However, more detailed primary base studies will need to be performed to further investigate this trend. The higher levels of Staphylococcal infections in some breeds of horses seem to suggest potential breed predisposition. However, the reason for this is unclear and no previous studies have reported this. Therefore, this warrants further investigations to establish the potential existence of breed predisposition. Although sex dimorphism of staphylococcal infections, especially methicillin resistant infections, have been observed in humans [32], no similar associations were observed in this study and to our knowledge, no studies have reported differences in staphylococcal infections in horses based on sex.

Coagulase positive *Staphylococcus* spp., especially *S. aureus* are responsible for a significantly large percentage of infections in horses as opposed to coagulase negative strains [1]. Therefore, the higher levels of resistance observed among *S. aureus* in this study is of concern, from a therapeutic point of view, due to the resulting potential treatment failures associated with the observed high levels of resistance. The relatively high levels of AMR and MDR observed in this study may suggest high selection pressure among *Staphylococcus* spp. isolates from horses treated at the veterinary teaching hospital. This may be due to the fact that most of the cases seen in the teaching hospital tend to be referral cases that may not have responded well to initial antimicrobial treatments by the primary care veterinarians. Thus, it is possible that most of these horses would have been on antibiotic treatment for prolonged periods before being transferred to the referral veterinary teaching hospital. Another plausible explanation for the high levels of antimicrobial resistance observed in the study could be the result of failure of horse owners to ensure that the animals complete the full course of prescribed antimicrobial therapy. This issue has been highlighted by some authors who reported that caretakers have a tendency to stop drug administration as soon as disease symptoms abate, a practice that has been incriminated in the development of antimicrobial drug resistance [17]. Transportation stress has also been incriminated in the high carriage of resistant *Staphylococcus* in equine patients admitted to clinics as a result of direct contact with referring veterinarians who might be carrying resistant *Staphylococcus* [4].

The high levels of antimicrobial resistance observed in this study is consistent with the observations in humans in South Africa by Essa et al. [12], who observed that up to 95.1% of the samples were MDR, and only 3.7% of the samples were susceptible to all antibiotics tested in the study. The very high levels of resistance to β-lactams observed in the current study is consistent with reports by Weese [1] who reported high levels of resistance to β-lactams among staphylococci and especially *S. aureus*. Some studies have reported that routine use of β-lactam antibiotics in prevention of surgical infections, predisposes horses to acquisition of methicillin resistant *S. aureus* [33, 34]. Therefore, the high levels of resistance to β-lactam antibiotics in the present study could signal the existence of methicillin resistance in staphylococcal infections in horses presented at the hospital under study. Unfortunately, methicillin was not routinely included in the susceptibility test panels used by the veterinary teaching hospital that supplied the data for the current study, and hence the levels of resistance to methicillin could not be assessed in the current study. However, it is encouraging to note that resistance to fluoroquinolones was relatively low implying that these antimicrobials are still relatively effective and therefore their use could more likely be associated with successful treatment outcomes compared to β-lactams. It is worth noting that in South Africa, some of the older antibiotics are readily available to farmers over the counter while the newer ones require prescription [35]. This may have impacted selection pressure for antimicrobial resistance especially influencing antimicrobials readily available over the counter.

The observed low levels of resistance towards aminoglycosides was not unusual. For instance, Abrahamsen [17] in a study conducted in Maine (USA), also observed that *Staphylococcus* spp. tended to be susceptible to both gentamicin and amikacin, both of which are aminoglycosides. Furthermore, a study by Schnellmann et al. [33], investigating emergence of resistance after hospitalization in Switzerland, found much lower levels of resistance to amikacin compared to other antimicrobials. However, it is worth noting that the level of resistance observed here may not be a true reflection of the level of resistance in the larger horse population. For example, Van den Eede et al. [4] observed a much lower level of resistance among horses on farms that were situated in a region surrounding an equine clinic in Belgium whereas much higher carriage rates of resistant *Staphylococcus* had been detected in horses presented at the clinic [4].

The significant differences in the percentage of MDR isolates across species, with *S. aureus* exhibiting higher levels of MDR compared to other species, was anticipated given that it is the most common species in horses and therefore more likely to be exposed to higher selection pressure during antibiotic treatments compared to the other less common species [30]. Worth noting was that MDR was frequently observed among isolates from horses less than 1 month old. This could be due to the fact that foals frequently require antimicrobial treatment to combat a variety of conditions. Moreover, the basic principle of antimicrobial treatment in neonatal foals is the use of broad-spectrum antimicrobials [36]. This practice potentially increases the selection pressure for antimicrobial resistance among foals. However, it is interesting to note that MDR isolates resistant to six or more drugs tended to occur in older horses, which suggests that the overall selection pressure for antimicrobial drug resistance could be higher in older horses. Some authors have indicated that after 3 days of hospitalization and treatment with penicillin, the percentage of *Staphylococcus* isolates showing antibiotic resistance dramatically increases in horses [33].

Although some authors have reported geographic differences in levels of AMR staphylococcal isolates [37], the current study did not identify significant geographic differences. This could most likely be due to the small samples sizes involved in some of the municipalities included in the study. Therefore, more detailed and larger studies need to be performed to more fully investigate geographic and other determinants of variations in AMR and MDR staphylococcal infections. Thus, our next set of studies will focus on these issues as well as investigating practices in the use of antimicrobials by both veterinary practitioners and animal owners.

A limitation of this retrospective laboratory-based study is that the source of samples (e.g. nasal, skin, etc) could not be assessed due to quality of these data. A positive outcome of this finding is that we will work with the laboratory to improve laboratory data capture. This will have a positive impact of improved data quality for similar studies in the future. Additionally, information on past antimicrobial use was not available and therefore we could not assess its associations with levels of AMR or MDR. Moreover, detailed analysis of the β-lactam resistant isolates were not performed and hence we could not assess their susceptibility to methicillin. Finally, it is possible that some of the isolates reported as *Staphylococcus* spp. may have belonged to *S. aureus*, *S. pseudintermedius*, *S. epidermidis* or *S. equinus*. Unfortunately, information was not available to elucidate this.

Conclusions

The above limitations notwithstanding, the study has shown evidence of seasonal patterns of staphylococcal infections and occurrence of AMR and MDR in horses. There is also evidence of differences in the occurrence of AMR and MDR by species of *Staphylococcus* and breed of horse. Resistance among *Staphylococcus* isolates was highest towards β-lactam antibiotics, but lowest towards amikacin. It should be pointed out that this was an exploratory descriptive study that did not lend itself to more detailed analyses such as use of multivariable models due to the small sample sizes involved. However, this being the first study of its kind in Africa, it provides useful descriptive information to guide future more detailed studies intended to address the problems of equine staphylococcal infections and antimicrobial resistance. Routine surveillance, prudent antimicrobial use and efficient infection control should be advocated as strategies to contain development of antimicrobial resistance in horse infections. Future studies will need to be primary-base involving large sample sizes to help understand specific local factors contributing to development of antimicrobial resistance so as to better guide treatment and control efforts.

Abbreviations

95% CI: 95% Confidence Interval; AMR: Antimicrobial Resistant; CoNS: coagulase-negative staphylococci; CoPS: coagulase-positive staphylococci; MDR: Multidrug Resistant; MRSA: Methicillin Resistant *Staphylococcus aureus*; p: *p*-value; *S. aureus*: *Staphylococcus aureus*; *S. epidermidis*: *Staphylococcus epidermidis*; *S. equinus*: *Staphylococcus equinus*; *S. hyicus*: *Staphylococcus hyicus*; *S. intermedius*: *Staphylococcus intermedius*; *S. pseudintermedius*: *Staphylococcus pseudintermedius*; spp.: Species; USA: United States of America; β-lactam: Beta-lactam

Acknowledgments

Carnegie African Diaspora Program and the University of South African Visiting Research Program are gratefully acknowledged for making it possible for Dr. Odoi to travel to South Africa to conduct the study.

Funding

This project was made possible by funding from the University of Tennessee Centers of Excellence, Carnegie African Diaspora Fellowship Program and the University of South Africa visiting research program that funded the research collaboration between Drs Odoi and Oguttu. The funders had no role in study design, data collection and analysis, decision to publish, or preparation of the manuscript.

Authors' contributions

JWO was involved in study design, results interpretation and editing of the manuscript. DNQ was involved in study design, data entry and manuscript writing. AO conceived the study idea, was involved in study design, analysed the data, interpreted the results and was involved in extensive editing of the manuscript. All authors read and approved the final manuscript

Consent for publication
Not applicable

Competing interests
The authors declare that they have no competing interests.

Author details
[1]Department of Agriculture and Animal Health, College of Agriculture and Environmental Sciences, University of South Africa, Florida Science Campus, Johannesburg, South Africa. [2]Section Veterinary Public Health, Department of Paraclinical Sciences, Faculty of Veterinary Sciences, University of Pretoria, Pretoria, South Africa. [3]Biomedical and Diagnostic Sciences, College of Veterinary Medicine, University of Tennessee, Knoxville, USA.

References

1. Weese JS. Staphylococcal infections. In: Sellon DC, Long M, editors. Equine Infect Dis Internet. Toronto: Elsevier Health Sciences; 2013. p. 664.
2. Devriese LA, Nzuambe D, Godard C. Identification and characteristics of staphylococci isolated from lesions and normal skin of horses. Vet Microbiol. 1985;10:269–77.
3. Busscher JF. Van Duijkeren E, Sloet van Oldruitenborgh-Oosterbaan MM. The prevalence of methicillin-resistant staphylococci in healthy horses in the Netherlands. Vet. Microbiol. 2006;113:131–6.
4. den Eede A, Martens A, Feryn I, Vanderhaeghen W, Lipinska U, Gasthuys F, et al. Low MRSA prevalence in horses at farm level. BMC Vet Res. 2012;8:213.
5. van Duijkeren E, Ten Horn L, Wagenaar JA, de Bruijn M, Laarhoven L, Verstappen K, et al. Suspected horse-to-human transmission of MRSA ST398. Emerg Infect Dis [Internet]. 2011;17:1137–9. Available from: http://www.ncbi.nlm.nih.gov/pmc/articles/PMC3358200/pdf/10-1330_finalL.pdf
6. van Duijkeren E, Moleman M, van Oldruitenborgh-Oosterbaan MM, Multem J, Troelstra A, Fluit AC, et al. Methicillin-resistant Staphylococcus Aureus in horses and horse personnel: an investigation of several outbreaks. Vet Microbiol. 2010; 141:96–102.
7. Weese JS, Caldwell F, Willey BM, Kreiswirth BN, McGeer A, Rousseau J, et al. An outbreak of methicillin-resistant Staphylococcus Aureus skin infections resulting from horse to human transmission in a veterinary hospital. Vet Microbiol. 2006;114:160–4.
8. Weese JS, Archambault M, Willey BM, Hearn P, Kreiswirth BN, Said-Salim B, et al. Methicillin-resistant Staphylococcus Aureus in horses and horse personnel, 2000-2002 141. EmergInfectDis Centers Dis Control Prev. 2005;11:430–5.
9. Perovic O, Koornhof H, Black V, Moodley I, Duse A, Galpin J. Staphylococcus Aureus bacteraemia at two academic hospitals in Johannesburg. South African Med J. 2006;96:714–7.
10. Magiorakos A-P, Srinivasan A, Carey RB, Carmeli Y, Falagas ME, Giske CG, et al. Multidrug-resistant, extensively drug-resistant and pandrug-resistant bacteria: an international expert proposal for interim standard definitions for acquired resistance. Clin. Microbiol. Infect. [Internet]. Blackwell Publishing Ltd; 2012 [cited 2016 Jun 24];18:268–81 Available from: http://linkinghub.elsevier.com/retrieve/pii/S1198743X14616323
11. Safdar N, Bradley EA. The risk of infection after nasal colonization with Staphylococcus Aureus. Am J Med [Internet]. 2008;121:310–5. Available from: http://www.sciencedirect.com/science/article/pii/S0002934307009746
12. Essa ZI, Connolly C, Essack SY. *Staphylococcus aureus* from Public Hospitals in Kwa-Zulu-Natal, South Africa–Infection Detection and Strain-Typing. South African J. Epidemiol. Infect. [Internet]. 2009 [cited 2016 Jun 24]; 24:4–7 Available from: http://www.sajei.co.za/index.php/SAJEI/article/viewFile/100/143.
13. Ruzauskas M, Couto N, Siugzdiniene R, Klimiene I, Virgailis M, Vaskeviciute L, et al. Methicillin-resistant coagulase-negative staphylococcus spp. prevalence in Lithuanian dogs: a cross-sectional study. Vet. Arh. 2015;85:175–87.
14. Kern A, Perreten V. Clinical and molecular features of methicillin-resistant, coagulase-negative staphylococci of pets and horses. J Antimicrob Chemother [Internet]. 2013;68:1256–66. Available from: http://jac.oxfordjournals.org/content/68/6/1256.full.pdf
15. Weese JS, Lefebvre SL. Risk factors methicillin-resistant staphylococcus aureus colonization in horses admitted to a veterinary teaching hospital. Can Vet J. 2007;48:921–6.
16. Bagcigil FA, Moodley A, Baptiste KE, Jensen VF, Guardabassi L. Occurrence, species distribution, antimicrobial resistance and clonality of methicillin- and erythromycin-resistant staphylococci in the nasal cavity of domestic animals. Vet Microbiol. 2007;121:307–15.
17. Abrahamsen K. Equine infectious diseases and microbial resistance to antibiotics. Dartmouth Undergradaute J Sci. 2004;1:37–41.
18. Oguttu WJ. Antimicrobial drug resistance of enteric bacteria from broilers fed antimicrobial growth enhancers and exposed poultry abattior workers. Pretoria: University of Pretoria; 2007.
19. Morton TM, Johnston JL, Patterson J, Archer GL. Characterization of a conjugative staphylococcal mupirocin resistance plasmid. DOI Antimicrob. Agents Chemother [Internet]. 1995 [cited 2017 Mar 4];39 Available from: http://aac.asm.org/content/39/6/1272.
20. Bjorland J, Steinum T, Sunde M, Waage S, Heir E. Novel plasmid-borne gene qacJ mediates resistance to quaternary ammonium compounds in equine *Staphylococcus aureus*, Staphylococcus simulans, and Staphylococcus intermedius. Antimicrob. Agents Chemother. [Internet]. 2003 [cited 2017 Mar 4];47:3046–52 Available from: http://aac.asm.org/cgi/doi/10.1128/AAC.47.10.3046-3052.2003.
21. Moodley A, Oosthuysen WF, Duse AG, Marais E, South African MSG. Molecular characterization of clinical methicillin-resistant Staphylococcus Aureus isolates in South Africa. J Clin Microbiol [Internet]. 2010;48:4608–11. Available from: http://www.ncbi.nlm.nih.gov/pmc/articles/PMC3008489/pdf/1704-10.pdf
22. Oosthuysen WF, Orth H, Lombard C, Sinha B, Wasserman E. In vitro characterization of representative clinical South African *Staphylococcus aureus* isolates from various clonal lineages. New microbes new Infect. [Internet]. Elsevier; 2014 [cited 2016 Jun 24];2:115–22. Available from: http://www.ncbi.nlm.nih.gov/pubmed/25356356.
23. SOUTHAFRICA.COM. Weather of Gauteng | By South Africa Channel [Internet]. South Africa Channels. 2017 [cited 2017 Mar 3] Available from: http://www.southafrica.com/gauteng/climate/.
24. World Weather Online. Weather Averages | Monthly Average High and Low Temperature | Average Precipitation and Rainfall days | World Weather Online [Internet]. 2012 [cited 2017 Mar 3]. Available from: https://www.worldweatheronline.com/johannesburg-weather-averages/gauteng/za.aspx.
25. Quinn PJ, Carter ME, Markey B, Carter GR. Clinical veterinary microbiology. Mosby Wolfe: Edinburgh, Scotland; 1994.
26. Clinical and Laboratory Standards Institute. Performance standards for antimicrobial susceptibility testing; eighteenth informational supplement. CLSI docum. Wayne, PA: Clinicall and Laboratory Standards Institute; 2008.
27. Dohne S, Merle R, Altrock AV, Waldmann KH, Verspohl J, Gruning P, et al. Antibiotic susceptibility of salmonella, campylobacter coli, and campylobacter jejuni isolated from northern German fattening pigs. J Food Prot. 2012;75:1839–45.
28. Royston P. A simple method for evaluating the Shapiro-Francia W' test for non-normality. Underst Stat. 1983;32:297–300.
29. Corporation STATA. Stata MP. Parallel E. 4905 Lakeway drive College Station. TX, USA: Stata Corporation; 2013.
30. Leekha S, Diekema DJ, Perencevich EN. Seasonality of staphylococcal infections. Clin Microbiol Infect [Internet]. 2012;18:927–33. Available from: http://onlinelibrary.wiley.com/doi/10.1111/j.1469-0691.2012.03955.x/pdf
31. Fisman DN. Seasonality of Infectious Diseases. https://doi.org/10.1146/annurev.publhealth.28.021406.144128. Annual Reviews; 2007;
32. Humphreys H, Fitzpatick F, Harvey, Brain J. Gender differences in rates of carriage and bloodstream infection caused by methicillin-resistant *Staphylococcus aureus*. Are they real, do they matter and why? Clin. Infect. Dis. [Internet]. 2015;61:1708–14. Available from: http://cid.oxfordjournals.org/content/early/2015/07/21/cid.civ576.full.pdf+html.
33. Schnellmann C, Gerber V, Rossano A, Jaquier V, Panchaud Y, Doherr MG, et al. Presence of New mecA and mph(C) Variants Conferring Antibiotic Resistance in Staphylococcus spp. Isolated from the Skin of Horses before and after Clinic Admission. J. Clin. Microbiol. [Internet]. American Society for Microbiology; 2006 [cited 2016 Jun 24];44:4444–54 Available from: http://jcm.asm.org/cgi/doi/10.1128/JCM.00868-06
34. Yah SC, Enabulele I, Eghafona NO. The screening of multi-drug resistance (MDR) susceptibilities of *Staphylococcus aureus* and *Staphylococcus epidermidis* to methicillin and vancomycin in teaching hospitals in Nigeria.

Sudan J. Med. Sci. [Internet]. Omdurman Islamic University; 2008 [cited 2016 Jun 24];2:257–62 Available from: http://www.ajol.info/index.php/sjms/article/view/38497.
35. Henton MM, Eagar HA, Swan GE, van Vuuren M. Part VI. Antibiotic management and resistance in livestock production. S. Afr. Med. J. [Internet]. 2011 [cited 2017 Jul 15];101:583–6. Available from: http://www.ncbi.nlm.nih.gov/pubmed/21920137.
36. Furr Martin O, Mogg T. Antimicrobial treatment of neonatal foals. Compedium. 2003;25:6.
37. Burton S, Reid-Smith R, McClure JT, Weese JS. *Staphylococcus aureus* colonization in healthy horses in Atlantic Canada. Can Vet J. 2008;49:797–9.

3

Relationship of diagnostic accuracy of renal cortical echogenicity with renal histopathology in dogs and cats

Tommaso Banzato[1], Federico Bonsembiante[2], Luca Aresu[2] and Alessandro Zotti[1*]

Abstract

Background: Renal cortical echogenicity is routinely evaluated during ultrasonographic investigation of the kidneys. Both in dog and cat previous *ex-vivo* studies have revealed a poor correlation between renal echogenicity and corresponding lesions. The aim of this study was to establish the in-vivo relationship between renal cortical echogenicity and renal histopathology.

Results: Thirty-eight dogs and fifteen cats euthanized for critical medical conditions were included in the study. Ultrasonographic images of both kidneys were acquired *ante mortem* at standardized ultrasonographic settings. The echogenicity was quantified by means of Mean Gray Value (MGV) of the renal cortex measured with ImageJ. A complete histopathological examination of both kidneys was performed. Five kidneys were excluded because histopathology revealed neoplastic lesions. Only samples affected by tubular atrophy showed statistically different values in dog, and histopathology explained 13% of the total variance. MGV was not correlated neither to the degeneration nor to the inflammation scores. However, significant differences were identified between mildly and severely degenerated samples. Overall, the classification efficiency of MGV to detect renal lesions was poor with a sensitivity of 39% and a specificity of 86%.
In cats, samples affected by both tubular vacuolar degeneration and interstitial nephritis were statistically different and histopathology explained 44% of the total variance. A linear correlation was evident between degeneration and MGV, whereas no correlation with inflammation was found. Statistically significant differences were evident only between normal and severely degenerated samples with a sensitivity of 54.17% and a specificity of 83.3% and MGV resulted scarce to discriminate renal lesions in this species.

Conclusions: Renal cortical echogenicity shows low relevance in detecting chronic renal disease in dog whereas it results worth to identify severe renal damage in cat.

Keywords: Kidney, Ultrasound, Image analysis, Pathology

Background

A thorough ultrasonographic inspection of the kidneys is mandatory in the clinical examination of dogs and cats with suspected or confirmed renal disease. The shape, size, contours, renal pelvis, renal medulla, corticomedullary distinction and renal cortical echogenicity are routinely evaluated [1, 2]. Focal renal diseases such as tumors, cysts or hematomas are readily detected using B-Mode ultrasound [1, 2], whereas the evaluation of diseases involving the entire kidney are more challenging since the relative ultrasonographic changes are usually subtle and non-specific. Increased renal cortical echogenicity was previously reported to be a common finding associated with renal insufficiency [1]. However, animals affected by severe renal insufficiency may show normal kidneys during ultrasonography [2].

* Correspondence: alessandro.zotti@unipd.it
[1]Department of Animal Medicine, Production and Health, Clinical Section, Radiology Unit, University of Padua, Viale dell'Università 16, Legnaro 35020, Padua, Italy
Full list of author information is available at the end of the article

To date, no in-vivo studies correlating renal cortical echogenicity and diffuse renal pathology in dogs and cats have been published. The relationship between renal cortical echogenicity and renal pathology was previously studied by the authors in a standardized *ex-vivo* study [3].

The aims of this present study are: 1) to describe in a standardized in-vivo operative conditions the relationship between renal cortical echogenicity and renal histopathology in dogs and cats; 2) to determine whether renal cortical echogenicity could be used to discriminate diffuse renal pathology.

Methods

Animals

All the animals included in this study were admitted for medical consult at the Veterinary Teaching Hospital, University of Padua, Italy, from January 2015 to May 2016. Ultrasonography was part of the routine clinical evaluation and was performed within 24 h prior to death. Written consent was obtained from the owners and a complete clinical history was obtained. All the animals were euthanized due to critical medical conditions unrelated to the purposes of the study.

A full necropsy was performed within 3 h from death on every cadaver and both kidneys were collected and formalin fixed.

Ultrasonographic procedures

All the ultrasounds were performed with a 4- to 9 MHz micro convex array transducer connected to a commercial sonographic scanner (Zonare, Zonare Medical Systems Inc, Mountain View, California, USA). The following ultrasonographic settings were selected in all the scans: abdominal preset, depth 4 cm, frequency 8.5 MHz, gain 90; time-gain-compensation control settings were maintained in a neutral position. Longitudinal and transversal scans were obtained for each kidney. Each scan included both the cortex and medulla.

Image analysis procedures

Images were stored in a digital imaging and communications in medicine format (DICOM) without compression. Mean Gray Value (MGV) calculated with an open-source sofware (ImageJ, 1.480 version, National Institutes of Health, Bethesda, USA) was used to quantify the echogenicity in three square 64x64 pixel region of interest (RoI) and then averaged. MGV is the sum of the pixel intensities within a given RoI divided by the number of pixels included in the RoI assuming a eight bit image with 256 possible shades of gray (2^8 combinations in binary code). The RoIs were always placed at about 1-cm depth within the cortical side proximal to the probe immediately under each kidney serosa. Care was taken to avoid focal lesions such as mineralizations or cysts.

Histological analysis

The kidney samples for histological analysis were processed routinely and paraffin embedded. Both right and left kidney were analyzed for each animal; serial 3 μm sections were obtained and stained routinely with specific renal stainings [3]. A set of morphological lesions was selected for the study including glomerulosclerosis, interstitial nephritis, glomerulonephritis, tubular atrophy, tubular necrosis, fibrosis, glomerular lipidosis, tubular vacuolar degeneration, amyloidosis. Additionally, the presence or absence of proximal tubular lipidosis was recorded in cat. Each kidney was considered as an independent sample. The samples revealing "no relevant findings" were considered as normal. Tumors were excluded from the study. All the histopathological lesions were recorded as present or absent and reported as a dichothomous variable. Furthermore, a 0 to 3 (0 = none, 1 = mild, 2 = moderate and 3 = severe) semi-quantitative degeneration (including glomerulosclerosis, tubular necrosis, fibrosis, glomerular and interstitial lipidosis, tubular atrophy, amyloidosis) and inflammation (including interstitial nephritis and glomerulonephritis) scores were assigned. The samples were analyzed in a blinded fashion by two veterinary pathologists (LA and FB), and differences in scores were resolved by consensus achieved through simultaneous viewing using a dual-headed microscope.

Statistical analysis

A commercially available software was used to perform the statistical analysis (IBM Corp. Released 2011. IBM SPSS Statistics for Windows, Version 20.0. Armonk, NY: IBM Corp.). The dog and cat data were analyzed separately. The variable MGV was tested for normality using the Shapiro-Wilk test. The MGV calculated on each kidney was included in the statistical analysis. The presence or absence of individual histopathological lesions was considered as a dichotomous variable and differences between groups were tested between samples showing a specific lesion and all the other samples. Analysis of variance (ANOVA) was used to calculate differences between groups for normally distributed data. Differences between groups in non-normally distributed data were investigated with the Mann-Whitney U test. A univariate analysis was performed to evaluate the variance of MGV explained by histological parameters.

Correlation between MGV and degeneration and inflammation score was tested by means of the Spearman rank-order test. Differences between inflammation and degeneration score groups in normally distributed data were calculated using ANOVA. Kruskal-Wallis H test was used to study differences between groups in non-normally distributed data. Multiple comparison tests were performed with the Tukey-Kramer method to test which of both the degeneration and inflammation score groups were significantly different from the others. The diagnostic performance of MGV in the detection of pathological samples (samples that were not classified as "no relevant findings") was tested by means of the receiver operating characteristic curve (ROC). In all the statistical analysis a $P < 0.05$ was considered significant.

Results

Dogs

Thirty-eight adult dogs (13 females and 25 males) weighing from 3 to 45 kg (mean age: 9.5 ± 4 years) were recruited for the study. Descriptive statistics of MGV in the dog samples classified by histopathological lesion are reported in Table 1. Twenty-one kidneys were classified as normal by optical microscopy examination. Five kidneys were classified as neoplastic and were excluded from further analyses. MGV resulted from the Shapiro-Wilk test as not normally distributed and therefore differences between groups were tested by means of the Mann-Whitney U test. Only the MGV calculated on samples affected by tubular atrophy resulted as significantly different ($U = 470$, $z = 2.74$, $p = 0.006$) between groups. The univariate analysis was performed with tubular atrophy as independent variable and MGV as dependent variable. The assumptions of linearity, independence of errors, homoscedasticity, unusual points and normality of residuals were met. Tubular atrophy accounted 13.4% of total MGV variability ($F(2–66) = 11.18$, $P = 0.001$, adj. $R^2 = 0.13$).

Descriptive statistics (Table 2) and box-and-whisker plots (Fig. 1) of MGV, classified on the basis of the degeneration and inflammation scores assigned by the pathologists, are reported. As a result of the Spearman rank-order correlation test there was no significant association between MGV and degeneration and inflammation scores. However, degeneration scores showed significant differences by Kruskal-Wallis H test ($\chi 2 = 8.55$; $p = 0.036$), more specifically post hoc test revealed significant differences between the grade 2 and grade 3 of the degeneration (Fig. 1). No significant results were evident for the inflammation score.

Finally, the ROC curve analysis showed a poor diagnostic performance of MGV (area under the receiver characteristics curve (AUROC) = 0.54; 95% confidence interval 0.32–0.60). Using a cut-off value of 35, sensitivity was 39% and specificity was 86% (Fig. 2).

Cats

Fifteen adult cats (five females and ten males) weighing from 3 to 9 kg (mean age 9.3 ± 4.1 years) were involved in the study. The descriptive statistics of MGV for cat are reported in Table 3. Six samples were classified as normal. A non-normal distribution of MGV was shown by Shapiro-Wilk test and therefore differences between groups were calculated by means of the Mann-Whitney U test. Differences between groups were evident for fibrosis ($U = 56$, $z = 2.33$, $p = 0.002$), tubular vacuolar degeneration ($U = 195$, $z = 6.43$, $p = 0.000$), interstitial nephritis ($U = 117$, $z = 3.04$, $p = 0.002$), and glomerulonephritis ($U = 0.5$, $z = -2.21$, $p = 0.005$). Since only two samples showed fibrosis and glomerulonephritis, these latter histological lesions were not considered in further analysis. Only histopathological lesions showing statistically significant differences were included in the univariate analysis. The assumptions of linearity, independence of errors, homoscedasticity, unusual points and normality of residuals were met. Both tubular vacuolar degeneration and interstitial nephritis were included in the model, $F(2–29) = 15.31$, $P < 0.000$, adj. $R^2 = 0.44$. Results of the univariate analysis are reported in Table 4.

Descriptive statistics and box-and-whisker plots (Fig. 3) for degeneration and inflammation are reported in Table 5. As a result of the Spearman rank-order correlation test, MGV and degeneration scores were significantly correlated ($r = 0.44$, $p = 0.014$), whereas MGV and inflammation scores were not correlated. Significant differences, calculated by means of the Kruskal-Wallis H test,

Table 1 Descriptive statistics and results of the Mann-Whitney U test of MGV calculated on the dog samples classified on the basis of histopathological lesions

		Presence of the considered lesion			Absence of the considered lesion		
Histological changes	No. of samples	Mean ± SD	Median	Range	Mean ± SD	Median	Range
No relevant findings	21	49.88 ± 18.7	41.24	26.9–93.8	47.96 ± 21.42	38.76	16.16–94.76
Glomerulosclerosis	33	47.79 ± 22.88	37.7	16.1–94.7	48,68 ± 18.67	41.36	25.47–93.08
Tubular atrophy*	11	66.8 ± 21.78	66.94	31.42–94.76	44.93 ± 18.63	37.77	16.13–93.08
Fibrosis	12	51.83 ± 27.68	44.54	20.23–94.76	47.53 ± 19.04	40.07	16.16–93.08
Glomerular atrophy	10	48.16 ± 20.94	41.16	25.69–77.35	48.29 ± 20.76	40.91	16.16–94.76
Interstitial nephritis	23	48.94 ± 22.61	44.03	20.23–94.76	47.96 ± 19.76	39.54	16.16–93.08
Glomerulonephritis	9	37.34 ± 8.75	35.52	25.69–49.36	49.83 ± 21.31	41.63	16.16–94.76
Neoplasia	5	33.05 ± 6.7	33.69	25.47–41.63	49.20 ± 20.81	44.03	16.16–94.76

*Statistically significant differences –$p < 0,05$

Table 2 Descriptive statistics of MGV of the dog samples classified on the basis of the degeneration and inflammation scores assigned by the pathologists

	Degeneration				Inflammation			
Score	No. of samples	Mean ± SD	Median	Range	No of samples	Mean ± SD	Median	Range
0	26	48.30 ± 19.25	40.91	21.61–93.08	44	51.1 ± 19.5	49.4	16.16–93.08
1	20	49.23 ± 21.32	38.26	25.69–92.41	13	42.45 ± 21.18	33.86	25.17–92.41
2	7	33.35 ± 15.5	30.30	16.16–58.57	5	45.76 ± 22.75	44.03	20.23–82.21
3	14	59.75 ± 21.21	61.47	31.42–94.76	5	56.25 ± 30.03	49.36	25.69–94.76

were evident between degeneration score groups ($\chi2 = 10.05$; $p = 0.018$); post-hoc test revealed significant differences between grade 0 and 3 and between grade 2 and 3 degeneration score groups (Fig. 1). No significant differences were evident between the inflammation score groups.

ROC curve analysis revealed that MGV had poor discriminating power between normal and pathological samples (AUROC = 0.65, 95% confidence interval 0.45–0.81). Choosing a cut-off value of 44% the sensitivity was 54% and specificity was 83% (Fig. 4).

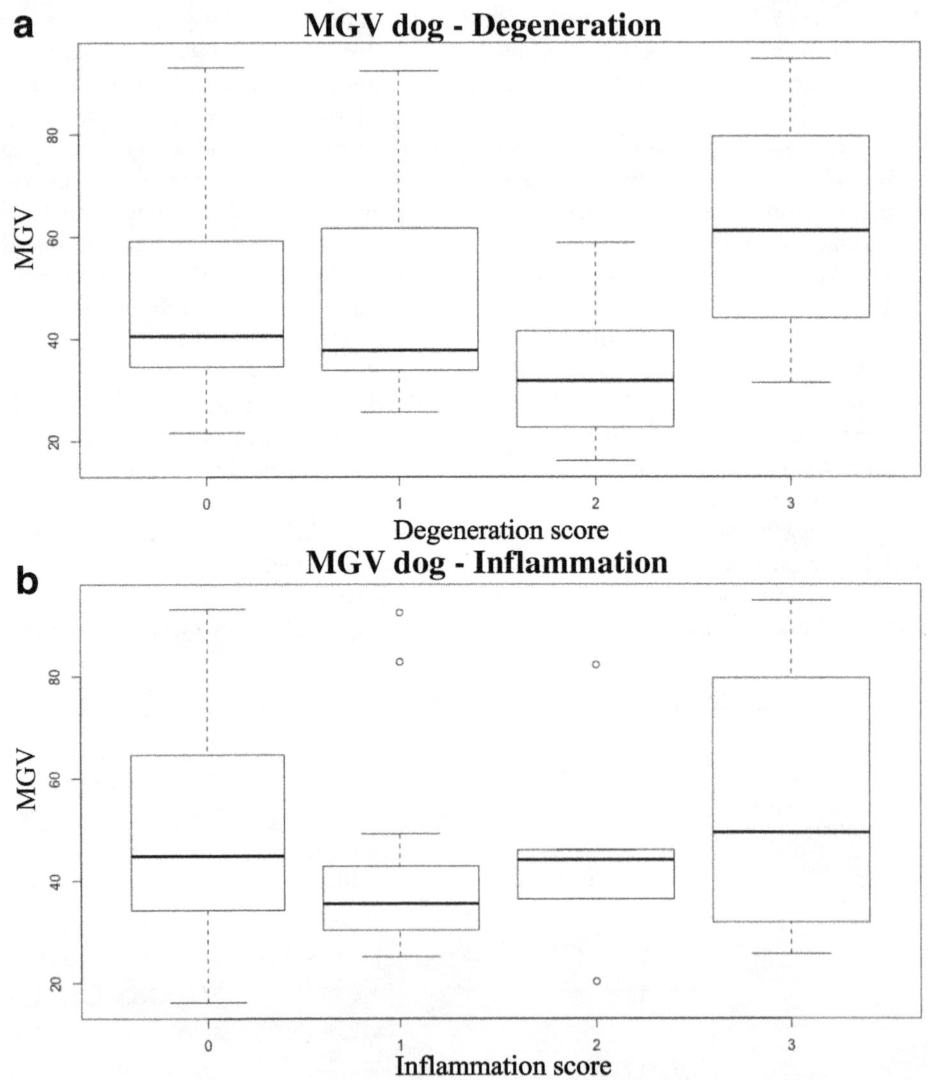

Fig. 1 Box-and-whisker plots of MGV in the dog samples classified on the basis of the degeneration (**a**) and inflammation (**b**) scores assigned by the pathologists

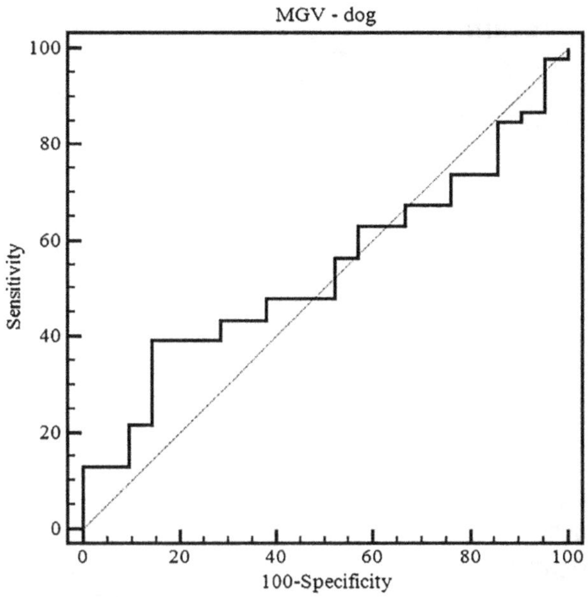

Fig. 2 ROC curve analysis of the dog samples classified as normal ("no relevant findings") and as pathological. (AUROC = 0.54; 95% confidence interval = 0.32–0.60). Choosing a cut-off value of 35 sensitivity was 39% and specificity was 86%)

Discussion

All previous in-vivo veterinary studies reported in the literature to objectively evaluate renal cortical echogenicity were performed in healthy animals [4–6]. These papers presented renal cortical echogenicity assessed by means of a tissue equivalent phantom [4] or in comparison to other organs [5, 6]. It is the authors' opinion that both these approaches have some limitations; comparison with a tissue equivalent phantom is a complicated and time consuming procedure [4]. On the other hand, comparison with other organs is unreliable because: 1) renal cortical echogenicity in dogs with normal renal function is reported to be hypo, iso- or hyper-echoic to

Table 4 Results of univariate analysis of the cat samples with MGV as dependent variable

Histological changes	B	Standard error	Beta
Constant	33.65	3.86	
Tubular vacuolar degeneration	13.329	6.11	0.321*
Interstitial nephritis	29.238	8.2	0.527*

B: unstandardized regression coefficient, Beta: standardized coefficient, *P value < 0.05

the liver [5]; 2) it assumes the spleen or the liver to be normal.

In the present work, the authors have identified the use of constant ultrasonographic settings (frequency, gain, time gain compensation, etc.) and sampling procedures to obtain comparable results. Interestingly, the variance expressed by the model was similar to a previous *ex-vivo* study [3] in dogs (12% in the *ex-vivo* study and 13% in the present in-vivo study) whereas it resulted higher in cats (23% in the *ex-vivo* study and 44% in the present in-vivo study). In our opinion, this might indicate that the patient related factors (such as body size, nutritional status) only actually accounts for a marginal part of the variability in kidney echogenicity. However, the diagnostic accuracy of MGV in the detection of pathological kidneys was lower in this in-vivo report than in our previous *ex-vivo* study, both for dogs and cats [3]. It is authors' opinion that the above differences might be, at least partially, explained by the smaller sample size of the present in-vivo study compared to that of the previous *ex-vivo* research [3].

The relationship between the MGV calculated in the dog samples and the degeneration score assigned by the pathologists was nonlinear, and statistically significant differences were evident only between grade 2 and 3 degeneration. Moreover, the mean MGV of the kidney samples graded as two on our degeneration score scale was lower than that of the remaining degeneration

Table 3 Descriptive statistics and results of the Mann-Whitney U test of MGV calculated on the cat samples classified on the basis of histopathological lesions

		Presence of the considered lesion			Absence of the considered lesion		
Histological changes	No. of samples	Mean ± SD	Median	Range	Mean ± SD	Median	Range
No relevant findings	6	36 ± 15.73	33.15	20.04–62.54	46.77 ± 22.05	46.43	17.86–110.97
Glomerulosclerosis	10	51.41 ± 32.67	49.92	17.86–110.97	41.23 ± 11.8	43.25	17.86–110.97
Proximal tubular lipidosis	24	47.79 ± 22,76	46.67	17.76–110.97	34.16 ± 10.57	33.83	22.94–48.57
Tubular atrophy	5	34.75 ± 7.87	34.19	24.5–46.67	46.6 ± 22.46	46.18	17.86–110.97
Fibrosis*	2	104.9 ± 8.52	104.9	98.84–110.97	40.32 ± 13.72	43.25	17.86–62.54
Tubular vacuolar *degeneration	15	56.18 ± 21.93	51.27	23.64–110.97	33.06 ± 12.54	34.06	17.86–62.54
Glomerular atrophy	9	41.6 ± 10.18	43.61	22.94–54.8	45.92 ± 24.5	44.13	17.86–110.97
Interstitial nephritis*	5	75.77 ± 27.24	60.01	49.67–110.97	38.39 ± 13.15	37.57	17.86–62.54
Glomerulonephritis*	2	18.76 ± 1.2	18.76	17.86–19.67	46.47 ± 20.64	45.15	20.05–110.97

*Statistically significant differences –p < 0,05

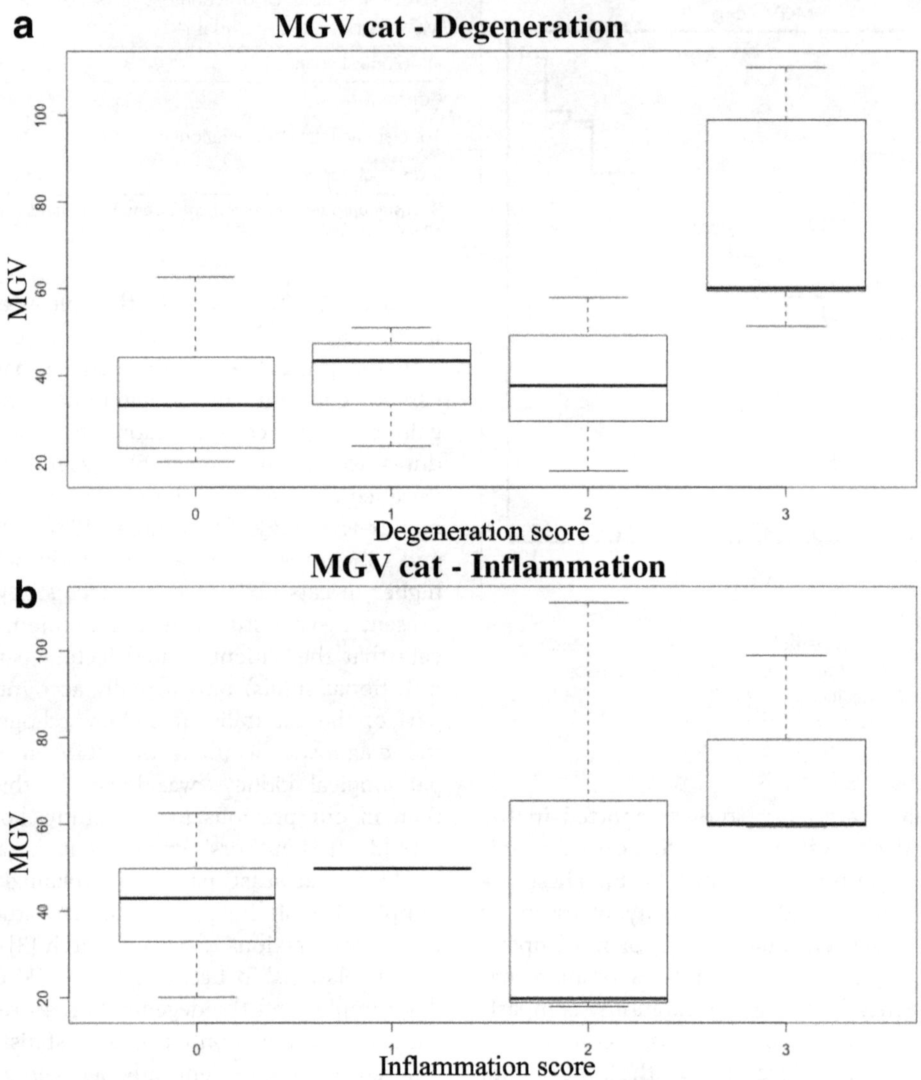

Fig. 3 Box-and-whisker plots of MGV in the cat samples classified on the basis of the degeneration (**a**) and inflammation (**b**) scores assigned by the pathologists

score groups. A similar relationship between MGV and degeneration was evident in the *ex-vivo* report [3].

ROC curve analysis calculated in order to detect pathological kidney changes shows a very low diagnostic accuracy of MGV. This is a partial consequence of the lack of correlation between degeneration and renal cortical echogenicity and the very high variability in the MGV calculated on normal samples (Tables 1 and 2).

MGV was always measured in the most proximal part of the renal cortex and focal hyperechoic areas caused by anisotropic ultrasound backscatter were carefully avoided. It is authors' opinion that, in the dog, at least

Table 5 Descriptive statistics of MGV of the cat samples classified on the basis of the degeneration and inflammation scores assigned by the pathologists

	Degeneration				Inflammation			
Score	No. of samples	Mean ± SD	Median	Range	No. of samples	Mean ± SD	Median	Range
0	6	36.03 ± 15.5	33.15	20.04–62.54	23	40.1 ± 12.27	42.88	20.04–62.54
1	4	40.25 ± 11.66	43.25	23.61–50.89	1	-	-	-
2	15	38.73 ± 13.23	37.57	17.86–57.81	3	49.5 ± 52.24	19.67	17.86–110.97
3	5	76.09 ± 26.87	60.01	51.26–110.97	3	72.74 ± 22.6	60.01	59.36–98.84

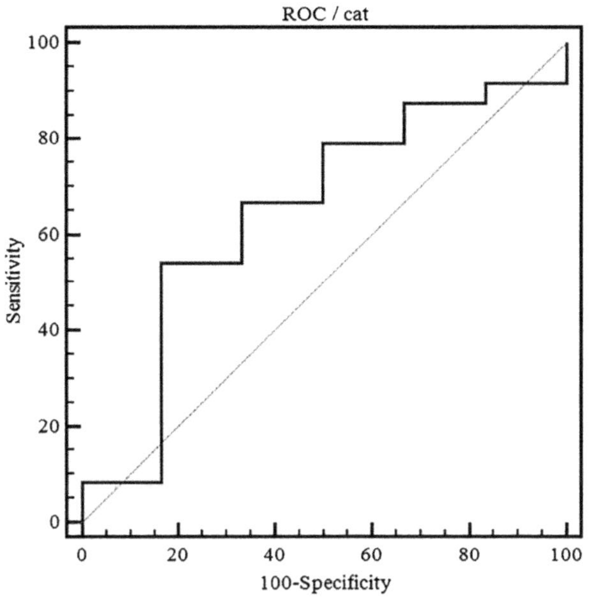

Fig. 4 ROC curve analysis of the cat samples classified as normal ("no relevant findings") and as pathological. (AUROC = 0.65, 95%; confidence interval:= 0.45–0.81). Choosing a cut-off value of 44 the sensitivity was 54% and the specificity was 83%)

part of the MGV variability in the normal samples could be explained by the anisotropic interaction between the ultrasound beam and the renal tubules [7].

The mean age of the dogs included in the present study was relatively high (9.5 ± 4 years) and all the histopathological lesions encountered were related to chronic rather than acute kidney disease; therefore, no data on the relationship between acute renal disease and renal echogenicity was available in this study. Some acute renal pathologies (e.g. ethylene glycol toxicity, leptospirosis) [1] are reported to dramatically increase renal cortical echogenicity; it is very likely that, in dogs, quantitative analysis of ultrasonographic images may be more accurate in the detection of acute rather than chronic renal disease. For this reason further studies, recording also clinical and biochemical data, are wished for the analysis of the relationship occurring between acute kidney disease and renal cortical echogenicity.

The results of this study revealed a significant linear correlation between the MGV calculated on the cat samples and the degeneration scores, whereas no correlation with the inflammation score was evident. Statistical analysis did not show any significant differences in the MGV of normal (grade 0) and mildly degenerated (grade 1 and 2) samples, whereas the MGV calculated on severely degenerated samples was significantly higher. On the other hand, the univariate analysis revealed a moderate influence of histopathological lesions on MGV (44% of MGV variance was explained by the model).

The poor diagnostic performance of MGV in the detection of pathological kidney changes in the cat – albeit higher than in the dog - is, in the authors' opinion, mostly associated to a large overlap between the MGV calculated in normal and pathological samples (Table 3).

In the cat, proximal tubular lipidosis is reported to increase renal cortical echogenicity in otherwise architecturally normal kidneys [8]. Interestingly, no statistically significant differences in the measured MGV associated with this anatomical variation were apparent in the present study. All the pathological samples in our study population presented a mixture of histological lesions, and no samples classified as "no relevant findings" showed significant proximal tubular lipidosis. Furthermore, no samples were classified as pathological only on the basis of the presence of proximal tubular lipidosis. Our results suggest that other morphological lesions such as fibrosis, tubular vacuolar degeneration, interstitial nephritis, glomerulonephritis rather than proximal tubular lipidosis have a direct influence on the echogenicity of pathological kidneys (Table 5).

Histopathological lesions were related to chronic rather than acute renal damage also in cats. Some forms of acute renal damages (e.g. lily intoxication) [1] are reported to significantly increase renal cortical echogenicity; it is beyond the authors' knowledge whether it would be possible to discriminate, by means of quantitative analysis of ultrasonographic images, between acute intoxication and severe degeneration.

In human medicine, a low correlation between renal lesions and ultrasonography has been established [9, 10] and the poor diagnostic value of renal cortical echogenicity in the detection of chronic renal disease has been clearly defined [11]. To the best of the authors' knowledge, this is the first in-vivo report in veterinary medicine to objectively evaluate renal cortical echogenicity in comparison to the detection of chronic renal damage through histopathology. Further studies involving a larger number of subjects are required to establish the relationship occurring between renal cortical echogenicity and acute renal disease in dogs and cats.

Conclusions

This is the first in-vivo report in veterinary medicine quantifying the changes in renal cortical echogenicity in relation to renal histopathology. In dogs, the high variability of the echogenicity in the normal kidney and the weak influence of pathological changes on renal cortical echogenicity reveal ultrasonography a poor test to discriminate between normal and chronically affected kidneys. In cats, despite the higher influence of renal damage on renal cortical echogenicity, pathological changes are evident only in chronic stages of disease thus limiting the usefulness of ultrasonography in detecting mild renal disease.

Abbreviations
ANOVA: Analysis of variance; DICOM: Digital imaging and communications in medicine format; MGV: Mean Gray Value; ROC: Receiver operator characteristics curve; RoI: Region of Interest

Funding
The present paper is part of a pilot study project funded by two research grants from the University of Padova, Italy (Grants #: CPDA124900/2012 and Junior Research Grant 2015) and by a research grant from Veneto Regional Council, Italy (Grant #: FSE 2105/201/27/1148/2013).

Authors' contributions
TB: conceived the study, performed the ultrasonographic examinations, drafted and revised the manuscript. FB: performed the histological examinations, drafted and revised the manuscript. LA: performed the histological examinations, drafted and revised the manuscript. AZ: conceived the study, performed the ultrasonographic examinations, drafted and revised the manuscript. All authors read and approved the final manuscript.

Competing interests
The authors declare that they have no competing interest.

Consent for publication
Not applicable.

Author details
[1]Department of Animal Medicine, Production and Health, Clinical Section, Radiology Unit, University of Padua, Viale dell'Università 16, Legnaro 35020, Padua, Italy. [2]Department of Comparative Biomedicine and Food Science, University of Padua, Viale dell'Università 16, Legnaro 35020, Padua, Italy.

References
1. D'Anjou MA, Penninck D. Kidneys and ureters. In: D'Anjou MA, Penninck D, editors. Atlas Small Animal Ultrasound, Second Ed. Ames: Wiley Blackwell; 2015. p. 331–61.
2. Nyland T, Widmer W, Mattoon JS. Urinary Tract. In: Nyland T, Mattoon JS, editors. Small Animal Diagnostic Ultrasound. 3rd ed. St. Luis: Elsevier; 2015. p. 557–607.
3. Zotti A, Banzato T, Gelain ME, Centelleghe C, Vaccaro C, Aresu L. Correlation of renal histopathology with renal echogenicity in dogs and cats: an ex-vivo quantitative study. BMC Vet Res. 2015;11:99.
4. Drost WT, Henry GA, Meinkoth JH, Woods JP, Lehenbauer TW. Quantification of hepatic and renal cortical echogenicity in clinically normal cats. AJVR. 2000;61:1016–20.
5. Ivancić M, Mai W. Qualitative and quantitative comparison of renal vs. hepatic ultrasonographic intensity in healthy dogs. Vet Radiol Ultrasound. 2008;49:368–73.
6. Yabuki A, Endo Y, Sakamoto H, Nagayoshi T, Matsumoto M, Suzuki S. Quantitative assessment of renal cortical echogenicity in clinically normal cats. Anat Hist Embryol. 2008;37:383–6.
7. Ruth JD, Heng HG, Miller MA, Constable PD. Effect of anisotropy and spatial compound imaging on renal cortical echogenicity in dogs. Vet Radiol Ultrasound. 2013;54:659–65.
8. Yeager AE, Anderson WI. Study of association between histologic features and echogenicity of architecturally normal cat kidneys. AJVR. 1989;50:860–3.
9. Quaia E, Bertolotto M. Renal parenchymal diseases: is characterization feasible with ultrasound? Europ Radiol. 2002;12:2006–20.
10. Rosenfield A, Siegel N. Renal parenchymal disease: histopathologic-sonographic correlation. Am J Roentgenol. 1981;137:793–8.
11. Moghazi S, Jones E, Schroepple J, McCleallan W, Hennigar RA, O'Neill WC. Correlation of renal histopathology with sonographic findings. Kidney Int. 2005;67:1515–20.

4

Salmonella serotypes and their antimicrobial susceptibility in apparently healthy dogs in Addis Ababa, Ethiopia

Bitsu Kiflu[1], Haile Alemayehu[2], Mukarim Abdurahaman[3], Yohannes Negash[2] and Tadesse Eguale[2*]

Abstract

Background: The close bond between pet animals and family members poses risk of infection with zoonotic bacterial pathogens such as *Salmonella*. No data is available on occurrence of *Salmonella* in dogs in Ethiopia. The aim of this study was therefore to determine the prevalence, serotype distribution and antimicrobial resistance of *Salmonella* from feces of apparently healthy dogs in Addis Ababa, Ethiopia.

Results: Of the total 360 dogs examined, 42 (11.7%; 95% Confidence limit of 8.5%–15.4%) were positive for *Salmonella*. Fourteen serotypes were detected and the predominant ones were *S.* Bronx ($n = 7$; 16.7%), *S.* Newport ($n = 6$; 14.3%), followed by *S.* Typhimurium, *S.* Indiana, *S.* Kentucky, *S.* Saintpaul and *S.* Virchow ($n = 4$; 9.5%) each. *Salmonella* infection status was significantly associated with history of symptom of diarrhea during the past 60 days (OR = 3.78; CI = 1.76–8.13; $p = 0$). Highest resistance rates were found for oxytetracycline (59.5%), neomycin (50%), streptomycin (38.1%), cephalothin (33.3%), doxycycline (30.9%), ampicillin (30.9%) and amoxicillin + clavulanic acid (26.2%). Thirty eight (90.5%) of the isolates were resistant or intermediately resistant to at least one of the 16 antimicrobials tested. Resistance to two or more antimicrobials was detected in 30 (71.4%) of the isolates. Resistance to three or more antimicrobials was detected in 19 (45.2%) of the isolates.

Conclusion: This study demonstrated high carriage rate of *Salmonella* serotypes known for causing human salmonellosis and large proportion of them were resistant to antimicrobials used in public and veterinary medicine for management of various bacterial infections, suggesting the possible risk of infection of human population in close contact with these dogs by drug resistant pathogens. Therefore, it is vital to work on raising public awareness on zoonotic canine diseases prevention measures and good hygienic practices.

Keywords: *Salmonella*, Serotype, Antimicrobial resistance, Dog, Zoonosis, Addis Ababa, Ethiopia

Background

Salmonellosis is an infectious disease of humans and animals caused by several serotypes of *Salmonella*. *Salmonella* is widespread in the environment and commonly found in farm effluents, human sewage and in any material subjected to fecal contamination [1]. *Salmonella* in animals are of major concern, because animals can serve as latent carriers of *Salmonella* serotypes and shed the organism into the environment without any apparent clinical signs posing risk of human infection [2]. Dogs are one of the important asymptomatic carriers of *Salmonella,* as they can harbour large bacterial load in the intestines and mesenteric lymph nodes which can be shed in their feces [3]. This could be of significant importance to public health as dogs have close contact with family members in households.

Antimicrobial resistant *Salmonella* and other zoonotic pathogens originating from companion animals have a great public health importance. The majority of studies on antimicrobial resistance in *Salmonella* focused on food animals and farm environments, since food animals are believed to be the major sources of resistant strains of non-typhoidal *Salmonella*. However, a few studies reported antimicrobial resistant *Salmonella* isolates, including multidrug resistant (MDR) ones from dogs

* Correspondence: tadesse.eguale@aau.edu.et
[2]Aklilu Lemma Institute of Pathobiology, Addis Ababa University, P.O. Box 1176, Addis Ababa, Ethiopia
Full list of author information is available at the end of the article

and other companion animals in different parts of the world [4–6].

In Ethiopia, no data is available on occurrence of zoonotic bacterial pathogens in dogs and possible risk of human infection with *Salmonella* from dogs. Majority of previous work focused mainly on food animals and food items [7, 8]. However, there is an increasing trend of keeping dogs in urban areas and demand for general veterinary services for dogs is also increasing [9]. The objectives of this study were therefore to investigate the prevalence, serotype distribution and antimicrobial susceptibility of *Salmonella* isolates from apparently healthy dogs in Addis Ababa, Ethiopia. In addition, various factors were also examined for the possible association of *Salmonella* occurrence in dogs.

Methods

Study area and study animals

The study was conducted from January to October, 2015 in Addis Ababa, which is the capital city and administration center for the Federal Democratic Republic of Ethiopia. Among ten sub-cities, four sub-cities namely, Gulele, Arada, Kirkos and Yeka were randomly selected. A total of 360 dogs were involved in this study. Those brought to veterinary clinics for anti-rabies vaccination (n = 264) were sampled. In addition, dogs (n = 96) were also sampled through door to door visit from households. Apparently healthy dogs of all age groups and both sexes were included in the study. Sick dogs and/or dogs treated recently with antimicrobials were not included in the study.

Sample and data collection

Rectal swab samples were collected with sterile cotton swab by rotating the swab inside the rectum of the dog and the swab was placed into screw caped test tubes containing 10 ml of sterile buffered peptone water (BPW) (Becton Dickinson, France). The test tubes were properly labeled and transported in ice box to Microbiology Laboratory of Aklilu Lemma Institute of Pathobiology, Addis Ababa University within 3–4 h of collection.

During sample collection, data was also collected from 252 households using a questionnaire that focused on assessing the possible risk factors of *Salmonella* infection. Possible risk factors considered for the presence of *Salmonella* including: age, sex, history of diarrhea during the last 2 months, purpose of dog ownership, type of food and source of food/meat provided to dog were among the questions included in the questionnaire.

Salmonella isolation and identification

Isolation and identification of *Salmonella* was conducted as described previously [7]. Briefly, fecal swabs in buffered peptone water (BPW) pre-enrichment broth were homogenized using vortex mixer for 30 s and incubated at 37 °C for 24 h. A 100 µl pre-enriched suspension was added into 9.9 ml of Rappaport-Vassiliadis enrichment Broth (RVB) (Oxoid, USA) and incubated at 42 °C for 24 h. At the same time, 1 ml of suspension was also transferred to 9 ml of Tetrathionate broth (TTB) (Oxoid, USA) and incubated for 24 h at 37 °C. It was then streaked from both RVB and TTB to Xylose Lysine Tergitol 4 (XLT-4) (Oxoid, USA) and Brilliant Green Agar (BGA) (Difco Becton Dickinson, USA) selective media and the plates were then incubated at 37 °C for 24 h. XLT-4 plates were incubated for additional 24 h and second reading was conducted at 48 h. Presumptive *Salmonella* colonies were further investigated biochemically using Triple Sugar Iron agar, Urea, Citrate and Lysine Iron Agar slants. Those colonies with typical *Salmonella* biochemical properties were then further confirmed by genus specific polymerase chain reaction (PCR) [10]. Reference strain of *S.* Typhimurium (ATCC 14028) was used as a positive control during biochemical analysis and PCR. Confirmed *Salmonella* isolates were stored at −80 °C in 20% glycerol until further testing.

Salmonella serotyping and phage typing

Salmonella isolates were serotyped and phage-typed at the Public Health Agency of Canada, World Organization for Animal Health (OIÉ) Reference Laboratory for Salmonellosis, Guelph, Ontario, Canada. Briefly, the somatic (O) antigens were determined by slide agglutination tests [11] and flagellar antigens were determined using a microplate agglutination technique [12]. The antigenic formulae of Grimont and Weill [13] were used to identify and assign the serotypes of the isolates. Phage typing of *S.* Typhimurium isolates was performed according to Anderson et al. [14] with reference phages obtained from the Public Health England, Gastrointestinal Bacteria Reference Unit, Colindale, England and the Public Health Agency of Canada, National Laboratory for Enteric Pathogens, Winnipeg, Canada. *Salmonella* isolates that reacted with the phages but did not conform to any recognized phage type were designated atypical (AT).

Antimicrobial susceptibility testing

Susceptibility of the isolates to 16 antimicrobials was determined using the disk diffusion method according to the guidelines of the Clinical and Laboratory Standards Institute [15]. Briefly, frozen isolates were subcultured on tryptic soy agar (Becton, Dickinson and Company, USA) from which 3 to 4 pure colonies were inoculated to a tube containing 5 ml of tryptic soy broth (TSB) (Becton, Dickinson and Company, USA) and mixed gently using sterile inoculating loop. It was then incubated at 37 °C for 4–5 h. The turbidity of the suspension was then adjusted to the optical density of a McFarland unit of 0.5 using sterile saline to standardize the inoculum size. Sterile cotton swab was dipped and rotated several times and pressed firmly on the inside wall of the tube above the fluid level to remove excess inoculum. It was then inoculated to Mueller Hinton Agar plate (Oxoid, Ltd) by streaking the swab over the entire surface of the plate. The inoculated plates were left at room temperature to dry for 5–10 min and antimicrobial discs were dispensed by pressing on the plate with sterile forceps and the plates were inverted and incubated at 37 °C overnight. Diameters of the zone of inhibition were measured to the nearest millimeter using a plastic transparent ruler. The interpretation of the categories of susceptible, intermediate or resistant was based on the CLSI guidelines [15]. The cut off points used for the interpretation is shown in Table 1. For the purpose of analysis, all readings classified as intermediate were considered as resistant unless indicated. Reference strain of *Escherichia coli* ATCC 25922 was used as a quality control. The list of antimicrobial discs (Sensi-Discs, Becton, Dickinson and Company, Loveton, USA) used in the study and their strength is shown in Table 1.

Statistical analysis

The data were computed by using statistical package for social sciences (SPSS version 20.0). The association between *Salmonella* occurrence and pre-specified categorical factors were compared using person's χ^2 test. The point prevalence was calculated as the number of infected individuals divided by the number of individual's sampled × 100. A p- value <0.05 was reported as statistically significant.

Results

Occurrence of *Salmonella* in dogs

Of the total 360 dogs examined, 42 (11.67%; 95% confidence limit of 8.5%–15.4%) were positive for *Salmonella*. There was no significant difference in prevalence of *Salmonella* among dogs from different sub-cities, purpose for which the dogs were kept and type and source of food/meat provided to dogs. Similarly, there was no significant difference in *Salmonella* carriage among age groups and sex ($p > 0.05$) (Table 2). Isolation of *Salmonella* was observed to be more common among dogs who had diarrhea within the past 2 months compared to those with no history of diarrhea (OR = 3.78, 95% CI = 1.76–8.13) (Table 3).

Salmonella serotype distribution

Overall, 14 different *Salmonella* serotypes were recovered, the predominant serotypes were *S.* Bronx (n = 7; 16.7%), *S.* Newport (n = 6; 14.3%), *S.* Typhimurium (n = 4; 9.5%), *S.* Indiana (n = 4; 9.5%), *S.* Kentucky (n = 4; 9.5%), *S.* Saintpaul (n = 4; 9.5%) and *S.* Virchow (n = 4; 9.5%). Other serotypes such as *S.* Anatum (n = 2), *S.* Haifa (n = 2), *S.* Braenderup (n = 1), *S.* Chailey (n = 1), *S.* Minnesota (n = 1), *S.* Muenchen (n = 1) and *S.* Tarshyne (n = 1) were also identified (Table 4). To our knowledge, *S.* Bronx, *S.* Chailey, *S.* Indiana, *S.* Minnesota and *S.* Tarshyne are reported for the first time in Ethiopia. Phagetyping of the

Table 1 List of antimicrobial discs used in the study, their strength and zone diameter interpretive cut off points in mm

Disk	Disc strength in µg	Resistant ≤ (mm)	Intermediate (mm)	Susceptible ≥ (mm)
Amikacin	30	14	15–16	17
Amoxicillin + clavulanic acid	20/10	13	14–17	18
Ampicillin	10	13	14–16	17
Cefoxitin	30	14	15–17	18
Ceftriaxone	30	19	20–22	23
Cephalothin	30	14	15–17	18
Chloramphenicol	30	12	13–17	18
Ciprofloxacin	5	20	21–30	31
Doxycycline	30	10	11–13	14
Gentamicin	10	12	13–14	15
Kanamycin	30	13	14–17	18
Nalidixic acid	30	13	14–18	19
Neomycin	30	12	13–16	17
Oxytetracycline	30	11	12–14	15
Streptomycin	10	11	12–14	15
Sulfamethoxazole and Trimethoprim	23.75 and 1.25	10	11–15	16

Table 2 Frequency of *Salmonella* carriage among apparently healthy dogs with respect to selected factors

Variables categories		Number examined	No. positive (%)	X^2(*p*-value)
Sub-cities	Gulele	137	16 (11.7)	2.1 (0.6)
	Arada	78	7 (9)	
	Kirkos	83	13 (15.7)	
	Yeka	62	6 (9.7)	
Sex	Male	291	35 (12.0)	0.2 (0.7)
	Female	69	7 (10.1)	
Age	Puppy (<6 month)	73	11 (15.0)	4.6 (0.3)
	>6 months - 2 yrs	84	9 (10.7)	
	>2 yrs. - 6 yrs	137	16 (11.7)	
	>6 yrs. to 10 yrs	46	2 (4.3)	
	Over 10 yrs	20	4 (20)	
Purpose of dog ownership	Guard	130	19 (14.7)	2.9 (0.2)
	Hobby	86	6 (6.9)	
	Guard + hobby	144	17 (11.8)	
Overall		360	42 (11.7)	

4 *S.* Typhimurium showed that two of the isolates were phage type 74 while the other two were atypical.

Antimicrobial susceptibility of *Salmonella* isolates

Frequency of isolates resistant or intermediately resistant to various antimicrobials is shown in Table 4. High resistance rate was recorded among isolates to oxytetracycline 25(59.5%), neomycin 21 (50%), streptomycin 16 (38.1%), cephalothin14 (33.3%), doxycycline 13 (30.9%), ampicillin 13 (30.9%), and amoxicillin + clavulanic acid 11(26.2%). All isolates were susceptible to ciprofloxacin and amikacin. Of the 42 *Salmonella* isolates, 38 (90.5%) were resistant to one or more of the antimicrobials tested. Resistance to two or more antimicrobials was detected in 30 (71.4%) of the isolates. Resistance to three or more antimicrobials was detected in 19 (45.2%) of the isolates. Resistance to five or more antimicrobials was detected in 10 (23.8%) of the isolates whereas 4 (9.5%) isolates were MDR to eight or more antimicrobials.

Different serotypes appeared to exhibit disparity in their susceptibility to some of the antimicrobials tested. For instance all *S.* Newport isolates were resistant to three or more antimicrobials. Likewise, 3 of the 4 *S.* Saintpaul isolates were resistant to five or more antimicrobials. On the other hand, strains belonging to *S.* Virchow, *S.* Typhimurium and *S.* Kentucky were resistant to relatively less number of antimicrobials (Table 5).

Discussion

Overall *Salmonella* prevalence of 11.7% in the current study is in line with the study conducted in Thailand in dogs which reported 13.2% of *Salmonella* carriage [16].

Table 3 Association of various factors with carriage of *Salmonella* among dogs in Addis Ababa

Variables	Categorical parameter	No. sampled	No. positive for *Salmonella* (%)	OR(95% CI)	X^2(*p*-value)
Diarrhea during the last months	Yes	62	16 (25.8)	3.8 (1.8–8.1)	(0.0)
	No	190	16 (8.4)		
Type of food provided to the dog	Meat	21	1 (4.8)	-	2.9 (0.3)
	Table scraps	17	4 (23.5)		
	Meat + table scraps	211	27 (12.8)		
	Commercial pet food	3	0		
Source of food/meat for dogs	Local unlicensed markets	198	24 (12.1)	-	0.9 (0.6)
	Licensed butchers	51	8 (15.7)		
	Supermarkets	3	0		
Overall		252	32		

Table 4 *Salmonella* serotype distribution and frequency of resistance to various antimicrobials

Antimicrobials tested	*Salmonella* serotypes and No.(%) of isolates [a]resistant to various antimicrobials ($n = 42$)														
	Bronx	Newport	Indiana	Kentucky	Saintpaul	Typhimurium	Virchow	Anatum	Haifa	Braenderup	Chailey	Minnesota	Muenchen	Tarshyne	No.(%) resistant
	$n = 7$	$n = 6$	$n = 4$	$n = 4$	$n = 4$	$n = 4$	$n = 4$	$n = 2$	$n = 2$	$n = 1$	$n = 1$	$n = 1$	$n = 1$	$n = 1$	
AM	2(28.6)	4(66.7)	1(25)	1(25)	3(75)	-	-	-	1(50)	-	1(100)	-	-	-	13(30.9)
AMC	1(14.3)	4(66.7)	1(25)	1(25)	3(75)	-	-	-	1(50)	-	-	-	-	-	11(26.2)
CF	1(14.3)	4(66.7)	1(25)	1(25)	3(75)	1(25)	1(25)	-	1(50)	-	1(100)	-	-	-	14(33.3)
CRO	-	-	-	-	-	-	-	-	1(50)	-	1(100)	-	-	-	2(4.8)
FOX	1(14.3)	-	1(25)	1(25)	-	-	-	-	1(50)	-	-	-	-	-	4(9.5)
AN	-	-	-	-	-	-	-	-	-	-	-	-	-	-	0
GM	1(14.3)	-	-	-	-	-	-	-	-	-	-	-	-	-	1(2.4)
K	-	-	-	-	-	-	-	-	-	1(100)	-	-	-	-	1(2.4)
N	5(71.4)	3(50)	1(25)	2(50)	2(50)	-	-	2(100)	2(100)	1(100)	1(100)	1(100)	1(100)	-	21(50)
S	3(42.9)	3(50)	4(100)	1(25)	1(25)	1(25)	-	1(50)	1(50)	-	1(100)	-	-	-	16(38.1)
SXT	-	-	1(25)	-	1(25)	-	-	-	1(50)	-	1(100)	-	-	-	4(9.5)
CIP	-	-	-	-	-	-	-	-	-	-	-	-	-	-	0
NA	-	-	1(25)	-	-	-	-	-	-	-	-	-	-	-	1(2.4)
DO	1(14.3)	5(83.3)	1(25)	-	3(75)	1(25)	-	1(50)	1(50)	-	-	-	-	-	13(30.9)
T	3(42.9)	5(83.3)	1(25)	3(75)	4(100)	2(50)	2(50)	2(100)	1(50)	1(100)	-	1(100)	-	-	25(59.5)
C	-	-	1(25)	-	1(25)	-	-	-	-	-	-	-	-	1(100)	3(7.1)

AN Amikacin, *AM* Ampicillin, *AMC* Amoxicillin-clavulanic acid, *C* Chloramphenicol, CF Cephalothin, *CRO* Ceftriaxone, *CIP* Ciprofloxcin, *FOX* Cefoxitin, *DO* Doxycycline, *GM* Gentamicin, *K* Kanamycin, *N* Neomycin, *NA* Nalidixic acid, *S* Streptomycin, *SXT* Sulfamethoxazole + Trimethoprim, *T* Oxytetracycline

[a]Isolates intermediately resistant were also considered resistant

Table 5 Antimicrobial resistance pattern of *Salmonella* serotypes isolated from dogs

Number	Serotypes	No.	Resistance pattern	
			Intermediate	Resistant
1	Anatum	1	N, T	-
2	Anatum	1	N	DO, S, T
3	Braenderup	1	K, N, T	-
4	Bronx	1	N, T	-
5	Bronx	1	T	-
6	Bronx	1	AMC, DO, N, S	AM, CF, FOX, GM
7	Bronx	1	N, T	AM
8	Bronx	2	N, S	-
9	Bronx	1	-	-
10	Chailey	1	N,S	AM, CF, CRO, SXT
11	Haifa	1	N	DO, T
12	Haifa	1	CRO, N, AM	AMC, CF, FOX, S, SXT
13	Indiana	1	N,S	-
14	Indiana	2	S	-
15	Indiana	1	DO, NA, T	AM, AMC, C, CF, FOX, S, SXT
16	Kentucky	1	-	AM, AMC,CF,FOX
17	Kentucky	1	S, T	-
18	Kentucky	2	N, T	-
19	Minnesota	1	N, T	-
20	Muenchen	1	N	-
21	Newport	1	CF, N	AM, AMC, DO, T
22	Newport	1	N	AM, AMC, CF
23	Newport	2	-	DO, S, T
24	Newport	1	AM, N	AMC, CF, DO, S, T
25	Newport	1	DO	AM, AMC, CF, T
26	Saintpaul	1	CF	AM, AMC, DO, T
27	Saintpaul	1	N	AM, AMC, CF, DO, T
28	Saintpaul	1	CF, S	AM, AMC, C, DO, SXT, T
29	Saintpaul	1	T, N	-
30	Tarshyne	1	-	C
31	Typhimurium Pt 74	1	-	-
32	Typhimurium Pt 74	1	CF, S, T	-
33	Typhimurium At	1	-	-
34	Typhimurium At	1	-	DO,T
35	Virchow	2	T	-
36	Virchow	1	-	-
37	Virchow	1	CF	-

Similarly, prevalence in dogs in Iran (13.2%), was comparable to the current finding [2]. However, studies in some developed countries showed much lower rates of *Salmonella* carriage compared to the present finding, for example, 0% in Canada [17]; 0.2% in UK [18], 1% in Turkey [19], and 2.3% in Colorado, USA [20]. The possible reason for the high prevalence of *Salmonella* in the current study and other previous studies compared to the ones conducted in developed countries could be due to differences in pet sanitary practices, feeding habit, difference in public awareness about dog zoonosis and socioeconomic status of the owners. Dog owners in developed countries are aware of the importance of hygiene and make use of the available veterinary care for their animals [21]. In addition, some factors such as difference in season of study, geographical areas and isolation methods employed might have also accounted for the observed difference [22]. In the current study, we used rectal swab samples instead of collection of larger volume of fecal samples which could have probably underestimated the true prevalence.

The association between *Salmonella* carriage and history of diarrhea during the past 2 months could presumably be due to *Salmonella* being one of the causes of clinical disease manifested by diarrhea in this dog population. In line to our finding, a study conducted in Texas, USA reported an association between diarrhea and positive *Salmonella* status in dogs [23]. Clinical salmonellosis is rare in dogs, but clinical signs including diarrhea, fever, anorexia, and abdominal pain are not uncommon [24].

A high degree of serotype diversity was observed among *Salmonella* isolates in the present study of which *S.* Bronx, *S.* Chailey, *S.* Indiana, *S.* Minnesota and *S.* Tarshyne had never been reported from Ethiopia. In related studies conducted in other countries, *S.* Newport and *S.* Typhimurium were reported from dogs [25–27] and pet food [28]. Lefebvre et al. [29] reported that *S.* Kentucky and *S.* Typhimurium were the most common serotypes recovered from dogs in Canada. Leonard et al. [30] also reported *S.* Kentucky as the second most dominant serotype isolated from dogs in Ontario, Canada. Some of the *Salmonella* serotypes isolated in the current study such as *S.* Bronx, *S.* Chailey and *S.* Tarshyne had not been previously reported from dogs. However, they were reported from other sources including humans in other countries. *S.* Chailey was isolated from human patients in Korea and New Zeland [31, 32], *S.* Tarshyne from antelope, ostrich and caracal [33]. *S.* Bronx, the predominant serotype in the current study was first isolated from diarrheic human patient in 1955 in USA [34] and our literature search showed no other report from any other source.

Some of the serotypes reported in this study were previously isolated from animals and animal products in the country. For instance: *S.* Newport, *S.*Typhimurium, *S.* Kentucky, *S.* Saintpaul, *S.* Virchow [7, 8, 35]. Moreover, majority of the serotypes identified in the current study such as *S.* Kentucky, *S.* Typhimurium, *S.* Virchow, *S.* Saintpaul were also isolated from diarrheic human patients in Addis Ababa in our recent study [36]. In this study, it was found that stool samples of 7.2% of the diarrheic human patients attending primary health centers in Addis Ababa were positive for *Salmonella.* The co-occurrence of similar serotypes in companion animals, food animals and humans suggests the circulation of these serotypes among various hosts in the study area.

Majority of the isolates in the current study were resistant or intermediately resistant to at least one antimicrobial and the prevalence of resistance was high to oxytetracycline, neomycin and streptomycin. Similarly, previous antimicrobial resistance studies on canine *Salmonella* in Trinidad [22] and Taiwan [37] reported higher levels of resistance. In contrast, a study conducted in Nigeria [38] in *Salmonella* isolates recovered from dogs demonstrated lower resistance rate to most of antimicrobials tested. The reason for difference in antimicrobial resistance profile between studies could be due to difference in serotypes involved and differences in the antimicrobial usage in humans, food animals as well as pets in respective study areas. The one possible reason for higher antimicrobial resistance in our finding could be, as feeding dogs with raw meat is common practice in Addis Ababa, there is a high chance of exposure to antimicrobial resistant *Salmonella* from different animal products used as pet food. High resistance rate to oxytetracycline and streptomycin in this study could be due to the fact that these drugs are the most commonly used antimicrobials in veterinary medicine in the country [7, 39], and as the majority of the dog owners in Addis Ababa feed raw animal products to their dogs [40], chance of being infected with resistant *Salmonella* from these raw animal products is very high. Previous work showed 71.3% of beef obtained from cattle slaughtered in central Ethiopia contained oxytetracycline residue [41]. Uncooked meat products such as head of cattle, sheep and goats, legs of slaughtered animals are the common food given for dogs in Addis Ababa.

S. Newport and *S.* Saintpaul showed high rate of resistance to many antimicorbials tested. This may be due to the fact that these serotypes were among the commonly isolated *Salmonella* serotypes from animal products in Ethiopia [42] and they might had possibly been subjected to various antimicrobials which might have rendered them to develop resistace and eventually got access to dogs through food.

Conclusion

This study showed high carriage rate of *Salmonella* serotypes commonly known for causing human salmonellosis and some of these isolates were resistant to antimicrobials used both in human and veterinary medicine for management of various bacterial infections, suggesting the possible risk of MDR *Salmonella* infection of human population in close contact with these dogs. Therefore, it is important to raise public awareness on zoonotic canine diseases prevention measures and good hygienic practices. Feeding dogs with cooked meat products, provision of clean water and improving hygiene of pet husbandry practices is therefore essential to prevent further spread of *Salmonella* and other foodborne zoonotic pathogens in dogs and people in close contact with dogs.

Abbreviations
BGA: Brilliant Green Agar; BPW: Buffered peptone water; MDR: Multi-drug resistance; RVB: Rappaport-Vassiliadis Broth; TTB: Tetrathionate broth; XLT-4: Xylose Lysine Tergitol 4

Acknowledgments
We would like to thank animal health professionals at various veterinary clinics in Addis Ababa and dog owners for their cooperation during sample collection. We are grateful to Dr. Roger P. Johnson, Dr. Linda Cole, Shaun Kernaghan, Ketna Mistry, Ann Perets and Betty Wilkie of the Public Health Agency of Canada, National Microbiology Laboratory at Guelph for serotyping and phagetyping of the *Salmonella* isolates.

Funding
This study was partly supported by Jimma University and Aklilu Lemma Institute of Pathobiology, Addis Ababa University.

Authors' contributions
TE was involved in conception of the study and preparation of the manuscript. BK was involved in sample collection, laboratory investigation and preparation of the draft manuscript. HA and YN participated in laboratory work. MA participated in preparation of the manuscript and data analysis. All authors read and approved the final manuscript.

Competing interests
The authors declare that they have no competing interests.

Consent for publication
Not applicable.

Author details
[1]Ministry of Livestock and Fisheries, P.O. Box 170042, Addis Ababa, Ethiopia. [2]Aklilu Lemma Institute of Pathobiology, Addis Ababa University, P.O. Box 1176, Addis Ababa, Ethiopia. [3]College of Agriculture and Veterinary Medicine, Jimma University, P.O.Box 307, Jimma, Ethiopia.

References
1. OIE. Report of the meeting of the OIE ad hoc group on Salmonellosis. May 2010 ed. Paris: World Organisation for Animal Health; 2010.
2. Salehi T, Badouei M, Madadgar O, Ghiasi S, Tamai I. Shepherd dogs as a common source for salmonella enterica serovar reading in Garmsar, Iran. Turk J Vet Anim Sci. 2013;37:102–5.
3. Hoelzer K, Moreno Switt AI, Wiedmann M. Animal contact as a source of human non-typhoidal salmonellosis. Vet Res. 2011;42:34.
4. Guardabassi L, Schwarz S, Lloyd DH. Pet animals as reservoirs of antimicrobial-resistant bacteria. J Antimicrob Chemother. 2004;54(2):321–32.
5. Lloyd DH. Reservoirs of antimicrobial resistance in pet animals. Clin Infect Dis. 2007;45(Suppl 2):S148–52.
6. Umber JK, Bender JB. Pets and antimicrobial resistance. Vet Clin North Am Small Anim Pract. 2009;39(2):279–92.
7. Eguale T, Engidawork E, Gebreyes AW, Asrat D, Alemayehu H, Medhin G, Johnson RP, Gunn JS. Fecal prevalence, serotype distribution and antimicrobial resistance of salmonellae in dairy cattle in central Ethiopia. BMC Microbiol. 2016;16(1):1–11.
8. Zewdu E, Cornelius P. Antimicrobial resistance pattern of salmonella serotypes isolated from food items and personnel in Addis Ababa, Ethiopia. Trop Anim Health Prod. 2009;41(2):241–9.
9. Atsbaha G, Hussien D, Cruz Cruz R. Assessment of major health problems of dogs in Mekelle City, Ethiopia. Global Veterinaria. 2014;12(2):176–80.
10. Cohen ND, Neibergs HL, McGruder ED, Whitford HW, Behle RW, Ray PM, Hargis BM. Genus-specific detection of salmonellae using the polymerase chain reaction (PCR). J Vet Diagn Investig. 1993;5(3):368–71.
11. Ewing. Serological Identificaiton of Salmonella. 1986.
12. Shipp CR, Rowe B. A mechanised microtechnique for salmonella serotyping. J Clin Pathol. 1980;33(6):595–7.
13. Grimont P, Weill F-X. Antigenic formulas of salmonella serotypes. 9th ed. France: WHO Collaborating Centre for Reference and Research on Salmonella; 2007.
14. Anderson ES, Ward LR, Saxe MJ, de Sa JD. Bacteriophage-typing designations of salmonella typhimurium. J Hyg (Lond). 1977;78(2):297–300.
15. CLSI: Performance standards for antimicrobial susceptibility testing; twenty-third informational SupplementM100-S23. Vol. 33; 2013.
16. Polpakdee A, Angkititrakul S, Suksawat F, Sparagano O, Kanistanon K. Epidemiology and antimicrobial resistance of salmonella sp. isolated from dogs and cats in northeastern Thailand. J Anim Vet Adv. 2012;11(5):618–21.
17. Murphy C, Reid-Smith RJ, Prescott JF, Bonnett BN, Poppe C, Boerlin P, Weese JS, Janecko N, McEwen SA. Occurrence of antimicrobial resistant bacteria in healthy dogs and cats presented to private veterinary hospitals in southern Ontario: a preliminary study. Can Vet J. 2009;50(10):1047–53.
18. Lowden P, Wallis C, Gee N, Hilton A. Investigating the prevalence of salmonella in dogs within the midlands region of the United Kingdom. BMC Vet Res. 2015;11:239.
19. Bagcigil AF, Ikiz S, Dokuzeylu B, Basaran B, Or E, Ozgur NY. Fecal shedding of salmonella spp. in dogs. J Vet Med Sci. 2007;69(7):775–7.
20. Hackett T, Lappin MR. Prevalence of enteric pathogens in dogs of north-central Colorado. J Am Anim Hosp Assoc. 2003;39(1):52–6.
21. Stull JW, Peregrine AS, Sargeant JM, Weese JS. Pet husbandry and infection control practices related to zoonotic disease risks in Ontario, Canada. BMC Public Health. 2013;13:520.
22. Seepersadsingh N, Adesiyun AA, Seebaransingh R. Prevalence and antimicrobial resistance of salmonella spp. in non-diarrhoeic dogs in Trinidad. J Vet Med B Infect Dis Vet Public Health. 2004;51(7):337–42.
23. Leahy AM, Cummings KJ, Rodriguez-Rivera LD, Rankin SC, Hamer SA. Evaluation of faecal salmonella shedding among dogs at seven animal shelters across Texas. Zoonoses Public Health. 2016;63(7):515–21.
24. Marks SL, Kather EJ. Bacterial-associated diarrhea in the dog: a critical appraisal. Vet Clin North Am Small Anim Pract. 2003;33(5):1029–60.
25. Morley PS, Strohmeyer RA, Tankson JD, Hyatt DR, Dargatz DA, Fedorka-Cray PJ. Evaluation of the association between feeding raw meat and salmonella enterica infections at a greyhound breeding facility. J Am Vet Med Assoc. 2006;228(10):1524–32.
26. McKenzie E, Riehl J, Banse H, Kass PH, Nelson S Jr, Marks SL. Prevalence of diarrhea and enteropathogens in racing sled dogs. J Vet Intern Med. 2010;24(1):97–103.
27. Ojo O, Ernest O, Adetosoye A. Salmonella Typhimurium infection in diarrhoeic and non-diarrhoiec dogs in Ibadan, Nigeria. Veterinarski Arhiv. 2009;79(4):371–7.
28. CDC. Human salmonellosis associated with animal-derived pet treats–United States and Canada, 2005, Centers for Disease Control and Prevention. MMWR Morb Mortal Wkly Rep. 2006;55(25):702–5.
29. Lefebvre SL, Reid-Smith R, Boerlin P, Weese JS. Evaluation of the risks of shedding salmonellae and other potential pathogens by therapy dogs fed raw diets in Ontario and Alberta. Zoonoses Public Health. 2008;55(8–10):470–80.
30. Leonard EK. What could your dog be carrying? – Zoonotic enteric bacteria in pet dogs in Ontario: prevalence, risk factors, and antimicrobial resistance. Ontario: The University of Guelph; 2014.
31. Kim S, Kim S, Shin J, Lee B, Park M. Occurrence and distribution of various genetic structures of class 1 and class 2 integrons in salmonella enterica isolates from foodborne disease patients in Korea for 16 years. Foodborne Path Dis. 2010;8(2):319–24.
32. Public Health Surveillance Information for New Zealand Public Health Action, Human *Salmonella* Isolates. 2012. No.12 December. https://surv.esr.cri.nz/enteric_reference/human_salmonella.php?we_objectID=3266. Accessed 10 Apr 2017.
33. Münch S, Braun P, Wernery U, Kinne J, Pees M, Flieger A, Tietze E, Rabsch W. Prevalence, serovars, phage types, and antibiotic susceptibilities of *Salmonella* strains isolated from animals in the United Arab Emirates from 1996 to 2009. Trop Anim Health Prod. 2012;44:1725–38.
34. Saphara I, Wasserman M, Friedman S. A new Salmonella type: Salmonella Bronex. J Bacteriol. 1955;69:447.
35. Alemu S, Zewde BM. Prevalence and antimicrobial resistance profiles of salmonella enterica serovars isolated from slaughtered cattle in Bahir Dar, Ethiopia. Trop Anim Health Prod. 2012;44(3):595–600.
36. Eguale T, Gebreyes WA, Asrat D, Alemayehu H, Gunn JS, Engidawork E. Non-typhoidal salmonella serotypes, antimicrobial resistance and co-infection with parasites among patients with diarrhea and other gastrointestinal complaints in Addis Ababa, Ethiopia. BMC Infect Dis. 2015;15:497.

37. Tsai HJ, Huang HC, Lin CM, Lien YY, Chou CH. Salmonellae and campylobacters in household and stray dogs in northern Taiwan. Vet Res Commun. 2007;31(8):931–9.
38. Jajere SM, Onyilokwu SA, Adamu NB, Atsanda NN, Saidu AS, Adamu SG, Mustapha FB. Prevalence of salmonella infection in dogs in maiduguri, northeastern Nigeria. Int J Microbiol. 2014;2014:392548.
39. Beyene T, Endalamaw D, Tolossa Y, Feyisa A. Evaluation of rational use of veterinary drugs especially antimicrobials and anthelmintics in Bishoftu, Central Ethiopia. BMC Res Notes. 2015;8:482.
40. Kiflu B, Abdurahaman M, Alemayehu H, Eguale T. Investigation on public knowledge, attitude and practices related to pet management and zoonotic canine diseases in Addis Ababa, Ethiopia. Ethiopian Vet J. 2016;20(1):67–78.
41. Bedada A, Molla B. Tetracycline residue levels in slaughtered beef cattle from three slaughter houses in Central Ethiopia. Global Veterinaria. 2012;8(6):546–54.
42. Tadesse G, Gebremedhin EZ. Prevalence of salmonella in raw animal products in Ethiopia: a meta-analysis. BMC Res Notes. 2015;8:163.

High prevalence of *Enterocytozoon bieneusi* zoonotic genotype D in captive golden snub-nosed monkey (*Rhinopithecus roxellanae*) in zoos in China

Fuchang Yu[1,2], Yayun Wu[1,2], Tongyi Li[3], Jianke Cao[1,2], Jiantang Wang[3], Suhui Hu[1,2], Huili Zhu[1,4], Sumei Zhang[1,2], Rongjun Wang[1,2], Changshen Ning[1,2] and Longxian Zhang[1,2*]

Abstract

Background: *Enterocytozoon bieneusi* is the dominant specie of microsporidia which can infect both anthroponotic and zoonotic species. The golden snub-nosed monkey is an endangered primate which can also infect by *E. bieneusi*. To date, few genetic data on *E. bieneusi* from golden snub-nosed monkeys has been published. Therefore, to clarify the prevalence and genotypes of *E. bieneusi* in captive golden snub-nosed monkeys is necessary to assess the potential for zoonotic transmission.

Result: We examined 160 golden snub-nosed monkeys from six zoos in four cities in China, using PCR and comparative sequence analysis of the ribosomal internal transcribed spacer (ITS). The overall prevalence of *E. bieneusi* was 46.2% (74/160); while the prevalence was 26.7%, 69.1%, 69.4% and 33.3% in Shanghai Zoo, Shanghai Wild Animal Park, Tongling Zoo, and Taiyuan Zoo respectively ($P = 0.006$). A total of seven *E. bieneusi* genotypes were found that included four known (D, J, CHG1, and CHG14) and three new (CM19–CM 21) genotypes. The most common genotype was D (54/74, 73.0%), followed by J (14/74, 18.9%); other genotypes were restricted to one or two samples. Phylogenetic analysis revealed that genotype D belonged to the previously-characterized Group 1, with zoonotic potential; whereas genotypes J, CHG1, CHG14 and CM19–CM 21 clustered in the previously-characterized Group 2, the so-called cattle host specificity group.

Conclusions: The findings of high prevalence of zoonotic *E. bieneusi* genotypes D and J in golden snub-nosed monkeys suggest that golden snub-nosed monkeys may be the reservoir hosts for human microsporidiosis, and vice versa.

Keywords: Microsporidia, Molecular characterization, Phylogeny, Nonhuman primates

Background

Microsporidia is a relatively diverse clade of unicellular fungi, living as obligate intracellular pathogens, comprising over 1300 species in at least 160 genera [1]. To date, 14 species of microsporidian pathogens have been diagnosed in humans [2], among which *Enterocytozoon bieneusi* is dominant [3]. Manifestations of microsporidiosis caused by *E. bieneusi* include stubborn chronic diarrhea, abdominal pain and weight loss, in immunocompromised people, such as those infected with HIV, organ transplant recipients, cancer patients, and diabetics; while in immunocompetent individuals *E. bieneusi* causes self-limiting diarrhea and malnutrition, and is sometimes asymptomatic [4–6]. *E. bieneusi* has also been detected in variety of animal hosts, including mammals, birds, rodents and reptiles [7, 8].

Since the first identification of *E. bieneusi* in an AIDS patient by Desportes and others in 1985, more than 240 genotypes of the species have been reported from numerous animal hosts, based on sequence analysis of the

* Correspondence: zhanglongxian8999@foxmail.com; zhanglx8999@henau.edu.cn; zhanglx8999@gmail.com
[1]College of Animal Science and Veterinary Medicine, Henan Agricultural University, Zhengzhou 450002, People's Republic of China
[2]International Joint Research Laboratory for Zoonotic Diseases of Henan, Zhengzhou 450002, People's Republic of China
Full list of author information is available at the end of the article

internal transcribed spacer (ITS) region of the ribosomal RNA (rRNA) gene [8–14]. Phylogenetic analysis of ITS sequences has revealed the presence of eight genotype groups [15]. More than 94% of the identified ITS genotypes of *E. bieneusi* constitute a large group with zoonotic potential, designated as Group 1, while the rest are divided into several host-adapted groups, designated as Groups 2 to 8 [10, 15, 16]. While the molecular phylogeny of these strains is well-studied, the full range of host diversity, including reservoirs and potential zoonotic transmission, remain unresolved issues [17].

The golden snub-nosed monkey is classified as a Category I protected species in China [18]. The species is listed as Category Endangered by the International Union for Conservation of Nature (IUCN), as its numbers have declined by more than 50% in the last 3 generations (approximately 40 years), because of habitat loss. This decline is continuing, though in some areas the populations are declining at a lower rate [19]. In an attempt to improve population numbers and protect the species' diversity, some golden snub-nosed monkeys have been captured and placed in zoos [20]. Several recent studies have focused on *E. bieneusi* in nonhuman primates (NHPs) in China and in Kenya, with 43 *E. bieneusi* ITS genotypes reported from various NHP species [15, 17, 21]. However, very limited genetic data are available on *E. bieneusi* from golden snub-nosed monkeys. The present study clarifies the prevalence of *E. bieneusi* in captive golden snub-nosed monkeys, as well as assessing the potential for zoonotic transmission.

Methods

Study sites and sampling

The study was conducted over a 5-month period (June to November 2015), during that period of time fecal specimens of golden snub-nosed monkeys were collected from Beijing Zoo (116°33′E, 39°94′N), Beijing Wildlife Park (116°33′E, 39°49′N), Shanghai Zoo (121°36′E, 31°19′N), Shanghai Wild Animal Park (121°72′E, 31°05′N), Taiyuan Zoo (112°57′E, 37°91′N) and Tongling Zoo (117°85′E, 30°82′N) (Fig. 1). Some of the monkeys live in single-individual cages; but the majority live as family units in large cages or houses, there are 2 to 4 monkeys in one family unit. The accommodation usually includes play equipment to occupy the animals. To avoid direct contact with visitors, cages are fenced and surrounded by ditches. All the monkeys are usually fed with multigrain bread twice a day, in the morning and afternoon, with eggs, nuts, seasonal fruits and vegetables as snacks.

A total of 160 fresh fecal specimens were collected from the six zoos in this study (Table 1 and Additional file 1: Table S1). All the specimens were collected with the help of local animal attendants, to minimize possible social disruption to the monkeys. Where monkeys were

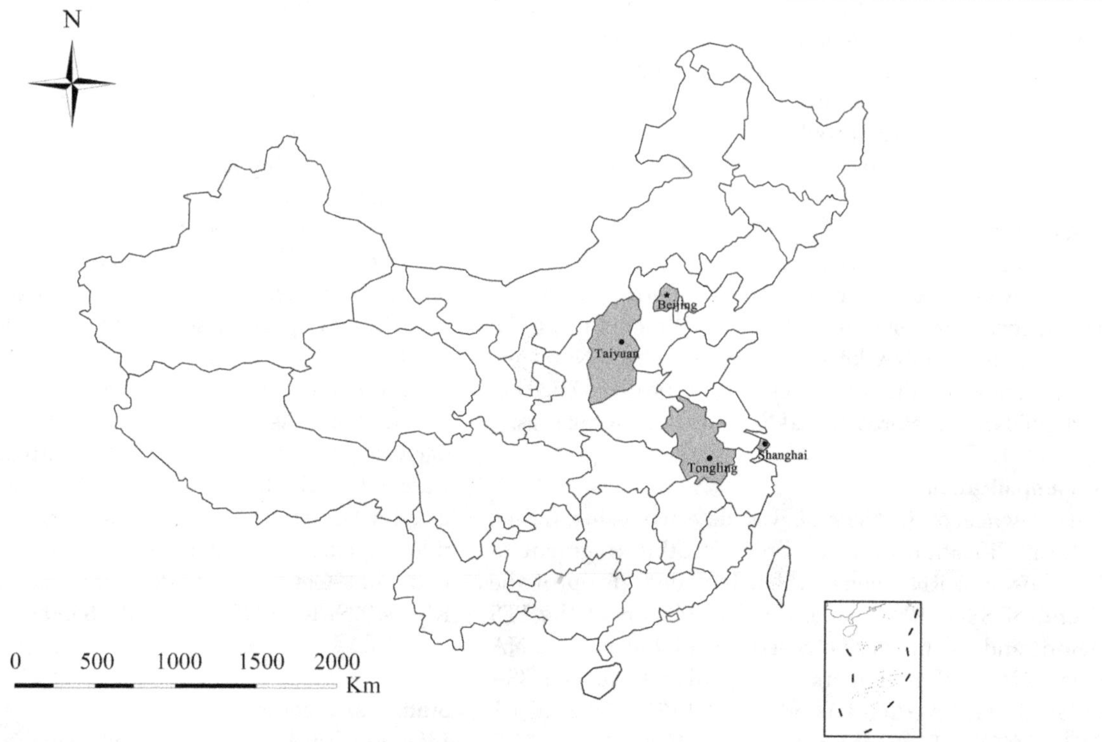

Fig. 1 Locations of zoos at which specimens were collected in this study. The figure was generated using the softwares of Chinamap 2.42, Microsoft PowerPoint 2003 and Adobe Photoshop CS6

Table 1 Prevalence and ITS genotype distribution of *E. bieneusi* in Golden snub-nosed monkeys in different zoos in China

Study location	No. of specimens	No. (%) of positive specimens	ITS genotypes (no. of specimens)	
			Known	Novel
Beijing Wildlife Park	25	0		
Beijing Zoo	8	0		
Shanghai Zoo	15	4(26.7)	J(2)	CM19(1), CM20(1)
Shanghai Wild Animal Park	55	38(69.1)	D(33), CHG1(1), J(3), CHG14(1)	
Tongling Zoo, Anhui Province	36	25(69.4)	D(21), J(3)	CM21(1)
Taiyuan Zoo, Shanxi Province	21	7(33.3)	J(6)	CM19(1)

housed individually, fresh fecal deposits were collected in the early morning, as the floors of animal houses were cleaned each evening. For monkeys that were kept in family units in houses during the day, fecal specimens were collected from houses where they spent the night. As the animal handlers described, almost all the monkeys only have one excretion during a whole night, and there are distinct differences among feces from different family members, such as color, smell, size, viscosity, hardness and so on. To avoid duplicate sampling of animals, the fecal deposits were collected for once according to their characteristics. All the specimens were placed into labeled clean zip-lock bags, transported to the Laboratory of Veterinary Parasitology, Henan Agricultural University, in a cooler with ice packs, transferred in water into a 50 ml centrifuge tube, sieved through a 6.5 cm diameter sieve with a pore size of 375 μm (to avoid cross-contamination between samples, the sieve was washed twice with distilled water), and then concentrated by centrifugation. The concentrated fecal specimens were stored in 2.5% potassium dichromate solution at 4 °C prior to DNA extraction.

DNA extraction

The stored fecal specimens were washed three times with distilled water after centrifugation, to remove the potassium dichromate. Genomic DNA was extracted using the *E.Z.N.A.R* Stool DNA kit (Omega Biotek Inc., Norcross, USA), following the manufacturer's protocol. The extracted DNA was stored at −20 °C prior to PCR analysis.

PCR amplification

The presence of *E. bieneusi* was detected using nested PCR amplification of a 389 bp nucleotide fragment of the ribosomal RNA gene, which included 76 bp of the 3′-end of SSU rRNA gene, the full 243 bp of the ITS region, and 70 bp of the 5′-region of the 5.8S rRNA gene [22]. Outer primers were EBITS3 (5′-GGTCA TAGGGATGAAGAG-3′) and EBITS4 (5′-TTCGAGTT CTTTCGCGCTC-3′); EBITS1 (5′-GCTCTGAATATC TATGGCT-3′) and EBITS2.4 (5′-ATCGCCGACGGAT CCAAGTG-3′) were used as nested primers for secondary PCR. The cycling parameters were as previously described [23]. Each specimen was analyzed twice, with 1 μl of extracted DNA as template for each PCR, using an Applied Biosystems 2720 Thermal Cycler (Applied Biosystems, Foster City, USA). KOD-Plus enzyme (Toyobo Co. Ltd., Osaka, Japan) was used for PCR amplification. A negative control without DNA was included in all PCRs. Secondary PCR products were examined after 1% agarose gel electrophoresis and staining with GelRed (Biotium Inc., Hayward, CA).

Nucleotide sequencing and genetic proximity analysis

All positive secondary PCR products were purified using Montage PCR filters (Millipore, Bedford, MA), and sequenced with the secondary PCR primers, by Sinogenomax Biotechnology Co. Ltd. (Beijing, China), using a BigDye Terminator v3.1 cycle sequencing kit (Applied Biosystems) on an ABI 3730 DNA analyzer (Applied Biosystems, Foster City, CA). The accuracy of nucleotide sequences was confirmed by bidirectional sequencing, and by sequencing additional PCR products if necessary.

Sequences were aligned with reference sequences that had been downloaded from GenBank, using Clustal × 2.1 (http://www.clustal.org/). To assess the phylogenetic relationships between ITS genotypes of *E. bieneusi* obtained in the present study and those downloaded from Genbank, a phylogenetic tree was constructed using the Neighbor-Joining(NJ) algorithm, based on a matrix of evolutionary distances calculated using the Kimura 2-parameter model, in MEGA 6.0 (http://www.megasoftware.net/). Confidence in the NJ tree was estimated using a bootstrap analysis with 1000 replicates. Nucleotide sequences obtained in this study have been deposited in GenBank under the accession numbers KU604929–KU604934 and KU685395.

Statistical analysis

Infection rates were compared using a chi-square test, with differences considered statistically significant at $P < 0.05$.

Results

Occurrence and genotypes of *E. bieneusi*

A total of 160 fecal specimens were examined for *E. bieneusi* by PCR, with 74 (46.2%) specimens being positive for *E. bieneusi*. The pathogen was detected in four zoos, including Shanghai Zoo (26.7% of specimens), Shanghai Wild Animal Park (69.1%), Tongling Zoo (69.4%), and Taiyuan Zoo (33.3%), of the six zoos enrolled in this study (Table 1). Differences in prevalence were statistically significant among different zoos ($P = 0.006$). Phylogenetic analysis showed the sequences came from seven distinct *E. bieneusi* genotypes, including four known genotypes (D, J, CHG1, and CHG14) and three new genotypes (named CM19, CM20 and CM21 in this study). As shown in Table 1, genotype D (54/74, 73.0%) was dominant, followed by genotype J (14/74,

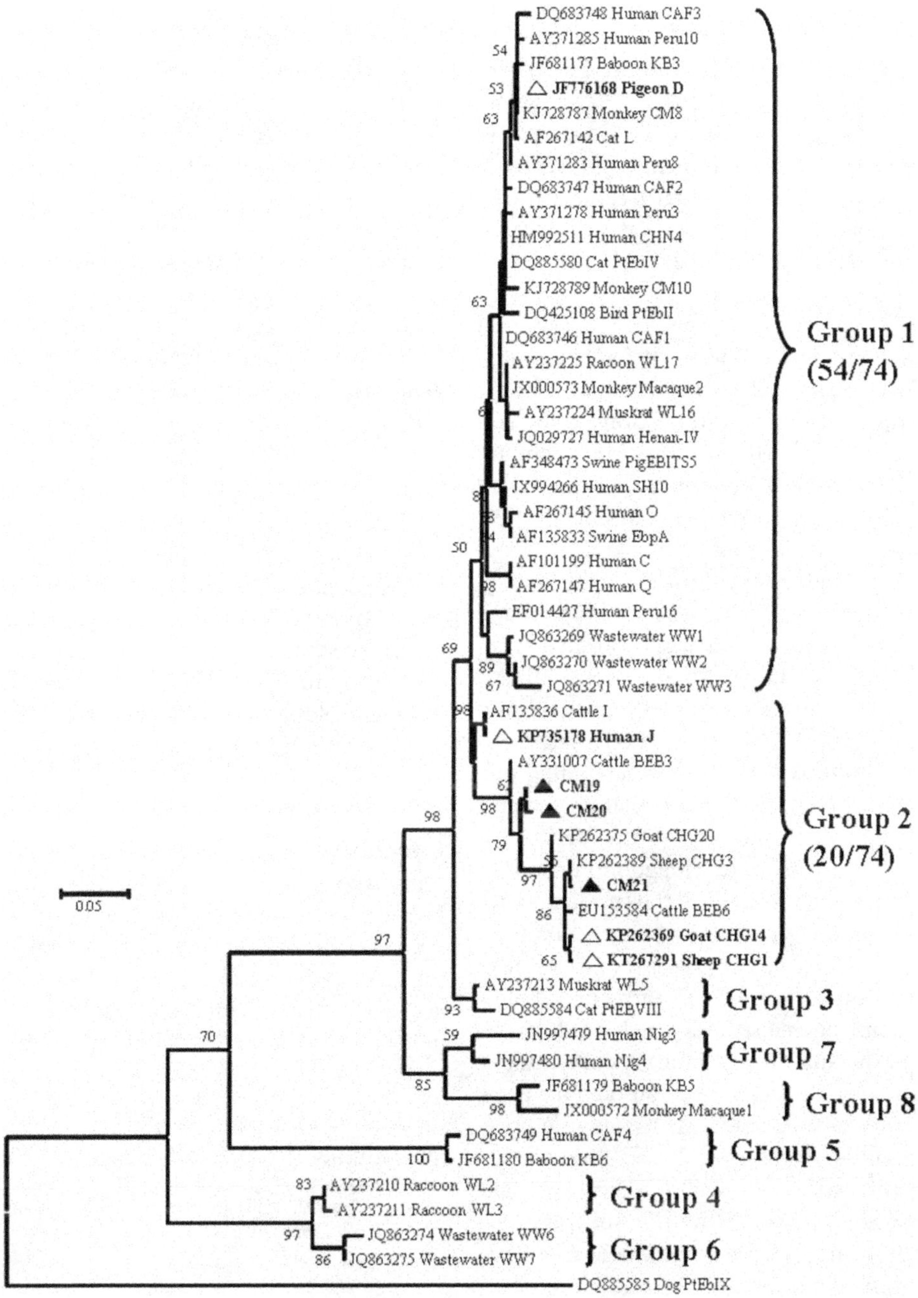

Fig. 2 Neighbor-Joining tree of *E. bieneusi* ITS genotypes. The tree was rooted with GenBank sequence DQ885585. Bootstrap values greater than 50% from 1000 replicates are shown on nodes. Each sequence from GenBank is identified by its accession number, host origin, and genotype designation. The group terminology for the clusters is based on previous papers by Thellier and Breton [6], and Karim et al. [15]. Known and new genotypes identified in this study are indicated by open and filled triangles, respectively

18.9%); CM19 was found in two specimens (2/74, 2.7%), while the remaining four genotypes were seen in only one specimen each (1/74, 1.4%).

Phylogenetic analysis and genetic proximity

Phylogenetic analysis revealed that genotype D belonged to the previously-described Group 1 (Fig. 2). New genotypes CM19 and CM20 differed from genotype CHG20 (KP262375) in Single Nucleotide Polymorphisms (SNPs) at ITS nucleotide positions 177 (an A to G change), 181 (T to C), 261 (G deletion), 268 (G insertion) and 270 (A to G); while CM20 has another SNP at position 177 (A to G). Compared to genotype CHG3 (KP262389), genotype CM21 had one SNP at position 265 (G to T). Genotypes J, CHG1, CHG14 and the three new genotypes (CM19, CM20, and CM21) formed Group 2 in our tree, which has previously been described as the so-called cattle host specificity group (Fig. 2 and Additional file 2: Table S2).

Discussion

In this study, *E. bieneusi* was found in 46.2% of golden snub-nosed monkeys examined in six zoos in China. The prevalence was higher than that previously reported for golden snub-nosed monkeys in Sichuan (3.5%, 1/29) and Shaanxi (9.5%, 6/63) provinces in China [21, 24]. All of the fecal specimens examined in this study were sampled from six zoos distributed in four locations (Beijing, Shanghai, Anhui Province and Shanxi Province). The infection rates of *E. bieneusi* in monkeys differed among the four zoos that included positive fecal samples. Similar results (11.4%–29.8% prevalence) have previously been reported in different NHP species from various parts of China [15, 17, 21, 24–26]. Perceived rates of infection are influenced by many factors, including the need for laboratory diagnosis, sample sizes, animal management practices, infection intensity of the pathogen, climate and geography. As a parasite with zoonotic potential, *E. bieneusi* has been proved to have the probability to transmit across different NHP species or between animals and animal handlers [27–29]. So the prevalence also maybe influenced by other NHPs living nearby or the animal handlers. As an endangered species which needs more care and protection, the snub-nosed monkeys are usually confined away from other NHP species in all the four zoos that included positive fecal samples. Thus an inference was made that the other NHPs contributed little to the high prevalence in this study. Although the fecal samples of animal handlers were not involved in this study, nevertheless, the transmission probability between monkeys and animal handlers is undeniable.

The zoonotic genotype D, which was the commonest in this study, has been observed frequently in other NHPs, including orangutan, gibbon, macaque and baboon [15, 17, 21, 24–26]. Genotype D has also been identified as the most prevalent genotype in humans, in human wastewater, and in many other animal species (cattle, pigs, sheep, dogs, cats, horses, beavers, otters, muskrats, raccoons, pigeons, falcons and foxes) worldwide [3, 8, 17, 29–34]. For example, a study examining 33 stool samples from human immunodeficiency virus (HIV)-infected adult patients in Thailand showed that genotype D was the most common, found in 36.4% (12 of 33) of the samples [29]. In a recent study, a total of 23 ITS genotypes were obtained from wastewater in Shanghai, Nanjing, Wuhan and Qingdao cities, with genotype D being the most prevalent, found in 279 of 338 (82.5%) positive samples [34]. These results demonstrate that interspecies transmission of genotype D poses a zoonotic risk, as well as being of public health significance already within the human population. The second commonest genotype found in this study, J, is most often found in cattle, though it has been reported as being in humans in Jilin province, China [35]. We have also found this genotype in patients from Henan Province, China (unpublished data). These findings suggest that genotype J may be transmissible from golden snub-nosed monkeys to humans, or vice versa.

The three new genotypes (CM19–CM21), CHG1 and CHG14 were all clustered in the previously-described Group 2, along with the zoonotic genotype J. Although these genotypes fall into a group that has previously been considered cattle-specific, genotype J clearly has the ability to infect humans. Thus, these three new genotypes belonging to Group 2 may also have the ability to cause human microsporidiosis.

Conclusion

Our study demonstrates a high prevalence of *E. bieneusi* genotypes D and J in golden snub-nosed monkey kept in zoos in China. As these genotypes are common to humans and animals, golden snub-nosed monkeys may serve as potential reservoir hosts for zoonotic *E. bieneusi* genotypes.

Abbreviations

HIV: Human immunodeficiency virus; ITS: Internal transcribed spacer; IUCN: The International Union for Conservation of Nature; NHPs: Nonhuman primates; rRNA: Ribosomal RNA

Acknowledgments

We want to thank all staffs who got involved in sample collection in this study at Beijing Zoo, Beijing Wildlife Park, Shanghai Zoo, Shanghai Wild Animal Park, Taiyuan Zoo and Tongling Zoo.

Funding
This study was supported, in part, by the National Natural Science Foundation of China (U1404327), the Key Program of the National Natural Science Foundation of China (31330079), and the Key National Science and Technology Specific Projects (2012ZX10004220-001).

Authors' contributions
Conceived and designed the experiments: LXZ. Performed the experiments: FCY, YYW, TYL, SMZ, RJW and SHH. Analyzed the data: FCY, JTW, HLZ and JKC. Wrote the manuscript: FCY, CSN and LXZ. All authors have read and approved the final manuscript.

Competing interests
The authors declare that they have no competing interests.

Consent for publication
Not applicable.

Author details
[1]College of Animal Science and Veterinary Medicine, Henan Agricultural University, Zhengzhou 450002, People's Republic of China. [2]International Joint Research Laboratory for Zoonotic Diseases of Henan, Zhengzhou 450002, People's Republic of China. [3]Zhengzhou Zoo, Zhengzhou 450000, People's Republic of China. [4]College of Animal Science, Henan Institute of Science and Technology, Xinxiang 453003, People's Republic of China.

References

1. Didier ES, Weiss LM. Microsporidiosis: current status. Curr Opin Infect Dis. 2006;19(5):485–92.
2. Didier ES, Weiss LM. Microsporidiosis: not just in AIDS patients. Curr Opin Infect Dis. 2011;24(5):490–5.
3. Matos O, Lobo ML, Xiao L. Epidemiology of *Enterocytozoon bieneusi* Infection in Humans. J Parasitol Res. 2012; doi:10.1155/2012/981424.
4. Mor SM, Tumwine JK, Naumova EN, Ndeezi G, Tzipori S. Microsporidiosis and malnutrition in children with persistent diarrhea. Uganda Emerg Infect Dis. 2009;15(1):49–52.
5. Sak B, Brady D, Pelikánová M, Květoňová D, Rost M, Kostka M, et al. Unapparent microsporidial infection among immunocompetent humans in the Czech Republic. J Clin Microbiol. 2011;49(3):1064–70.
6. Thellier M, Breton J. *Enterocytozoon bieneusi* in human and animals, focus on laboratory identification and molecular epidemiology. Parasite. 2008;15(3):349–58.
7. Karim MR, Yu F, Li J, Li J, Zhang L, Wang R, et al. First molecular characterization of enteric protozoa and the human pathogenic microsporidian, *Enterocytozoon bieneusi*, in captive snakes in China. Parasitol Res. 2014;113(8):3041–8.
8. Santín M, Fayer R. Microsporidiosis: *Enterocytozoon bieneusi* in domesticated and wild animals. Res Vet Sci. 2011;90(3):363–71.
9. Desportes I, Charpentier YL, Galian A, Bernard F, Cochand-Priollet B, Lavergne A, et al. Occurrence of a New Microsporidan: *Enterocytozoon bieneusi* ng, n. sp., in the Enterocytes of a Human Patient with AIDS1. J Protozool. 1985;32(2):250–4.
10. Henriques-Gil N, Haro M, Izquierdo F, Fenoy S, del Águila C. Phylogenetic approach to the variability of the microsporidian *Enterocytozoon bieneusi* and its implications for inter-and intrahost transmission. Appl Environ Microbiol. 2010;76(10):3333–42.
11. Zhang Z, Huang J, Karim MR, Zhao J, Dong H, Ai W, et al. Zoonotic *Enterocytozoon bieneusi* genotypes in Pere David's deer (*Elaphurus davidianus*) in Henan. China Exp Parasitol. 2015;155:46–8.
12. Zhao W, Zhang W, Yang D, Zhang L, Wang R, Liu A. Prevalence of *Enterocytozoon bieneusi* and genetic diversity of ITS genotypes in sheep and goats in China. Infect Genet Evol. 2015;32:265–70.
13. Zhao Z, Wang R, Zhao W, Qi M, Zhao J, Zhang L, et al. Genotyping and subtyping of *Giardia* and *Cryptosporidium* isolates from commensal rodents in China. Parasitology. 2015;142(6):800–6.
14. Fiuza VR, Oliveira FC, Fayer R, Santin M. First report of *Enterocytozoon bieneusi* in pigs in Brazil. Parasitol Int. 2015;64(4):18–23.
15. Karim MR, Wang R, Dong H, Zhang L, Li J, Zhang S, et al. Genetic polymorphism and zoonotic potential of *Enterocytozoon bieneusi* from nonhuman primates in China. Appl Environ Microbiol. 2014;80(6):1893–8.
16. Guo Y, Alderisio KA, Yang W, Cama V, Feng Y, Xiao L. Host specificity and source of *Enterocytozoon bieneusi* genotypes in a drinking source watershed. Appl Environ Microbiol. 2014;80(1):218–25.
17. Karim MR, Dong H, Li T, Yu F, Li D, Zhang L, et al. Predomination and new genotypes of *Enterocytozoon bieneusi* in captive nonhuman primates in zoos in China: high genetic diversity and zoonotic significance. PLoS One. 2015;10(2):e0117991.
18. Wen R. Research for the Species of *Rhinopithecus* and Their Distribution in Ancient and Modern Times. Chinese J Nature. 2003;25(1):41–8.
19. Yongcheng L, Richardson M. *Rhinopithecus roxellana*. In: The IUCN Red List of Threatened Species 2008. the International Union for Conservation of Nature. 2008. http://www.iucnredlist.org/details/39829/0. Accessed 18 Feb 2016.
20. Yu Z. A Comparative Analysis of the Reproductive Fitness of a Captive Population of Golden Snub-Nosed Monkey. Chinese J Wildlife. 2011;32(2):69–72.
21. Du SZ, Zhao GH, Shao JF, Fang YQ, Tian GR, Zhang LX, et al. Qi M, Yu SK. *Cryptosporidium* spp., *Giardia intestinalis*, and *Enterocytozoon bieneusi* in Captive Non-Human Primates in Qinling Mountains. Korean J Parasitol. 2015; 53(4):395–402.
22. Sulaiman IM, Fayer R, Lal AA, Trout JM, Schaefer FW, Xiao L. Molecular characterization of microsporidia indicates that wild mammals harbor host-adapted *Enterocytozoon* spp. as well as human-pathogenic *Enterocytozoon bieneusi*. Appl Environ Microbiol. 2003;69(8):4495–501.
23. Buckholt MA, Lee JH, Tzipori S. Prevalence of *Enterocytozoon bieneusi* in Swine: an 18-Month Survey at a Slaughterhouse in Massachusetts. Appl Environ Microbiol. 2002;68(5):2595–9.
24. Karim MR, Wang R, He X, Zhang L, Li J, Rume FI, et al. Multilocus sequence typing of *Enterocytozoon bieneusi* in nonhuman primates in China. Vet Parasitol. 2014;200(1–2):13–23.
25. Li W, Kiulia NM, Mwenda JM, Nyachieo A, Taylor MB, Zhang X, et al. *Cyclospora papionis*, *Cryptosporidium hominis*, and human-pathogenic *Enterocytozoon bieneusi* in captive baboons in Kenya. J Clin Microbiol. 2011;49(12):4326–9.
26. Ye J, Xiao L, Li J, Huang W, Amer SE, Guo Y, et al. Occurrence of human-pathogenic *Enterocytozoon bieneusi*, *Giardia duodenalis* and *Cryptosporidium* genotypes in laboratory macaques in Guangxi. China Parasitol Int. 2014; 63(1):132–7.
27. Karim MR. Molecular epidemiology and multilocus typing of *Croptosporidium* spp., *Giardia duodenalis* and *Enterocytozoon bieneusi* in nonhuman primates in China. Zhengzhou: Henan Agricultural University; 2014.
28. Ye P. The Research on Gastrointestinal Parasites in Provisioned and Wild-raiding in Sichuan Snub-nosed monkeys (*Rhinopithecus roxellanain*) in Autumn and Winter. Changsha: South University of Forestry and Technology; 2013.
29. Wan Q, Xiao L, Zhang X, Li Y, Lu Y, Song M, et al. Clonal Evolution of *Enterocytozoon bieneusi* Populations in Swine and Genetic Differentiation in Subpopulations between Isolates from Swine and Humans. PLoS Negl Trop Dis. 2016;10(8):e0004966.
30. Leelayoova S, Subrungruang I, Suputtamongkol Y, Worapong J, Petmitr PC, Mungthin M. Identification of genotypes of *Enterocytozoon bieneusi* from stool samples from human immunodeficiency virus-infected patients in Thailand. J Clin Microbiol. 2006;44(8):3001–4.
31. Mori H, Mahittikorn A, Thammasonthijarern N, Chaisiri K, Rojekittikhun W, Sukthana Y. Presence of zoonotic *Enterocytozoon bieneusi* in cats in a temple in central Thailand. Vet Parasitol. 2013;197(3–4):696–701.
32. Mori H, Mahittikorn A, Watthanakulpanich D, Komalamisra C, Sukthana Y. Zoonotic potential of *Enterocytozoon bieneusi* among children in rural communities in Thailand. Parasite. 2013;20:14.
33. Santín M, Cortés Vecino JA, Fayer R. A zoonotic genotype of *Enterocytozoon bieneusi* in horses. J Parasitol. 2010;96(1):157–61.
34. Zhao W, Zhang W, Yang Z, Liu A, Zhang L, Yang F, et al. Genotyping of *Enterocytozoon bieneusi* in Farmed Blue Foxes (*Alopex lagopus*) and Raccoon Dogs (*Nyctereutes procyonoides*) in China. PLoS One. 2015;10(11):e0142611.
35. Li N, Xiao L, Wang L, Zhao S, Zhao X, Duan L, et al. Molecular surveillance of *Cryptosporidium* spp., *Giardia duodenalis*, and *Enterocytozoon bieneusi* by genotyping and subtyping parasites in wastewater. PLoS Negl Trop Dis. 2012;6(9):e1809.

6

Comprehensive genomic characterization of five canine lymphoid tumor cell lines

Sarah C. Roode[1], Daniel Rotroff[2], Kristy L. Richards[3,4,5,11], Peter Moore[6], Alison Motsinger-Reif[2,4], Yasuhiko Okamura[7], Takuya Mizuno[8], Hajime Tsujimoto[9], Steven E. Suter[4,5,10*] and Matthew Breen[1,4,5*]

Abstract

Background: Leukemia/lymphoma cell lines have been critical in the investigation of the pathogenesis and therapy of hematological malignancies. While human LL cell lines have generally been found to recapitulate the primary tumors from which they were derived, appropriate characterization including cytogenetic and transcriptional assessment is crucial for assessing their clinical predictive value.

Results: In the following study, five canine LL cell lines, CLBL-1, Ema, TL-1 (Nody-1), UL-1, and 3132, were characterized using extensive immunophenotyping, karyotypic analysis, oligonucleotide array comparative genomic hybridization (oaCGH), and gene expression profiling. Genome-wide DNA copy number data from the cell lines were also directly compared with 299 primary canine round cell tumors to determine whether the cell lines represent primary tumors, and, if so, what subtype each most closely resembled.

Conclusions: Based on integrated analyses, CLBL-1 was classified as B-cell lymphoma, Ema and TL-1 as T-cell lymphoma, and UL-1 as T-cell acute lymphoblastic leukemia. 3132, originally classified as a B-cell lymphoma, was reclassified as a histiocytic sarcoma based on characteristic cytogenomic properties. In combination, these data begin to elucidate the clinical predictive value of these cell lines which will enhance the appropriate selection of in vitro models for future studies of canine hematological malignancies.

Background

Hematological diseases in humans are widely heterogeneous including numerous molecular subtypes with wide ranging prognoses and therapeutic responses. Oncogenesis is well understood for some subtypes, while the molecular changes leading to other subtypes remain unknown [1]. A similar level of molecular heterogeneity likely exists in the >1000 leukemia/lymphoma (LL) cell lines that have been described to date [2].

Although the use of cell lines provides numerous advantages, including ease of handling and manipulation, high homogeneity, provision of a continuous source of sample material, and accessibility to the scientific community [3], detailed characterization is crucial before they are used as an in vitro preclinical cancer models. Nearly 100 % of examined human LL cell lines carry stable genetic alterations and karyotypic changes that maintain the major features of the original cells [2] while a number of other human LL cell line studies have provided evidence that these cell lines have a high clinical predictive value that may translate into a favorable response rates in Phase II clinical trials [4, 5].

Cell line characterization minimally requires that a comprehensive set of immunophenotyping and cytogenetic data have been published [6]. However, with the recent explosion of advances in the genomics field, it is now possible to provide a more in-depth assessment of cytogenetic and transcriptional characteristics of cell lines that can provide further insight into biological processes including chromosomal translocations, signaling pathways, mutational analysis, gene dysregulation, and RNAi gene silencing [2]. Of the >1000 human LL cell lines described, ~40 % have been characterized in sufficient detail for accurate classification as discrete LL subtypes [6].

Spontaneously occurring lymphoid malignancies in dogs share the same histopathological and clinical features of

* Correspondence: steven_suter@ncsu.edu; Matthew_Breen@ncsu.edu
[4]Comparative Medicine Institute, North Carolina State University, Raleigh, NC, USA
[1]Department of Molecular Biomedical Sciences, College of Veterinary Medicine, North Carolina State University, CVM Research Building - Room 348, 1060 William Moore Drive, Raleigh 27607, NC, USA
Full list of author information is available at the end of the article

their human couterparts, in addition to evolutionarily conserved chromosome aberrations and mutations, indicating shared pathogenesis across species [7–9]. There are only a small number of established canine LL cell lines, six of which have already been characterized at the genomic level [10, 11]. Similar to human LL cell lines, the importance of detailed genomic and phenotypic characterization in an effort to define a framework to assess their clinical predictive value was recently emphasized [12]. Five additional canine LL cell lines, CLBL-1, Ema, UL-1, TL-1 (Nody-1), and 3132, have been used previously in in vitro studies [13–21]. These cell lines have varying levels of characterization, none of which includes an in-depth genomic and transcriptomic approach [22–24].

We present a comprehensive characterization of five canine LL cell lines starting with an extended panel of immunophenotyping. High resolution oligonucleotide array comparative genomic hybridization (oaCGH) was performed to assess genome-wide copy number status, and multicolor fluorescence in situ hybridization (FISH) analysis was used to further identify copy number imbalances and structural changes in karyotype architecture. Transcription status of each cell line was investigated using high-density array based gene expression profiling (GEP) and quantitative reverse transcriptase polymerase chain reaction (qRT-PCR). Additionally, genome wide copy number data of each cell line were compared with data from primary canine round cell tumors to further confirm their classification and relevance as in vitro pre-clinical models of lymphoid neoplasia for canine and comparative medicine.

Methods

Canine LL cell lines

Five previously established canine LL cell lines with varying levels of initial characterization were included in this study: CLBL-1 [22] (kind gift from Dr. Barbara Rutgen, University of Veterinary Medicine Vienna, Austria, Ema [23] (kind gift from Dr. Takuya Mizuno, Yamaguchi University, Japan), TL-1 [23] (Nody-1, kind gift from Dr. Yasuhiko Okamura, Iwate University, Japan), UL-1 [23] (kind gift from Dr. Hajime Tsujimoto, University of Tokyo, Japan), and 3132 [24, 25] (kind gift from Dr. Mark Holmes, University of Cambridge, UK). All cell lines were maintained at 37 °C and 5 % CO_2 in RPMI-1640 culture medium (Mediatech, Hendon, VA) supplemented with 10 % fetal bovine serum (FBS, Mediatech), 2 mM Glutamax (Life Technologies, Grand Island, NY), and 100 μg/ml Primocin (Invivogen, San Diego, CA) and tested negative using a PCR Mycoplasma test kit (Applichem, Cheshire, CT).

Immunophentyping

Immunophenotyping of each line was completed using flow cytometry as previously described [11, 26] at the UC Davis Leukocyte Antigen Biology Laboratory using a panel of monoclonal antibodies reactive with canine leukocyte antigens, including CD1a, CD1c, CD3, CD4, CD5, CD8α, CD8β, CD11a, CD11b, CD11c, CD11d, CD14, CD18, CD21, CD34, CD45, CD45RA, CD49a, CD54, CD79α, CD80, CD86, DM5, MHC-II, 5G2, AG5, TCRαβ, TCRγδ, TCRαβ, TCRCCγδ, and Thy-1 (CD90). Analysis at the NCSU Clinical Immunology Laboratory was also performed using a smaller number of antibodies, including CD3, CD4, CD5, CD8α, CD21, CD34, and CD79α/β.

PARR

Polymerase chain reaction for antigen receptor rearrangement (PARR) was completed as previously described [27, 28] to assess clonality and, possibly lineage. PCR products were separated using capillary gel electrophoresis (QIAxcel Electrophoresis System, Qiagen, Valencia, CA). A clonal sample was determined if one or more discrete bands were seen on the gel, and a polyclonal sample was determined if multiple bands or a smear of amplicons were seen. A negative sample was determined if no bands were seen.

Isolation of cell line DNA and RNA and generation of metaphase preparations

Aliquots of 1×10^7cells were removed from the same culture flask at the same time point for isolation of DNA and RNA and preparation of metaphase chromosome preparations to ensure consistency in downstream analyses. DNA was isolated using the DNeasy Blood and Tissue kit (Qiagen, Valencia, CA) and manufacturer's protocol, and quantity and quality of DNA were evaluated using spectrophotometry (260/280 > 1.8) and gel electrophoresis. RNA was isolated using the RNeasy Plus Mini Kit (Qiagen) and manufacturer's protocol, and assessed using the 2100 Bioanalyzer RNA 6000 Nano Kit (Agilent Technologies, Santa Clara, CA) to confirm an RNA integrity number (RIN) >9.0. Metaphase chromosome preparations were prepared from each cell line as previously described [29] using conventional techniques of colcimid arrest (final concentration of 50 ng/ml for 1 h), hypotonic treatment, and methanol-glacial acetic acid fixation prior to being dropped onto glass slides.

Identification of copy number aberrations (CNAs) using oaCGH

oaCGH was completed as previously described using a 180,000 feature canine oligonucleotide array (Agilent Technologies) with repeat-masked 60mer oligonucleotides spaced ~13 kb across the genome [30]. An equimolar pool of DNA from 25 clinically healthy female dogs was used as a common reference for all cell lines. Cell line and reference DNA was labeled with Cyanine 3-dUTP and

Cyanine 5-dUTP, respectively, using the Agilent Enzymatic Labeling Kit, and probe hybridization, array washing, and scanning was performed as described elsewhere [30].

Scan data were processed using Feature Extraction v.10.10 software (Agilent Technologies) and imported into Nexus Copy Number v7.5 (Biodiscovery, Hawthorne, CA). Raw data were evaluated to identify and exclude probes displaying non-uniform hybridization or signal saturation, and copy number calls were made using Biodiscovery's FASST2 segmentation algorithm. Copy number calls were based on a minimum of three consecutive probes per segment, and mean log2 cell line:reference thresholds of +/− 0.2 were used to define gain and loss, respectively. Genes within the defined intervals were identified using the UCSC canine genome browser (CanFam2 assembly; http://genome.ucsc.edu/) and the NCBI gene database (http://www.ncbi.nlm.nih.gov/gene). Genes previously associated with cancer were based on those reported in the Cancer Gene Census (http://cancer.sanger.ac.uk/cosmic/census) [31].

Further statistical analyses using the Feature Extraction data were performed using R [32]. The signals (rProcessedSignal and gProcessedSignal) were normalized using the following equations:

$$a = \log_2(rprocessedSigna/gProcessedSignal) \quad (1)$$

$$ProcessedRatio = [a\text{–}mode\ (a)]/MAD(a) \quad (2)$$

Where, *Processed ratio* is the centered and normalized ratio of the Agilent processed fluorescent signals. Segmentation was performed across all chromosomes using circular binary segmentation [33]. Data were further dichotomized as gain (1), no change (0), or loss (−1), based on segments that were +/− 3 MAD (mean absolute deviation) from the median of each sample's response across all chromosomes. Hierarchical clustering of the five cell lines was performed using dichotomous data using Euclidean distance and Ward's method. Additionally, hierarchical clustering of the cell lines with 299 canine primary round cell tumors including 123 leukemias [34], 106 lymphomas (Thomas et al., in preparation), and 70 histiocytic malignancies (Kennedy et al., in preparation) was performed using segmented data using Euclidean distance and Ward's method. Tumor type and subtype were both annotated on the heatmap.

FISH analysis

FISH of all cells lines was performed as previously described [29] to evaluate structural changes and verify oaCGH copy number data using panels of clones from the CHORI-82 dog bacterial artificial chromosome (BAC) library (www.chori.org). Initially, two clones (326 K03 and 330E21), previously determined to hybridize to the centromeric regions of canine autosomes [35], were fluorescently labeled and hybridized to metaphase preparations of each cell line. Centromeric signals were used to properly orient the chromosomes, aid in confirming modal chromosome count, and identify bi-armed chromosomes.

Twenty additional BAC clones were selected to contain known oncogenes and tumor suppressor genes that met two of the three following criteria: (1) located in a region of CNA in at least one of the five cells lines, (2) displayed differential expression between cell lines based on the GEP, and (3) have been associated with human and/or canine lymphoid malignancies in prior studies [8, 9, 36, 37, 38, 39, 40, 41, 42, 43, 44, 45, 46]. The BAC clones selected represented the following genes: *BCL11B, IGH, VEGFA, CCNC, FOXO3A, CDKN2A, MYC, KIT, CDK6, EZH2, MYCBP2, FLT3, PTEN, HEY1, E2F5, NFKB2, ERG, MLLT2, CD83,* and *DEK* (Table 1). The 20 clones were divided into four panels of five for multicolor FISH, and each panel was hybridized to metaphase spreads of each cell line and healthy dog controls. Copy number status of each probe was scored in at least 50 cells of each cell line and normal controls.

GEP analysis

Total RNA from each cell line was used to perform gene expression profiling (GEP) as described elsewhere [11, 47] using the GeneChip Canine Genome 2.0 array (Affymetrix, Santa Clara, CA) which is comprised of 18,000 *Canis familiaris* mRNA transcripts and over 20,000 non-redundant predicted genes. Additionally, total RNA was isolated as described from lymph nodes harvested from six healthy mixed breed dogs that showed no evidence of lymphoid neoplasia at necropsy [11]. Microarrays were processed by the Lineberger Functional Genomic Core Facility at the University of North Carolina Chapel Hill. Total RNA (1 µg) was processed for microarray hybridization using the MessageAmp II-Biotin Enhanced Kit (Ambion, Life Technologies, Grand Island, NY) and hybridization was performed according to Affymetrix technical protocols. GEP analysis was performed using GeneSpring GX v12 (Agilent Technologies). Expression array data were normalized using the GC-RMA procedure [48] and signals were median-centered across all arrays. Data were filtered to remove probe sets with limited variation (standard deviation <2) across all arrays, and fold change analysis was performed for each cell line using the averaged expression data from the normal lymph node controls as baseline. Additionally, unsupervised hierarchical clustering analysis was performed across all cell lines and controls using the filtered probe set. Functional analysis was performed by evaluating for enrichment in genes that were up- or down-regulated in each cell line by >5-fold compared to normal lymph node controls. Enrichment analysis in Gene Ontology (GO) biological processes and Kyoto Encyclopedia of Genes and Genome

Table 1 BAC clones from CHORI-82 dog library selected to represent 20 cancer-related genes for FISH analysis. Chromosome locations based on the CanFam2 genome assembly are noted

Gene	BAC clone	Chromosome	Start (bp)	Stop (bp)
BCL11B	326-K01	8	70,661,395	70,752,579
IGH	027-N17	8	75,997,304	76,191,846
VEGFA	152-L05	12	15,212,673	15,228,610
CCNC	268-D08	12	60,739,913	60,764,849
FOXO3A	048-I05	12	68,583,078	68,701,688
CDKN2A	325-C12	11	44,255,629	44,256,009
MYC	335-M01	13	28,238,008	28,242,545
KIT	98-B16	13	50,017,518	50,212,194
CDK6	181-D14	14	21,147,772	21,367,160
EZH2	300-P18	16	4,905,169	4,971,032
MYCBP2	216-G13	22	33,561,172	33,820,510
FLT3	062-D23	25	14,581,755	14,658,045
PTEN	521-G14	26	40,921,802	40,981,821
HEY1	484-E08	29	30,184,049	30,186,972
E2F5	157-A19	29	34,748,851	34,758,529
NFKB2	001-D14	28	17,903,193	17,910,910
ERG	100-F17	31	35,578,420	35,760,306
MLLT2	468-E14	32	13,354,180	13,586,952
CD83	127-B24	35	16,354,899	16,533,175
DEK	517-A02	35	20,035,294	20,172,093

(KEGG) Pathways was completed using the Database for Annotation, Visualization, and Integrated Discovery (DAVID) v 6.7 [49, 50].

qRT-PCR analysis

One ug of total RNA from each cell line and two normal lymph node controls was used to perform qRT-PCR to validate GEP as previously described [11]. qRT-PCR was performed using Applied Biosystems OneStepPlus Real-Time PCR system (Life Technologies) and a cycling protocol with an initial denaturation at 95 °C for 3 min; followed by 40 cycles of 95 °C for 3 s, 62 °C for 20 s, and 72 °C for 15 s; with a final extension at 72 °C for 5 min, followed by a melt curve analysis. All assays were performed in triplicate.

Primers were designed using NCBI Primer-BLAST as previously described [11] for *MYC, KIT, FLT3, PTEN*, and *RPL32* (Table 2). Relative quantification using the comparative Ct method ($\Delta\Delta C_T$) was performed as described previously using normal lymph node as the baseline for comparisons. *RPL32* was used as the reference gene based on its stable expression across all samples in GEP analysis and previous identification as a suitable qRT-PCR reference gene for canine lymphoid neoplasia [51].

Table 2 Primer sequences and associated cDNA amplicons length used for qRT-PCR analysis

Primer	Sequence	Amplicon length
MYC-F	5′-TCGCCTATTTGGGAAGACAC-3′	141
MYC-R	5′-AAGCTGACGTTGAGAGGCAT-3′	
KIT-F	5′-CGAAGATGTGTGAAGCAGGA-3′	126
KIT-R	5′-GTGTCCGCTACCCTGGAATA-3′	
PTEN-F	5′-ACTTTGAGTTCCCTCAGCCA-3′	141
PTEN-R	5′-AGGTTTCCTCTGGTCCTGGT-3′	
FLT3-F	5′-CAGAGGCAGTGTATGGAGCA-3′	129
FLT3-R	5′-GGCAATTCAGGGAACTGTGT-3′	
RPL32-F	5′-ATGCCCAACATTGGTTATGG-3′	180
RPL32-R	5′-CTCTTTCCACGATGGCTTTG-3′	

Results

Immunophenotyping

Flow cytometry data are presented in Table 3. All cell lines expressed CD45 and CD45RA, and 4/5 expressed CD18, which verifies a leukocytic origin. CLBL-1 displayed positive staining for CD1a, CD1c, CD11a, CD11b, CD54, CD79α, CD80, CD86, and MHC-II and no staining for CD3, CD4, CD5, CD8, and Thy-1 indicating a mature B-cell origin, which is further supported by a monoclonal product resulting from PCR analysis of the *IGH* gene. Ema was positive for Thy-1, a T-cell marker. TL-1 cells were negative for most antigens, however weak expression of MHCII was observed, which may indicate a T-cell phenotype as MHCII is expected to have high intensity on B cells and antigen presenting cells, with much weaker expression observed on T cells [52]. TL-1 and Ema both were found to have rearrangement of *TCRG* gene (oligoclonal for TL-1), further supporting a mature T-cell phenotype for both cell lines. UL-1 expressed most antigens including CD34, which indicates an immature precursor phenotype. Positive expression for CD3, CD4, CD5, CD8α, CD8β, CD11d, and Thy-1 all support a T-cell phenotype. UL-1 is also positive for CD14, which is normally a marker for myeloid cells; however, expression is also demonstrated in B and T cell precursors but not mature cells [52], further supporting an immature phenotype. Additionally, PCR of *TCRG* indicated a monoclonal product further supporting T-cell phenotype. 3132 is most likely of dendritc/histiocytic origin based on the positive expression of CD1a and CD11c, which is characteristic of histiocytic diseases [53] and a combination not found in other cell lines of lymphoid origin in this or previous studies [10, 11]. Additionally, strong intensity for MHC-II further supports dendritic cell origin. However, a T-cell origin cannot be completely ruled out based on expression of CD4, CD8α, and a monoclonal product resulting from PCR of *TCRG*.

Table 3 Phenotypic characteristics of canine LL cell lines based on flow cytometry analysis

Cell line Antigen	CLBL-1	Ema	TL-1	UL-1	3132
CD1a	++	–	–	+	+
CD1c	++	–	–	+	++
CD3	–	–	–	+	–
CD4	–	–	–	+	+
CD5	–	–	–	+	–
CD8α	–	–	–	++	++
CD8β	–	–	–	+	–
CD11a	+	+	–	–	+
CD11b	+	–	–	–	++
CD11c	–	–	–	–	++
CD11d	–	–	–	+	–
CD14	–	–	–	+	+
CD18	++	++	–	++	++
CD21	–	–	–	+	–
CD34	–	–	–	+	–
CD45	++	++	++	+	++
CD45RA	++	+	+	+	+
CD49α	++	++	–	++	++
CD54	++	–	–	+	++
CD79α/β	++	–	–	–	–
CD80	+	++	++	+	++
CD86	+	–	–	+	++
DM5	–	–	–	+	–
MHC-II	++	–	+	+	++
TCRαβ	–	–	–	+	–
TCRγδ	–	–	–	+	+
Thy-1 (CD90)	–	++	–	+	–

Strong expression (++), intermediate expression (+), or no expression (–) of each antigen is indicated

Karyotype architecture

Chromosome enumeration and centromere localization via FISH of metaphase chromosomes was used to assess the gross karyotypic architecture of each cell line. The normal dog karyotype includes 38 pairs of acrocentric autosomes, a large sub-metacentric X chromosome and a small metacentric Y chromosome [54]. Enumeration of chromosomes from 30 metaphase spreads of each cell line indicated varying levels of aneuploidy (Fig. 1). CLBL-1, Ema, and 3132 were all hypodiploid, while TL-1 and UL-1 contained normal modal chromosome counts (Table 4).

Genome wide copy number imbalance

oaCGH analysis revealed varying levels of genomic imbalance in each of the cell lines with detected CNAs ranging in size from 19.5 Mb to entire chromosomes (Fig. 2). Large differences in the number of aberrations (Fig. 3a) and the percent of the genome impacted by regions of imbalance (Fig. 3b) were also noted. CLBL-1, TL-1, and UL-1 have a similar and even distribution of the number of aberrant gains and losses; whereas Ema was skewed towards an increase in the number of losses, and 3132 was skewed towards regions of copy number gain. When the cumulative size of CNAs and the percent of the genome impacted by imbalance were assessed, Ema and TL-1 were minimally changed which is reiterated from the oaCGH profiles in which both cell lines had less visually obvious CNAs. CLBL-1 and UL-1 had similar total percent of the genome changed, but CLBL-1 had a greater percent of the genome with imbalances of loss and UL-1 had a greater percent of the genome gained. 3132 had the greatest percent of the genome changed which was expected given the number of aberrations detected and the extensive genomic complexity visualized in the oaCGH profile. Cancer-associated genes in regions of imbalance were identified and are detailed in Additional file 1: Table S1. Cell lines were clustered to determine their relatedness to each other based on genome-wide copy number assessment (Fig. 4). 3132 branched away from the other four, and Ema and TL-1, the two mature T-cell neoplasms based on immunophenotyping, were the most closely related.

FISH analysis

FISH analysis was completed for 20 genes relevant to lymphoid neoplasia to verify oaCGH data, enumerate the level of imbalance at each locus, and investigate any structural aberrations associated with the selected genes of interest. The 20 genes were divided into four panels of five for multicolor FISH analysis. Each of the four FISH panels is identified in the insets of Fig. 5 with control chromosomes from clinically healthy dogs indicating the appropriate localization of each BAC clone. A representative metaphase spread with CNAs or structural changes in one of the cell lines is shown in each panel.

Structural changes were identified in each cell line. CLBL-1 contains a derivative 13 chromosome that appears to include two copies of *Canis familiaris* 13 (CFA 13) joined by the centromere resulting in the formation of a metacentric chromosome (Fig. 5b), in addition to a grossly normal copy of CFA 13 based on the location of the 2 probes on CFA 13. A similar abnormality occurred in UL-1 with chromosome 25, as is evidenced by 2 copies of *FLT3* forming a metacentric chromosome in addition to an acrocentric chromosome with *FLT3* placement in the expected location on CFA 25 (Fig. 5c). Both Ema and *CLBL-1* contained a derivative metacentric chromosome resulting from the apparent fusion of CFA 28 and CFA 35 (Fig. 5d). Ema

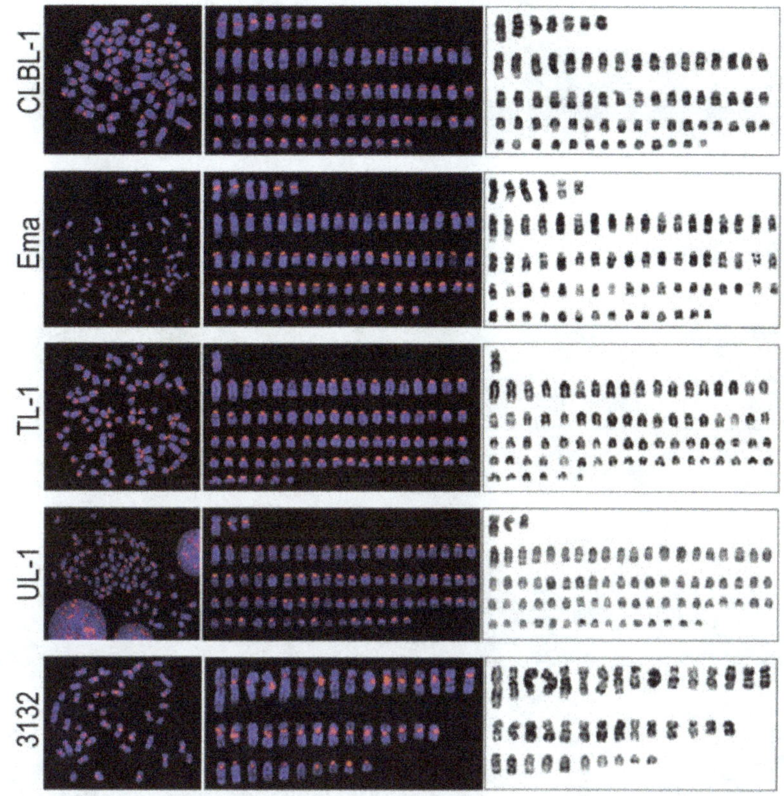

Fig. 1 Karyotypic organization of each canine LL cell line. Centromeric regions were visualized through the use of two BAC clones, and used to orient the chromosomes. Images of DAPI stained metaphase spreads (left panel) were used to prepare rudimentary karyotypes (middle and right panels). Chromosomes were arranged by descending size of bi-armed chromosomes followed by single-armed chromosomes

contained additional copies of CFA 28 and CFA 35, while *CLBL-1* contained another CFA 28 and a heterozygous loss of CFA 35. Numerous structural aberrations occurred in 3132, and appeared to be random from cell to cell. Further detail of these structural changes was difficult to ascertain given the heterogeneity observed in the metaphase spreads.

A summary of the frequency of CNA at each of the 20 investigated loci is presented in Fig. 6. Ema and TL-1 showed grossly normal copy number changes, as was seen in the oaCGH; however, both were found to have a homozygous deletion of *CDKN2A*. Ema also had a heterozygous loss of *MLLT2* in 100 % of cells and a heterozygous loss of *FLT3* in 15 % of cells which was detected via oaCGH. Additionally, TL-1 had three copies of *E2F5* and *HEY1*, both located on CFA 30, in 100 % of cells. UL-1 and CLBL-1 showed copy number changes in nine and 10 of the loci evaluated, respectively. CLBL-1 exhibited heterozygous losses of *CCNC, FOXO3A, CDK6, MYCBP2, PTEN, CD83,* and *DEK*, and a copy number of three for *MYC* and *KIT* (both located on CFA 13) in the majority of cells (>87 %). UL-1 had more genes gained, with three copies of *BCL11B, IGH, VEGFA, CCNC, FOXO3A, FLT3,* and *NFKB2* in the vast majority (>93 %) of cells. Additionally, 50 % of cells gained an extra copy of *CDK6*. FISH analysis of 3132 showed copy number changes at 19/20 loci, many of which were strikingly heterogeneous. *MYC, KIT,* and *CD83* each have proportions of cells with normal copy number and gains of 3, 4, and >4 copies. Losses of *ERG* and *EZH2* were

Table 4 Chromosome enumeration of five canine LL cell lines based on evaluation of 30 metaphase spreads

Cell line	Ploidy	Modal chromosome number	Chromosome range	Bi-armed chromosomes
CLBL-1	Hypodiploid	70	66–72	4–7 per cell
Ema	Hypodiploid	73	70–76	5–7 per cell
TL-1	Normal	78	76–82	1 per cell
UL-1	Normal	78	76–80	1–3 per cell
3132	Hypodiploid	40	37–42	25–34 per cell

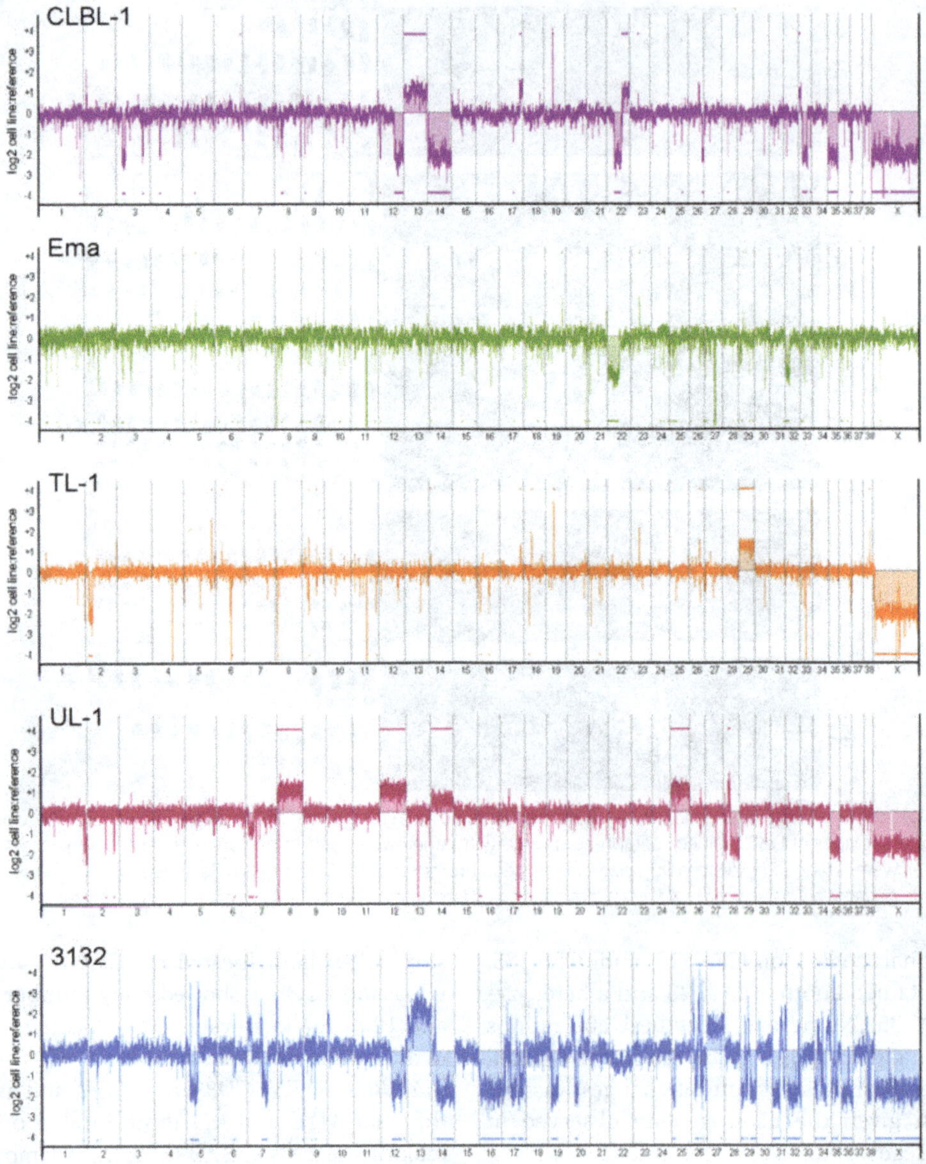

Fig. 2 oaCGH profiles of each of the five canine LL cell lines. Each oaCGH profile includes the chromosomes (1–38,X) on the x-axis and log2 cell line:reference ratio on the y-axis with copy number gains and losses indicated by the horizontal bars above and below the midline, respectively

identified in all or nearly all 3132 cells, with proportions (10–23 %) of cells displaying homozygous deletion.

Gene expression analysis

GEP data were filtered to remove probe sets with limited variation (standard deviation <2) across the five cell lines and six non-neoplastic lymph nodes resulting in 1153 probe sets used for subsequent analyses. Unsupervised clustering resulted in immediate branching of 3132 from the other 10 samples. The remaining samples were then separated into two discrete groups including the four cell lines, and the six control lymph nodes (Fig. 7). Normal lymph nodes unsurprisingly display greater transcription conservation across biological replicates compared with the cell lines as indicated by their shorter connecting branches. The cell lines displaying the greatest transcriptional similarity were Ema and TL-1, the two mature T-cell lines, as reiterated from the oaCGH clustering analysis. UL-1, most likely an immature T-cell phenotype, is also more similar to Ema and TL-1 than CLBL-1, a B-cell line.

Fold change analysis was also completed by comparing each cell line with the mean expression of the non-neoplastic lymph nodes. Fold changes of known cancer related genes and the transcripts with the 50 largest absolute fold changes (up or down) in each cell line are listed in Additional file 1: Tables S2 and S3, respectively,

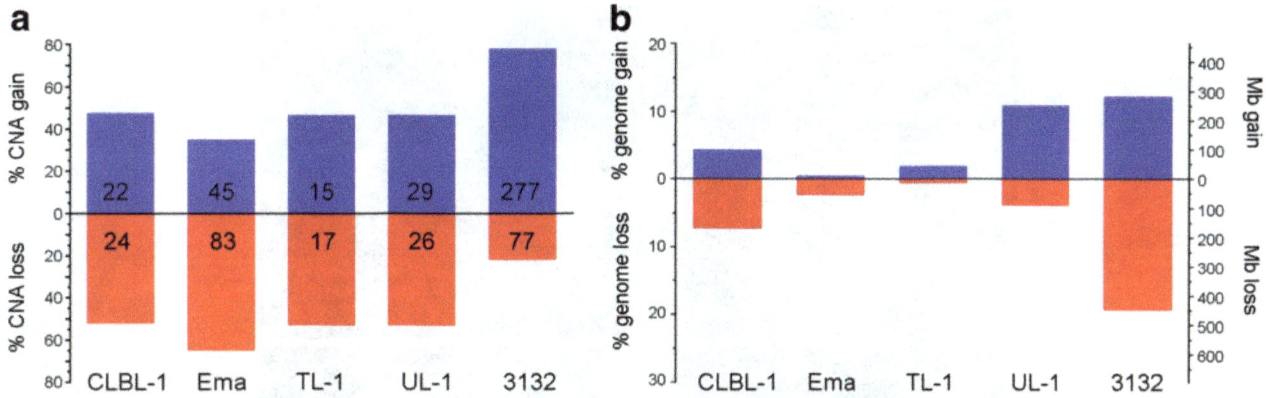

Fig. 3 Genomic imbalances identified in the five canine LL cell lines. **a** Percentage of CNAs detected as gain or loss via oaCGH analysis, with the total number indicated on each column. **b** Genomic imbalances in each cell line expressed as percent genome changed and the total number of megabases (Mb) within regions of copy number change. Copy number changes on the X chromosome were omitted from these analysis as the reference was sex mismatched in 4/5 cell lines

as genes that may have functional relevance. Additionally, genes with a fold change >5 were further assessed in functional gene-annotation enrichment analysis. Due to limited functional annotation of canine genes, official gene symbols were used for enrichment analysis based on human gene annotations. Up to the top ten enriched GO biological processes and KEGG pathways are listed in Additional file 1: Tables S4 and S5, respectively. All five cell lines exhibited upregulation of genes associated with the GO biological processes of cell proliferation and division, and three of five exhibited upregulation of genes involved in metabolic processes (e.g. sterol biosynthetic process, glucose metabolic process, cholesterol metabolic process). All five cell lines also exhibited downregulation of genes involved in immune response and leukocyte activation. When the KEGG pathways were assessed, four of the cell lines exhibited upregulation of metabolic and biosynthesis pathways (e.g. steroid

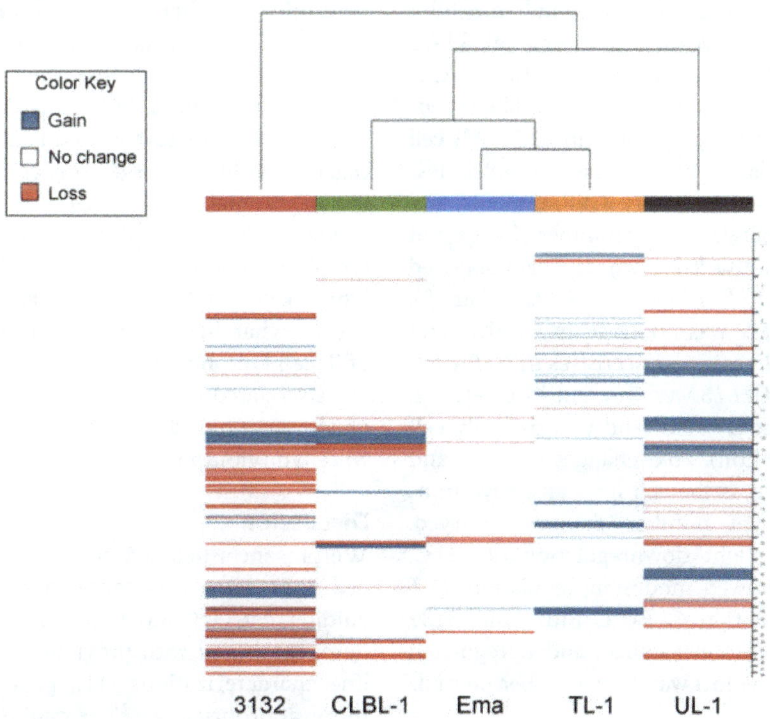

Fig. 4 Hierarchical clustering of canine LL cell lines based on genome wide copy number status. Dichotomous data was clustered using Euclidian distance and Ward's method. Columns represent the individual cell lines and rows represent individual regions along the genome. Blue indicates a region of gain and red indicates a region of loss

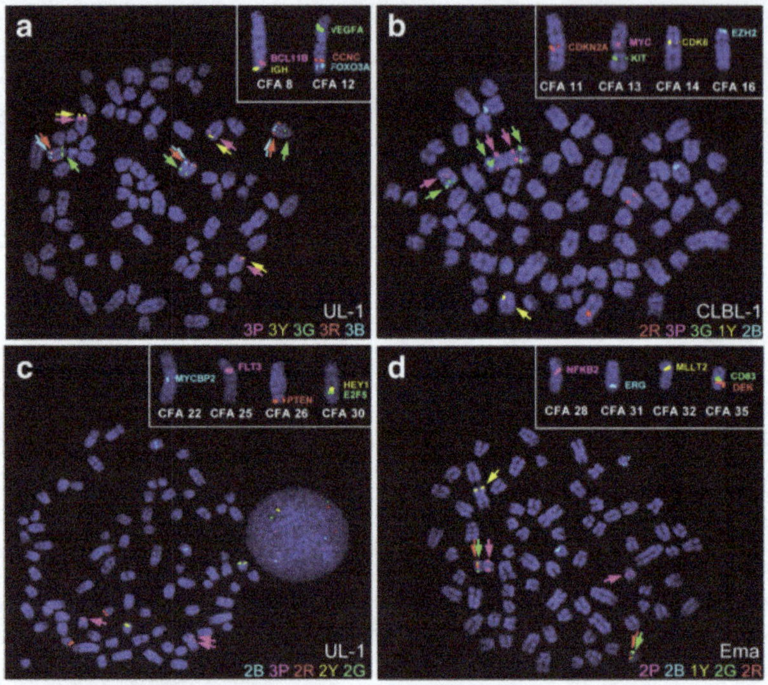

Fig. 5 FISH analysis of 20 cancer-related genes in each canine LL cell line verifies and enumerates oaCGH findings and identifies structural aberrations. The 20 genes were divided into four panels of five genes each for multicolor FISH (**a-d**). In each panel, individual chromosomes from clinical healthy control dogs are included in the inset to show normal probe placement. For each gene panel, a representative metaphase spread showing copy number or structural aberrations (arrows) is included. Cell line and copy number of each probe are denoted in each panel

biosynthesis, pyruvate metabolism) as similarly identified in the GO term analysis. TL-1 was also found to exhibit upregulation of genes in both the ERBB and Jak-STAT signaling pathways; while genes involved in the MAPK signaling pathways and the NOD-like and Toll-like receptor signaling pathways were upregulated in 3132. All cell lines exhibited downregulation of cell adhesion molecules.

qRT-PCR was performed to verify GEP findings and analyze the relationship between copy number change and expression change in four well known cancer associated genes including *MYC, KIT, FLT3*, and *PTEN* (Fig. 8). Homozygous loss of *PTEN* was observed in CLBL-1 and 3132, which both show the greatest decreases in *PTEN* expression. Three copies of *FLT3* were present in UL-1, and this gene was upregulated 17 fold (and was the only cell line to show an upregulation). Fold changes in *MYC* and *KIT* are more variable across the cell lines and have minimal correlation with copy number changes observed. CLBL-1 and Ema had slight downregulation of *MYC*, while the other three showed modest upregulation. *KIT* was largely downregulated in CLBL-1, Ema, and 3132 (two of which had copy number gains), and upregulated 8-fold in TL-1 in which the loci was copy number neutral.

Genome-wide CNA comparison with primary tumors

Finally, we compared the five cell lines with genome wide copy number data generated in our laboratory from 299 primary round cell tumors via clustering analysis to determine whether the cell lines represented primary tumors, and, if so, what subtype each most closely resembled (Fig. 9). All cell lines were found to cluster within the primary tumors, indicating they are more closely related to primary tumors than other cell lines. 3132 segregated within a large cluster composed of primarily histiocytic malignancies. CLBL-1 branches from a cluster of mature B-cell neoplasms consisting primarily of B-cell lymphomas with a smaller subset of B-cell chronic lymphocytic leukemias. TL-1 and Ema both clustered in a somewhat heterogeneous grouping comprised chiefly of T-cell lymphomas, and both these cell lines were most closely related to a T-cell lymphoma. UL-1 grouped in a cluster composed of acute leukemias, most of which were lymphoid in origin.

Discussion

We present a detailed characterization of five canine LL cell lines using a genome-wide molecular approach including oaCGH and GEP analysis. The data presented here, combined with previously published canine LL cell line characterizations [11], provides the opportunity to more appropriately select canine LL cell lines for preclinical in vitro studies. Overall, our data suggests that CLBL-1 represents a mature B-cell lymphoma as previously reported [22], and Ema and TL-1 both represent

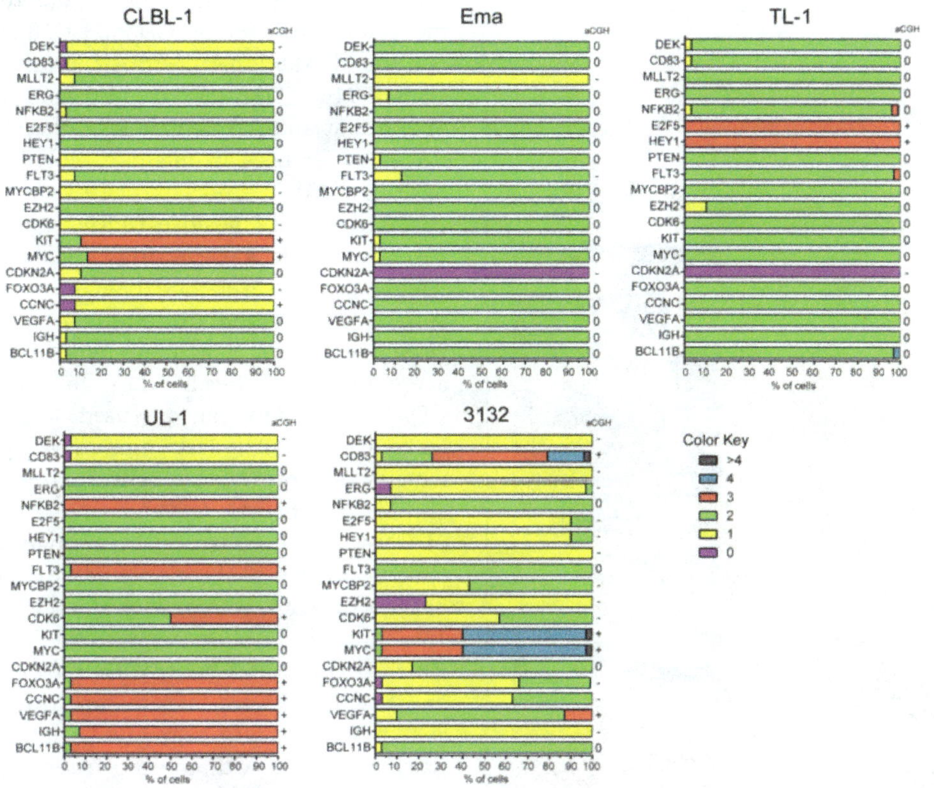

Fig. 6 Summary of CNAs identified in FISH analysis of 20 cancer-related genes in each canine LL cell line. Each chart shows the distribution of copy number for each probe, based on the analysis of 50 cells from each cell line. Data are stacked to represent the percentage of cells displaying copy numbers 0 to >4 as indicated by the color key. To the right of each chart, dichotomized oaCGH data as gain (+), loss (–) or no change (0) is notated

T-cell lymphomas as previously reported [23]. In contrast, UL-1 should be reclassified as T-cell acute lymphoblastic leukemia (instead of a T-cell lymphoma) and 3132 should be reclassified as a histiocytic sarcoma (instead of a B-cell lymphoma).

CLBL-1 immunophenotyping in this study agreed with the immunophenotyping published when the cell line was initially established. Positive expression of CD11a, CD79α, CD45, CD45RA, and MHCII and no expression of CD3, CD4, CD5, CD8, CD11d, CD14, CD21, CD34, and CD56 classifies it as a B-cell lymphoma. Additionally, B-cell PARR revealed a monoclonal rearrangement, which we also found [22]. CLBL-1 was the only cell line in this dataset that had been previously karyotyped [55]. It was found to be hypodiploid with a modal chromosome number of 70–71, which matches our findings. There was only one biarmed chromosome mentioned, derivative chromosome 13, which we also identified via FISH analysis. Since centromere visualization was not previously completed, and a non-standard canine chromosome nomenclature was used, correlation of further previously identified chromosome aberrations with our findings via DAPI banding, FISH, and oaCGH was not possible. Numerous CNAs identified in CLBL-1 via oaCGH are shared with primary canine B-cell lymphomas (B-LSA). Gain of CFA 13 has been identified in 25 % of B-LSA. Loss of CFA14 and loss of the proximal region of CFA 3 have also been found to occur in ~10 % of B-LSA [8]. Additionally, CLBL-1 clustered with primary mature B-cell lymphoid neoplasia when clustered with 299 primary canine round cell tumors, further supporting the classification of CLBL-1 as a B-cell lymphoma.

Ema immunophenotyping, at the time of establishment, was positive for CD3, CD45, CD45RA, and Thy-1. In our assessment, Ema was also positive (intermediate signal) for CD11a and CD18 and negative for CD3. Similarly, TL-1 was originally positive for CD3, CD18, CD45, CD45RA, and MHC11 while our immunophenotyping indicated no expression of CD3 and CD18. The slight differences in the immunophenotyping data may be due to factors that can influence flow cytometry data including, the amount of antibody used, the call threshold of positive versus negative, instrumentation, and other reagents. Alternatively, it's possible that the loss or gain of antigens on the cell surface occurred while in culture. Both Ema and TL-1 were previously T-cell PARR positive, which is consistent with our PARR data. Overall, the changes observed in immunophenotype did not impact the overall interpretation of the classification of both these cell lines as mature T-cell lymphoid neoplasia.

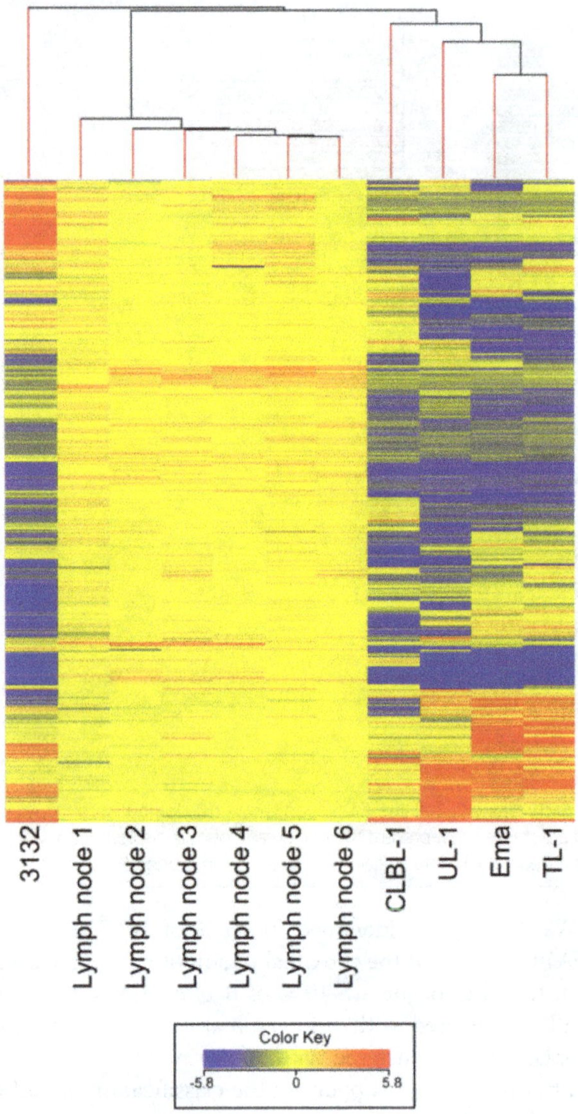

Fig. 7 Unsupervised hierarchical clustering of gene expression data from five canine LL cell lines and six non-neoplastic control lymph nodes. Data were filtered to remove transcripts displaying limited variability (standard deviation <2) resulting in 1153 probe sets used for clustering analysis using Euclidian distance and Ward's method

Both Ema and TL-1 were found to have a copy number loss in the region containing *CDKN2A* in oaCGH analysis, which was further confirmed to be a homozygous loss of the gene loci in FISH analysis. *CDKN2A* loss occurs in >55 % of T-cell lymphomas (T-LSA) and <2 % of other subtypes of canine leukemia and lymphoma [8, 34]. Ema was also found to have a loss of the proximal half of CFA 22, which occurs in 20 % of T-LSA, and TL-1 had a gain of CFA 29 previously identified in 40 % of T-LSA [8]. Ema and TL-1 were also the cell lines most closely related in clustering analyses using both the oaCGH and GEP data, and both segregated with primary T-LSA when clustered with primary canine round cell tumors.

UL-1 immunophenotyping at the time of establishment was positive for CD8α, CD18, CD45, CD45RA. We found additional positive expression of CD3, CD4, CD5, CD14, CD21, CD34, Thy-1, and MHC-II. All were detected at an intermediate level therefore, as discussed earlier, differences in methods and data analysis could have resulted in previous negative findings. UL-1 was also T-cell PARR positive which agrees with our PARR findings. UL-1 was previously classified as a T cell lymphoma; however, based on expression of CD34, a surface glycoprotein expressed on hematopoietic stem cells, we suggest it is more representative of a T-cell acute leukemia (T-cell ALL). In veterinary medicine, CD34 expression can be used to suggest an acute leukemia since it is less commonly expressed in malignancies of more mature cells, such as lymphomas and chronic lymphocytic leukemias [26, 56]. Several regions of CNA are also shared with primary canine ALLs including the loss of the distal end of CFA 1 which occurs in 20 % of ALLs, gain of CFA 12 and 25 which occurs in 15 and 10 % of ALLs, respectively, and loss of CFA 35 which occurs in 15 % of ALLs. Of the CNAs identified in UL-1, more were in common with ALLs than other subtypes. UL-1 also segregated with a group of ALLs when clustered with primary round cell tumors. Together, these findings support the classification of UL-1 as a T-cell ALL.

3132 immunophenotyping in our laboratory, in conjunction with the original description of the cells (cellular pleomorphism, multinucleated giant cells, numerous mitotic figures, extreme variations in nuclear:cytoplasm ratio) suggests this cell line is representative of a disseminated histiocytic sarcoma (HS). No immunophentypic or genomic analysis of this cell line has been previously reported, although it was later described as a B-cell lymphoma based on detectable surface immunoglobulins [24], and it has since been cited in the literature as a B-cell lymphoma [21]. Our immunophenotyping revealed expression of CD1, CD11c, CD18, and MHCII which is the characteristic immunophenotype of canine HS [53, 57]. Since the cells also exhibit low and intermediate expression of CD4 and TCRδγ, respectively, we could not completely rule out a T-cell lymphoma with aberrant expression of CD11c [52, 53], although subsequent genomic results further supported HS. 3132 cells were also T-cell PARR positive, although rearrangements of both T-cell receptor and immunoglobulin genes have been previously identified in human histiocytic sarcomas [1, 58] and in canine histiocytomas [53]. Finally, our karyotypic, CNA, and GEP data also suggests that 3132 cells represent a histiocytic sarcoma. Metaphase spreads from primary cases contain highly variable chromosome numbers with a range of 42–53 and an abundance of aberrant bi-armed chromosomes which is comparable to

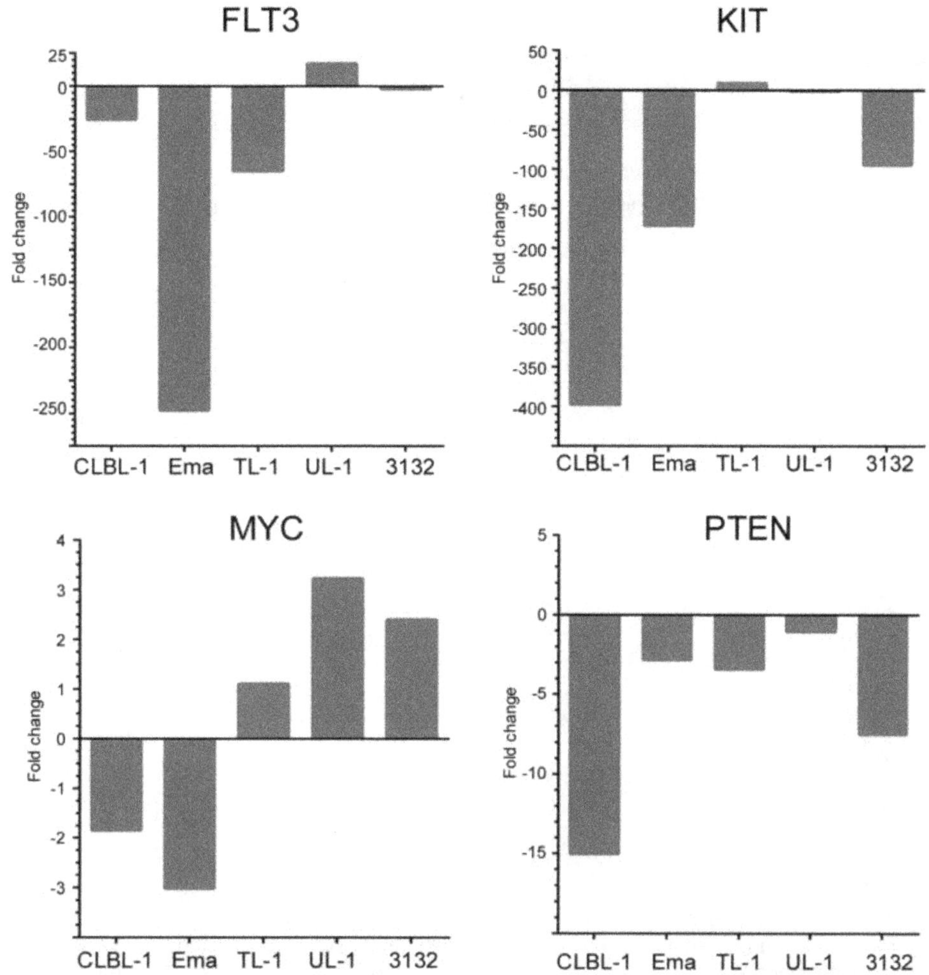

Fig. 8 qRT-PCR analysis of gene expression in five canine LL cell lines. Transcriptional levels of *FLT3*, *PTEN*, *MYC*, and *KIT* were assessed to verify microarray changes and further analyze the relationship between copy number change and expression change. *RPL32* was used as a reference gene to normalize expression levels between samples, and fold changes were calculated relative to the average expression in two non-neoplastic lymph nodes

karyotypic findings of 3132. oaCGH of 3132 cells was indicative of high genomic instability based on the number of CNAs identified, the percentage of the genome involved in regions of CNA, and the observation that several chromosomes include numerous of gains and losses across the chromosome, all of which have been found in primary HS [59]. Several specific CNAs are also shared with primary HS, including loss of CFA 16 and loss of CFA 31. Loss of CFA 12, 14, and 36 and gain of CFA 13 are also conserved with CNAs in primary canine HS [59]. When examining cluster analysis of GEP data with primary canine round cell tumors, 3132 segregated with a large group of histiocytic malignancies.

Dysregulation of several genes previously associated with canine diffuse large B-cell lymphoma in the NF-kB signaling and B-cell receptor signaling pathways shared conserved expression in CLBL-1 including the following: *KRAS, NRAS, PIK3R5, PLCG2, TGFBR2, TNFAIP3, TRADD, BCL2A1, CAMK2D, NFATC2* [48], *BUB1B, PRKCD, CD83, CXCL13, CD36, IL8, IL2, CD40LG, LCK, LTBR*, and *TNFSF11* [21]. Similarities were also noted between CLBL-1 and other targeted B-cell lymphoma gene expression studies, including *KIT* (almost 400-fold based on qRT-PCR) [60] and *ZAP70* downregulation (decreased 10 fold) [61].

There are less reported data regarding gene expression changes in other canine hematopoietic malignancies. *KIT* expression is decreased in canine T-cell LSA [62], and was decreased three fold in the TL-1 cell line. *SYK* expression is downregulated in canine T cell malignancies [61] and was downregulated 12–14 fold in all three T-cell cell lines (Ema, TL-1, and UL-1). *MMP9* and *TIMP1* expression is significantly upregulated in canine T-cell lymphomas [13], and was upregulated in both Ema and TL-1 cells. UL-1 was the only cell line to

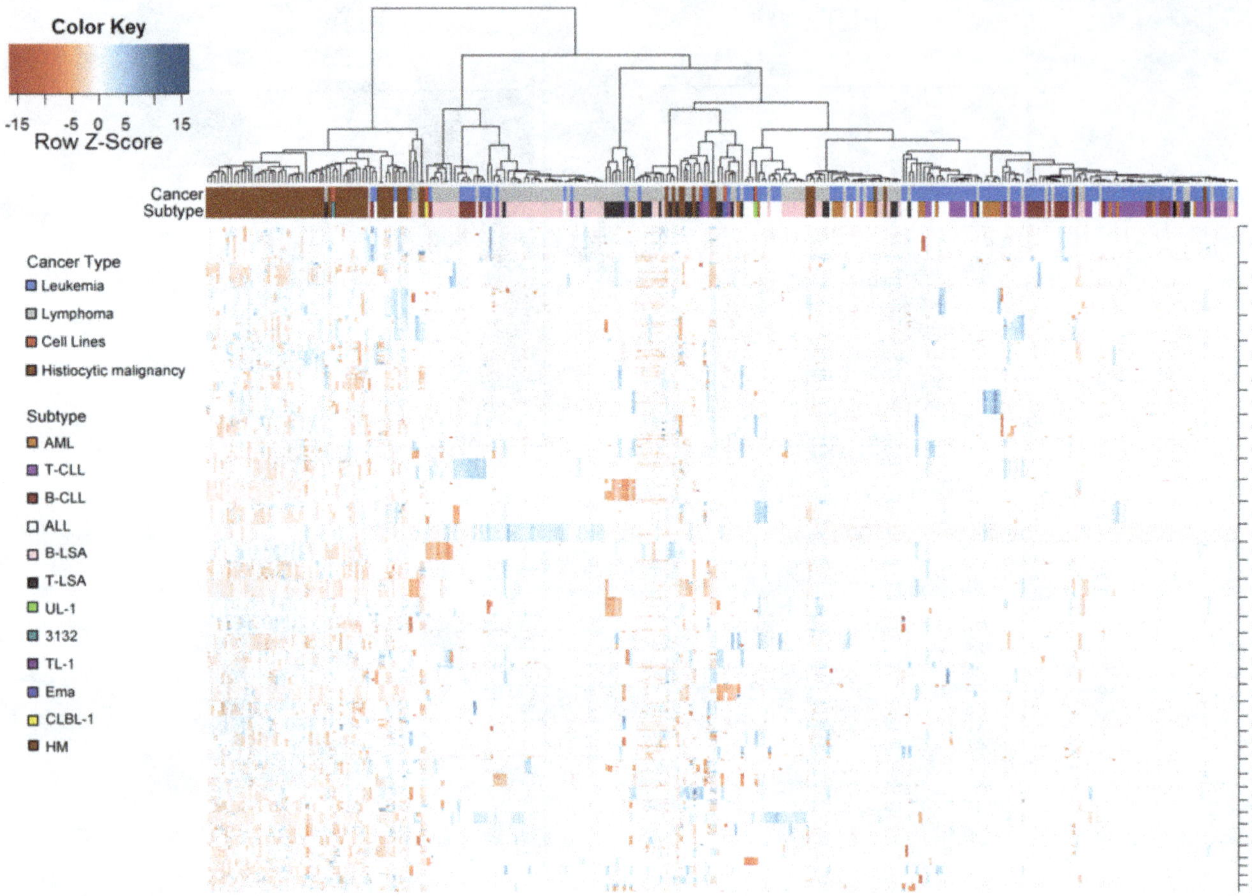

Fig. 9 Hierarchical clustering of canine LL cell lines with 299 primary canine round cell tumors including 123 leukemias, 106 lymphomas, and 70 histiocytic malignancies based on genome wide copy number status. Data consisted of segmented values that were scaled and clustered using Euclidian distance and Ward's method. Columns represent individual patients and rows represent individual markers along the genome. Blue indicates a region of gain and red indicates a region of loss. Cancer type and Subtype metadata is annotated for each column. Abbreviations are as follows: Acute myeloid leukemia (AML), T-cell chronic lymphocytic leukemia (T-CLL), B-cell chronic lymphocytic leukemia (B-CLL), acute lymphoblastic leukemia (ALL), B-cell lymphoma (B-LSA), T-cell lymphoma (T-LSA), and histiocytic malignancy (HM)

upregulate *FLT3*, and increased *FLT3* expression has been previously identified in canine a subset of acute lymphocytic leukemias and the GL-1 cell line [9]. Upregulation of *VEGFA* was also found in UL-1 and has been previously reported in canine ALL [62]. Finally, upregulation of *GTSF1*, *LUM*, and *PYPH* and downregulation of *CLEC12A* and *CD9* in primary canine histiocytic sarcomas [63, 64] were found to be dysregulated similarly in 3132 cells.

Cross contamination of cell lines is a common issue in the scientific community with ~19 % of human LL cell lines being cross contaminated [6]. This problem is further evidenced by the identification of human cells in five recently characterized canine B-cell lymphoma cell lines [65]. Our cytogenetic analysis of chromosomal architecture, in conjunction with oaCGH and FISH analysis, proves none of the examined cell lines are cross contaminated with other canine or human cells.

Conclusion

In summary, we present the comprehensive immunophenotypic and genomic characterization of 5 canine LL cell lines that confirms their cell of origin in 3 cell lines (CLBL-1, Ema, and TL-1) and refutes their cell of origin in 2 cell lines (UL-1 and 3132). These data provide valuable information that can be used to select cell lines for preclinical in vitro studies based on the presence or absence of particular immunophenotypic and/or genomic characteristics of interest, which will enhance their clinical predictive value. The generation of integrated molecular profiling of cell lines and comparison with primary tumors will allow further exploration into their biology and clinical utility in veterinary medicine and contribute to comparative and translational studies of hematopoietic malignancies in dogs and humans.

Additional file

Additional file 1: Table S1. Known cancer-associated genes located in regions of genomic imbalance in each of the five cell lines. **Table S2.** Summary of fold changes of cancer-associated genes for each cell line when normalized expression level was compared with mean normalized expression levels of non-neoplastic lymph nodes. **Table S3.** List of 50 transcripts from each cell line with the largest absolute fold changes when normalized expression level was compared with mean normalized expression levels of non-neoplastic lymph nodes. **Table S4.** Gene ontology (GO) biological processes enriched for genes upregulated or downregulatued by >5 fold in each cell line when compared with non-neoplastic lymph nodes. The top ten terms associated with up and down regulated genes are listed. **Table S5.** KEGG pathways associatated with genes upregulated or down-regulated by >5 fold in each cell line when compared with non-neoplastic lymph node. Up to the top ten pathways associated with up or down regulated genes are listed.

Abbreviations

CNA: Copy number analysis; FISH: Fluorescent in situ hybridization; GEP: Gene expression profiling; LL: Leukemia/lymphoma; oaCGH: Oligonucleotide array comparative genomic hybridization; PARR: Polymerase chain reaction for antigen receptor rearrangement

Acknowledgements

We thank Dr. Rachael Thomas and Katie Kennedy for providing oaCGH data for primary canine lymphomas and histiocytic sarcomas, and Linda English (NCSU Clinical Immunology Laboratory) for flow cytometry data.

Funding

This study was funded in part by awards made by the North Carolina University Cancer Research Fund administered by the Lineberger Comprehensive Cancer Center and the Comparative Medicine Institute (SES), AKC-Canine Health Foundation (Grant number 01843, MB) and the NCSU Cancer Genomics Fund (MB). SCR was supported in part by an NCSU Comparative Biomedical Science DVM-PhD training fellowship and a NIH T35 training grant.

Authors' contributions

SRC, MB, and SES conceived, designed, and performed the experiments. DR, AMR, and KLR provided statistical analysis. PM performed the immunophenotypic analysis. SCR, KLR, YO, TM, HT, SES, and MB wrote and edited the manuscript. All authors read and approved the final manuscript.

Competing interests

The authors declare that they have no competing interests.

Consent for publication

Not applicable.

Author details

[1]Department of Molecular Biomedical Sciences, College of Veterinary Medicine, North Carolina State University, CVM Research Building - Room 348, 1060 William Moore Drive, Raleigh 27607, NC, USA. [2]Bioinformatics Research Center, Department of Statistics, North Carolina State University, Raleigh, NC, USA. [3]Department of Medicine, University of North Carolina, Chapel Hill, NC, USA. [4]Comparative Medicine Institute, North Carolina State University, Raleigh, NC, USA. [5]Cancer Genetics Program, Lineberger Comprehensive Cancer Center, University of North Carolina, Chapel Hill, NC, USA. [6]Department of Pathology, Microbiology, and Immunology, College of Veterinary Medicine, University of California, Davis, CA, USA. [7]Veterinary Teaching Hospital, Faculty of Agriculture, Iwate University, Morioka, Japan. [8]Laboratory of Veterinary Internal Medicine, Faculty of Agriculture, Yamaguchi University, Yamaguchi, Japan. [9]Graduate School of Agricultural and Life Sciences, University of Tokyo, Bunkyo, Japan. [10]Department of Clinical Sciences, College of Veterinary Medicine, North Carolina State University, CVM Research Building - Room 308, 1051 William Moore Drive, Raleigh, NC 27607, USA. [11]KLR current address: Department of Biomedical Sciences, Cornell University, Ithaca, NY, USA.

References

1. Swerdlow S, Campo E, Harris NL. WHO classification of tumours of haematopoietic and lymphoid tissues. France: IARC Press; 2008.
2. MacLeod RA, Nagel S, Scherr M, Schneider B, Dirks WG, Uphoff CC, Quentmeier H, Drexler HG. Human leukemia and lymphoma cell lines as models and resources. Curr Med Chem. 2008;15(4):339–59.
3. Ferreira D, Adega F, Chaves R. The importance of cancer cell lines as in vitro models in cancer methylome analysis and anticancer drugs testing. In: López-Camarillo C, Aréchaga-Ocampo E, editors. Oncogenomics and cancer proteomics - novel approaches in biomarkers discovery and therapeutic targets in cancer, InTech. 2013.
4. Rücker FG, Sander S, Döhner K, Döhner H, Pollack JR, Bullinger L. Molecular profiling reveals myeloid leukemia cell lines to be faithful model systems characterized by distinct genomic aberrations. Leukemia. 2006;20(6):994–1001.
5. Andersson A, Edén P, Lindgren D, Nilsson J, Lassen C, Heldrup J, Fontes M, Borg Å, Mitelman F, Johansson B. Gene expression profiling of leukemic cell lines reveals conserved molecular signatures among subtypes with specific genetic aberrations. Leukemia. 2005;19(6):1042–50.
6. Drexler HG, Matsuo Y, MacLeod RA. Continuous hematopoietic cell lines as model systems for leukemia–lymphoma research. Leuk Res. 2000;24(11): 881–911.
7. Breen M, Modiano JF. Evolutionarily conserved cytogenetic changes in hematological malignancies of dogs and humans – man and his best friend share more than companionship. Chromosom Res. 2008;16(1):145–54.
8. Thomas R, Seiser EL, Motsinger-Reif A, Borst L, Valli VE, Kelley K, Suter SE, Argyle D, Burgess K, Bell J, et al. Refining tumor-associated aneuploidy through 'genomic recoding' of recurrent DNA copy number aberrations in 150 canine non-Hodgkin's lymphomas. Leuk Lymphoma. 2011;52(7):1321–35.
9. Suter S, Small G, Seiser E, Thomas R, Breen M, Richards K. FLT3 mutations in canine acute lymphocytic leukemia. BMC Cancer. 2011;11(1):38.
10. Kisseberth WC, Nadella MVP, Breen M, Thomas R, Duke SE, Murahari S, Kosarek CE, Vernau W, Avery AC, Burkhard MJ. A novel canine lymphoma cell line: a translational and comparative model for lymphoma research. Leuk Res. 2007;31(12):1709–20.
11. Seiser E, Thomas R, Richards K, Kathryn Kelley M, Moore P, Suter S, Breen M. Reading between the lines: molecular characterization of five widely used canine lymphoid tumour cell lines. Vet Comp Oncol. 2011;11(1):30–50.
12. Comazzi S, Guscetti F, Marconato L. First meeting of the European canine lymphoma group. Workshop: state of the art and comparative aspects in canine lymphoma. CH-Lugano, 22 June 2013. Hematol Oncol. 2013;32(2):68–71.
13. Aricò A, Giantin M, Gelain ME, Riondato F, Comazzi S, Rütgen BC, Essler SE, Dacasto M, Castagnaro M, Aresu L. The role of vascular endothelial growth factor and matrix metalloproteinases in canine lymphoma: in vivo and in vitro study. BMC Vet Res. 2013;9(1):94.
14. Fujiwara-Igarashi A, Goto-Koshino Y, Mochizuki H, Sato M, Fujino Y, Ohno K, Tsujimoto H. Inhibition of p16 tumor suppressor gene expression via promoter hypermethylation in canine lymphoid tumor cells. Res Vet Sci. 2014;97(1):60–3.
15. Fujiwara N, Kawasaki H, Yabe R, Christensen DJ, Vitek MP, Mizuno T, Sato K, Ohama T. A potential therapeutic application of SET/I2PP2A Inhibitor OP449 for Canine T-cell lymphoma. J Vet Med Sci. 2013;75(3):349–54.
16. Kojima K, Fujino Y, Goto-Koshino Y, Ohno K, Tsujimoto H. Analyses on activation of NF-kB and effect of bortezomib in canine neoplastic lymphoid cell lines. J Vet Med Sci. 2012;75(6):727–31.
17. Shiomitsu K, Xia X, Waite K, Sehgal I, Li S. Evaluation of the aurora kinase inhibitor, ZM447439, in canine malignant lymphoid cells in vitro. Open J Vet Med. 2013;3:29.
18. Tomiyasu H, Goto-Koshino Y, Fujino Y, Ohno K, Tsujimoto H. Antitumour effect and modulation of expression of the ABCB1 gene by perifosine in canine lymphoid tumour cell lines. Vet J. 2014;199(1):103–9.

19. Tomiyasu H, Goto-Koshino Y, Fujino Y, Ohno K, Tsujimoto H. The regulation of the expression of ABCG2 Gene through mitogen-activated protein kinase pathways in canine lymphoid tumor cell lines. J Vet Med Sci. 2013;76(2):237–42.
20. Tomiyasu H, Goto-Koshino Y, Fujino Y, Ohno K, Tsujimoto H. Epigenetic regulation of the ABCB1 gene in drug-sensitive and drug-resistant lymphoid tumour cell lines obtained from canine patients. Vet J. 2014;199(1):103–9.
21. Mudaliar MA, Haggart RD, Miele G, Sellar G, Tan KA, Goodlad JR, Milne E, Vail DM, Kurzman I, Crowther D. Comparative gene expression profiling identifies common molecular signatures of NF-kB activation in canine and human diffuse large B cell lymphoma (DLBCL). PLoS One. 2013;8(9):e72591.
22. Rütgen BC, Hammer SE, Gerner W, Christian M, De Arespacochaga AG, Willmann M, Kleiter M, Schwendenwein I, Saalmüller A. Establishment and characterization of a novel canine B-cell line derived from a spontaneously occurring diffuse large cell lymphoma. Leuk Res. 2010;34(7):932–8.
23. Umeki S, Ema Y, Suzuki R, Kubo M, Hayashi T, Okamura Y, Yamazaki J, Tsujimoto H, Tani K, Hiraoka H. Establishment of five canine lymphoma cell lines and tumor formation in a xenotransplantation model. J Vet Med Sci. 2012;75(4):467–74.
24. Holmes MA, Duffus W, Gorman N. Natural cytotoxicity in the dog: description of two new allogeneic tumour targets. Vet Immunol Immunopathol. 1989;23(1):161–70.
25. Strandstrom H, Rimaila-Parnanen E. Canine atypical malignant lymphoma. Am J Vet Res. 1979;40(7):1033.
26. Vernau W, Moore P. An immunophenotypic study of canine leukemias and preliminary assessment of clonality by polymerase chain reaction. Vet Immunol Immunopathol. 1999;69(2):145–64.
27. Burnett R, Vernau W, Modiano J, Olver C, Moore P, Avery A. Diagnosis of canine lymphoid neoplasia using clonal rearrangements of antigen receptor genes. Vet Pathol. 2003;40(1):32–41.
28. Thalheim L, Williams L, Borst L, Fogle J, Suter S. Lymphoma immunophenotype of dogs determined by immunohistochemistry, flow cytometry, and polymerase chain reaction for antigen receptor rearrangements. J Vet Intern Med. 2013;27(6):1509–16.
29. Breen M, Hitte C, Lorentzen TD, Thomas R, Cadieu E, Sabacan L, Scott A, Evanno G, Parker HG, Kirkness EF, et al. An integrated 4249 marker FISH/RH map of the canine genome. BMC Genomics. 2004;5(1):65.
30. Thomas R, Borst L, Rotroff D, Motsinger-Reif A, Lindblad-Toh K, Modiano JF, Breen M. Genomic profiling reveals extensive heterogeneity in somatic DNA copy number aberrations of canine hemangiosarcoma. Chromosom Res. 2014;22(3):305–19.
31. Futreal PA, Coin L, Marshall M, Down T, Hubbard T, Wooster R, Rahman N, Stratton MR. A census of human cancer genes. Nat Rev Cancer. 2004;4(3): 177–83.
32. R Core Team. R: A language and environment for statistical computing. Vienna: R Foundation for Statistical Computing; 2013.
33. Olshen AB, Venkatraman E, Lucito R, Wigler M. Circular binary segmentation for the analysis of array-based DNA copy number data. Biostatistics. 2004; 5(4):557–72.
34. Roode SC, Rotroff D, Avery AC, Suter SE, Bienzle D, Schiffman JD, Motsinger-Reif A, Breen M. Genome-wide assessment of recurrent genomic imbalances in canine leukemia identifies evolutionarily conserved regions for subtype differentiation. Chromosom Res. 2015;23(4):681–708.
35. Thomas R, Duke SE, Karlsson EK, Evans A, Ellis P, Lindblad-Toh K, Langford CF, Breen M. A genome assembly-integrated dog 1 Mb BAC microarray: a cytogenetic resource for canine cancer studies and comparative genomic analysis. Cytogenet Genome Res. 2008;122(2):110–21.
36. Kapushesky M, Adamusiak T, Burdett T, Culhane A, Farne A, Filippov A, Holloway E, Klebanov A, Kryvych N, Kurbatova N. Gene expression atlas update—a value-added database of microarray and sequencing-based functional genomics experiments. Nucleic Acids Res. 2012;40(D1):1077–81.
37. Wall M, Campbell L. Cytogenetics of Lymphomas. In: Wiernik PH, Goldman J, Dutcher J, Kyle R, editors. Neoplastic Diseases of the Blood. 5th ed. New York: Springer Science; 2013. p. 945–84.
38. Zhao W-L, Mourah S, Mounier N, Leboeuf C, Daneshpouy ME, Legrès L, Meignin V, Oksenhendler E, Le Maignin C, Calvo F. Vascular endothelial growth factor-A is expressed both on lymphoma cells and endothelial cells in angioimmunoblastic T-cell lymphoma and related to lymphoma progression. Lab Investig. 2004;84(11):1512–9.
39. van Delft FW, Horsley S, Colman S, Anderson K, Bateman C, Kempski H, Zuna J, Eckert C, Saha V, Kearney L. Clonal origins of relapse in ETV6-RUNX1 acute lymphoblastic leukemia. Blood. 2011;117(23):6247–54.
40. Li Z, Zhang H, Chen Y, Fan L, Fang J. Forkhead transcription factor FOXO3a protein activates nuclear factor kB through B-cell lymphoma/leukemia 10 (BCL10) protein and promotes tumor cell survival in serum deprivation. J Biol Chem. 2012;287(21):17737–45.
41. Li H, Lahti JM, Valentine M, Saito M, Reed SI, Look AT, Kidd VJ. Molecular Cloning and Chromosomal Localization of the Human Cyclin C (CCNC) and Cyclin E (CCNE) genes: deletion of the CCNC gene in human tumors. Genomics. 1996;32(2):253–9.
42. Simon C, Chagraoui J, Krosl J, Gendron P, Wilhelm B, Lemieux S, Boucher G, Chagnon P, Drouin S, Lambert R. A key role for EZH2 and associated genes in mouse and human adult T-cell acute leukemia. Genes Dev. 2012;26(7): 651–6.
43. Fujiwara S, Yamashita Y, Nakamura N, Choi Y, Ueno T, Watanabe H, Kurashina K, Soda M, Enomoto M, Hatanaka H. High-resolution analysis of chromosome copy number alterations in angioimmunoblastic T-cell lymphoma and peripheral T-cell lymphoma, unspecified, with single nucleotide polymorphism-typing microarrays. Leukemia. 2008;22(10):1891–8.
44. Costello R, Sanchez C, Le Treut T, Rihet P, Imbert J, Sébahoun G. Peripheral T-cell lymphoma gene expression profiling and potential therapeutic exploitations. Br J Haematol. 2010;150(1):21–7.
45. Nagel S, Venturini L, Przybylski GK, Grabarczyk P, Meyer C, Kaufmann M, Battmer K, Schmidt CA, Drexler HG, Scherr M. NK-like homeodomain proteins activate NOTCH3-signaling in leukemic T-cells. BMC Cancer. 2009; 9(1):371.
46. Abdelali RB, Asnafi V, Leguay T, Boissel N, Buzyn A, Chevallier P, Thomas X, Lepretre S, Huguet F, Vey N. Pediatric-inspired intensified therapy of adult T-ALL reveals the favorable outcome of NOTCH1/FBXW7 mutations, but not of low ERG/BAALC expression: a GRAALL study. Blood. 2011;118(19):5099–107.
47. Richards KL, Motsinger-Reif AA, Chen H-W, Fedoriw Y, Fan C, Nielsen DM, Small GW, Thomas R, Smith C, Dave SS. Gene profiling of canine B-cell lymphoma reveals germinal center and postgerminal center subtypes with different survival times, modeling human DLBCL. Cancer Res. 2013;73(16): 5029–39.
48. Wu Z, Irizarry RA, Gentleman R, Murillo FM, Spencer F. A model based background adjustment for oligonucleotide expression arrays. In: Johns Hopkins University, Dept of Biostatistics Working Papers. 2004. Working Paper 1.
49. Dennis Jr G, Sherman BT, Hosack DA, Yang J, Gao W, Lane HC, Lempicki RA. DAVID: database for annotation, visualization, and integrated discovery. Genome Biol. 2003;4(5):3.
50. Huang DW, Sherman BT, Lempicki RA. Systematic and integrative analysis of large gene lists using DAVID bioinformatics resources. Nat Protoc. 2008;4(1): 44–57.
51. Tsai P-C, Breen M. Array-based comparative genomic hybridization–guided identification of reference genes for normalization of real-time quantitative polymerase chain reaction assay data for lymphomas, histiocytic sarcomas, and osteosarcomas of dogs. Am J Vet Res. 2012;73(9):1335–43.
52. Ortolani C. Flow cytometry of hematological malignancies. Wiley; 2011.
53. Moore P. A review of histiocytic diseases of dogs and cats. Vet Pathol. 2014; 51(1):167–84.
54. Breen M. Canine cytogenetics–from band to basepair. Cytogenet Genome Res. 2008;120(1–2):50–60.
55. Rütgen BC, Willenbrock S, Reimann-Berg N, Walter I, Fuchs-Baumgartinger A, Wagner S, Kovacic B, Essler SE, Schwendenwein I, Nolte I. Authentication of primordial characteristics of the CLBL-1 cell line prove the integrity of a canine B-cell lymphoma in a murine in vivo model. PLoS One. 2012;7(6): e40078.
56. Reggeti F, Bienzle D. Flow cytometry in veterinary oncology. Veterinary Pathology. 2011;48(1):223–35.
57. Affolter V, Moore P. Localized and disseminated histiocytic sarcoma of dendritic cell origin in dogs. Vet Pathol. 2002;39(1):74–83.
58. Hanson CA, Jaszcz W, Kersey JH, Astorga MG, Peterson BA, Gajl-Peczalska KJ, Frizzera G. True histiocytic lymphoma: histopathologic, immunophenotypic and genotypic analysis. Br J Haematol. 1989;73(2):187–98.
59. Hedan B, Thomas R, Motsinger-Reif A, Abadie J, Andre C, Cullen J, Breen M. Molecular cytogenetic characterization of canine histiocytic sarcoma: A spontaneous model for human histiocytic cancer identifies deletion of tumor suppressor genes and highlights influence of genetic background on tumor behavior. BMC Cancer. 2011;11(1):201.
60. Giantin M, Aresu L, Aricò A, Gelain M, Riondato F, Comazzi S, Dacasto M. Evaluation of tyrosine-kinase receptor c-kit mutations, mRNA and protein

expression in canine lymphoma: might c-kit represent a therapeutic target? Vet Immunol Immunopathol. 2013;154(3):153–9.

61. Mortarino M, Gelain M, Gioia G, Ciusani E, Bazzocchi C, Comazzi S. ZAP-70 and Syk expression in canine lymphoid cells and preliminary results on leukaemia cases. Vet Immunol Immunopathol. 2009;128(4):395–401.
62. Aricò A, Giantin M, Gelain M, Riondato F, Mortarino M, Comazzi S, Dacasto M, Castagnaro M, Aresu L. Matrix metalloproteinases and vascular endothelial growth factor expression in canine leukaemias. Vet J. 2013;196(2):260–2.
63. Boerkamp KM, van der Kooij M, van Steenbeek FG, van Wolferen ME, Koerkamp MJG, van Leenen D, Grinwis GC, Penning LC, Wiemer EA, Rutteman GR. Gene expression profiling of histiocytic sarcomas in a canine model: the predisposed flatcoated retriever dog. PLoS One. 2013;8(8):e71094.
64. Boerkamp KM, van Steenbeek FG, Penning LC, Koerkamp MJG, van Leenen D, Vos-Loohuis M, Grinwis GC, Rutteman GR. The two main forms of histiocytic sarcoma in the predisposed flatcoated retriever dog display variation in gene expression. PLoS One. 2014;9(6):e98258.
65. Zwingenberger AL, Vernau W, Sh C, Yan W, Chen X, Gordon IK, Kent MS. Corrigendum to "Development and characterization of 5 canine B-cell lymphoma cell lines" [Leuk. Res. 36 (5)(2011) 601–606]. Leuk Res. 2013;37(1):120.

A description of the gross pathology of drowning and other causes of mortality in seabirds

Victor R. Simpson[1*] and David N. Fisher[2,3]

Abstract

Background: Mortality of seabirds due to anthropogenic causes, especially entrapment in fishing gear, is a matter of increasing international concern. This study aimed at characterising the gross pathology of seabirds that drowned in fishing nets and comparing it with that in other common causes of mortality.

Results: Post-mortem examinations were performed on 103 common guillemots, 32 razorbills, 37 shags and 5 great northern divers found stranded in Cornwall during 1981–2016. Pathology in birds that died in confirmed incidents of drowning in fishing nets (n = 95) was compared with that in cases of suspected drowning (n = 6), oil (n = 53) and polyisobutylene (PIB) (n = 3) pollution, adverse weather (n = 6) and stranding of unknown cause (14). The majority of drowned birds were in good nutritional state, freshly dead and approximately 50% had freshly ingested fish in their proximal gut. Principle lesions were: gross distention of the heart and major veins with dark blood, intensely congested, swollen and oedematous lungs which released white frothy fluid when excised, watery fluid in the air sacs that ranged from clear to deep red depending on state of carcase preservation. PIB-affected birds were in good nutritional state; their pathology was largely consistent with that in confirmed drowning cases; it is likely that drowning was the ultimate cause of death. Birds affected by oil, adverse weather or that stranded due to unknown cause were all in poor or emaciated condition, the mean body mass of the guillemots and razorbills being, respectively, 53 and 57% of those that drowned. They had little or no food in their alimentary tracts and many showed evidence of enteric inflammation, haemorrhage and ulceration. None had fluid in their air sacs and none showed significant cardio-respiratory system lesions.

Conclusions: Drowned birds consistently showed a distinctive set of gross pathological lesions. When combined with contemporaneous observations, the pathology may be sufficient to permit a diagnosis of drowning, especially where a batch of freshly dead birds are examined. The observations in this study are likely to be of value when investigating stranding incidents, particularly where it is suspected that legislation aimed at protecting seabirds is not being complied with.

Keywords: Seabird, Auk, Stranding, Drowning, Bycatch, Pathology, Air sac, Oil, Polyisobutylene

Background

In recent decades there has been increasing international concern over the level of seabird mortality caused by human activities, the most significant of which are entrapment in fishing gear (bycatch) and oil pollution. Global estimates of mortality caused by the fishing industry are imprecise but it is suggested that 400,000 birds die annually in gill nets and 320,000 in longline fisheries [1]. In the North Sea and Baltic it is believed that at least 90,000 waterbirds drown in nets annually and that the true number could be as high as 200,000 [2]. Major oil spill incidents, which often affect tens or even hundreds of thousands of birds, are well publicised. However, innumerable small oil spills go largely unrecorded but are believed to be responsible for greater mortality. In Newfoundland alone the mortality from repeated low level inputs of oil, so-called chronic pollution, is estimated to average 315,000 birds annually [3]. Chronic oil pollution is also a major concern in Europe, especially in the North West European waters [4]; these include the English Channel and the Celtic sea.

* Correspondence: vic@wildlifevic.org
[1]Wildlife Veterinary Investigation Centre, Chacewater, Truro, Cornwall TR4 8PB, UK
Full list of author information is available at the end of the article

Cornwall is a maritime county in south-west England where commercial fishing, shipping and tourism are major contributors to the local economy. It is also rich in marine wildlife and the relatively natural 700 Km coastline, bounded by the English Channel to the south and the Celtic sea to the north, supports large populations of seabirds. Incidents of stranded dead or dying birds are common and post-mortem examinations frequently identify anthropogenic factors as the cause. The purpose of this report is to characterise the gross pathology seen in common guillemots (*Uria aalge*), razorbills (*Alca torda*), shags (*Phalacrocorax aristotelis*) and great northern (GN) divers (*Gavia immer*) that had drowned and to compare this with the pathology seen in birds that died due to oil pollution or other causes.

Methods

This was an opportunistic study of seabirds submitted for post-mortem examination by the Royal Society for the Prevention of Cruelty to Animals (RSPCA), various conservation bodies, government agencies and members of the public. The birds had either been found dead, moribund or sick along the coast of Cornwall. Dead and moribund birds were sent directly for post-mortem examination whilst sick birds, many of which showed clear evidence of oil pollution, were treated at a wildlife hospital; those that died or were euthanased due to a poor prognosis were normally submitted for post-mortem examination within 24 h. In incidents involving large numbers of birds a representative sample, usually of ten to fifteen birds, was examined. Between 1981 and 2001 the post-mortems were performed at the Veterinary Laboratories Agency (VLA), Truro, and thereafter, until 2016, at the Wildlife Veterinary Investigation Centre. In most incidents the birds were examined within 24 h of them being found but in a few cases carcases were either submitted frozen or a proportion were frozen on receipt for logistical reasons.

Each bird was given a unique reference number and examined following a standard protocol [5]. The body mass, excluding ingesta mass, was recorded in all cases. Liver mass was recorded in most cases and pectoralis muscle mass in drowning cases; however, in some incidents constraints on time prevented all these parameters from being recorded. Age class was determined as sub-adult or adult by the degree of gonad development. In selected cases parasites were submitted to Dr. E. Harris at the Natural History Museum, London for identification. Samples of watery fluid were taken from the air sacs of selected drowned birds and examined by direct light microscopy for the presence of plankton, diatoms or other marine contaminants.

Statistical analyses were performed in the software R ver. 3.1.2 [6]. Only birds with a known cause of death were included in the analyses. To determine whether birds differed in body mass due to cause of death, sex and species, a linear model (LM) was used with the log of body mass as a response (this was necessary to achieve normality), and age (adult or sub-adult), sex, species and cause of death (either drowned or non-drowned) as predictor variables. The LM also included a sex-species interaction, a species-age interaction, and an age-cause of death interaction, to account for any differences between the species in sexual dimorphism, variation in the difference between age classes between the species, and variation in the difference between drowned and non-drowned masses between age classes respectively.

Linear models were also used to analyse organ mass relative to body mass, as it might be expected that when a bird loses condition its organs may not regress in the same way. Therefore, for each of liver and pectoral muscle mass, LMs were used with organ mass set as a response and body mass, sex, age, and species as predictor variables. The cause of death was included as a predictor in the model for liver mass but could not be included in the model for pectoral muscle mass as this was only recorded in those birds that had drowned. The model for liver mass included an interaction between mass and cause of death (to determine whether birds that died in a certain way had different body mass-liver mass relationships). These LMs used a normal error structure.

In all cases, terms were removed and resulting models tested for significant differences with the previous model using F tests. The first terms to be removed were those with the highest *p*-values. Single terms were not tested until any interactions involving them had been removed. If species, or an interaction involving it, was found to be significant, we conducted pair-wise comparisons for each species pair by removing the other species from the dataset and re-analysing the subset with the final model. This allowed us to directly compare one species against another, while controlling for other factors e.g. cause of death or body mass (for organ mass).

Results

Post-mortem examinations were performed on 177 birds. More than half of these (n = 95) came from eight observed drowning incidents. The rest were from four suspected but unconfirmed drowning incidents, 15 oil pollution incidents, a single confirmed incident of polyisobutylene (PIB) pollution and a suspected 'storm wreck' (mass death of debilitated birds due to extreme weather conditions). There were six incidents where birds became stranded for no obvious reason and where their gross appearance, and the circumstances, such as location and weather conditions, did not suggest a likely cause. This category of mortality is hereafter referred to as unknown cause. The species and number of birds examined in each type of incident are summarised in Table 1.

Table 1 The number of mortality incidents by category of death and the species and numbers of birds examined in each category

Incident type & number	Number & species of birds examined	Total
Drowning, confirmed *n* = 8	39 guillemots, 25 razorbills, 26 shags, 5 GN divers	95
Drowning, unconfirmed, 4	1 guillemot, 3 razorbills, 2 shags	6
PIB pollution, *n* = 1	3 guillemots	3
Oil pollution, *n* = 15	48 guillemots, 3 razorbills, 2 shags	53
Unknown cause, *n* = 6	12 guillemots, 1 razorbill, 1 shag	14
Storm wreck, n = 1	6 shags	6

Gross pathology in each category of death

Confirmed drowning

External features

Five of the eight observed incidents of drowning in fishing nets involved guillemots or razorbills, either together or as a single species. The birds ranged from freshly dead to slightly autolysed. Their plumage was usually wet but in good condition and a few birds had slight scavenger damage. Body condition in the great majority of cases was good with well-developed muscles and good to excellent subcutaneous fat deposits. A sixth confirmed incident involved 26 shags, two guillemots and a razorbill. Their plumage was in good condition, although very wet and contaminated by sand; two shags showed signs of scavenger damage and some birds showed evidence of mild autolysis. Two of the shags and a guillemot were examined within 24 h of submission and the rest after being stored at minus 20° C. The majority of the shags and the razorbill were in good muscular condition with good to excellent subcutaneous fat deposits but the guillemots were only in poor to fair condition. Thirteen of the shags and one guillemot had localised dark red, irregular, subcutaneous areas of suspected bruising, often with associated oedema. These lesions were mostly around the neck but also over the shoulders, sternum or the lateral aspect of the thighs. Large numbers of subcutaneous mites (*Laminosioptes* sp.) were present in the shags, particularly in the precrural area. Five GN divers died in the other two confirmed incidents. All were submitted freshly dead and the plumage in each case was in good condition. One diver had monofilament nylon net enclosing the left carpal joint and another had net around the joints of both wings which prevented them from being extended; the right hock joint of the latter bird was dislocated. Muscle condition was good in all five birds and subcutaneous fat deposits ranged from fair to excellent. Three divers were examined in fresh condition and two after being stored at minus 20° C.

Internal features

The skin over the ventro-lateral surface of the neck and body was reflected and in every case the jugular veins were observed to be greatly distended with dark blood. Care was taken not to puncture the exposed clavicular air sac and, with the exception of the divers, when slight fluctuating pressure was applied to the abdomen, fluid was observed moving in the distended air sac of most birds (Fig. 1). In divers, the clavicular air sac appeared to be bi-lobed but did not extend far enough forward in the interclavicular space to be properly visualised; however, applying pressure to the abdomen did cause distention of subcutaneous air sacs in the axillae, presumed to be extra-thoracic diverticula of the clavicular air sacs. In all species, when the carcase was opened, watery fluid was also frequently seen in the other air sacs, in particular the abdominal air sacs. An example of this can be viewed in an additional movie file [see Additional file 1]. In freshly dead or slightly autolysed specimens the fluid was normally watery, non-frothy and completely clear or slightly blood-tinged. In birds that had been refrigerated for 24 h it was usually slightly more blood-tinged whereas in birds that had been frozen it ranged from blood-tinged to dark red (Fig. 2). Watery fluid was recorded in the air sacs of over 86% (82/95) of cases; it may also have been present in some of the early incidents but not specifically noted. The volume of water varied from case to case but it was not considered practical to try to quantify it. A small amount of

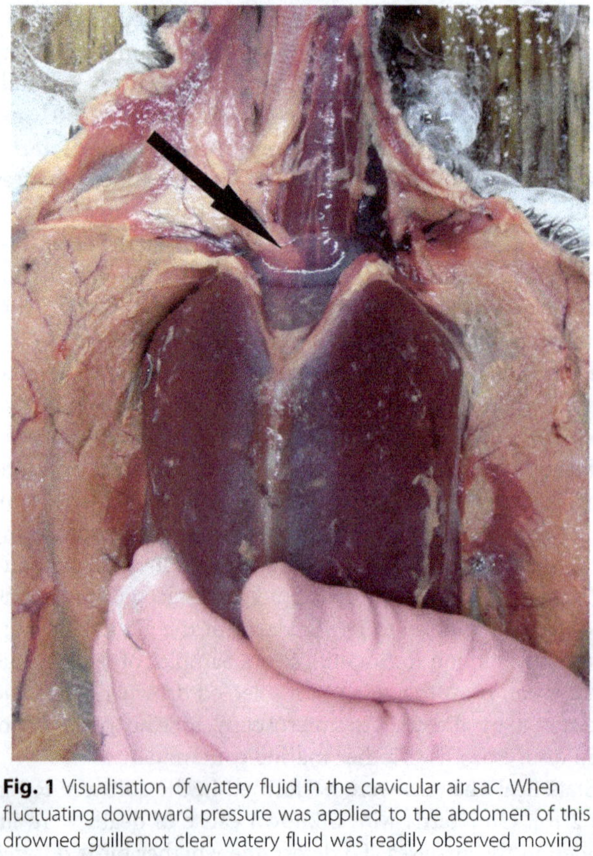

Fig. 1 Visualisation of watery fluid in the clavicular air sac. When fluctuating downward pressure was applied to the abdomen of this drowned guillemot clear watery fluid was readily observed moving in the distended clavicular air sac (arrow)

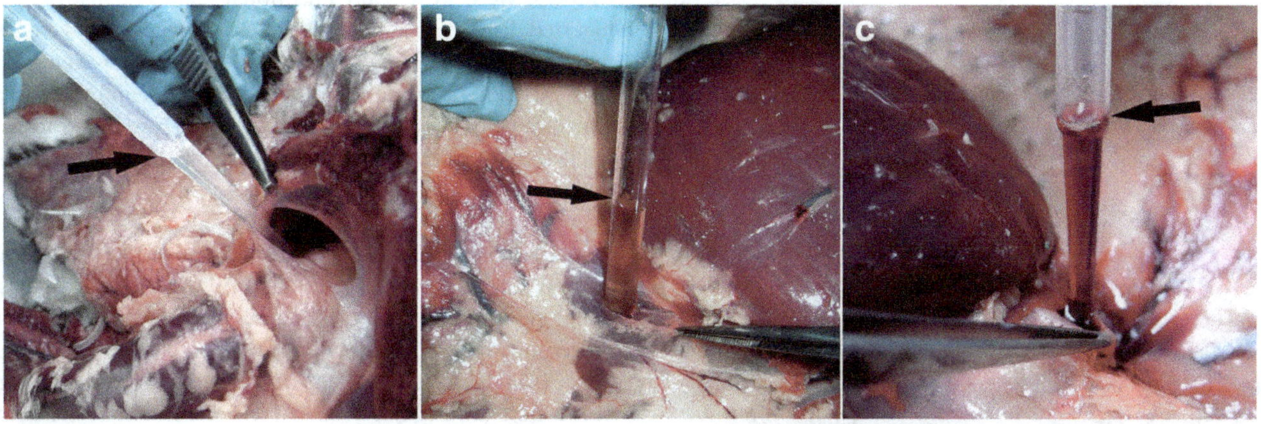

Fig. 2 Variation in appearance of the fluid in the air sacs of drowned birds. These three GN divers died in the same incident and were submitted freshly dead. **a**: clear fluid is drawn from the clavicular air sac of a freshly dead bird. **b**: This bird had been held at 4° C for 24 h. The fluid is blood tinged and is being aspirated from the axillary diverticulum of the left clavicular air sac. **c**: This bird had been stored at minus 20° C for two months; the fluid is being drawn from the axillary diverticulum of the right clavicular air sac and is dark red

fluid, either clear or blood tinged, but not frothy, was occasionally seen in the lower trachea and bronchi; this was most marked in the GN divers.

The lungs in all the confirmed drowned birds were swollen, intensely congested and oedematous and, when excised or sectioned, fluid exuded from cut surfaces. The fluid in freshly dead birds was usually white and frothy (Fig. 3). It was blood tinged in slightly autolysed ones and deeper red and less frothy in birds that had been frozen. In all cases, the cranial and caudal venae cavae and the chambers of the heart, especially the right atrium, were grossly distended with dark blood (Fig. 4).

Congestion of the kidneys, and to a lesser degree the liver, was common. In the incident involving 26 shags, the heads of four shags, the two guillemots and the razorbill were cut in the mid sagittal plane and in each case the space between the dorsal surface of the cerebellum and the cranium, believed to be the occipital sinus, was distended with dark blood (Fig. 5). Removal of the cranium showed the other dural venous sinuses over the caudal brain to be markedly congested with blood.

Approximately half the birds in each of the confirmed drowning incidents had small fish, mostly Clupeid or Ammodytes-type, in their oesophagus, proventriculus and gizzard and these varied from being freshly ingested to partly digested. Otoliths were often present in otherwise empty gizzards. Large pale nematodes, identified as *Contracaecum rudolphi*, were frequently present in the proventriculus and gizzard of the shags, often in large numbers. No lesions were seen in the intestines. Overall, there were no notable differences between the species in the pathology due to drowning, although the distension of the venae cavae was more pronounced in the auks.

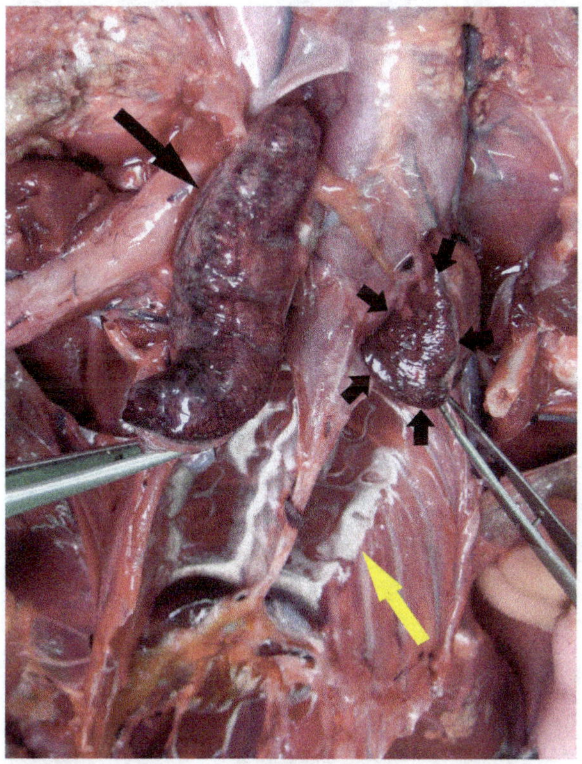

Fig. 3 Thoracic cavity of a drowned shag showing swollen and intensely congested lungs. The lungs have been excised and moved cranially for examination. The right lung is shown intact (black arrow) but the left lung was bisected and the cranial half removed; the cut surface of the caudal half (small arrows) shows that the intense congestion extends evenly throughout the parenchyma. The white frothy fluid adjacent to the spine (yellow arrow) was released from the lungs when they were excised

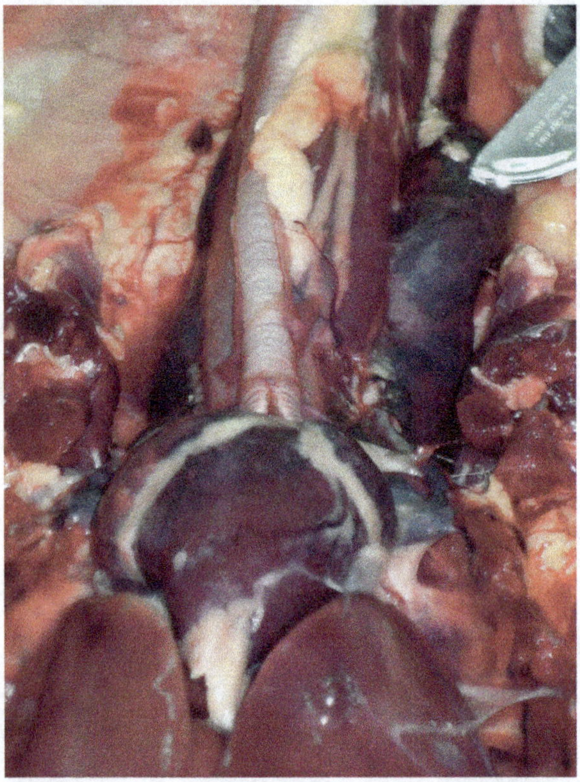

Fig. 4 Ventral view of the organs at the base of the neck and cranial thorax of a drowned guillemot. The heart and cranial venae cavae are markedly distended with dark blood. The scalpel points to the distended left cranial vena cava. The right cranial vena cava is partially obscured

Unconfirmed drowning

Six birds were examined from four unconfirmed drowning incidents. In the most significant of these 39 dead razorbills washed ashore at the fishing port of Mevagissey. Two were submitted for examination. Both birds had waterlogged feathers, were in a good nutritional state and had freshly ingested fish in the proventriculus. Their lungs were intensely congested but the possible presence of water in air sacs was not recorded. The other three unconfirmed incidents were of a minor nature involving just four birds, a guillemot, a razorbill and two shags. Both the shags were in a good nutritional state and one had freshly ingested fish in the proventriculus and gizzard. The lungs in both birds were intensely congested and produced white frothy fluid when excised. There was subcutaneous bruising around the base of the neck of one shag. The razorbill was in fair body condition and had a moderate quantity of part-digested sand eels (*Ammodytes* sp.) in the stomach. It had several large blood clots around the base of the neck and cranial thorax. Meaningful examination of the internal organs was not possible due to autolysis. The guillemot was in excellent body condition with congested lungs and watery fluid in the air sacs. As the birds in the unconfirmed drowned category had post-mortem lesions that were largely consistent with those in the confirmed drowning category, both groups are classed as drowned birds in the rest of this paper.

PIB pollution

Three frozen guillemots from a confirmed PIB spill were examined. The entire body surface of all three birds was coated in a thick layer of the whitish, glue-like, material; adhering to this were numerous stones, fragments of plastic and other marine debris (Fig. 6). The extreme stickiness of the coating meant that the birds' limbs could not be extended or moved freely away from their body. The carcases showed mild autolysis, their subcutaneous fat deposits were good to moderate and muscular condition was good. In each case, the chambers of the heart and the cranial and caudal venae cavae were greatly distended with dark blood and the lungs were swollen and intensely congested. There was a moderate to large amount of dark

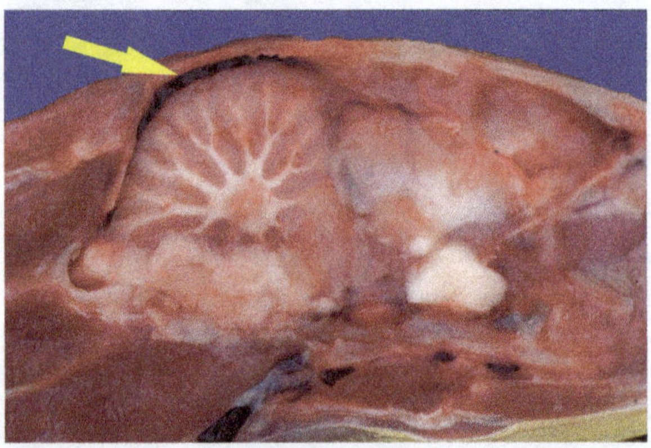

Fig. 5 Sagittal section of the head of a drowned shag. The occipital sinus is greatly distended with dark blood (arrow). Reflection of the cranium showed widespread congestion of the caudal dural venous sinuses with dark blood

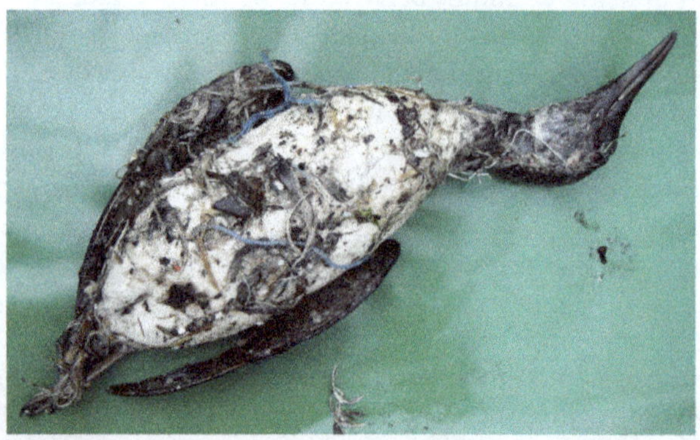

Fig. 6 Ventral view of a guillemot contaminated by PIB. There is a thick layer of the gluey compound coating the whole body surface adherent to which are small stones and a variety of marine debris. The bird was in good muscular condition and had excellent subcutaneous fat deposits

blood-stained fluid throughout the body cavity but, due to changes caused by autolysis and freezing, it was not possible to say whether there may have been fluid in the air sacs ante-mortem. The livers appeared normal or slightly congested but the kidneys were markedly congested. Chronic granulomatous lesions up to 15 × 20 mm were present in the mucosa of the upper or mid in oesophagus of two birds; beneath the granulomatous layer there was ulcerated tissue in which was embedded unidentified small nematodes. One of the birds had four small sprat-like fish in the proventriculus and approximately 20 g of digested food in the gizzard but neither of the other birds had a significant amount of food in the upper alimentary tract. The post-mortem findings in the PIB-affected birds were largely consistent with those seen in confirmed cases of drowning and it was concluded that the ultimate cause of death was drowning, probably because the PIB had prevented the birds from moving their limbs. However, they could also have been affected to some degree by hypothermia and starvation.

Oil pollution

All but five of the 53 birds that died following exposure to oil were guillemots, the others being three razorbills and two shags. Most of the oiled birds showed a consistent pattern of lesions, irrespective of whether they had been examined immediately after being found stranded or after they had died or been euthanased in rehabilitation centres. There were no significant differences in the post-mortem findings between the species. Subcutaneous fat deposits were either minimal or absent and skeletal muscles were wasted. The heart and major blood vessels were unremarkable. In most cases the respiratory system appeared normal but two guillemots had lesions in the thoracic air sacs consistent with aspergillosis; both of these birds had been in extended hospital care. The livers of oiled birds were noticeably small and gall bladders were often distended with bile. There was normally no food in the upper alimentary tract but in some hospitalised birds there was a small amount fish in the proventriculus and gizzard. In almost half (20/45) of recorded cases, the mucosal surface of the isthmus, at the junction between the proventriculus and gizzard, showed changes that ranged from reddish brown discolouration (Fig. 7) to marked inflammation, haemorrhage and ulceration: nematode worms were sometimes observed in the submucosa beneath the lesion. In most instances the lesion was associated with blackish or reddish-black fluid that extended from the proventriculus and gizzard to the intestines. Severe inflammation and thickening of the small intestine was also common. There were no consistent lesions in other organs but the adrenal glands in some birds appeared enlarged.

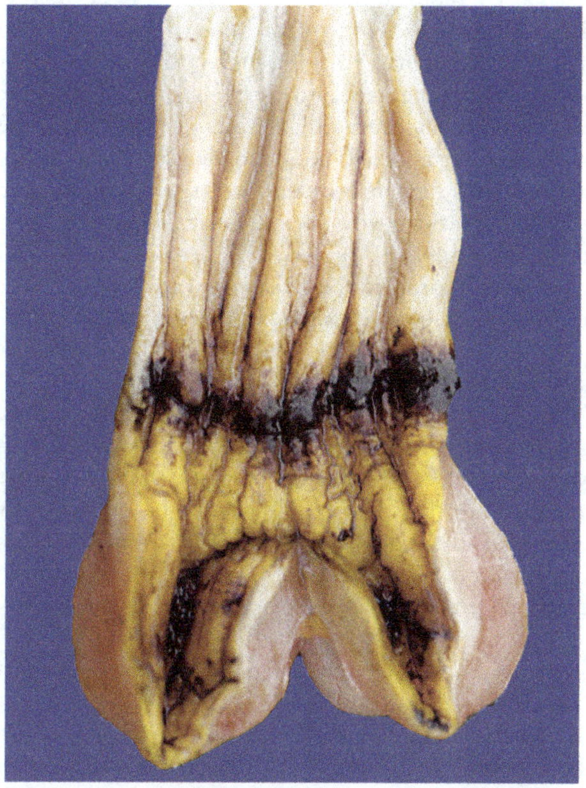

Fig. 7 The opened proventriculus and gizzard of an oiled guillemot. The mucosa over the isthmus region is discoloured dark reddish brown and ulcerated. There was blackish, thick fluid in the lumen of the gizzard and this extended into the intestines

Unknown cause

Fourteen birds, 12 guillemots, one shag and one razorbill were submitted in six stranding incidents where the cause was not apparent. The post-mortem lesions in the guillemots were largely the same as those seen in the oiled birds. They were in poor muscular condition with no significant subcutaneous fat deposits and little of no food in their alimentary tracts. In one incident, which involved around 30 guillemots, three out of the four birds examined had caseous, necrotic ulcers in the oesophagus associated with fourth stage larvae of *Contracaecum* sp. Three guillemots in another incident had lesions of the isthmus consistent with those seen in many oiled birds. The shag had died in emaciated condition with yellowish jelly in the proventriculus and the razorbill had extensive respiratory lesions indicative of aspergillosis. However, this bird had been hospitalised and the lesions could have been of a secondary nature.

Storm wreck

The single storm wreck incident involved six shags that were found dead together on a sheltered beach following a period of extremely stormy weather. Their plumage was clean with no evidence of oil. All six birds were in poor muscular condition with no subcutaneous fat. Several had subcutaneous masses of *Laminosioptes* sp. mites. Two had extensive haemorrhages around the upper neck and puncture wounds to the neck and chest consistent with attack by a mammalian predator. The alimentary tracts were empty save for a small amount of blackish bloody fluid and numerous nematodes identified as *C. rudolphi* in the gizzards. No lesions were seen in heart, kidneys or spleen but the livers appeared regressed. In five birds the respiratory tract appeared normal but one bird had extensive lung and air sac lesions consistent with aspergillosis.

Examination of air sac fluid

Watery fluid taken from the air sacs of two razorbills that died in a confirmed drowning incident showed unlysed erythrocytes and unidentified, motile, plankton-type organisms. However, fluid samples taken from the air sacs of two guillemots and a razorbill that died in a second confirmed incident and of a guillemot and a shag in third confirmed incident all proved negative for marine organisms.

Relationship between body and organ weights and cause of death

Most of the birds that died due to drowning had good subcutaneous fat deposits, well developed muscles and were heavier than birds that died of other causes (LM, $F_{1127} = 565.7$, $p < 0.001$). (Figure 8, see also Table 2). In all species males were heavier than females (LM, $F_{1127} = 7.4$, $p = 0.008$), with the sex-species interaction being non-significant (LM, $F_{2,124} = 1.7$, $p = 0.196$). Adults were heavier than immature birds in all species (LM, $F_{1127} = 6.9$, $p = 0.01$), with the species – age interaction being non-significant (LM, $F_{2122} = 0.4$, $p = 0.656$; Table 3). There were differences among the species in body mass (LM, $F_{2,127} = 333.0$, $p < 0.001$). Shags were heavier than guillemots (LM, $F_{1,105} = 391.7$, $p < 0.001$), and razorbills (LM, $F_{1,50} = 600.7$, $p < 0.001$), and guillemots were heavier than razorbills (LM, $F_{1,96} = 92.1$, $p < 0.001$). Pectoralis muscle mass was only recorded only in drowned birds and, as this did not assist in comparison with other causes of death, the data are shown in Additional file 2 and Figure S1.

Where birds died in poor or emaciated condition a low body mass was not due solely to reduced or absent fat deposits and regressed skeletal muscles but to regressed internal organs such as the liver. It was noticeable when examining oiled or unknown cause guillemots, for example, that their livers often appeared small and weighing confirmed this, their mean mass being 22.8 g and 24.3 g respectively compared with 50.6 g in those that had drowned (Table 2). Liver mass was positively related to body mass (LM, $F_{1,98} = 14.6$, $p < 0.001$) and birds that died of drowning had heavier livers for a given body mass (LM, $F_{1,98} = 18.3$, $p < 0.001$) (Figs. 9 and 10). Liver mass was not influenced by age class (LM, $F_{1,91} = 0.3$, $p = 0.590$) or

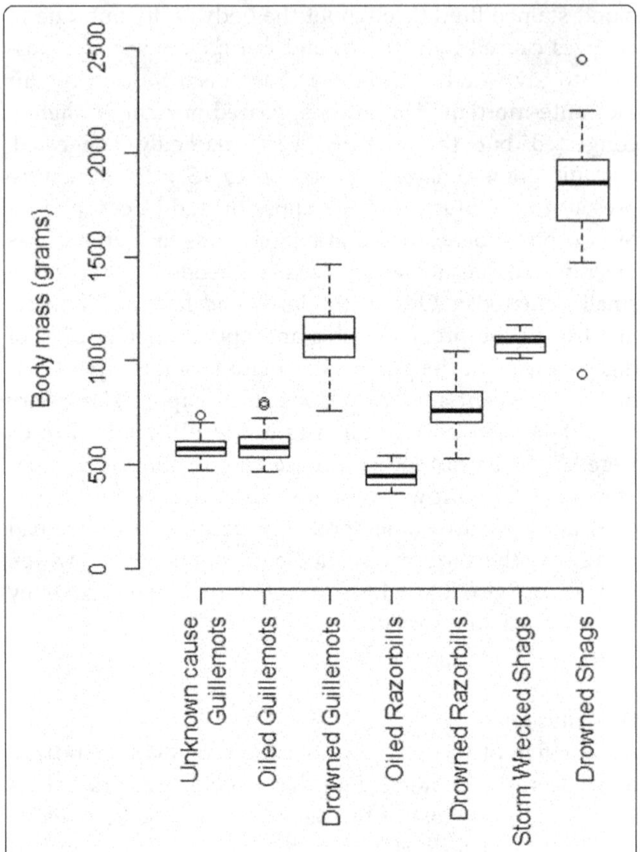

Fig. 8 Variation of body mass in relation to cause of death. The body mass (Q1 and Q3, inter quartile range and median values) of birds that drowned was significantly greater than that of birds dying of other causes. Combinations of species and cause of death not plotted if there were less than three individuals

sex (LM, $F_{1,97} = 1.0$, $p = 0.325$). Birds that died of drowning did not have a different relationship between body and liver mass to those who died of other causes (LM, $F_{1,96} = 0.7$, $p = 0.418$). Controlling for body mass, there were species differences in liver masses (LM, $F_{2,98} = 5.1$, $p = 0.007$). Razorbills had smaller livers for a given body mass than guillemots (LM, $F_{1,69} = 4.1$, $p = 0.047$) and shags (LM, $F_{1,37} = 9.8$, $p = 0.003$), which were not different (LM, $F_{1,88} = 0.5$, $p = 0.477$).

All data used in statistical analysis is included in Additional file 3.

Discussion

Much of the recorded pathology relating to drowning and other causes of mass mortality of seabirds is derived from studies where specimens were frozen prior to post-mortem examination and where, in many cases, the birds were affected by a variable degree of autolysis [7–11]. A consequence of this is that some lesions, especially those affecting the respiratory system, become obscured by artefactual changes. Descriptions of lesions in birds known to

Table 2 The body mass, liver mass and pectoral muscle mass of the different species within the various categories of death

Species	Mean body mass g (Range, sd, n)			
	drowned	oiled	Unknown cause	Storm wreck
guillemots	1112.4 (760–1461, 157.3, 43)	592.5 (468–800, 73.6, 48)	586.2 (470–740, 76.2, 12)	NA
shags	1814.7 (930–2448, 272.9, 27)	NA	1046 (NA, NA, 1)	1086.3 (1010–1168, 56.3, 6)
razorbills	783.7 (530–1045, 125.2, 26)	448.3 (360–542, 91.1, 3)	455 (NA, NA, 1)	NA
	Mean liver mass g (Range, sd, n =)			
guillemots	50.6 (28.8–75, 10.3, 35)	22.8 (11.4–43, 9.0, 21)	24.3 (14–41.7, 10.0, 6)	NA
shags	72.4 (55.8–102, 10.5, 26)	NA	NA	30.6 (26.6–33.1, 2.6, 5)
razorbills	33.3 (20–51.4, 9.6, 10)	19.4 (NA, NA, 1)	NA	NA
	Mean pectoral mass g (Range, sd, n =)			
guillemots	156.2 (127.2–177, 17.1, 11)	NA	NA	NA
shags	180.8 (136.2–236.4, 22.2, 25)	NA	NA	NA
razorbills	95.1 (82.3–103, 9.13, 4)	NA	NA	NA

NA No data obtained

have drowned and where at least some of the carcases were examined in fresh, unfrozen, condition are uncommon. In this study, the majority of the 95 birds known to have drowned were examined in fresh condition. The changes seen in the respiratory system showed a high level of uniformity and were considered to be entirely consistent with the inhalation of seawater.

When a bird inhales under normal circumstances, fresh air passes along the primary bronchi and enters, via openings known as ostia, directly in to the caudal air sacs (caudal thoracic and abdominal sacs); air from some secondary bronchi and parabronchi also passes, via the ostia, in to the caudal air sacs. On exhalation, most of the air (more than 88%) in the caudal air sacs passes, via secondary bronchi and their parabronchi, in to the lung parenchyma; only a small amount (less than 12%) escapes via the primary bronchi and trachea [12]. During the next phase of inhalation, the air in the parabronchi and the parenchyma, having undergone gaseous exchange, is drawn via secondary bronchi, in to the cranial air sacs (cervical, clavicular, and cranial thoracic air sacs). Fresh air is prevented from entering the cranial air sacs directly from the primary or secondary bronchi due to a system of valves [12, 13]. Assuming that inhaled seawater behaves in much the same way as air, most of the water found in the cranial air sacs of the known or suspected drowned birds in the present study must have passed through the pulmonary parenchyma after being expelled from the caudal air sacs.

It might be argued that if a bird had died at sea from causes other than drowning water could have entered the respiratory system, and in particular the air sacs, after it had died. The evidence does not support this. Many of the oiled and unknown cause birds in this study appeared to have died at sea yet none had anything more than a small amount of water beyond the proximal trachea. None had water in their air sacs. Even if water was able to passively enter the air sacs post-mortem, this would not result in the pathological changes seen in the lungs and cardiovascular system of drowned birds. As part of the standard post-mortem protocol followed in this study [5], all the birds were thoroughly washed in warm water and detergent and this included immersion of their head; despite this, watery fluid was only seen in the air sacs of the drowned or suspected downed birds.

The presence of a large amount of froth or frothy fluid around the nose, mouth and/or in the airways is a well-recognised feature of humans and other mammals that have drowned in sea water; however, it is not considered to be pathognomonic for drowning [14, 15]. A small amount of watery, clear, slightly frothy fluid was occasionally present in the lower trachea and bronchi of the drowned birds but, in contrast to what often happens in drowned mammals, it never extended up the trachea or

Table 3 The body mass by age class and sex of drowned and non-drowned guillemots and shags

	Mean body mass g. (Range, sd, n =)		
	Drowned Guillemots	Non-drowned Guillemots	Drowned Shags
Adult males	1148.3 (1002–1354, 118.9, 11)	613.6 (468–800, 96.2, 9)	1965.9 (1794–2448, 152, 14)
Adult females	1124.1 (794–1461, 167.0, 14)	577.2 (483–740, 68.14, 17)	1687.6 (1563–1798, 87.3, 7)
Immature males	1042.3 (851–1214, 121.1, 6)	599.5 (528–713, 53.3, 11)	1915.3 (1694–2200, 258.9, 3)
Immature females	1070.4 (810–1320, 233.5, 5)	558.8 (470–615, 54.1, 5)	1492.5 (1466–1519,37.5, 2)

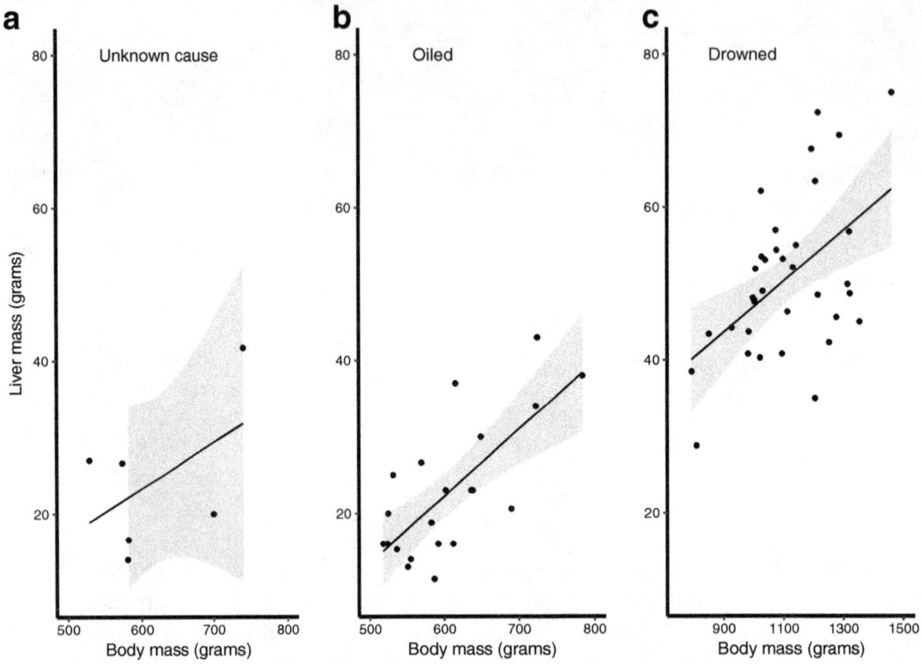

Fig. 9 Body to liver mass relationship in guillemots dying of different causes. Plots show the significant, positive relationship between body and liver mass. Light grey areas indicate standard errors around the regression line. Birds that died of drowning had heavier livers than other birds for a given body mass, while the body mass – liver mass relationship did not differ between birds that died of drowning compared to other causes

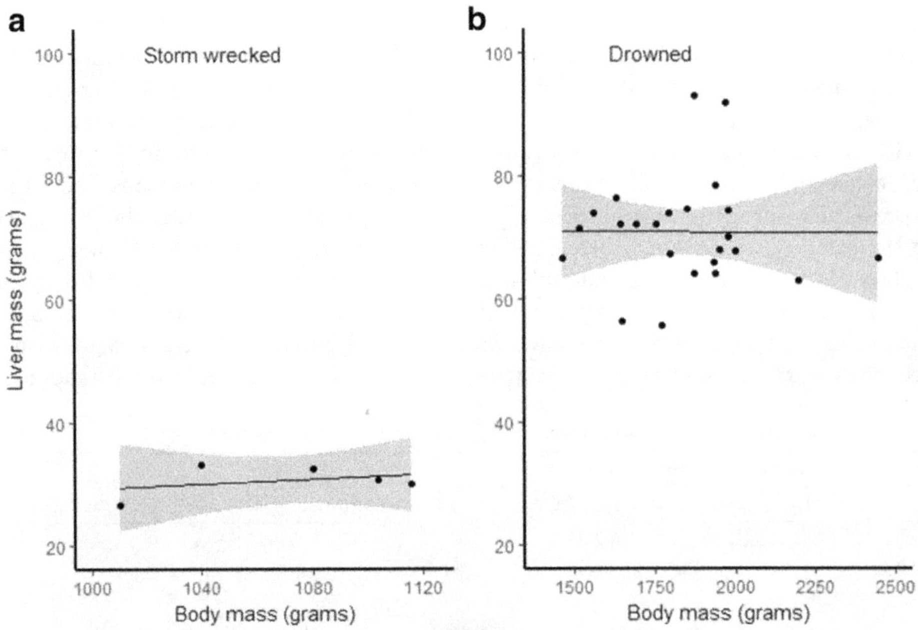

Fig. 10 The plots show the relationship between liver and body mass in storm-wrecked shags compared with that in drowned shags

into the mouth and nares. In mammals, when sea water enters airways it destroys the surfactant coating and, because it is hypertonic to plasma, water is drawn, together proteinaceous fluid, from the lung parenchyma in to the alveoli; this results in haemoconcentration and hypovolaemia [14]. In birds, surfactant occurs mostly lining the walls of the parabronchial atria and the air capillaries. It is presumed that it is this, admixed with seawater and protein-rich fluid released from the parenchyma, that forms the white frothy fluid seen when the lungs of drowned birds are excised or bisected. The release of this fluid from the lungs, together with gross pulmonary congestion and oedema, was a constant feature in the drowned birds. However, in drowned birds affected by autolysis, and especially those that had been frozen prior to examination, the normally white fluid ranged from blood tinged to deep red and tended to be less frothy.

In all the drowned birds, including the PIB affected guillemots but not those birds dying of other causes, the major veins and the chambers of heart, especially those on the right side, were markedly distended with dark blood. It is considered that these changes could be indicative of acute circulatory failure and hypoxaemia, possibly as a result of back pressure on the pulmonary arteries due to a combination of extreme pulmonary congestion, oedema and haemoconcentration. The marked congestion of the occipital and other dural venous sinuses observed in drowned birds is, in the authors' experience, unusual and is not normally seen in birds dying of other causes. However, as the dural venous sinuses drain via the caudal cephalic veins directly in to the jugular veins [16], the congestion of the sinuses is likely to be a result of drowning.

In the oiled birds, the predominant post-mortem lesions of emaciation, blackish fluid in empty or near-empty alimentary tracts and enteritis were consistent with those recorded in birds known to have been exposed to oil [7, 17–19]. However, the same or very similar lesions were also frequently seen in the non-oiled, unknown cause, birds in the present study and they cannot be considered specific for oil exposure. The nature and origin of the blackish fluid is not clear. In a study of oiled rhinoceros auklets (*Cerorhinca monocerata*) blackish fluid in the gut was shown not to be ingested oil [7]. Similarly, analysis of black fluid in the intestines of oiled guillemots and razorbills proved negative for hydrocarbons but positive for occult blood [19]. In ducks experimentally dosed with oil, the dark gut fluid also proved positive for occult blood: no discrete focal lesions were present and the authors concluded that blood had entered the gut by diapedesis [18]. In the present study it is likely that the blackish fluid in the gut was, at least in part, due occult blood as a result of haemorrhage from an inflamed or ulcerated isthmus or, where there were no visible haemorrhagic lesions, as a result of diapedesis. Blackish-red fluid is commonly present in the gut of birds of prey dying of starvation where it is believed to be stress-related [20]. Stress was thought to be responsible for histological lesions in the adrenal glands of birds experimentally dosed with crude oil [21]. It is suggested that stress may also contribute to the formation of blackish fluid in the gut of oiled or debilitated sea birds.

Birds exposed to oil, whether by contamination of plumage or by ingestion, suffer severe weight loss [7, 22, 23], in part due to hypothermia, impaired mobility, starvation and stress but also due to the direct toxic effect of oil on internal organs [21, 22, 24]. The oiled birds in this study were almost all in debilitated condition with nil or negligible amounts of subcutaneous fat, wasted muscles and regressed internal organs. Both their mean body mass and liver mass was significantly lower than that in drowned birds which, in almost every case, had good subcutaneous fat, well-developed muscles and normal looking internal organs. However, the condition of birds that had died due to adverse weather or that had become stranded due to unknown cause was not significantly different from that of the oiled birds. The mean body mass of oiled and unknown cause guillemots (592.5 g and 586.2 g respectively) was approximately half that of the drowned birds (1111.6 g). The fact that the emaciated, non-drowned birds had lighter livers than expected for a given body weight suggests that liver atrophy started to occur at an early stage of illness. This has been recognised in debilitated waterfowl elsewhere [25]. Although the body mass of the drowned guillemots would have been influenced to some degree by the fact that their plumage was often wet, and possibly by the presence of some residual ingesta, the mean was very similar to that of healthy adults (1107 g) and immatures (877 g) wintering in Scotland [26]. It is considered unlikely that the volume of water in the air sacs of drowned birds relative to their body mass would have significantly affected these results.

The post-mortem lesions in the oiled birds and the unknown cause birds in the present study were similar to those reported in two studies of guillemots that stranded dead in Belgium [8, 9]. In both the Belgian studies, weight loss, cachexia and haemorrhagic gastroenteritis were the most common findings but there was no clear correlation between these lesions and the presence of oil, either on the plumage or in the gut [8, 9]. In one study [8] the mean body mass of the cachectic birds was 708 g compared with 781 g in birds considered non-cachectic. Although oiling was considered to be the main cause of death, no cause was determined in the 45% of birds that were not oiled, many of which had haemorrhagic enteropathy lesions [8]. In the other Belgian study [9] birds showing cachexia and haemorrhagic gastroenteritis had lower a body mass than non-lesioned birds; however, although the authors classed the non-lesioned birds as 'normal', they acknowledged that their mean body mass was around 25% less than the mean of 1031 g seen in healthy guillemots shot in Scotland [27]. The non-oiled, cachectic birds in both these studies would appear similar to the unknown cause birds in the present study. The authors of both the Belgian studies suggest that the emaciated state of the non-oiled birds could have been due to a variety of factors including food deprivation, adverse weather and mild chronic exposure to oil [8, 9]; however both studies were carried out during the winter months when the body mass of guillemots should have be at their maximum [26, 27]. Another possible explanation for some of the unknown cause deaths in both the present study and those in Belgium is that they were originally oiled birds which had been treated in a rehabilitation centre but had then died post release. Various organisations regularly treat oiled seabirds in Cornwall but is well recognised that the post release survival rate in auks is poor [28].

The six shags diagnosed as storm wrecked were found in the sheltered Helford creek during the so-called 'Burns Day Storm' in January 1990. The storm affected most of north-western Europe and is one of the strongest European windstorms on record. Storm wrecked birds are typically in poor emaciated condition and have little or no fat deposits, presumably because of difficulty in feeding in turbulent, often turbid, water and also prolonged physical exertion [29]. Two of the Helford shags had bite wounds and subcutaneous haemorrhage to the upper neck and pectoral muscles. It seems likely that in their weakened state they had been killed by a predator, possibly an American mink (*Mustela vison*). Although storm wrecks have long been recognised as natural events [30], incidents such as the one in 1969 which killed around 17,000 guillemots in the Irish Sea, led to research which also implicated the possible role of pollutants, in particular polychlorinated biphenyls [31, 32]. Subsequent studies have also shown that storm-wrecked birds often have high tissue levels of heavy metals, in particular mercury, and as a result may be less able to cope with adverse weather [33]. However, despite much research, the role, if any, played by pollutants in seabird wrecks is not clear.

Exposure of birds to PIB contrasts with that due to oil in that PIB is relatively nontoxic; it is a synthetic polymer used to make many products including sealants, chewing gum, cosmetics and adhesive tape. In its raw state is hydrophobic but when mixed with sea water it forms a viscous glue-like layer that floats just beneath the surface. As with oil, birds become exposed to PIB when it is discharged from ships' tanks. The body condition of the PIB-contaminated birds in this study was good and this is consistent with the observation in a previous PIB incident, in the Netherlands in 2010 where the birds died in *"excellent physical condition (large deposits of fat, muscular breast, good organ condition, full stomachs), indicating rapid death"* [34]. The rapidity of death is almost certainly a result of the immobilising effect of a heavy coating of PIB.

Conclusion

The lesions in drowned birds in this study were mostly similar to those reported in three earlier studies [10, 34, 35] but were probably more easily recognised as the majority were examined in fresh condition whereas the birds in the previous studies were mostly frozen. One notable difference was that skeletal fractures and haemorrhages, which were common features of drowned birds in North America and New Zealand [35, 36], were rarely seen in this study. In human and veterinary mammalian pathology it is generally accepted that there are no post-mortem lesions that are pathognomonic for the diagnosis of drowning [14, 37]. However, it is perhaps pertinent to question whether this should be applied to avian pathology, especially when birds drown in seawater. In the author's experience the presence of a significant amount of clear watery fluid in the air sacs is only seen in cases of drowning. Whilst other causes of mortality such as asphyxia due smothering, polytetrafluorethylene (PTFE) toxicity, chemical irritation or acute infections such as yersiniosis may result in pulmonary lesions that can resemble, to some degree, those of drowning, none are associated with a significant amount of clear watery fluid free in the air sacs. The authors accept, however, that where carcases are autolysed or have been frozen, or both, it may be difficult or impossible to distinguish fluid arising from inhalation of water from that arising as a result of inflammatory or toxic lesions, or as artefacts caused by autolysis, freezing and thawing. Nevertheless, in freshly dead birds, the combination of watery fluid in air sacs, lungs that are extremely congested, oedematous and releasing white frothy fluid, and marked distension of the heart and major veins, should be taken as strong indication of death from drowning. If, in addition, the bird is one of a batch that died in good physical condition with freshly ingested fish in their upper alimentary tract, it is the authors' opinion that a diagnosis of drowning may be made with a degree of confidence. The pathologist might wish to try to confirm the diagnosis by demonstrating plankton, diatoms or other contaminants in the respiratory system. However, water taken from the air sacs of several confirmed drowning cases in the present study gave conflicting results. These results tend to support the widely held view among forensic pathologists that diatom testing to confirm death by drowning is unreliable [14, 15, 38, 39].

Public anger and distress following major wildlife mortality incidents, together with concern over declining fish stocks, undoubtedly act as drivers for increased protection of marine species. Following a series of bycatch incidents at St Ives, Cornwall, a byelaw was made in 1999 which allows the imposition of a temporary - but significant - ban on all fishing in the event of more than a specified number of birds being caught in nets [40]. The discharge of PIB along the coast of Cornwall and Devon in 2013 caused the death of at least 4200 birds. Previous incidents had occurred elsewhere in Europe in 1994, 1998 and 2010 but no action against the polluters was possible as it was legal at that time for ships to discharge at sea. The 2013 incident led to concerted lobbying of the UK Government by a range of conservation organisations and public groups and resulted in the International Maritime Organisation of the UN imposing an international ban in 2014 on the discharge of high viscosity PIB [41]. These two examples demonstrate what can happen when there is a very public mortality incident and where the cause is proven. By contrast, chronic low level mortality, irrespective of the cause, tends to attract little media attention and as a result no action is taken.

Seabirds face ever increasing threats from human activities and in the European Union (EU) there have been recent moves aimed at providing more protection. One of the requirements of the EU Birds Directive (2009/147/EC) is that Member States designate as Special Protection Areas (SPAs) the most suitable territories for rare or vulnerable species (as listed in Annex I of the Directive, Article 4.1) and for all regularly occurring migratory species (Article 4.2) [42]. In a second piece of legislation aimed at protecting marine wildlife, the European Commission stated its intention to impose a complete ban on the use of drift nets in EU waters in 2015 [43]. However, neither piece of legislation imposes any requirement on Member States to systematically look for and examine stranded seabirds. Fishermen are not required to report bycatch and, without data on the frequency or causes of mortality and the species involved, the regulatory authorities are unlikely to have the evidence needed to enforce controls on human activities that are harmful to birds. It is apparent that if the legislation is to be properly implemented there needs to be systematic collection and meaningful examination of stranded seabirds. By providing a clear description of the lesions that characterise death by drowning it is hoped this report will assist anyone performing post-mortem examinations, whether veterinarians, zoologists or ecologists, to determine whether or not the birds have drowned.

Additional files

Additional file 1: Gt N Diver B2337 Water in abdominal air sacs. In this movie, fluctuating pressure is being applied to the caudal abdominal wall of a GN Diver. The air sacs are distended with air and watery fluid can be seen moving within the bird's right abdominal air sac.

Additional file 2: Relationship of pectoral muscle mass to body mass in drowned birds by species. These data allow comparison of pectoral muscle mass to body mass in apparently healthy birds. **Figure S1** Correlation between body mass and pectoral mass. Description: Correlation between body mass and pectoral mass of guillemots, razorbills and shags that had drowned. (DOCX 883 kb)

Additional file 3: This file shows all the raw data used in statistical analyses in this study.

Acknowledgements
The authors wish to thank the many people who supported this study over many years, in particular Rex Harper and Leslie Sutton of the RSPCA for submitting many of the specimens and Beverly Rule, Nick Davison and Philip Booth at VLA Truro for their laboratory support. Thanks also go to David Couper of RSPCA, Mark Grantham of British Trust for Ornithology, Helene Jessop of Royal Society for the Protection of Birds, Luke Marsh at Falmouth Marine School and Jean Bradford at South Devon Seabird Trust for their advice and providing data. Jeff and Jan Loveridge, Matt Slater, Jessica Hirons, Alison Fogg, Cornwall Marine Strandings Group, and Colin Trundle, Cornwall Inland Fisheries Conservation Authority, kindly collected and submitted corpses. The authors thank Eileen Harris, Natural History Museum, London, for identifying parasites and Hazel Selley, Natural England, for fish identification. Grateful thanks also to Mark Stidworthy, International Zoo Veterinary Group, for advice on pathology, Thijs Kuiken, Erasmus University, who kindly commented on an earlier draft manuscript and Richard Cook, Natural England for advice on legislation. Jane Simpson is thanked for clerical and laboratory assistance and Zoe Greatorex for assistance with formatting the manuscript.

Funding
Contributions to the cost of post-mortem examinations were made to VRS by Natural England and by Cornwall Wildlife Trust Marine Strandings Group. The funders had no role in study design, data collection and analysis, decision to publish, or preparation of the manuscript.

Authors' contributions
VS conceived and coordinated the study, performed the post-mortem examinations and drafted the preliminary manuscript. DF performed the statistical analyses and contributed to discussions. Both authors contributed to writing the draft manuscript and read and approved the final manuscript.

Ethics approval
Not applicable. All the birds examined in this study were either found dead or were euthanased on welfare grounds. The euthanasia of a wild animal to relieve suffering is not subject to the Animals (Scientific Procedures) Act 1986 and is permitted under the Royal College of Veterinary Surgeons, Guide to Professional Conduct, section 8 Euthanasia.

Consent for publication
Not applicable.

Competing interests
The authors declare they have no competing interests.

Author details
[1]Wildlife Veterinary Investigation Centre, Chacewater, Truro, Cornwall TR4 8PB, UK. [2]Centre for Ecology and Conservation, University of Exeter, Penryn, Cornwall TR10 9FE, UK. [3]Present Address: Department for Integrative Biology, University of Guelph, Guelph, ON N1G 2W1, Canada.

References
1. Birdlife International. Seabirds and Marine - Seabird Bycatch. 2015. Available from: http://www.birdlife.org/sites/default/files/attachments/key_threats_bycatch.pdf. Accessed 6 Apr 2017.
2. Žydelis R, Bellebaum J, Österblom H, Vetemaa M, Schirmeister B, Stipniece A, et al. Bycatch in gillnet fisheries — an overlooked threat to waterbird populations. Biol Conserv. 2009;142:1269–81.

3. Wiese FK, Robertson GJ: Assessing seabird mortality from chronic oil discharges at sea. J Wildlife Manage 2004; 68(3):627-638. Available from: 10.2193/0022-541X(2004)068[0627:ASMFCO]2.0.CO;2. Accessed 6 Apr 2017.
4. MARPOL. Special areas under MARPOL. International Convention for the Prevention of Pollution from Ships. 2016. Available from: http://www.imo.org/en/OurWork/Environment/SpecialAreasUnderMARPOL/Pages/Default.aspx Accessed 6 Mar 2017.
5. Simpson VR. Post-mortem examination. In: Beynon PH, Forbes NA, Lawton MPC, editors. BSAVA Manual of Psittacine Birds. Cheltenham: British Small Animal Veterinary Association; 1996. p. 69–86.
6. R Core Team: R: A language and environment for statistical computing. R Foundation for Statistical Computing, Vienna: 2016. URL: http://www.R-project.org/. Accessed 6 Mar 2017.
7. Oka N, Okuyama M. Nutritional Status of Dead Oiled Rhinoceros Auklets (*Cerorhinca monocerata*) in the Southern Japan Sea. Mar Pollut Bull. 2000;40: 340–7. 10.1016/S0025-326X(99)00223-4.
8. Debacker V, Holsbeek L, Tapia G, Gobert S, Joiris CR, Jauniaux T, et al. Ecotoxicological and pathological studies of common guillemots *Uria aalge* beached on the Belgian coast during six successive wintering periods (1989-90 to 1994-95). Dis Aquat Org. 1997;29:159–68.
9. Jauniaux T, Brosens L, Meire P, Offringa H, Coignoul F. Pathological investigations on guillemots (*Uria aalge*) stranded on the Belgian coast during the winter of 1993-94. Vet Rec. 1998;143:387–90. 10.1136/vr.143.14.387.
10. Hocken AG. Necropsy findings in yellow-eyed penguins (*Megadyptes antipodes*) from Otago, New Zealand. New Zeal J Zool. 2005;32(1):1–8. 10.1080/03014223.2005.9518391.
11. Camphuysen CJ, Bao R, Fortin M, Roselaar CS, Heubeck M. Post-mortem examination of Great Northern Divers *Gavia immer* killed in the Prestige oil spill, Galicia, Spain, 2002/03. Seabird. 2010;23:53–65.
12. King AS, McLelland J. Respiratory system in birds, their structure and function. 2nd ed. London: Baillière Tindall; 1984. p. 110–44.
13. Worden AN: Respiratory System. In *Functional anatomy of birds*. London: Cage Birds, Dorset House, Stamford St, London; 1956:55–62.
14. Farrugia A, Ludes B: Diagnostic of Drowning in Forensic Medicine. In: Forensic Medicine - From Old Problems to New Challenges. Edited by Vieira DN. InTech; Croatia. 2011:53-55. ISBN: 978–953–307-262-3. http://www.intechopen.com/books/forensic-medicine-from-old-problems-to-newchallenges/diagnostic-of-drowning-in-forensic-medicine Accessed 6 Apr 2017.
15. Anon. Forensic medicine for medical students. 2015. Available from: http://www.forensicmed.co.uk/pathology/bodies-recovered-from-water/. Accessed 6 Apr 2017.
16. Baumel JJ. Systema Cardiovasculare, Venae. In *Handbook of Avian Anatomy*. 2nd Edition. Edited by Baumel JJ. Cambridge: Nuttall Ornithological Club; 1993:445–475.
17. Keeble E. Seabirds: gulls, auks, gannets, petrels. In: Mullineaux E, Best R, Cooper JE, editors. BSAVA manual of wildlife casualties. Quedgeley: British Small Animal Veterinary Association; 2003. Chapter 18.
18. Harthung R, Hunt GS. Toxicity of some oils to waterfowl. J Wildlife Manage. 1966;30:564–70.
19. Holmes JP. Health of free-living guillemots *Uria aalge* and razorbills *Alca torda*: the value of detailed post mortem examinations in a sample of beached seabird carcases. Project submitted in part fulfilment or the requirements for the Master of Science Degree in Wild Animal Health, University of London. 1995.
20. Simpson VR, Harris EA. *Cyathostoma lari* (Nematoda) Infection in Birds of Prey. J Zool. 1992;227:655–9.
21. Leighton FA. Clinical, Gross, and Histological Findings in Herring Gulls and Atlantic Puffins that Ingested Prudhoe Bay Crude Oil. Vet Pathol. 1986;23:254–63.
22. Peakall DB, Hallet D, Miller DS, Butler RG, Kinter WB. Effects of ingested crude oil on black guillemots: a combined field and laboratory study. Ambio. 1980;9:28–30.
23. Khan RA, Ryan P. Long term effects of crude oil on common murres (*Uria aalge*) following rehabilitation. B Environ Contam Tox. 1991;46:216.
24. Leighton FA. The toxicity of petroleum oils to birds. Environ Rev. 1993;1(2): 92–103. 10.1139/a93-008.
25. Wobeser GA. Malnutrition-starvation. In: Diseases of wild waterfowl. New York and London: Plenum Press; 1981. p. 201–3.
26. Harris MP, Wanless S, Webb A. Changes in body mass of Common Guillemots *Uria aalge* in southeast Scotland throughout the year: Implications for the release of cleaned birds. Ringing Migr. 2000;20(2):134–42. 10.1080/03078698.2000.9674235.
27. Furness RW, Thompson DR, Harrison N. Biometrics and seasonal changes in body composition of Common Guillemots *Uria aalge* from north-west Scotland. Seabird. 1994;16:22–9.
28. Wernham CV, Peach WJ, Browne S: Survival Rates of Rehabilitated Guillemots. BTO Research Report No. 186 for the Countryside Council for Wales. BTO, Thetford; 1997.
29. Underwood LSA, Stowe TJ. Massive wreck of seabirds in eastern Britain in 1983. Bird Study. 1984;31:79–88.
30. Newton A. A dictionary of birds. London: A & C Black; 1896. p. 399.
31. Natural Environment Research Council (Great Britain), and MW Holdgate. *The seabird wreck of 1969 in the Irish Sea*. Natural Environment Research Council; 1971.
32. Bourne WRP. The mass mortality of common murres in the Irish Sea in 1969. J Wildlife Manage. 1976;40:4,789–92.
33. Fort J, Lacoue-Labarthe T, Nguyen HL, Boué A. Mercury in wintering seabirds, an aggravating factor to winter wrecks? Sci Total Environ. 2015; 427-428:448–54.
34. Camphuysen CJ, Schouten S, Gronert A. Mystery spill of polyisobutylene $(C_4H_8)_n$ off the Dutch coast affecting seabirds in March 2010. Seabird. 2010;23:143–5.
35. Hamel NJ, Burger AE, Cherleton K, Davidson P, Lee I, Bertram DF, et al. Bycatch and beached birds: assessing mortality impacts in coastal net fisheries using marine bird strandings. Mar Ornithol. 2009;37:41–60.
36. Darby JT, Dawson SM. Bycatch of yellow-eyed penguins (*Megadyptes antipodes*) in gillnets in New Zealand waters 1979-1997. Biol Conserv. 2000;93:327–32.
37. Merck M. Patterns of non-accidental injury: asphyxia and drowning. In: Merck MD, editor. Veterinary forensics: animal cruelty investigations. 1st ed. Iowa: Blackwell, Ames; 2007. p. 163–8.
38. Sauko P, Knight B: Immersion deaths. In Knights forensic pathology. 3rd Edition. Edited by Sauko P, Knight B. London; Edward Arnold: 2004:395-411. https://www.google.co.uk/search?q=knight%27s+forensic+pathology+pdf&ie=utf-8&oe=utf-8&gws_rd=cr&ei=GnJzWOLIJIX4aOPSi4gD. Accessed 6 Apr 17.
39. Lunetta P, Modell JH: Macroscopical, microscopical, and laboratory findings in drowning victims- A comprehensive review. In *Forensic pathology reviews*, Volume 3. Edited by Tsokos, M. Humana Press; 2005:3–77. https://link.springer.com/book/10.1007/978-1-59259-910-3 Accessed 6 Apr 17.
40. CIFCA: Cornwall sea fisheries District St Ives Bay Gill net fishery Byelaw, 2011. Available from: https://secure.toolkitfiles.co.uk/clients/17099/sitedata/Byelaws%20and%20orders/Cornwall_SFC/St-Ives-Bay-Gill-net-fishery.pdf. Accessed 6 Apr 17.
41. RSPB: PIB and other Hazardous and Noxious Substances (HNS) A serious hazard to the marine environment. RSPB briefing; 2014. Available from: https://www.rspb.org.uk/Images/PIB_and_seabirds_RSPB_Briefing_tcm9-344511.pdf. Accessed 6 Apr 17.
42. JNCC.:Directive 2009/147/EC on the conservation of wild birds (codified version). Available from: http://jncc.defra.gov.uk/page-1373. Accessed 6 Apr 17.
43. Anon: Fisheries: European Commission proposes full ban on driftnets. European Commission press release; 2014. Available from: http://europa.eu/rapid/press-release_IP-14-563_en.htm. Accessed 6 Apr 17.

8

Molecular characterization of hemotropic mycoplasmas (*Mycoplasma ovis* and '*Candidatus* Mycoplasma haemovis') in sheep and goats in China

Xiaoxing Wang, Yanyan Cui, Yan Zhang, Ke Shi, Yaqun Yan, Fuchun Jian, Longxian Zhang, Rongjun Wang and Changshen Ning*

Abstract

Background: Hemotropic mycoplasmas (hemoplasmas) are emerging zoonotic pathogens with a worldwide distribution that can cause mild to severe hemolytic anemia, icterus, ill-thrift, infertility, and poor weight gain. However, understanding of the molecular epidemiology of hemoplasmas (*Mycoplasma ovis* and '*Candidatus* Mycoplasma haemovis') is limited in sheep and goats, and the hemoplasma strain/species/variant '*Candidatus* M. haemovis' was poorly studied throughout the world and had never been detected in China until now. Thus, the aim of the present study was to determine the molecular prevalence of hemoplasmas, including *M. ovis* and '*Candidatus* M. haemovis' in sheep and goats from seven provinces and one autonomous region of China.

Methods: A total of 1364 blood samples were collected from sheep and goats in seven provinces and one autonomous region of China. All blood samples were tested for hemoplasmas (*M. ovis* and '*Candidatus* M. haemovis') by nested PCR amplification based on 16S rRNA gene. Positive specimens underwent nucleotide sequencing and phylogenetic analysis.

Results: Overall, 610 specimens (44.7%, 610/1364) were shown to be hemoplasmas (*M. ovis* and '*Candidatus* M. haemovis') -positive by nested PCR amplification based on 16S rRNA gene. The prevalence in goats was 44.1% (379/860), and 45.8% (231/504) in sheep, while that in grazing small ruminants was 54.4% (396/728) and 33.6% (214/636) in house feeding small ruminants. Sequencing of the nearly complete 16S rRNA gene was successful for the 103 randomly selected positive specimens from different farms in different sampling sites of China. Among them, analysis of the 16S rRNA gene sequences identified *M. ovis* (n = 56) and '*Candidatus* M. haemovis' (n = 47). Two (KU983740 and KU983746) of the four novel genotypes obtained in this study were closely related to *M. ovis*, while the other two genotypes (KU983748 and KU983749) had high identity with '*Candidatus* M. haemovis'. Remarkably, the genotype (KU983740) of *M. ovis* in sheep and goats in this study fell in a clade with two human hemoplasmas from USA (KF313922 and GU230144) and shared 99.8%–99.9% with them.

Conclusions: In this study, '*Candidatus* M. haemovis' was first detected in Chinese sheep and goats and hemoplasmas (*M. ovis* and '*Candidatus* M. haemovis') are highly prevalent, and widely distributed in China.

Keywords: Hemoplasmas, *Mycoplasma ovis*, '*Candidatus* Mycoplasma haemovis', Small ruminants, 16S rRNA gene

* Correspondence: nnl1986@163.com
College of Animal Science and Veterinary Medicine, Henan Agricultural University, Zhengzhou 450002, People's Republic of China

Background

Hemotropic mycoplasmas (hemoplasmas, formerly classified as *Haemobartonella* and *Eperythrozoon* spp.) are uncultivated, small, pleomorphic, wall-less bacteria that parasitize on the surface of animal erythrocytes [1–3]. Hemoplasmas have now been reclassified into the *Mycoplasma* genus based on 16S rRNA gene sequence. These pathogens can cause mild to severe hemolytic anemia, icterus, ill-thrift, infertility, and poor weight gain, but death is rare in infected adults [1, 4–6]. Worldwide, hemoplasmas have been reported to affect livestock [2, 7–10], companion animals [11–17], wildlife [5, 18, 19], and humans [20–23].

Mycoplasma ovis (formerly *Eperythrozoon ovis*), which could elicit major health problems and high mortality in lambs, has been identified in sheep and goats [8, 24–26]. In 2009, a novel hemoplasma, a 17 bp long deletion and an overall the 16S RNA gene sequence identity of only 97% compared to *M. ovis*, has been detected in Hungary. Subsequent studies identified this new hemoplasma as '*Candidatus* M. haemovis' [24]. Subsequently, complete genome sequencing conducted by Deshuillers et al. revealed that *M. ovis* strain Michigan contains two copies of 16S rRNA gene, one corresponding to *M. ovis*, and the other to '*Candidatus* M. haemovis' [27]. Therefore, Deshuillers et al. and other researchers can speculate that *M. ovis* and '*Candidatus* M. haemovis' may exist as a single species with two copies of 16S rRNA gene or as two different species [27].

With an increasing number of hemoplasmosis clinical cases, many countries have suffered extensive losses of livestock. However, few epidemiological surveys on hemoplasmosis in sheep and goats have been conducted during the last decade. The prevalence of *M. ovis* was 6.3% (36/573) in small ruminants in North Africa [28], 20% (4/20) in goats in Switzerland [25], 87% (27/31) in captive cervids in Brazil [26] and 26.3% (5/19) in free-living Japanese serows [18]. Surprisingly, a 49-year-old veterinarian from Texas of USA was found to be co-infected by two *M. ovis* variants, *M. ovis* and '*Candidatus* M. haemovis'. In China, *M. ovis* was found in 41.0% (151/371) and 16.1% (192/1191) in small ruminants from Hubei province and Chongqing city, respectively [29, 30]. However, understanding of the molecular epidemiology of hemoplasmas (*M. ovis* and '*Candidatus* M. haemovis') is limited in sheep and goats. And '*Candidatus* M. haemovis' was poorly studied throughout the world and had never been detected in China until now. Thus, the aim of the present study was to determine the molecular prevalence of hemoplasmas, including *M. ovis* and '*Candidatus* M. haemovis' in sheep and goats from seven provinces and one autonomous region of China.

Methods

Specimen collection

A total of 1364 EDTA-anticoagulated blood samples were collected from jugular vein of sheep and goats in Henan, Guizhou, Shanxi, Shaanxi, Yunnan, Qinghai, Heilongjiang provinces and the Inner Mongolia autonomous region from March 2012 to May 2015 (Fig. 1 and Additional file 1: Figure S1).

For each animal, one blood sample was collected into an EDTA tube marked with breed, gender, age, and

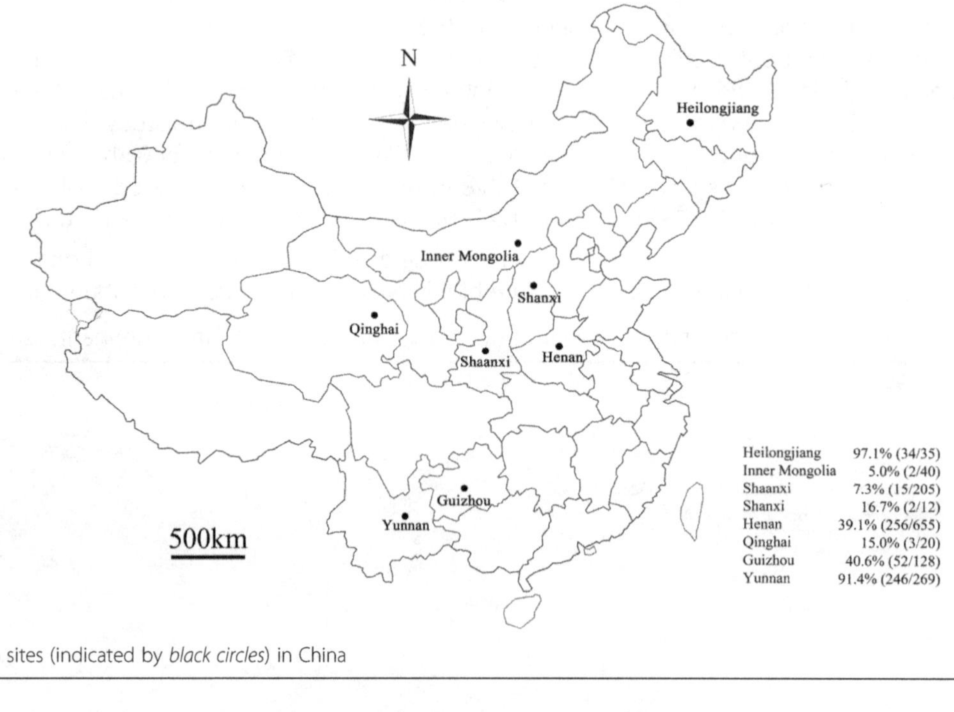

Fig. 1 Collection sites (indicated by *black circles*) in China

feeding habit of the animal. The animals have no obvious clinical symptoms during blood sampling. The specimens were then transported in an ice box to the laboratory for further processing and analysis.

DNA extraction

For each specimen, DNA was extracted from 500 μl of anticoagulated whole blood using a Genome DNA Extraction Kit (LifeFeng, Shanghai, China) according to the manufacturer's instructions. DNA was eluted from the column with 200 μl Tris-EDTA buffer. After DNA extraction, DNA concentration and quality was measured using absorbance ratio between 260/280 nm (Nanodrop, Thermo Scientific, USA). And all the specimens were subjected to a GAPDH gene conventional PCR assay as described previously to confirm the presence of amplifiable DNA and exclude PCR inhibition [31]. DNA was stored at −20 °C until PCR amplification.

Nested PCR

All samples were tested at least three times for hemoplasmas (*M. ovis* and '*Candidatus* M. haemovis') DNA using a nested PCR assay that amplified an approximately 500 bp fragment of the 16S rRNA gene [32]. The base sequences of four primers (A1/A2 and B1/B2) are shown in Table 1 and the binding sites of four primers are shown in Additional file 1: Figure S2. First-round PCR was performed in a total volume of 25 μl, containing 2.5 μl of 10 × LA PCR Buffer II (Mg^{2+} plus), 4.0 μl of dNTP mixture (2.5 mM each dNTP), 0.5 μl of each A1 and A2 primer (25 μM), 1.25 U of LA *Taq* polymerase (TaKaRa, Dalian, China), 16.25 μl of double distilled water, and 1.0 μl of DNA template. Cycling conditions were: 94 °C for 5 min, followed by 30 cycles of 94 °C for 30 s, 61 °C for 30 s, and 72 °C for 1 min, with a final extension at 72 °C for 7 min. Second-round nested PCR contained 2.5 μl of 10 × PCR Buffer, 2.0 μl of dNTP mixture (2.5 mM each dNTP), 0.5 μl of each B1 and B2 primer (25 μM), 0.75 U of r *Taq* polymerase (TaKaRa), 18.35 μl of double distilled water, and 1.0 μl of the first-round PCR product (diluted 10-fold). Cycling conditions were: 94 °C for 5 min, followed by 35 cycles of 94 °C for 30 s, 59 °C for 30 s, and 72 °C for 45 s, with a final extension at 72 °C for 7 min. A positive control for *M. ovis* from a naturally infected Boer goat preserved by our laboratory was used in all reactions, while double distilled water was used as a negative control. Secondary PCR products were examined by 1% agarose gel electrophoresis and visualized after GelRed (Biotium Inc., Hayward, CA) staining.

PCR for 16S rRNA gene and sequencing

One hundred three positive specimens representative of different hosts, farms/flocks and geographic locations were selected and the nearly complete 16S rRNA gene sequences were amplified using the protocol described by Grazziotin et al. [26]. Primers are shown in Table 1. The 25 μl PCR mixture is the same as first-round PCR mixture of the nested PCR. PCR products were purified using Montage PCR filters (Millipore, Bedford, MA) and sequenced using a BigDye Terminator v3.1 cycle sequencing kit (Applied Biosystems, Foster City, CA) on an ABI 3730 DNA analyzer (Applied Biosystems). The nucleotide sequences were confirmed by bidirectional sequencing and by sequencing a new PCR product if necessary.

Phylogenetic analysis

Nucleotide sequences of the nearly complete 16S rRNA gene together with reference sequences downloaded from GenBank were aligned using ClustalX 2.0 (http://www.clustal.org/) with further adjustments made manually as necessary. And then Mega 5.05 (http://www.megasoftware.net/) software was applied to conduct phylogenetic and molecular evolutionary analysis. A bootstrap phylogenetic tree demonstrating the relationship of *M. ovis* and '*Candidatus* M. haemovis' genotypes to other hemoplasma species was created by the neighbor-joining method using a distance matrix corrected for nucleotide substitutions based on the Kimura 2-parameter model. A bootstrap analysis was used to assess the robustness of the clusters using 1000 replicates.

Statistical analysis

Positive rates were compared using the chi-square test. Differences were considered statistically significant at $P < 0.05$. Analyses were performed using QuickCalcs

Table 1 Primers used for amplification of the 16S rRNA gene of hemoplasmas (*Mycoplasma ovis* and '*Candidatus* Mycoplasma haemovis')

Primers	Nucleotide sequences	Target fragment/bp	Remarks
A1	5′-GGATAGCAGCCCGAAAGG-3′	1060	1st PCR
A2	5′-GCAGCCCAAGGCATAAGG-3′		
B1	5′-CTACGGGAAGCAGCAGTG-3′	506 or 489	Nested PCR [32]
B2	5′-CTCGACCTAACATCAAATACCT-3′		
16S Fw	5′-ATGCAAGTCGAACGAGTAGA-3′	1341	Conventional PCR [26]
16S Rv	5′-TGATACTTTCTTTCATAGTTTG-3′		

software (GraphPad Software Inc., La Jolla, CA). The odds ratios (ORs) of the univariate analysis were calculated using measures of association along with 95% confidence intervals (CIs).

Nucleotide sequence accession numbers

The four novel sequences determined in this study were deposited in GenBank under accession numbers: KU983740, KU983746, KU983748 and KU983749.

Results

Molecular prevalence of hemoplasmas (*M. ovis* and '*Candidatus* M. haemovis') in sheep and goats

As shown in Fig. 1, of the 1364 blood specimens from sheep and goats, 610 (44.7%) were found to be positive for hemoplasmas (*M. ovis* and '*Candidatus* M. haemovis') by PCR amplification of the 16S rRNA gene. And the positive samples distributed in 49 studied farms from seven provinces and one Aut. Reg.. In the 35 sheep and goats from Heilongjiang province, 34 (97.1%) were identified as hemoplasmas (*M. ovis* and '*Candidatus* M. haemovis') -positive, while just two (5.0%) of the 40 animals in the Inner Mongolia Aut. Reg. was positive. On the other hand, the animals in three farms, including one in Henan province and two from Yunnan province were 100% positive for hemoplasmas (*M. ovis* and '*Candidatus* M. haemovis') (Additional file 1: Table S1).

The infection rates of hemoplasmas (*M. ovis* and '*Candidatus* M. haemovis') in sheep and goats in Heilongjiang (34/35, 97.1%) and Yunnan (246/269, 91.4%) were significantly higher than that of other provinces/ Aut. Reg.. A higher prevalence was observed in grazing sheep and goats (54.4%) than household sheep and goats (33.6%). Male animals had significantly higher hemoplasmas (*M. ovis* and '*Candidatus* M. haemovis') infection rates, at 60.0%, than females (41.6%). There were no significant differences between prevalence in different age groups of sheep and goats as well as that between sheep (45.8%) and goats (44.1%) (Table 2). The potential risk factors associated to percentage of infection with hemoplasmas were determined by statistical calculations. Among animal age, gender, species and feeding habits, gender (OR = 2.10, CI = 1.58–2.81) and the use of grazing (OR = 2.35, CI = 1.89–2.93) were identified as potential risk factors for hemoplasmas infection ($P < 0.001$) (Table 2).

Sequence analysis of 16S rRNA gene

Sequencing of the nearly complete 16S rRNA gene was successful for the 103 randomly selected positive specimens. Among them, analysis of the 16S rRNA gene sequences identified *M. ovis* (n = 56) and '*Candidatus* M. haemovis' (n = 47). The origin of the 103 positive specimens was shown in Additional file 1: Table S2. After alignment, the obtained 103 16S rRNA gene sequences formed four sequence clusters KU983740, KU983746, KU983748 and KU983749.

KU983740 (n = 50) and KU983746 (n = 6) genotypes had 99.7% and 99.6% identity, respectively, to *M. ovis* from sheep in the USA (AF338268), and 99.9% and 99.8% identity, respectively, to a human *M. ovis* isolate form USA (KF313922). Both genotypes shared a high degree of identity (99.8%) with another human *M. ovis* isolate (GU230144), while, lower identity of them with sheep '*Candidatus* M. haemovis' genotypes from Japan (AB617737) (97.3% and 97.4%, respectively) were identified. However, the other two genotypes KU983748 (n = 21) and KU983749 (n = 26) were closely related to '*Candidatus* M. haemovis' (AB617737), with 99.5% and 99.4% identities, respectively, yet, their identities with *M. ovis* (AF338268) were 97.4% and 97.5%, respectively. Based on the 16S rRNA gene sequence analysis, the four

Table 2 Factors associated with positive hemoplasmas (*Mycoplasma ovis and 'Candidatus* Mycoplasma haemovis') infection in sheep and goats in China

Factor	No. positive/No. examined	Infection rate (%)	OR (95% CI)	χ^2	*p*
Age group					
< 1 year	205/450	45.6	1.05 (0.84–1.32)	0.19	0.664
≥ 1 year	405/914	44.3			
Gender					
Male	138/230	60.0	2.10 (1.58–2.81)	26.12	<0.001
Female	472/1134	41.6			
Species					
Sheep	231/504	45.8	1.07 (0.86–1.34)	0.40	0.527
Goat	379/860	44.1			
Feeding habits					
Grazing	396/728	54.4	2.35 (1.89–2.93)	59.11	<0.001
Household	214/636	33.6			

novel genotypes in this study differed from *M. ovis* (AF338268) at several nucleotide positions along the full-length of the gene (Table 3).

Phylogenetic analysis

Phylogenetic analysis revealed that the four novel genotypes accompanied by five other '*Candidatus* M. haemovis' (AB617737, AB617736, EU828580, EU828581 and JF931131), six other *M. ovis* (GU230144, JF931135, FJ440328, KF313922, AF338268 and EU828582) as well as one *Mycoplasma* spp. (FJ824847) formed a separate clade. In addition, '*Candidatus* M. haemovis' and *M. ovis* genotypes fell into two different groups. The two genotypes KU983740 and KU983746, representing 56 *M. ovis* sequences from the present study, were grouped in the same clade with two human genotypes from USA (GU230144 and KF313922) (Fig. 2).

Discussion

Globally, hemotropic *Mycoplasma* spp. are emerging or re-emerging zoonotic pathogens that affect numerous animal species including humans, potentially causing loss of livestock and public health concern. *M. ovis* is prevalent worldwide, and is causative of hemolytic anemia in sheep and goats [4].

In the present study, the prevalence of hemoplasmas (*M. ovis* and '*Candidatus* M. haemovis') in sheep and goats was found to be 44.7% (610/1364). A similar prevalence of *M. ovis* was previously reported in goats in Hubei, China (41.0%, 151/371) [29], while a lower rate was detected in sheep in Tunisia (6.3%, 36/573) [28]. A higher *M. ovis* prevalence was previously found in sheep in Malaysia (94.0%, 47/50) [33], Argentina (81.8%, 9/11) [9], and Hungary (51.5%, 17/33) [24]. The differences in prevalence between this study and others [9, 24, 28, 29, 33] may be caused by discrepancy in the age groups studied, as well as the number of animals, detection methods, and geographic and ecological environments. In this study, there is a striking difference in prevalence between the north-central sampling sites (Qinghai, 15.0%; Shanxi, 16.7%; Shaanxi, 7.3% and Inner Mongolia, 5.0%) versus the southern and eastern sites (Guizhou, 40.6%; Yunnan, 91.4%; Heilongjiang, 97.1% and Henan, 39.1%). The climate type of north-central sampling sites is monsoon climate of medium latitudes, whereas southern sites are subtropical monsoon climate. Invertebrate vector abundance and vegetation species in north-central sampling sites is relatively lower than southern sites. Therefore, we speculated the different climates, vegetation species and invertebrate vector abundance factors that may contribute to the apparent difference in prevalence in different provinces.

It was reported that the *M. ovis* prevalence was significantly higher in young sheep than adults ($P < 0.001$) by Rjeibi et al. [28]. However, in the present study, there was no significant difference in hemoplasmas (*M. ovis* and '*Candidatus* M. haemovis') infection rates between different age groups of sheep and goats. Nevertheless, significant differences were detected among the prevalence of hemoplasmas (*M. ovis* and '*Candidatus* M. haemovis') according to animal gender and feeding habits of the host animals, although no differences were observed between samples obtained from different genders by Song et al. [29]. In this study, potential risk factors were identified as animal gender and feeding habits of the host animals, providing useful information for control of the hemoplasmosis. Grazing flocks are more likely to be exposed to blood-sucking arthropods than household flocks. Household flocks received good feeding and management, which were thought to be important for the prevention from various diseases. Therefore, infections of hemoplasmas may be transmitted by blood-sucking arthropods and reusing needles during herd immunization in China.

'*Candidatus* M. haemovis' was first demonstrated in a sheep flock with fatal hemolytic anemia in Hungary [24], following studies reported the presence of both *M. ovis* and '*Candidatus* M. haemovis' DNAs in sheep in Hungary [24], Japan [8], and the USA [27], in goats in Switzerland [25], and in *Capricornis crispus* in Japan [18]. However, there was no report documented the existence of *M. ovis*

Table 3 16S rRNA gene alignment from two *M. ovis* genotypes (KU983740 and KU983746) and two '*Candidatus* M. haemovis' genotypes (KU983748 and KU983749) and their comparison with two hemotropic mycoplasma sequences

Position[a]	101	118	120	125	188	201	266	272	319	340	439–455	464	466	475	507	510	570	635	648	763	1183	1274
M. ovis (AF338268)	G	T	G	G	G	G	T	G	C	G	AA...TG	T	G	A	C	C	G	C	G	C	C	C
KU983740($n = 50$)	A	C	*	T	*	*	*	*	*	*	**...**	*	*	*	*	*	*	*	*	*	T	*
KU983746($n = 6$)	A	C	*	T	*	*	*	*	*	*	**...**	*	*	*	*	*	T	*	*	*	T	*
Candidatus M. haemovis (AB617737)	A	C	T	T	T	A	C	A	T	A	–...–	C	T	C	T	T	T	T	A	T	T	T
KU983748($n = 21$)	A	C	*	T	T	*	*	A	T	A	–...–	*	*	*	T	T	T	T	A	T	T	T
KU983749($n = 26$)	A	C	*	T	T	*	*	A	T	A	–...–	*	*	*	T	T	*	T	A	T	T	T

[a]position numbers given with respect to *M. ovis* (GenBank accession number: AF338268)
*identical to the reference sequence; –, base deletion

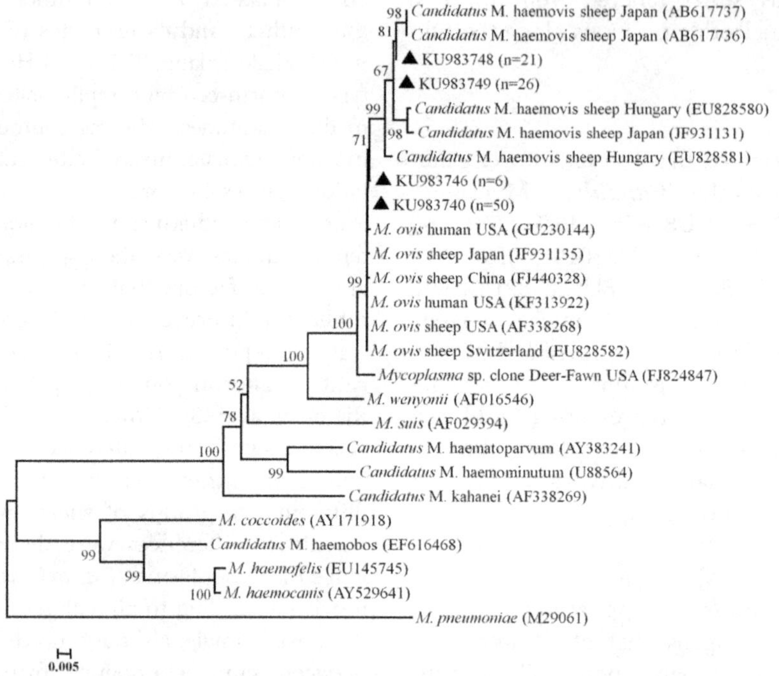

Fig. 2 Phylogenetic relationships of *Mycoplasma ovis* and '*Candidatus* M. haemovis' genotypes identified here and other hemotropic mycoplasmas. Phylogeny was inferred with a neighbor-joining analysis of the nearly complete 16S rRNA gene sequences based on distances calculated with the Kimura 2-parameter model. *Mycoplasma pneumoniae* was used as an outgroup. Bootstrap values >50% from 1000 replicates are shown on the nodes. The genotypes detected in this study are shown as *triangles*

and '*Candidatus* M. haemovis' in sheep and goats in China. Therefore, detection of hemoplasmas (*M. ovis* and '*Candidatus* M. haemovis') by nested PCR and sequence analyses in the present study represents the first molecular evidence of the occurrence of '*Candidatus* M. haemovis' in sheep and goats in China.

Phylogenetic analysis revealed that '*Candidatus* M. haemovis' and *M. ovis* belong to the same clade. 16S rRNA gene homology between *M. ovis* and '*Candidatus* M. haemovis' in this study was very high, at 97.3–97.5% (data not shown), revealing the close genetic relationship between them, which suggested that '*Candidatus* M. haemovis' might not be a new hemoplasma species, but another copy of *M. ovis* 16S rRNA gene, which was validated by Deshuillers et al.'s report that *M. ovis* strain Michigan has two different copies of the 16S rRNA gene. The detection of multiple different 16S rRNA gene sequences in a veterinarian in Texas [22], in a severe anemia sheep in Japan [8], in goats in Switzerland [25] and in sheep in Hungary [24], might also be explained by the existence of multiple copies of the 16S rRNA gene within a single strain of *M. ovis*, each having a variable genetic composition, as reported for other bacteria [34].

In previous studies, only five hemotropic *Mycoplasma* spp., *M. haemofelis*-like [21], *M. suis*-like [35], *M. ovis* [22], '*Candidatus* Mycoplasma haemohominis' [36], and '*Candidatus* Mycoplasma haematoparvum' [37] organisms, were described to be infected by human beings. Sykes et al. reported the first case of human infection with hemotropic mycoplasma (*M. ovis* and '*Candidatus* M. haemovis') in a veterinarian in Texas. Additionally, among the 11 hemotropic *Mycoplasma* spp. identified from 489 patients, *M. ovis*-like organism was the most prevalent [23], a species which was mainly found in small ruminants, such as deer [26, 38, 39], goats [4, 25, 33], sheep [4, 8, 24, 28, 40], and Japanese serows [18]. It is noteworthy that the nucleotide sequences of *M. ovis* (KU983740 and KU983746) in the present study had highest homology with *M. ovis* (GU230144 and KF313922) from humans (99.8% and 99.8–99.9%). The high homology of the *M. ovis* genotypes obtained in the present study with human genotypes observed here may provide additional evidence for the zoonotic potential of *M. ovis*, which were raised by Sykes et al. and then verified by Maggi et al.

Conclusions

This study provides further evidence about the prevalence of hemoplasmas (*M. ovis* and '*Candidatus* M. haemovis'), and presents the first detection of '*Candidatus* M. haemovis' in sheep and goats in China. Our data showed a high prevalence and widespread distribution of hemoplasmas (*M. ovis* and '*Candidatus* M. haemovis') in sheep and goats. Further studies are needed to evaluate the pathogenicity of '*Candidatus* M. haemovis' in sheep and goats, as well as the zoonotic potential of *M. ovis*.

Abbreviations

'*Candidatus* M. haemovis': '*Candidatus* Mycoplasma haemovis'; 16S rRNA: 16S ribosomal RNA; Aut. Reg.: Autonomous region; *B. henselae*: *Bartonella henselae*; DNA: Deoxyribonucleic acid; EDTA: Ethylenediaminetetraacetic acid; HIV: Human immunodeficiency virus; *M. haemofelis*: *Mycoplasma haemofelis*; *M. ovis*: *Mycoplasma ovis*; *M. suis*: *Mycoplasma suis*; PCR: Polymerase chain reaction

Acknowledgements

Veterinary officers and farmers are appreciated for helping with sample collection in China. We are grateful to Dr. Junqiang Li and Fuchang Yu for their constructive comments during initiation of the study.

Funding

This work was supported by the Earmarked Fund for China Modern Agro-Industry Technology Research System (nycytx-39) and the Collaborative Innovation Center of Modern Animal Husbandry, Henan Province, China.

Authors' contributions

CSN conceived and designed the experiments; XXW, YYC, YZ and KS performed the experiments; XXW, YZ, KS and YQY analyzed the data; XXW, FCJ, LXZ, RJW, and CSN wrote the manuscript. All the authors have read and approved the final version of the manuscript.

Competing interests

The authors declare that they have no competing interests.

Consent for publication

Not applicable.

References

1. Messick JB. Hemotrophic mycoplasmas (hemoplasmas): a review and new insights into pathogenic potential. Vet Clin Pathol. 2004;33:2–13.
2. Hoelzle L. Haemotrophic mycoplasmas: recent advances in *Mycoplasma suis*. Vet Microbiol. 2008;130:215–26.
3. Biondo AW, Dos Santos AP, Guimarães AM, Vieira RF, Vidotto O, Macieira Dde B, et al. A review of the occurrence of hemoplasmas (hemotrophic mycoplasmas) in Brazil. Rev Bras Parasitol Vet. 2009;18:1–7.
4. Neimark H, Hoff B, Ganter M. *Mycoplasma ovis* comb. nov. (formerly *Eperythrozoon ovis*), an epierythrocytic agent of haemolytic anaemia in sheep and goats. Int J Syst Evol Microbiol. 2004;54:365–71.
5. Mascarelli PE, Keel MK, Yabsley M, Last LA, Breitschwerdt EB, Maggi RG. Hemotropic mycoplasmas in little brown bats (*Myotis lucifugus*). Parasit Vectors. 2014;7:117.
6. Willi B, Meli ML, Luthy R, Honegger H, Wengi N, Hoelzle LE, et al. Development and application of a universal Hemoplasma screening assay based on the SYBR green PCR principle. J Clin Microbiol. 2009;47:4049–54.
7. Dieckmann SM, Winkler M, Groebel K, Dieckmann MP, Hofmann-Lehmann R, Hoelzle K, et al. Haemotrophic Mycoplasma infection in horses. Vet Microbiol. 2010;145:351–3.
8. Tagawa M, Takeuchi T, Fujisawa T, Konno Y, Yamamoto S, Matsumoto K, et al. A clinical case of severe anemia in a sheep coinfected with *Mycoplasma ovis* and *Candidatus* Mycoplasma haemovis' in Hokkaido, Japan. J Vet Med Sci. 2012;74:99–102.
9. Aguirre D, Thompson C, Neumann R, Salatin A, Gaido A, de Echaide S. Clinical mycoplasmosis outbreak due to *Mycoplasma ovis* in sheep from Shalta, Argentina. Clinical, microbiological and molecular diagnosis. Rev Argent Microbiol. 2008;41:212–4.
10. Fujihara Y, Sasaoka F, Suzuki J, Watanabe Y, Fujihara M, Ooshita K, et al. Prevalence of hemoplasma infection among cattle in the western part of Japan. J Vet Med Sci. 2011;73:1653–5.
11. Torkan S, Aldavood SJ, Rafie SM, Hejazi H, Shirani D, Momtaz H. Prevalence and risk factor analysis of *Haemobartonella felis* in cats using direct blood smear and PCR assay. Comp Clin Pathol. 2013;22:1103–9.
12. Sykes JE. Feline hemotropic mycoplasmas. Vet Clin North Am Small Anim Pract. 2010;20:62–9.
13. Compton S, Maggi RG, Breitschwerdt EB. *Candidatus* Mycoplasma haematoparvum and *Mycoplasma haemocanis* infections in dogs from the United States. Comp Immunol Microbiol Infect Dis. 2012;35:557–62.
14. Willi B, Novacco M, Meli M, Wolf-Jäckel G, Boretti F, Wengi N, et al. Haemotropic mycoplasmas of cats and dogs: transmission, diagnosis, prevalence and importance in Europe. Schweiz Arch Tierheilkd. 2010;152:237.
15. Roura X, Peters IR, Altet L, Tabar M-D, Barker EN, Planellas M, et al. Prevalence of hemotropic mycoplasmas in healthy and unhealthy cats and dogs in Spain. J Vet Diagn Investig. 2010;22:270–4.
16. Sykes JE, Ball LM, Bailiff NL, Fry MM. 'Candidatus Mycoplasma haematoparvum', a novel small haemotropic mycoplasma from a dog. Int J Syst Evol Microbiol. 2005;55:27–30.
17. Hornok S, Meli M, Gönczi E, Ignits É, Willi B, Lutz H, et al. First molecular identification of '*Candidatus* mycoplasma haemominutum' from a cat with fatal haemolytic anaemia in Hungary. Acta Vet Hung. 2008;56:441–50.
18. Ohtake Y, Nishizawa I, Sato M, Watanabe Y, Nishimura T, Matsubara K, et al. *Mycoplasma ovis* detected in free-living Japanese serows, *Capricornis crispus*. J Vet Med Sci. 2011;73:371–3.
19. Maggi RG, Mascarelli PE, Balakrishnan N, Rohde CM, Kelly CM, Ramaiah L, et al. "*Candidatus* Mycoplasma haemomacaque" and *Bartonella quintana* Bacteremia in Cynomolgus Monkeys. J Clin Microbiol. 2013;51:1408–11.
20. Hu Z, Yin J, Shen K, Kang W, Chen Q. Outbreaks of hemotrophic mycoplasma infections in China. Emerg Infect Dis. 2009;15:1139.
21. dos Santos AP, dos Santos RP, Biondo AW, Dora JM, Goldani LZ, de Oliveira ST, et al. Hemoplasma infection in HIV-positive patient, Brazil. Emerg Infect Dis. 2008;14:1922–4.
22. Sykes JE, Lindsay LL, Maggi RG, Breitschwerdt EB. Human coinfection with *Bartonella henselae* and two hemotropic mycoplasma variants resembling *Mycoplasma ovis*. J Clin Microbiol. 2010;48:3782–5.
23. Maggi RG, Compton SM, Trull CL, Mascarelli PE, Mozayeni BR, Breitschwerdt EB. Infection with hemotropic Mycoplasma species in patients with or without extensive arthropod or animal contact. J Clin Microbiol. 2013;51:3237–41.
24. Hornok S, Meli ML, Erdos A, Hajtos I, Lutz H, Hofmann-Lehmann R. Molecular characterization of two different strains of haemotropic mycoplasmas from a sheep flock with fatal haemolytic anaemia and concomitant *Anaplasma ovis* infection. Vet Microbiol. 2009;136:372–7.
25. Hornok S, Hajtos I, Meli ML, Farkas I, Gonczi E, Meili T, et al. First molecular identification of *Mycoplasma ovis* and '*Candidatus* M. haemoovis' from goat, with lack of haemoplasma PCR-positivity in lice. Acta Vet Hung. 2012;60:355–60.
26. Grazziotin AL, Santos AP, Guimaraes AMS, Mohamed A, Cubas ZS, De Oliveira MJ, et al. *Mycoplasma ovis* in captive cervids: prevalence, molecular characterization and phylogeny. Vet Microbiol. 2011;152:415–9.
27. Deshuillers PL, Santos AP, do Nascimento NC, Hampel JA, Bergin IL, Dyson MC, et al. Complete genome sequence of *Mycoplasma ovis* strain Michigan, a hemoplasma of sheep with two distinct 16S rRNA genes. Genome Announc. 2014;2:e01235–13.
28. Rjeibi MR, Darghouth MA, Omri H, Souidi K, Rekik M, Gharbi M. First molecular isolation of *Mycoplasma ovis* from small ruminants in North Africa. Onderstepoort J Vet Res. 2015;82:912.
29. Song W, Song Q, He L, Zhou Y, Zhao J. The establishment and application of a semi-nested PCR assay for the detection of *Mycoplasma ovis*. Small Rumin Res. 2014;119:176–81.
30. ZuoYong Z, Kui N, Shi Jun H, Hong Lin L, Ming T, You Lan H, et al. Infection rate and risk factors analysis of Haemotrophic Mycoplasma (formerly *Eperythrozoon ovis*) in Chongqing area. Chinese Journal of Preventive Veterinary Medicine. 2010;32:563–6.
31. Frota IM, Leitão CC, Costa JJ, Brito IR, Van dHR SJR. Stability of housekeeping genes and expression of locally produced growth factors and hormone receptors in goat preantral follicles. Zygote. 2011;19:71–83.
32. Xiaoxing WANG, Yanyan CUI, Fuchun JIAN, Zhongyi ZHANG, Jianfeng NING, Longxian ZHANG, et al. Establishment and application of a nested-PCR method assay for detection of *Mycoplasma ovis*. J Henan Agricultural University. 2016;50:506–11.
33. Jesse FFA, Jazid NHBA, d Mohamme K, Tijjani A, ELT C, Abba Y, et al. Hemotropic Mycoplasma ovis infection in goats with concurrent gastrointestinal parasitism in Malaysia. J Adv Vet Anim Res. 2015;2:464–8.

34. Michon A-L, Aujoulat F, Roudiere L, Soulier O, Zorgniotti I, Jumas-Bilak E, et al. Intragenomic and intraspecific heterogeneity in *rrs* may surpass interspecific variability in a natural population of *Veillonella*. Microbiology. 2010;156:2080–91.
35. Yuan CL, Liang AB, Yao CB, Yang ZB, Zhu JG, Cui L, et al. Prevalence of *Mycoplasma suis* (*Eperythrozoon suis*) infection in swine and swine-farm workers in Shanghai, China. Am J Vet Res. 2009;70:890–4.
36. Steer JA, Tasker S, Barker EN, Jensen J, Mitchell J, Stocki T, et al. A novel hemotropic Mycoplasma (hemoplasma) in a patient with hemolytic anemia and pyrexia. Clin Infect Dis. 2011;53:e147–e51.
37. Maggi RG, Mascarelli PE, Havenga LN, Naidoo V, Breitschwerdt EB. Co-infection with *Anaplasma platys*, *Bartonella henselae* and *Candidatus* Mycoplasma haematoparvum in a veterinarian. Parasit Vectors. 2013;6:103.
38. Maggi RG, Chitwood MC, Kennedy-Stoskopf S, DePerno CS. Novel hemotropic Mycoplasma species in white-tailed deer (*Odocoileus virginianus*). Comp Immunol Microbiol Infect Dis. 2013;36:607–11.
39. Boes KM, Goncarovs KO, Thompson CA, Halik LA, Santos AP, Guimaraes A, et al. Identification of a *Mycoplasma ovis*-like organism in a herd of farmed white-tailed deer (*Odocoileus virginianus*) in rural Indiana. Vet Clin Pathol. 2012;41:77–83.
40. Suzuki J, Sasaoka F, Fujihara M, Watanabe Y, Tasaki T, Oda S, et al. Molecular identification of '*Candidatus* Mycoplasma haemovis' in sheep with hemolytic anemia. J Vet Med Sci. 2011;73:1113–5.

9

The nutritional status affects the complete blood count of goats experimentally infected with *Haemonchus contortus*

S. Cériac[1], C. Jayles[2], R. Arquet[2], D. Feuillet[1], Y. Félicité[1], H. Archimède[1] and J.-C. Bambou[1*]

Abstract

Background: Gastrointestinal nematode (GIN) remains the most important pathogenic constraint of small ruminant production worldwide. The improvement of the host immune response against GIN though breeding for improved animal resistance, vaccination and nutritional supplementation appear as very promising methods. The objective of this study was to investigate the effect of four nutritional status differing in protein and energy levels (Hay: 5.1 MJ/Kg of dry matter (DM) and 7.6% of crude protein (CP), Ban: 8.3 MJ/Kg of DM and 7.5% of CP, Soy: 7.6 MJ/Kg of DM and 17.3% of CP, BS: 12.7 MJ/Kg of DM and 7.4% of CP) on the haematological disturbances due to *Haemonchus contortus* infection in Creole kid goats.

Results: No significant effect of the nutritional status was observed for faecal egg count (FEC) but the experimental infection induced haematological disturbances whose intensity and lengthening were dependent on the nutritional status. A transient marked regenerative macrocytic hypochromic anaemia as revealed by a decrease of packed cell volume (PCV), red blood cells (RBC) and hemoglobin and an increase of reticulocytes was observed in all infected groups except Hay. In this latter, the anaemia settled until the end of the experiment. Furthermore, *H. contortus* induced a thrombocytopenia significantly more pronounced in the group under the lowest nutritional status in term of protein (Hay and Ban). A principal component analysis revealed that the variables that discriminated the nutritional status were the average daily gain (ADG) and the PCV, considered as measures of the level of resilience to *H. contortus* infection. Moreover, the variables that discriminated infected and non-infected animals were mostly related to the biology of RBC (i.e. size and hemoglobin content) and they were correlated with FEC.

Conclusions: The severity and the lengthening of the regenerative anaemia and the thrombocytopenia induced by *H. contortus* have been affected by the nutritional status. The protein enriched diets induced resilience to the infection rather than resistance. This suggests that resilience is associated with an improved regenerative capacity of the bone marrow. However, this needs to be further investigated to understand the relationships between resistance, resilience and dietary supplementation.

Keywords: Blood cells, Gastrointestinal nematode, Goats, Nutrition

Background

Gastrointestinal nematode (GIN) infection remains the most important pathogenic constraint of small ruminant production worldwide. The use of chemical drugs as the unique control method is compromised due to the widespread development of anthelmintic resistant GIN populations throughout the world [1, 2]. In addition, the negative possible environmental impacts of anthelmintic residues and the growing consumer demand for chemical-free animal products increase the need for alternative and/or complementary control strategies [3]. The integrated management of GIN infection aims to better control the GIN populations in order to reach a favourable equilibrium for animal production between host and parasites. Thus, numerous axes of research have been developed to control the parasite population both during the host and the free living stages. The improvement of the host immune response against GIN

* Correspondence: jean-christophe.bambou@inra.fr
[1]URZ, INRA, 97170 Petit-Bourg, Guadeloupe, France
Full list of author information is available at the end of the article

though breeding for improved animal resistance, vaccination and nutritional supplementation appear as very promising methods [4, 5].

Nutritional management of small ruminants has long been considered as a tool for the control of GIN infections [6, 7]. It has been suggested that the nutritional status and the capacity of the host to mount an efficient immune response against invading pathogens are closely associated [8, 9]. Indeed, mounting an immune response is both expensive, in terms of proteins, and calories, because of the metabolic requirement of immune cells, the synthesis of proteinaceous immune mediators and the repairing of damaged tissue [10]. Minerals, trace elements and vitamins are also required for the development of immunity [11, 12]. However, numerous studies have shown that the level of nutrition of the host improve either the resilience or the resistance to GIN infections [13, 14]. The resistance is considered as the capacity of the host to develop an efficient protective response and limit the level of parasitism and the resilience as the capacity to limit the pathophysiological consequences of the infection and maintain the level of production. The expression of resilience or resistance would depend on the host genotype, the physiological stage and the quality of the diet mainly in term of protein [15, 16].

Studies that investigate the impact of the nutritional status of infected small ruminants on the interaction between the GIN parasitism and the physiological disturbances are lacking. Therefore the objective of this study was to investigate the effect of the nutritional status on the haematological disturbances due to *Haemonchus contortus* infection in Creole kid goats.

Methods

Animals, management and experimental design

This experiment was conducted at the Institut National de la Recherche Agronomique Animal Production Unit (INRA-PTEA, Guadeloupe, French West Indies) experimental facilities (16°N16' latitude, 61°W30' longitude). The Creole goat kids (n = 60, 18.88 ± 3.54 kg body weight (BW); 7 months old) had experienced GIN infection at pasture before been randomly placed indoors in four collective pens (n = 15 kids/pen) corresponding to the experimental groups, 1 month before the experimental infection. The animals were drenched with moxidectine (Cydectine®, Fort Dodge Veterinaria S.A., Tours, France, 300 μg/kg BW) and toltrazuril (Baycox Ovis, Bayer HealthCare, Loos, France, 20 mg/kg BW) and housed under worm-free conditions. During this period, nematode faecal egg counts (FEC) remained at zero. Each group was placed under one of 4 distinct dietary status: Hay (Hay ad libitum non supplemented), Ban (Hay ad libitum + 1250 g of Fresh unripe banana/kids), Soy (Hay +250 g Soybean Meal/kids) and BS (Hay ad libitum + 125 g of Soybean Meal +625 g of Fresh unripe banana/kids). The composition and nutritional values of the diets is shown in Table 1. The supplement, fresh banana (cut into thin slices each day) and/or soybean meal were distributed first and individually with the help of yoke traps during the time of diet consumption.. Thereafter, the hay was distributed ad libitum and animals have free-choice access to fresh water. Feeding stalls were long enough to avoid competition for hay between the kids. The offered hay was adjusted to the groups BW (120% of the maximum intake capacity). After a 1 month period of adaptation to the collective pens and the diet conditions, a total of 10 kids/pen in each group were experimentally infected with a single oral dose of 10,000 *H. contortus* third-stage infective larvae (L3) and 5 kids/pen remain non-infected (infected and non-infected groups on the same diet remained in the same collective pen). The L3 were obtained 35 days before challenge from coproculture of monospecifically infected donor Creole goats with isolates previously obtained from Creole goats reared on pasture in different farms in Guadeloupe [17].

Growth measurements

The animals were weighed weekly from the day of infection until the end of the experiment to adjust the offered quantities at 120% of the maximum intake capacity according to BW changes and to measure the individual growth rates.

Faecal egg count

Approximately 10 g of faeces were weekly collected during experimental infection directly from the rectum of each animal to determine the FEC. The faeces were kept

Table 1 Composition and nutritional values of diets

	Nutritional conditions			
	Hay	Ban	Soy	BS
Ingredients (g/Kg DM)				
Hay	1000	750	780	762.5
Fresh banana	0	250	0	125
Soybean meal	0	0	220	112.5
Chemical composition (%)				
OM[a]	88.2	92.9	94.2	94.7
CP[b]	7.6	8.3	17.3	12.7
NDF[c]	65.9	50.8	46.3	45.0
ADF[d]	32.2	25.8	23.2	21.8
ADL[e]	4.6	3.0	2.2	2.7
ME[f] (MJ/Kg DM)	5.1	7.5	7.6	7.4

[a]*OM* Organic Matter, [b]*CP* Crude protein, [c]*NDF* Neutral Detergent Fiber, [d]*ADF* Acid Detergent Fiber, [e]*ADL* Acid Detergent Lignin, [f]*ME* Metabolizable Energy

in plastic tubes to avoid contamination and immediately transported from the experimental facility to the laboratory in refrigerated vials. All samples were individually analyzed using a modified McMaster method for rapid determination and FEC was expressed as the number of eggs/g faeces [18].

Blood cell counts

During the experimental infection, blood samples were individually collected once a week by jugular venipuncture on each animal by using disposable syringes and 20-Ga needles. A 4 mL portion of each blood sample was placed in commercial anticoagulant tubes (ethylenediamine tetraacetic acid K_3, EDTA tubes; Becton Dickinson, Plymouth, UK). Blood samples previously placed in EDTA coated tubes were analyzed for a standard haematological profil using a MS4-e (Melet Schloesing Pharmaceuticals s.a., Rue du Collège 90 CH-2300, La Chaux de Fonds, Suisse). The number of circulating eosinophils was determined according to the method of Dawkins et al. [19] with a Malassez cell counter.

Calculation and statistical analysis

All the animal variables were analyzed by a linear mixed model using the PROC MIXED of SAS (Version 9, SAS Inst., Inc., Cary, NC, 1999). Because of skewed distributions, FEC and eosinophilia variables were logarithm transformed (ln (FEC + 15), ln (Blood eosinophils + 1) respectively) and the other haematological data were square-root transformed, to normalise residual variances. The model included fixed effects of the days post-infection (T), the dietary status (D), the infection status (I) and the significant interaction between D and I and T as defined below:

$$y_{ijklm} = \mu + Di + Ij + T_k + (D \times I \times T)_{ijk} + a_{ijl} + + \varepsilon_{jklm}.$$

where y is the observed values; μ the overall mean; D_i the fixed effect of the ith dietary condition (i = 1 to 4), I_j the fixed effect of the jth infection status (infected vs non-infected), T_k the fixed effect of the kth day post-infection (k = 0 to 49), $(D \times I \times T)_{ijk}$ the interaction of the dietary condition, the infection status and the days post-infection, a_{ijl} is the random effect associated with the lth animal in dietary condition i and infection status j; and $_{ijklm}$ the random error. All the interactions were initially tested for all variables and only the $(D \times I \times T)_{ijk}$ was statistically significant ($P < 0.05$) and retained in the model. An unstructured variance-covariance structure was used to model the covariance between two observations on the same animal. The same model was applied for all the animal variables except growth rate (Average Daily Gain, ADG). The ADG of the animals were estimated by adjusting the weight curve with a linear model. Significance was declared at ≤5% of probability. A principal component analysis (PCA) was performed using the FactoMineR package [20] in R version 3.3.2 (R Cor Team, 2016). The PCA allows to explore the relationships between all the variables (zootechnical, parasitological and haematological) and to describe similarities and differences between animals and associations between variables, to better defined the nutritional and the infection status respectively. The PCA was done with the 13 variables (2 parasitological and zootechnical variables and 11 haematological variables) as active variables and the animals as individuals, ignoring the infection status (I) and the dietary conditions (D). The interaction D × I was included in the PCA analysis as illustrative variable to obtain their coordinates on the different principal components. The two first principal components were then used to plot each animal individually from 28 to 49 days post-infection (d.p.i). corresponding to the period of eggs excretion in the faeces.

Results

Parasitological and zootechnical parameters

In the experimentally infected animals, the FEC remained at zero until 28 d.p.i. (Fig. 1). Thereafter FEC increased significantly whatever the dietary status until 49 d.p.i. No significant effect of the dietary status was observed for FEC ($P > 0.05$). No faecal egg excretion was observed in the non-infected animals during the study (data not shown).

A significant interaction was observed between the dietary and the infection status for the ADG ($P < 0.001$, Fig. 2). The ADG was significantly higher in the Soy and the BS groups whatever the infection status ($P < 0.01$). No significant difference was observed between the non-supplemented groups (Hay) whatever the infection status and the non-infected kids of the Ban group ($P > 0.05$). A significant negative effect of the infection status was observed only in the Soy and the Ban groups (−12% and −76% between non-infected and infected kids respectively, $P < 0.05$). The ADG of infected kids was significantly higher in the Hay group compared with the Ban group (48.5 vs. 8.05 g/day respectively, $P < 0.01$). No effect of the infection status was observed in the Hay and the BS groups ($P > 0.05$).

Haematological parameters

Significant interactions were observed between the dietary and the infection status and the time (d.p.i.) for all the haematological parameters ($P < 0.01$, Fig. 3). A higher variability of the measured parameters was observed in the infected animals. The packed cell volume (PCV), the red blood cells concentration (RBC), the blood hemoglobin concentration, the mean corpuscular hemoglobin concentration (MCHC) and the platelets

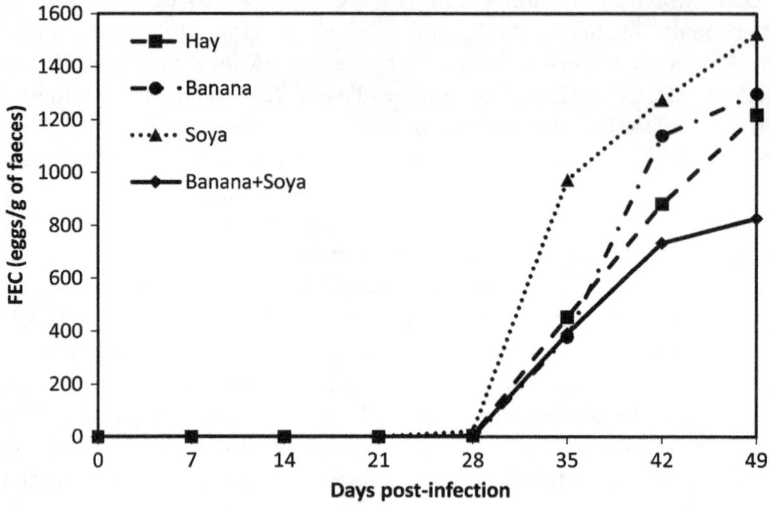

Fig. 1 Least square means of Faecal egg counts (FEC) according to the nutritional status: Ban: Banana (•, Infected and gray circle, Non-Infected); Hay (■, Infected and gray square, Non-Infected); Soy: Soybean Meal (▲, Infected and gray triangle, Non-Infected); BS: Soybean Meal + Banana (♦, Infected and gray diamond, Non-Infected)

concentration significantly decreased in the infected animals but not in the non-infected ones. In the infected animals, at 21 d.p.i. the Hay group reached the lowest values for these haematological parameters except MCHC and it remained significantly lower than the Ban, Soy and BS groups ($P < 0.01$, Fig. 3). The mean corpuscular volume (MCV) increased significantly ($P < 0.01$) in the infected animals whatever the dietary status. No interaction between time and the dietary status was observed for MCV in the non-infected animals ($P > 0.05$).

Circulating immune cells

The results for circulating basophils were negligible whatever the dietary or the infection status (data not shown). A significant interaction between the dietary and the infection status and the time was observed for the circulating immune cells except for circulating monocytes ($P < 0.01$, Fig. 4). Circulating lymphocytes and neutrophils decreased slightly but significantly in infected animals ($P < 0.05$). No variation of the circulating monocytes was observed during the course of the experiment whatever the dietary and the infection status ($P > 0.05$). The circulating eosinophils were significantly higher in the infected animals from 14 to 35 d.p.i. ($P < 0.001$). At 35 d.p.i. the circulating eosinophils decreased to the level of non-infected animals in all dietary status except for Hay.

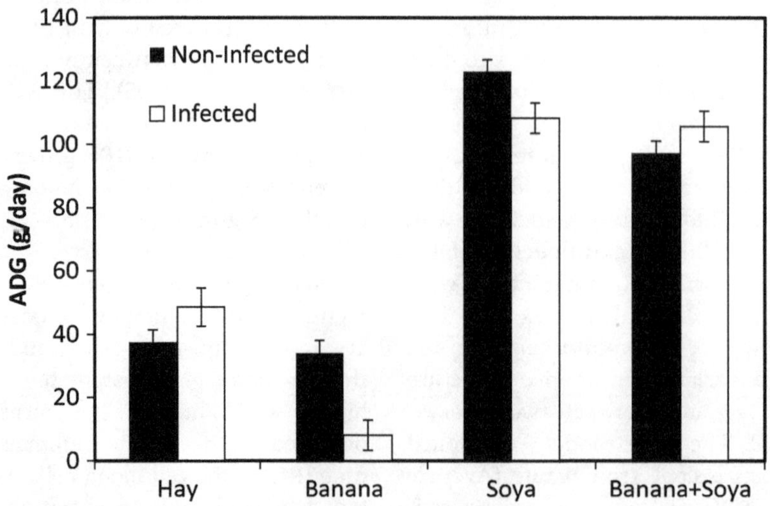

Fig. 2 Means and standard errors of Average Daily Gain (ADG) according to the nutritional and the infection status

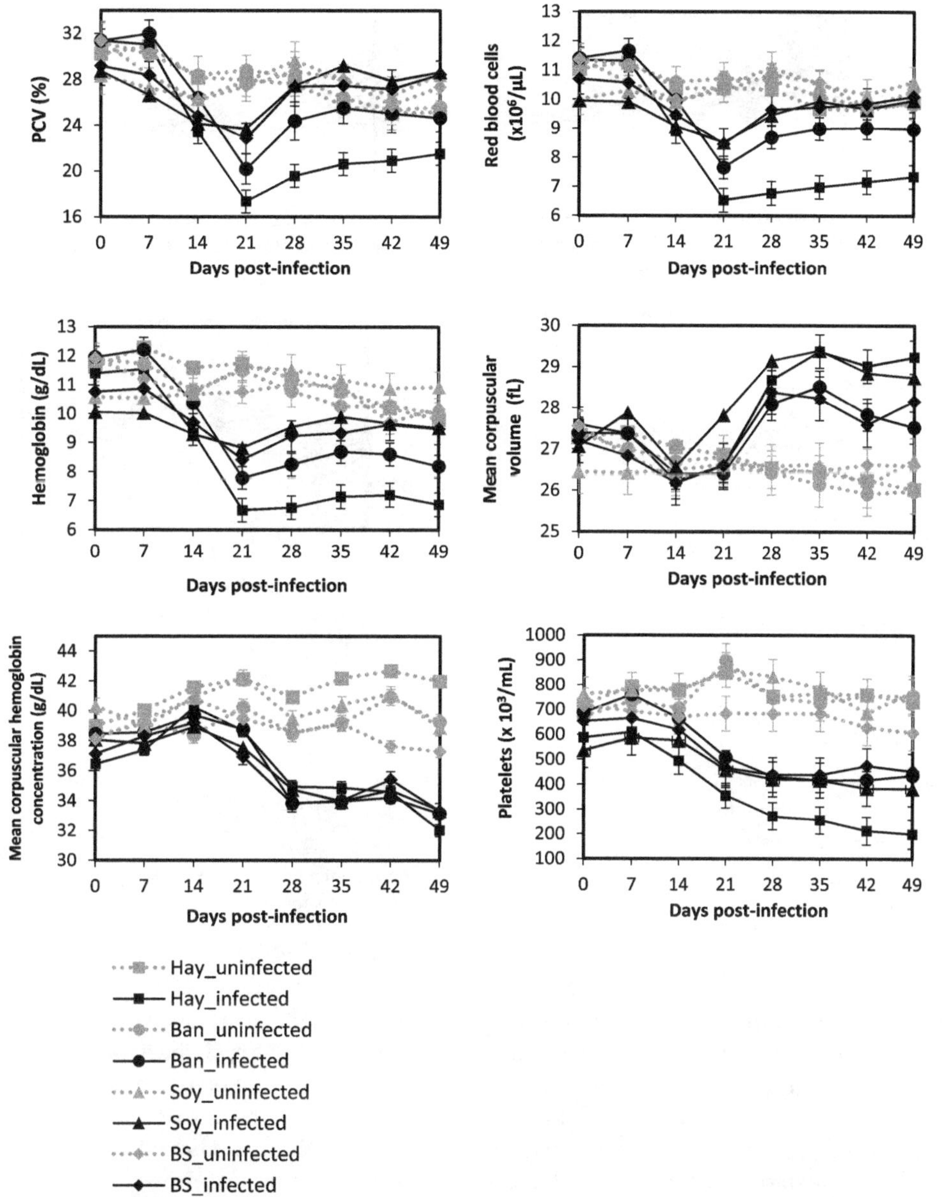

Fig. 3 Least square means of haematological parameters according to the nutritional and the infection status: Ban: Banana (•, Infected and gray circle, Non-Infected); Hay (■, Infected and gray square, Non-Infected); Soy: Soybean Meal (▲, Infected and gray triangle, Non-Infected); BS: Soybean Meal + Banana (♦, Infected and gray diamond, Non-Infected)

Principal component analysis of the haemotological, parasitological and zootechnical parameters

The first three principal components of the PCA explained 70.3% of the total variation (34.1%, 19.5% and 16.6% respectively, Table 2). The Fig. 5a shows the contribution of each parameter to the first and the second principal component. The first principal component seemed to contrast FEC, MCV with Platelets, MCH and MCHC. The second principal component seemed to be mainly defined by the contrast between PCV, RBC ADG, and monocytes, lymphocytes and eosinophils. Each animal at each time point, from 28 to 49 d.p.i. was projected on the scatter plot using the two first principal components (Fig. 5b). The infection status (infected and non-infected) was mainly described by the first principal component and the dietary status (Hay, Ban, Soy and BS) by the second principal component.

Discussion

The nutritional status is closely associated with the intensity of the pathological impact of GIN infection in small ruminants. It has been shown that an improved nutritional status can reduce significantly production losses due to GIN infection by reducing both morbidity

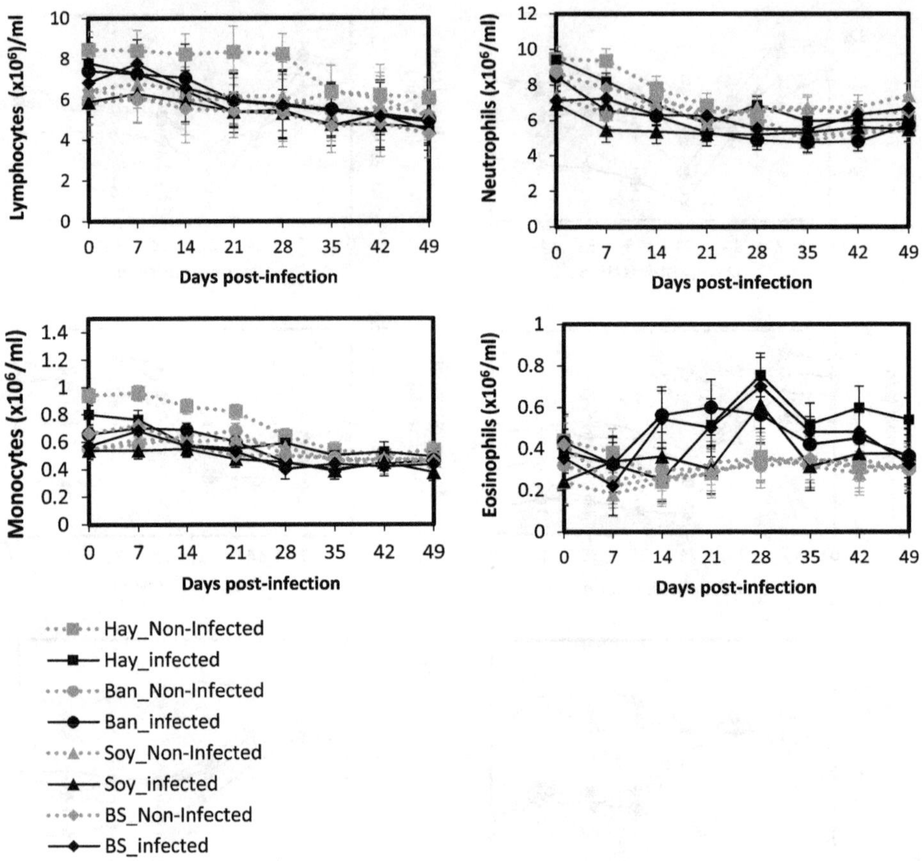

Fig. 4 Least square means of blood immune cells according to the nutritional and the infection status: Ban: Banana (•, Infected and gray circle, Non-Infected); Hay (■, Infected and gray square, Non-Infected); Soy: Soybean Meal (▲, Infected and gray triangle, Non-Infected); BS: Soybean Meal + Banana (♦, Infected and gray diamond, Non-Infected)

and mortality [21, 22]. In *H. contortus* infection, morbidity and mortality are mainly caused by the haematophagous activity of both larval and adult stages of the parasite whose consequence is an irreversible loss of protein. The objective of this study was to investigate the effect of the nutritional status on the haematological disturbances due to *H. contortus* infection in Creole kid goats. No significant effect of the nutritional status was observed for FEC. In accordance with a previous study, a single bolus oral experimental infection of Creole kid goats that previously experienced natural GIN infection at pasture induce a low level of parasitism measured through the FEC and the lengthening of the prepatent period [17]. Nonetheless, we showed a significant interaction between the nutritional and the infection status on the growth rate. The animal placed under the lowest nutritional status in term of protein (i.e. Hay and Ban) showed the lowest growth rate and the experimental infection reduced the growth rate only for animals placed in the Ban and the Soy groups. Furthermore, the experimental infection induced haematological disturbances whose intensity and lengthening were dependent on the

Table 2 Estimate of eigenvalues (λj), percentage of variance (λ%), and cumulative variance and eigenvectors associated to the three first principal components of the animal responses during an experimental *H. contortus* infection (from 28 to 49 days post-infection)

F[a]	λj	λ(%)	Cumulative variance (%)	Associated eigenvectors[b]												
				ADG[b]	FEC[c]	PCV[d]	RBC[e]	Hgb[f]	MCV[g]	MCH[h]	MCHC[i]	Plat[j]	Lym[k]	Mon[l]	Neut[m]	Eos[n]
1	4.78	34.14	34.14	0.26	−0.36	0.48	0.66	0.84	−0.50	0.63	0.71	0.80	0.67	0.55	0.50	0.24
2	2.73	19.49	53.63	0.59	0.03	0.76	0.67	0.52	0.25	−0.13	−0.23	0.13	−0.48	−0.56	−0.29	−0.31
3	2.33	16.63	70.27	0.31	0.31	0.37	0.18	−0.02	0.55	−0.44	−0.61	−0.44	0.54	0.42	0.53	0.16

[a]*F* Functions (Principal components), [b]*ADG* Average Daily Gain, [c]*FEC* Feacal Egg counts, [d]*PCV* Packed Cell Volume, [e]*RBC* Red Blood Cells, [f]*Hgb* Hemoglobin, [g]*MCV* Mean Corpuscular Volume, [h]*MCH* Mean Corpuscular Hemoglobin, [i]*MCHC* Mean Corpuscular Hemoglobin Concentration, [j]*Plat* Platelets, [k]*Lym* Lymphocytes, [l]*Mon* Monocytes, [m]*Neut* Neutrophiles, [n]*Eos* Eosinophils

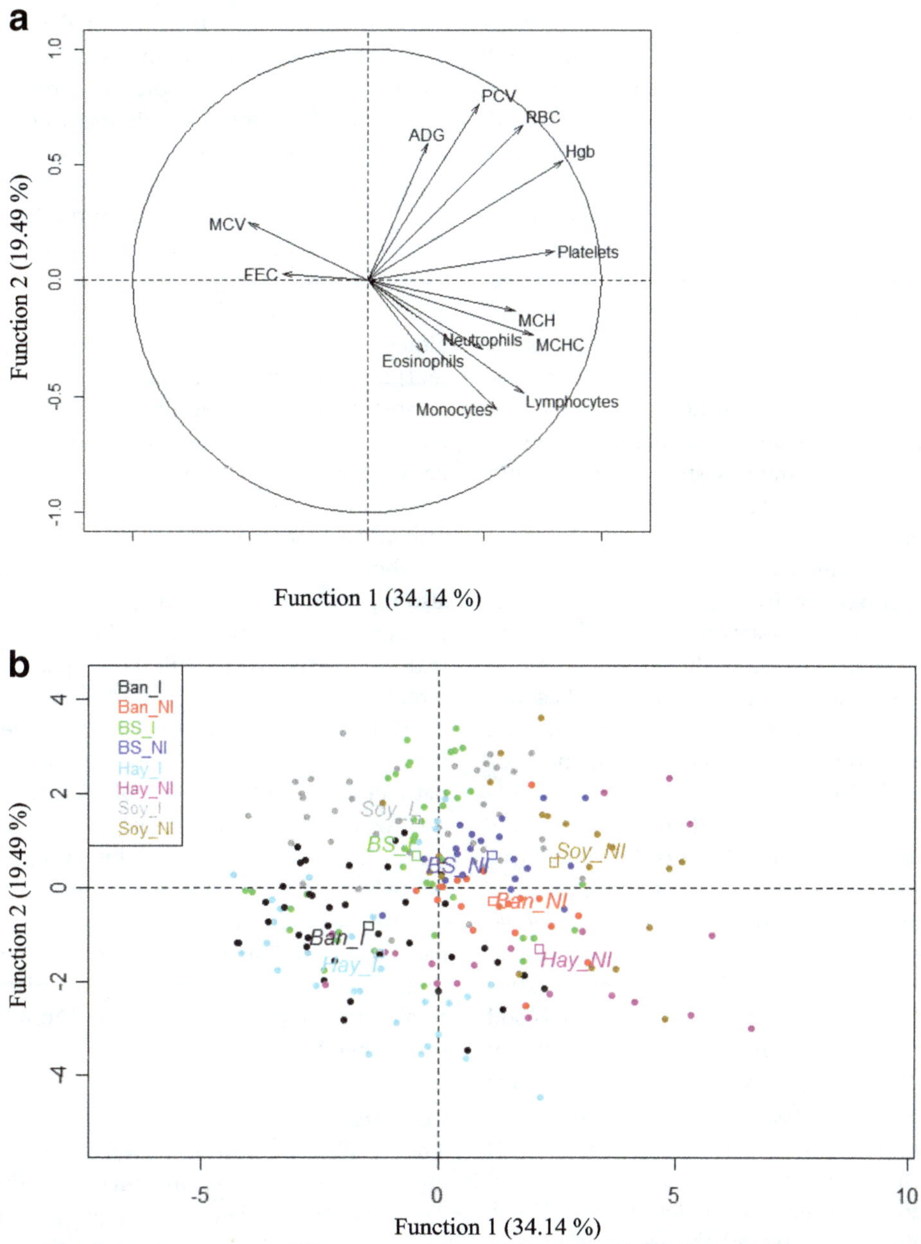

Fig. 5 Principal component analysis of the haematological, parasitological and zootechnical parameters. **a** Mapping of the parameters and (**b**) Representation of the animals according to the dietary (Ban: Banana; Hay; Soy: Soybean Meal; BS: Soybean Meal + Banana) and the infection (I: experimentally infected with *Haemonchus contortus*; NI: Non-infected) status from 28 until 49 days post-infection on two-dimensional scatter plot. FEC: Faecal egg counts; MCV: Mean Cell Volume; ADG: Average Daily Gain; PCV: Packed Cell Volume; RBC: Red Blood Cells; Hgb: Hemoglobin; MCH: Mean Corpuscular Hemoglobin; MCHC: Mean Corpuscular Hemoglobin Concentration

nutritional status. A transient marked anaemia as revealed by a decrease of PCV, RBC and hemoglobin concentrations was observed in all infected groups except Hay. In this latter, the anaemia settled until the end of the experiment. Interestingly, the concentration of hemoglobin (MCHC) did not increase proportionally with the increase in RBC size (MCV). These RBC with a larger volume and a lower hemoglobin concentration were probably reticulocytes (i.e. immatures RBC) as previously shown [23]. These results were in accordance with previous studies conducted in sheep, characterizing the type of anaemia induced by *H. contortus* as regenerative macrocytic hypochromic anaemia [24, 25]. Indeed, the pathogenesis of regenerative anaemia includes external hemorrhage which is chronic in the case of *H. contortus* infection. Furthermore, in the present experiment the number of platelets decreased in all infected animals. This thrombocytopenia was significantly more pronounced in the Hay group, as for PCV, RBC and hemoglobin. Similarly, it has been shown in *H. contortus* infected sheep that the number of platelets decreased progressively during the course of *H. contortus* infection [23]. To our knowledge, besides this study in sheep and ours in goats, this result has never been described in the literature. However, a platelet aggregation and adhesion inhibitor from adults *H. contortus* has been identified and characterized in vitro [26]. It must be emphasized that the host blood taken from the abomasal mucosa is the main nutrient source of the parasitic stage of *H. contortus*. Altogether, these results strongly suggested that *H. contortus* has developed a broad-spectrum strategy to manipulate the host's hemostatic system, which would target especially the blood platelets.

With the exception of eosinophils, the blood leucocytes counts were not affected by the infection and the nutritional status. Indeed, many studies showed significant correlations between resistance/susceptibility to GIN infection and the magnitude of the peripheral blood eosinophil [27]. Even though this relationship has not been observed in all studies, it is largely admitted that peripheral blood eosinophil plays a key role in the protective response to GIN [28–30]. In contrast with a previous study in Creole goat [31], blood eosinophil counts were not affected by the nutritional status. In the present study the nutritional status were not as contrasted as it was previously. On the other hand, it has been shown that peripheral blood lymphocytes are also involved in the protective response to GIN. A significant negative phenotypic correlation has been found between blood lymphocyte counts and *H. contortus* fecundity [32]. In contrast, in another sheep breed, lymphopenia was observed in *H. contortus* infected lambs [33]. However, the close association between the resistance to GIN infection and the host immune response has been demonstrated in a study showing that depletion of CD4+ T lymphocytes significantly increased the parasitic load in a resistant sheep breed [28]. In Creole goats experimentally infected, we have showed that the level of circulating activated CD4+ and CD8+ T lymphocytes were higher in susceptible animals compared with resistant [34]. Altogether these results obtained in different sheep breeds and goats, with different level of parasitism confirmed the effective role of lymphocytes in the host response against GIN, but also emphasize the need to better investigate this relationship.

The comparison between the Hay and the Ban groups showed that infected animals in the Hay groups prioritize growth at the expense of a marked pathological impact while the reverse was observed in the Ban group. These results were partly in keeping with previous studies suggesting that an improved nutritional status (here Soy and BS compared to Hay and Ban) induced resilience rather than resistance to the experimental *H. contortus* infection (i.e. reduced pathological impact for the same parasitic load) [25, 35, 36]. Interestingly, the PCA revealed that in our study the variables that discriminated the nutritional status were ADG and PCV, considered as measures of the level of resilience to *H. contortus* infection, and eosinophils. Moreover, the variables that discriminated infected and non-infected animals at the cellular level were mostly related to the biology of red blood cells (i.e. size and hemoglobin content) and they were correlated with FEC. The association of eosinophils with resilience was not surprising in our animal model since we had previously shown that, in contrast with numerous studies in sheep, blood eosinophil counts were associated with the level of infection rather than the protective response in goats [34].

Otherwise, other studies including one of ours, have also reported resistance to GIN (i.e. reduced pathological impact and parasitic load) induced by an improved nutritional status [31, 37, 38]. Discrepancy between the different studies could be attributed to the animals physiological stage which would influenced the trade-offs between the immune response against invading pathogens and others physiological functions [39]. The quality of the metabolizable protein arising from the rumen (microbial protein vs by-pass protein), could also be an explanation since the amino acid composition of immune proteins is more compatible with that of by-pass proteins [16]. Further research is needed to better understand the nutrition × parasitism interaction in small ruminant for a better fine tuning of the technical recommendations to breeders.

Conclusions

The results showed that infection with *H. contortus* induced a regenerative anaemia and a thrombocytopenia. The severity and lengthening of these pathological disturbances have been affected by the nutritional status, the protein enriched diets induced resilience to the infection rather than resistance. This suggests that resilience is associated with an improved regenerative capacity of the bone marrow. However, further investigation to understand the relationships between resistance, resilience and dietary supplementation.

Acknowledgments

The authors want to give thanks to the Gardel team for care and handling of the animals: T. Kandassamy, W. Troupé, J. Gobardhan and S.-A. Matou.

Funding

This study was funded by the Project Agroecodiv (La Région Guadeloupe and Fonds Européens FEDER) and the INRA métaprogramme GISA (Gestion Intégrée de la Santé Animale) Project Strep (drastic and Sustainable Treatment Reduction against Parasitism in livestock). S. Ceriac was supported by a doctoral fellowship from la Région Guadeloupe and the division of animal genetics of INRA.

Authors' contributions

JCB, HA and SC conceived and designed the experiments, CJ and RA and the Gardel team collected samples for the haematological and parasitological analysis. DF and YF performed the haematological and parasitological analysis. JCB and SC performed the statistical analysis and wrote the paper. All authors read and approved the final manuscript.

Competing interest

The authors declare that they have no competing interests.

Consent for publication

Not applicable.

Author details

[1]URZ, INRA, 97170 Petit-Bourg, Guadeloupe, France. [2]PTEA, INRA, 97170 Le Moule, Guadeloupe, France.

References

1. Bishop SC, Morris CA. Genetics of disease resistance in sheep and goats. Small Rumin Res. 2007;70(1):48–59.
2. Papadopoulos E. Anthelmintic resistance in sheep nematodes. Small Rumin Res. 2008;76(1-2):99–103.
3. Beynon SA. Potential environmental consequences of administration of anthelmintics to sheep. Vet Parasitol. 2012;189(1):113–24.
4. Baker RL, Gray GD. Worm control for small ruminants in tropical Asia. Australian Centre for International Agricultural Research (ACIAR). 2003; Monograph 113:63–95.
5. van Wyk JA, Bath GF. The FAMACHA((c)) system for managing haemonchosis in sheep and goats by clinically identifying individual animals for treatment. Vet Res. 2002;33(5):509–29.
6. Clunies Ross I, Gordon H. McL.: nutritional factors affecting reistance to haemonchosis. Aust Vet J. 1933;9:100–7.
7. Gibson TE. The influence of nutrition on the relationships between gastro-intestinal parasites and their hosts. Proc Nutr Soc. 1963;22:15–20.
8. Adams CA. Nutrition-based health in animal production. Nutr Res Rev. 2006;19(1):79–89.
9. Colditz IG. Six costs of immunity to gastrointestinal nematode infections. Parasite Immunol. 2008;30(2):63–70.
10. Lochmiller RL, Deerenberg C. Trade-offs in evolutionary immunology: just what is the cost of immunity? Oikos. 2000;88(1):87–98.
11. Koski KG, Scott ME. Gastrointestinal nematodes, trace elements, and immunity. J Trace Elem Exp Med. 2003;16(4):237–51.
12. McClure SJ. How minerals may influence the development and expression of immunity to endoparasites in livestock. Parasite Immunol. 2008;30(2):89–100.
13. Torres-Acosta JFJ, Sandoval-Castro CA, Hoste H, Aguilar-Caballero AJ, Camara-Sarmiento R, Alonso-Diaz MA. Nutritional manipulation of sheep and goats for the control of gastrointestinal nematodes under hot humid and subhumid tropical conditions. Small Rumin Res. 2012;103(1):28–40.
14. Walkden-Brown SW, Kahn LP. Nutritional modulation of resistance and resilience to gastrointestinal nematode infection - a review. Asian-Australas J Anim Sci. 2002;15(6):912–24.
15. Knox MR, Torres-Acosta JFJ, Aguilar-Caballero AJ. Exploiting the effect of dietary supplementation of small ruminants on resilience and resistance against gastrointestinal nematodes. Vet Parasitol. 2006;139(4):385–93.
16. Houdijk JGM. Differential effects of protein and energy scarcity on resistance to nematode parasites. Small Rumin Res. 2012;103(1):41–9.
17. Bambou JC, de la Chevrotiere C, Varo H, Arquet R, Kooyman FNJ, Mandonnet N. Serum antibody responses in Creole kids experimentally infected with Haemonchus contortus. Vet Parasitol. 2008;158(4):311–8.
18. Aumont G, R. Pouillot, Mandonnet N: Le dénombrement des éléments parasitaires: Un outil pour l'étude de la résistance génétique aux endo-parasites chez les petits ruminants. Workshop final de l'AT CIRAD-MIPA 72/94, Guadeloupe 1997.
19. Dawkins HJS, Windon RG, Eagleson GK. Eosinophil responses in sheep selected for high and low responsiveness to Trichostrongylus colubriformis. Int J Parasitol. 1989;19(2):199–205.
20. Le S, Josse J, Husson F. FactoMineR: an R package for multivariate analysis. J Stat Softw. 2008;25(1):1–18.
21. Sykes AR, Coop RL. Interaction between nutrition and gastrointestinal parasitism in sheep. New Zeal Vet J. 2001;49(6):222–6.
22. Walkden-Brown SW, Kahn LP: Nutritional modulation of resistance and resilience to gastrointestinal nematode infection - a review. In: International symposium on new challenges for animal science in a new century 2001; Sendai, Japan; 2001: 912-924.
23. Andronicos NM, Henshall JM, Le Jambre LF, Hunt PW, Ingham AB. A one shot blood phenotype can identify sheep that resist Haemonchus contortus challenge. Vet Parasitol. 2014;205(3–4):595–605.
24. Khan FA, Sahoo A, Sonawane GG, Karim SA, Dhakad S, Pareek AK, Tripathi BN. Effect of dietary protein on responses of lambs to repeated Haemonchus contortus infection. Livest Sci. 2012;150(1–3):143–51.
25. Abbott EM, Parkins JJ, Holmes PH. The effect of dietary-protein on the pathogenesis of acute ovine haemonchosis. Vet Parasitol. 1986; 20(4):275–89.
26. Crab A, Noppe W, Pelicaen C, Van Hoorelbeke K, Deckmyn H. The parasitic hematophagous worm Haemonchus contortus inhibits human platelet aggregation and adhesion: partial purification of a platelet inhibitor. Thromb Haemost. 2002;87(5):899–904.
27. Meeusen E, Balic A, Bowles V. Cells, cytokines and other molecules associated with rejection of gastrointestinal nematode parasites. Vet Immunol Immunopathol. 2005;108(1–2):121–5.
28. Gill HS. Genetic control of acquired resistance to haemonchosis in merino lambs. Parasite Immunol. 1991;13:617–28.
29. Adams DB. Systemic responses to challenge infection with Haemonchus contortus in immune merino sheep. Vet Res Commun. 1993;17(1):25–35.
30. Woolaston RR, Manueli P, Eady SJ, Barger IA, LeJambre LF, Banks DJD, Windon RG. The value of circulating eosinophil count as a selection criterion for resistance of sheep to trichostrongyle parasites. Int J Parasitol. 1996;26(1):123–6.
31. Bambou JC, Archimede H, Arquet R, Mahieu M, Alexandre G, Gonzalez-Garcia E, Mandonnet N. Effect of dietary supplementation on resistance to experimental infection with Haemonchus contortus in Creole kids. Vet Parasitol. 2011;178(3–4):279–85.
32. Rowe A, McMaster K, Emery D, Sangster N. Haemonchus contortus infection in sheep: parasite fecundity correlates with worm size and host lymphocyte counts. Vet Parasitol. 2008;153(3–4):285–93.
33. Ortolani EL, Leal MLD, Minervino AHH, Aires AR, Coop RL, Jackson F, Suttle NF. Effects of parasitism on cellular immune response in sheep experimentally infected with Haemonchus contortus. Vet Parasitol. 2013;196(1–2):230–4.
34. Bambou JC, Gonzalez-Garcia E, de la Chevrotiere C, Arquet R, Vachiery N, Mandonnet N. Peripheral immune response in resistant and susceptible Creole kids experimentally infected with Haemonchus contortus. Small Rumin Res. 2009;82(1):34–9.
35. Wallace DS, Bairden K, Duncan JL, Fishwick G, Holmes PH, McKellar QA, Murray M, Parkins JJ, Stear M: Influence of soyabean meal supplementation on the resistance of Scottish blackface lambs to haemonchosis. Res Vet Sci 1996, 60(2):138-143.
36. Datta FU, Nolan JV, Rowe JB, Gray GD. Protein supplementation improves the performance of parasitised sheep fed a straw-based diet. Int J Parasitol. 1998;28(8):1269–78.
37. Louvandini H, Veloso CFM, Paludo GR, Dell'Porto A, Gennari SM, McManus CM. Influence of protein supplementation on the resistance and resilience on young hair sheep naturally infected with gastrointestinal nematodes during rainy and dry seasons. Vet Parasitol. 2006;137(1–2):103–11.
38. Nnadi PA, Kamalu TN, Onah DN. The effect of dietary protein on the productivity of west African dwarf (WAD) goats infected with Haemonchus contortus. Vet Parasitol. 2009;161(3–4):232–8.
39. Rauw W. Immune response from a resource allocation perspective. Front Genet. 2012;3(267)

10

Pharmacokinetic and pharmacodynamic modeling of sarafloxacin against avian pathogenic *Escherichia coli* in Muscovy ducks

Yang Yu[1,2,3], Yu Feng Zhou[1,2,3], Jian Sun[1,2,3], Wei Shi[1,3], Xiao Ping Liao[1,2,3] and Ya Hong Liu[1,2,3,4*]

Abstract

Background: This study focused on utilizing pharmacokinetics/pharmacodynamics (PK/PD) modeling to optimize therapeutic dosage regimens of sarafloxacin against avian pathogenic *Escherichia. coli* O78 strain in Muscovy ducks. The ex vivo PK/PD study of sarafloxacin was conducted in Muscovy ducks after intravenous (i.v.) and oral (p.o.) administrations at a single dose of 10 mg/kg bodyweight (BW). The serum samples were analyzed by reverse phase high-performance liquid chromatography (RP-HPLC) using a fluorescence detection method. Sarafloxacin PK data were analyzed by a non-compartmental method using Winnonlin software.

Results: Calculations of the area under the concentration-time curves ($AUC_{0\text{-}24h}$) were 8.57 ± 0.59 and 8.37 ± 0.29 μg · h/ml following i.v. and p.o. administration, respectively. Elimination half-lives ($t_{1/2\beta}$) were 6.11 ± 0.99 h and 8.21 ± 0.64 h for i.v. injection and p.o. administration, respectively. The mean in vitro plasma protein binding of sarafloxacin was 39.3%. Integration using the sigmoid E_{max} model, the mean values of $AUC_{0\text{-}24h}$/MIC needed for bacteriostatic, bactericidal and bacterial eradication action were 25.4, 40.6, and 94.4 h, respectively.

Conclusions: Sarafloxacin administered at a 10 mg/kg dose may be insufficient for treatment of *E. coli* O78 infections with an MIC equally to or over 0.125 μg/ml. Furthermore, higher doses of sarafloxacin are required to minimize antimicrobial resistance considering the MPC theory.

Keywords: Dosage regimens, Muscovy ducks, Mutant prevention concentration, Pharmacokinetics/pharmacodynamics, Sarafloxacin, Avian pathogenic *Escherichia Coli*

Background

The minimum inhibitory concentration (MIC) and minimum bactericidal concentration (MBC) were used to evaluate the efficacy of antimicrobial drugs to eradicate the entire pathogen population [1]. The mutant prevention concentration (MPC) has been proposed to evaluate the ability of antimicrobial agents to prevent the emergence of antibacterial resistance [2]. Pharmacokinetics/pharmacodynamics (PK/PD) principles may provide an effective way to control the occurrence and dissemination of bacterial resistance [3, 4]. For fluoroquinolones, the PK/PD indices are calculated by the ratio of area under the concentration-time curve to MIC (AUC/MIC) and the ratio of peak drug concentration to MIC (C_{max}/MIC) [3, 5]. Recently, the values of AUC/MPC and C_{max}/MPC were determined to minimize the occurrence of the antibacterial resistance [1, 6, 7].

Muscovy ducks are reared for their distinctive taste, high yield of breast meat and low calorie content [8]. Colibacillosis is the most common disease in the poultry industry causing serious death and economic losses worldwide, e.g. in China [9]. Birds infected with Avian pathogenic *Escherichia coli* (APEC) are more likely to

* Correspondence: lyh@scau.edu.cn
[1]National Risk Assessment Laboratory for Antimicrobial Resistance of Animal Original Bacteria, South China Agricultural University, Guangzhou 510642, China
[2]Guangdong Provincial Key Laboratory of Veterinary Pharmaceutics Development and Safety Evaluation, South China Agricultural University, Guangzhou 510642, China
Full list of author information is available at the end of the article

develop infectious bursal disease, mycoplasmosis, coccidiosis, Newcastle Disease, infectious bronchitis, and nutritional deficiencies [10]. APEC are responsible for aerosacculitis, polyserositis, pericarditis, yolk sac infection, respiratory tract infection, septicemia and other extra-intestinal diseases in chickens, turkeys, ducks and other avian species [11–13]. Serotype O78 is recognized as one of the most common and prevalent serogrouping of APEC isolates [11, 12]. *E. Coli* strains with the O78 serotype are highly pathogenic and commonly exist in poultry industry. Therefore, treatment of colibacillosis caused by APEC O78 demands far more attention in poultry farming. However, current vaccines have poor efficacy, and therapy is mainly based on antimicrobial therapy.

Sarafloxacin, a second generation fluoroquinolone antibiotic exclusively developed for veterinary use, shows excellent antimicrobial activity [14–16], and is mainly used to treat colibacillosis by binding to topoisomerase II in Gram-negative bacteria [17–19]. In the European Union, sarafloxacin was proposed for use in poultry and fish in 1998 [20]; and difloxacin (whose primary metabolite is sarafloxacin) was authorized in 1998 but in the meantime the marketing authorization was withdrawn [21].

Publications have reported the pharmacokinetics of sarafloxacin in several animals and birds [15, 22]; however, few studies focused on the PK/PD modeling of sarafloxacin in Muscovy ducks. The aims of this work are to: 1) study the PK/PD modeling of sarafloxacin; 2) optimize the clinical dosage regimens for treatment of colibacillosis in Muscovy ducks particularly against the *E.coli* O78 strains; and 3) assess the risks of using sarafloxacin employing the MPC theory.

Methods

Bacterium and reagents

The experiments were performed using an APEC O78 strain (identified by a serum agglutination test) isolated from ducks colibacillosis and stored in our laboratory. Phylogenetic grouping of this strain was B_2 type and determined by multiplex PCR using specific primers from *chuA*, *yjaA* genes and TSPE4.C2 fragment. *E. coli* ATCC 25922 (China Institute of Veterinary Drug Control, Beijing, China) was used for the quality control purpose. Sarafloxacin was purchased from Unichna Bio-technology of Zhengzhou Co., LTD, Zhengzhou, China.

Animals and experimental design

Twenty-four healthy Muscovy ducks (purchased from the Jiangcun poultry market in Baiyun district, Guangzhou, China) of 100–120 days old and weighing 2.4–2.6 kg were used. Ducks were fed commercial drug-free food. All ducks were examined daily, adapted well to the environment, and were clinically healthy prior to the study. All protocols were approved by the Animal Research Committees of South China Agricultural University. All experiments were conducted using the guidelines of the American Association for Accreditation of Laboratory Animal Care (AAALAC) [23].

Animals were randomly divided into two groups of 12/group. Feed was eliminated for 12 h before and 6 h post-administration. Sarafloxacin (2.5%) was injected intravenously into the left brachial vein at 10 mg/kg body weight (BW). For oral administration, a soluble powder (5%), was directly administered into the crop at 10 mg/kg BW. Blood samples were collected from the right brachial vein at 0, 5, 15, 30, 45 min, and 1, 1.5, 2, 3, 4, 6, 8, 12, 16, 24, 36 h post-i.v. administration. For p.o. administration, the time points for blood collection were at 0, 10, 20, 30, 45 min, and 1, 1.5, 2, 3, 4, 6, 8, 12, 16, 24, 36 h. The serum samples were obtained by centrifugation at 2000 g for 10 min and stored at – 20 °C until analyses within 2 weeks.

Sarafloxacin analysis

A total of 0.1 mL acetonitrile was added into 0.1 mL of serum sample. The mixture was rigorously vortexed for 1 min, and then centrifuged at 15,000 g for 5 min. The supernatant was filtered through a 0.22 μm cellulose membrane, and 10 μL were injected into the reverse phase high-performance liquid chromatography (RP-HPLC) system. This RP-HPLC includes a 2695 Waters Alliance system (Milford, MA, USA), a HYPERSIL BDS C_{18} Column (5, USA), and a HYPERS. The mobile phase consisted of acetonitrile and 0.1% trifluoroacetic acid (29:71, v: v) at 1 mL/min flow rate. A Waters 2475 fluorescence detector operated at an excitation wavelength of 280 nm and an emission wavelength of 460 nm.

The retention time of sarafloxacin in the serum was 4.9 ± 0.2 min. The standard curve of sarafloxacin was linear in the range of 0.02–10 μg/mL with correlation coefficient (R) of 0.994. The recovery of sarafloxacin from serum ranged from $96.5 \pm 1.45\%$ to $104 \pm 0.76\%$. The limit of detection (LOD) and limit of quantitation (LOQ) were 0.01 and 0.02 μg/mL, respectively.

Protein binding

In vitro protein binding was determined using an ultracentrifugation method [24]. Sarafloxacin was added to blank plasma samples to produce concentrations of 0.1, 1 and 10 μg/mL. After 1 h incubation at 37 °C, 0.5 mL of each sample was placed in a Microcon YM-10 centrifugal filter device (Millipore, USA), and centrifuged at 1500 g for 20 min at 4 °C. Nonspecific binding of the drug to the ultrafiltration membrane was also determined. The drug concentrations in drug-free plasma samples and ultrafiltrate samples were determined as described above. The in vitro plasma protein binding of sarafloxacin was calculated using the following equation:

$$BP\% = [1 - C_U/C_T] \times 100\%$$

where C_U is the concentration in the ultrafiltrate, and C_T is the total drug concentration.

MIC, MBC and MPC

The MIC and MBC were determined in both Mueller Hinton Broth (MHB) and drug-free serum using a standard broth micro-dilution method [25]. MPC was determined as previously described with slight modifications [26]. A single colony was grown overnight in 10 mL MHB, and 1 mL of this culture was then transferred to 100 mL MHB for 24 h incubation. The culture was washed twice with PBS and centrifuged at 4000 g for 20 min at 4 °C. The precipitate was re-suspended in 10 mL of MHB to obtain a 10^{10} CFU/mL bacterial load. Aliquots of 100 μL were re-suspended and applied to MHA plates containing sarafloxacin at concentrations of 1× to 128× MIC. MPC was recorded as the lowest concentration that prevented bacterial growth after 72 h incubation.

Time-killing curves

In vitro time-killing curve experiments were conducted in MHB and blank serum using drug concentrations ranged from 0.25 × to 16 × MIC. Serum samples obtained at 0, 0.5, 1, 2, 4, 6, 8, 12 and 24 h post-p.o. administration were used to measure the ex vivo time-killing curves. The initial bacterial counts were about 10^6 CFU/mL. The 50 μL aliquot was diluted appropriately, and 100 μL of each dilution were applied onto MHA plates at 0, 3, 6, 9 and 24 h. All agar plates were incubated at 37 °C for 18 h. The limit of detection (LOD) was 100 CFU/mL.

PK analysis

Pharmacokinetic data were analyzed using the Winnonlin Program (version 5.1; Pharsight, St. Louis, MO, USA) based on a non-compartmental model. The bioavailability was estimated by the following equation:

$$F\% = AUC_{PO}/AUC_{IV} \times 100\%$$

where AUC_{PO} is the AUC after p.o. administration, and AUC_{IV} is the AUC after i.v. injection.

PK/PD integration and modeling

The PK/PD modeling was analyzed by the Sigmoid E_{max} model of Winnonlin Software. The equation was defined as:

$$E = E_{max} - (E_{max} - E_0) \times C^N/(C^N + EC_{50}{}^N)$$

Where E is the antibacterial effect. E_{max} is the $\log_{10}$ difference in bacterial counts between 0 and 24 h in the control sample. E_0 is the $\log_{10}$ difference in bacterial counts between 0 and 24 h in the sample containing sarafloxacin when the LOD of 100 CFU/mL is reached. C is the PK/PD indexes. EC_{50} is the PK/PD surrogate parameters producing 50% of the maximal antibacterial. N is the Hill coefficient which describes the slope of the sigmoid curves.

The PK/PD surrogate markers of antibacterial activity, including C_{max}/MIC, $AUC_{0\text{-}24h}$/MIC, C_{max}/MPC and $AUC_{0\text{-}24h}$/MPC, were determined using in vitro PD data and in vivo PK values post-i.v. and -p.o. administration of sarafloxacin. In this model, $AUC_{0\text{-}24h}$/MIC values were calculated according to the four levels of antibacterial effectiveness: a bacteriostatic action (i.e., no change in colony counts, $E = 0$), a 50% reduction in colony counts, a bactericidal action (i.e., a 99.9% reduction in bacterial counts, $E = -3$), and a bacterial elimination effect (i.e., a 99.99% reduction in bacterial counts, $E = -4$) [27].

Evaluation of dosage regimens

Optimal dosage providing a specific antibacterial effect was calculated using the following equation:

$$\text{Dose (per day)} = Cl_{(\text{per hour})} \times (AUC_{0\text{-}24h}/MIC) \times MIC/(F \times fu)$$

Where Cl is the clearance, $AUC_{0\text{-}24h}$/MIC is the ratio of the area under serum concentration-time curve over a 24 h period to MIC value achieved from PK/PD integration, F is the bioavailability, *fu* is the unbound fraction of sarafloxacin.

Statistical analysis

The PK and ex vivo PK/PD data are presented as mean ± SD. All the data are conducted using the SPSS 16.0 software package (SPSS Inc., Chicago, IL).

Results

Pharmacokinetic profiles

A Semi-logarithmic plot of serum concentrations of sarafloxacin following i.v. and p.o. administrations is presented in Fig. 1 and PK parameters calculated by Winnonlin using a non-compartmental model are shown in Table 1. Initial drug concentration in serum for i.v. injection was about 7.53 μg/mL, and it rapidly decreased to approximately 0.2 μg/mL at 12 h. For oral administration, a rapid absorption, with a time of peak concentration (T_{max}) of 0.44 ± 0.16 h, was observed and the C_{max} was 2.03 ± 0.73 μg/mL. The half-lives of elimination ($t_{1/2\beta}$) were 6.11 ± 1.97 and 8.21 ± 2.31 h

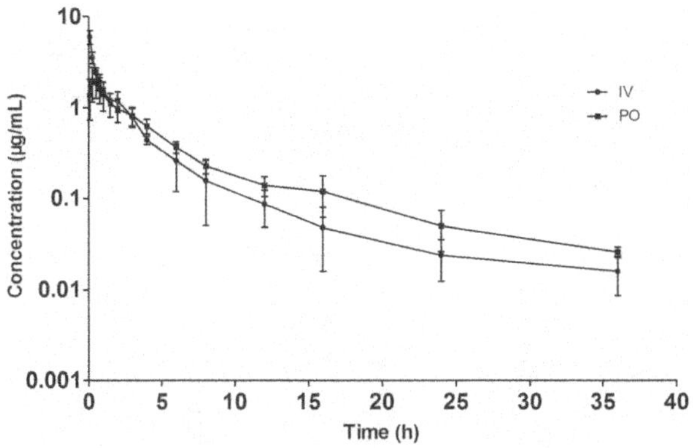

Fig. 1 Semi-logarithmic plot of serum concentrations *v.s.* time of sarafloxacin in Muscovy ducks ($n = 12$) following a single i.v. and p.o. administration at a single dose of 10 mg/kg BW. Bars represent standard deviations

following i.v. and p.o. administrations, respectively and the $AUC_{0\text{-}24h}$ were 8.43 ± 1.06 and 8.26 ± 1.08 μg · h/mL, respectively. Bioavailability (F%) for oral dosing route was 97.6 ± 5.32%. Drug concentrations of both routes of administration were below the LOD level at 48 h after a single dose of sarafloxacin in Muscovy ducks.

Protein binding

The percent of sarafloxacin recovery from ultrafiltration membrane exceeded 95%, suggesting that the ultrafiltration membrane had no specific adsorption of the drug. Table 2 shows the protein binding rates of sarafloxacin. Bound fraction of sarafloxacin ranged from 24.5 to 56.1% for drug concentrations varied from 0.1 to 10 μg/mL with a mean binding rate of 39.3%.

Table 1 Pharmacokinetic parameters of sarafloxacin after a single i.v. and p.o. administration at a dose of 10 mg/kg BW to Muscovy ducks ($n = 12$) using a non-compartmental model

Parameter	Unit	IV	PO
$T_{1/2\beta}$	h	6.11 ± 1.97	8.21 ± 2.31
T_{max}	h	—	0.44 ± 0.16
C_{max}	μg/mL	—	2.03 ± 0.73
$AUC_{0\text{-}24\ h}$	μg/mL · h	8.43 ± 1.06	8.26 ± 1.08
V_Z	L/kg	10.4 ± 3.32	—
Cl	L/kg · h	1.18 ± 0.16	—
V_Z/F	L/kg	—	14.1 ± 3.55
Cl/F	L/kg · h	—	1.21 ± 0.17
$MRT_{0\text{-}24\ h}$	h	4.17 ± 1.04	7.75 ± 1.86
F	%	—	97.6 ± 5.32

$T_{1/2\beta}$ elimination half-life, *AUC* area under the curve, T_{max} time for peak concentration, C_{max} peak concentration, V_Z/F apparent volume of distribution, *Cl/F* overall body clearance, *MRT* mean residence time, *AUMC* area under the moment curve, *F* bioavailability

Table 2 Plasma protein binding of sarafloxacin at three spiked levels

Spiked levels (μg/mL)	Protein binding rate (%)
0.1	56.1 ± 4.58
1	37.4 ± 2.07
10	24.5 ± 0.90

MIC, MBC and MPC values

The MIC, MBC and MPC of sarafloxacin are presented in Table 3. The MPC value for sarafloxacin was 1 μg/mL. The ratio of MBC/MIC was 2 μg/mL either in MH broth or in serum, and MPC/MIC value was 8 in MH broth medium.

Time-killing curves

In vitro time-killing curves of sarafloxacin against are shown in Fig. 2. Bacterial growth was inhibited obviously at drug concentration at 1 × MIC, but re-growth was observed after 9 h of incubation. However, the number of bacteria after incubation for 24 h was still below the initial load. For exposure at drug concentration at 2 × MIC, a bactericidal activity was observed in 24 h, but bacterial cells were not eradicated in the serum samples. When drug concentration was raised from 4 × to 16 × MIC, better antibacterial effectiveness was achieved, showing both bactericidal and eradication effect in 3 h of incubation.

Figure 3 shows the ex vivo time-killing curves, in which sarafloxacin concentrations in serum samples obtained at 0, 0.5, 1, 2, 4, 6, 8, 12 and 24 h after p.o. administration were 0, 2.22, 1.68, 1.32, 0.75, 0.37, 0.27, 0.13, and 0.04 μg/mL, respectively. A rapid bactericidal or elimination action was observed after 3 h of incubation and no re-growth was seen after 24 h for all serum samples collected between 0.5 and 6 h. A bacteriostatic action could be observed from serum samples collected at 8 h, whereas the serum sampling at 12 h and 24 h exhibited almost non-inhibitory effect.

Table 3 MIC, MBC and MPC values of sarafloxacin against *E. coli* O78 in MHB and serum medium

Parameter	Values (μg/mL)	Parameter	Values (μg/mL)
In MH broth		*In serum*	
MIC	0.125	MIC	0.25
MBC	0.25	MBC	0.5
MPC	1	MBC/MIC	2
MBC/MIC	2		
MPC/MIC	8		

MIC minimum inhibitory concentration, *MBC* minimum bactericidal concentration, *MPC* mutant prevention concentration, *MBC/MIC* ratio of in vitro MBC to MIC, *MPC/MIC* ratio of in vitro MPC to MIC

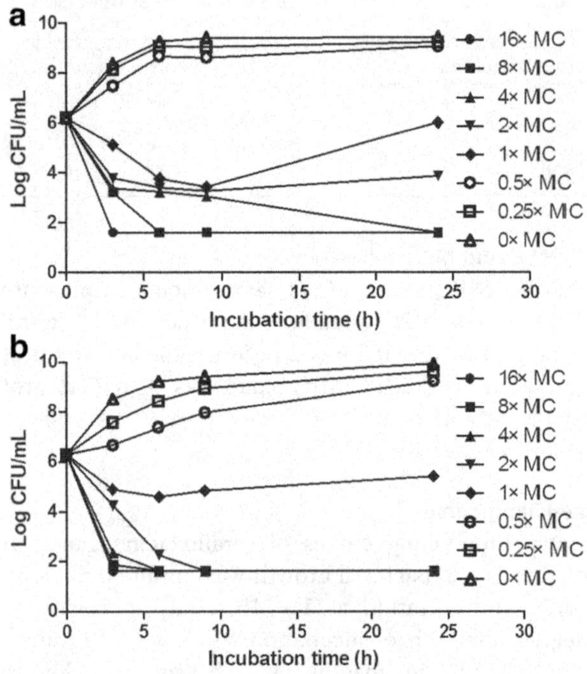

Fig. 2 In vitro time-kill curves of sarafloxacin against the *E. coli* O78 strain in serum (**a**) and MHB (**b**). Numerical values on the right represent sarafloxacin concentrations

PK/PD integration and modeling

PK/PD parameters from the study are summarized in Table 4. The values of $AUC_{0\text{-}24h}$/MIC and C_{max}/MIC were 33.4 ± 4.44 h and 8.12 ± 2.92. Table 5 shows the indexes of PK/PD integration from Sigmoid E_{max} model. The relationship between antibacterial effectiveness and PK/PD parameter of $AUC_{0\text{-}24h}$/MIC is exhibited in Fig. 4. The mean values of $AUC_{0\text{-}24h}$/MIC that produced bacteriostatic action, bactericidal activity and bacterial eradication effect were 25.4, 40.6 and 94.5 h, respectively.

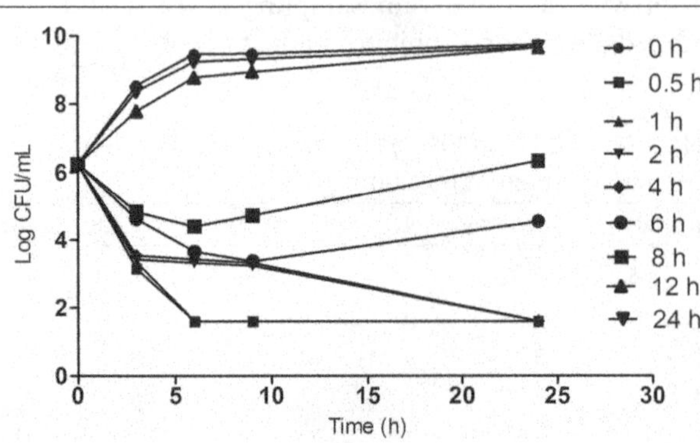

Fig. 3 Ex vivo time-kill curves of sarafloxacin against the *E. coli* O78 strain after p.o. administration of sarafloxacin at a dose of 10 mg/kg BW. Values are the means (*n* = 12) and the SD values are excluded for clarity

Table 4 Integration of PK/PD parameters of sarafloxacin against *E. coli* O78 after i.v. and p.o. administration (10 mg/kg) in ducks

Parameter	IV	PO
$AUC_{0\text{-}24\ h}$/MIC (h)	34.3 ± 4.72	33.5 ± 4.44
C_{max}/MIC	-	8.12 ± 2.92
$AUC_{0\text{-}24\ h}$/MBC (h)	17.2 ± 2.36	16.7 ± 2.23
C_{max}/MBC	-	4.06 ± 1.45
$AUC_{0\text{-}24\ h}$/MPC (h)	8.57 ± 1.18	8.37 ± 1.11
C_{max}/MPC	-	2.03 ± 0.73

Discussion

Sarafloxacin MICs in MHB or serum against the *E. coli* O78 strain used in this study were 0.125 ~ 0.25 μg/mL, which is moderate susceptible comparing with previous reports [14, 28]. In this study, a low ratio of MBC/MIC suggests that sarafloxacin has bactericidal activity against the *E. coli* O78 strain. In addition, the MPC/MIC ratio for sarafloxacin was in agreement with the values calculated for fluoroquinolones from previous reports [29].

In Muscovy ducks, sarafloxacin was rapidly and extensively distributed into body fluids and tissues after i.v. administration. A calculated distribution volume was 10.04 ± 3.32 L/kg, which is higher than that in broilers [15]. The $t_{1/2\beta}$ after i.v. injection of sarafloxacin was estimated to be 6.11 ± 1.97 h, much higher than those reported in pigs and chickens [15], and a slightly higher than that of marbofloxacin in ducks [30]. Therefore, a longer withdrawal time may be required in Muscovy ducks than in other food-producing animals for consideration of residue food safety concerns. A maximum concentration (C_{max}) of 2.03 ± 0.73 μg/mL following p.o. administration of sarafloxacin in this study was observed at 0.44 ± 0.16 h. Bioavailability was 97.6% in ducks, which was much higher than the previously reported values of 42.6% in pigs, 59.6% in chickens [15], but similar to that of marbofloxacin and moxifloxacin in ducks [30, 31], indicating a rapid and

Table 5 Parameters of PK/PD modeling based on ex vivo serum data after p.o. administration of sarafloxacin in muscovy ducks (*n* = 12)

Parameter	Unit	*E. coli* O78
Log E_0	CFU/mL	3.58 ± 0.27
Log E_0 − Log E_{max}	CFU/mL	8.31 ± 0.28
Slope(*N*)	—	3.42 ± 0.15
$AUC_{0\text{-}24\ h}$/MIC for bacteriostatic action	h	25.4 ± 1.68
$AUC_{0\text{-}24\ h}$/MIC EC_{50}	h	27.5 ± 1.86
$AUC_{0\text{-}24\ h}$/MIC for bactericidal action	h	40.6 ± 2.46
$AUC_{0\text{-}24\ h}$/MIC for bacterial eradication	h	94.5 ± 7.70

E_0: difference in bacterial count in control sample between time 0 and 24 h; E_{max}: difference in bacterial count in sample containing sarafloxacin between time 0 and 24 h, when limit of detection is reached; *N*: the Hill coefficient; $AUC_{0\text{-}24\ h}$/MIC EC_{50}: $AUC_{0\text{-}24\ h}$/MIC of drug producing 50% of the maximum antibacterial effect

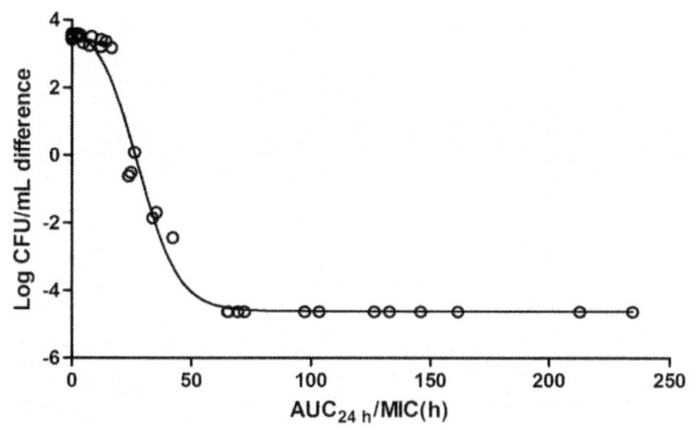

Fig. 4 Plots of the ex vivo $AUC_{0\text{-}24h}$/MIC ratios versus the difference of bacterial counts (log $_{10}$ CFU/mL) between 0 and 24 h for *E. coli* O78 strain

almost complete absorption following p.o. administration. Total body clearance was 1.18 L/kg/h, similarly to that in broilers [15]. The AUCs after i.v. and p.o. administrations were comparable with the results obtained from chickens and pigs [15].

It is recognized that only the unbound fraction of the drug has the antibacterial activity [27]. The plasma protein binding of sarafloxacin was 39.3%, consistent with previous reports [24]. Based on the time-killing curves, antibacterial activity of sarafloxacin against the *E. coli* strains was concentration-dependent. Similar to other fluoroquinolones and aminoglycosides, the ratios of $AUC_{0\text{-}24h}$/MIC and C_{max}/MIC were key PK-PD parameters correlating with clinical efficacy in target animals [3]. Attainment target of $AUC_{0\text{-}24h}$/MIC of 100–125 h or C_{max}/MIC of 8–10 should be obtained for fluoroquinolones in order to exert great bacteriological and treatment effects against Gram-negative bacterial pathogens; on the contrary, $AUC_{0\text{-}24h}$/MIC of 30 h should be achieved against Gram-positive pathogens [5, 32, 33]. However, optimal PK/PD endpoints for fluoroquinolones were not fixed dependent upon combinations of drug, pathogen and target species, as described in previous reports [16, 28]. Thus, appropriate endpoints of PK/PD parameters should be established for specific drug against specific pathogen in given target animal species. In the present study, the values of $AUC_{0\text{-}24h}$/MIC theoretically needed for bacteriostatic, bactericidal and eradication activity were calculated using the sigmoid E_{max} model. The value calculated for eradication activity against the *E. coli O78* strain (94.5 h) was smaller than the literature value of 125 h [32]. At a dosage of 10 mg/kg BW administered p.o., the in vivo $AUC_{0\text{-}24h}$/MIC ratio for the *E. coli* O78 strain (33.5 h) was slightly lower than the ex vivo $AUC_{0\text{-}24h}$/MIC ratio required for bactericidal action (40.6 h). These results indicated that the dosage of 10 mg/kg BW was not high enough to cure colibacillosis caused by *E. coli* O78 (MIC = 0.125 μg/mL). Thus, daily dosage regimens for sarafloxacin following p.o. administration to achieve bacteriostatic, bactericidal and eradicaton effects were calculated as 6.30, 10.1 and 23.6 mg/kg BW, respectively for dose optimization. Considering that sarafloxacin is concentration dependent antibiotic and convenience of clinical application, single dose administration daily is recommended.

As described in other previous reports [1, 6, 7], the MPC theory is also taken into consideration when optimizing the sarafloxacin dosage regimens in ducks. Traditional PK/PD modeling regards MIC and MBC as the major PD parameters; however, they may have only considered antibacterial activity against pathogenic population [1]. With the increasing of antimicrobial resistance, the MPC and mutant prevention window (MSW, defined as the concentration range between MIC and MPC in which the resistant mutants are selectively enriched [2]) have been used to evaluate antibacterial activity to prevent selection and development of antibacterial resistant mutants. The new PK/PD parameters, including $AUC_{0\text{-}24h}$/MPC, C_{max}/MPC and T > MPC, were used for the optimization of dosage regimens in the current study. In this study the values of $AUC_{0\text{-}24h}$/MPC and C_{max}/MPC (8.37 h and 2.03, respectively) for sarafloxacin against the *E. coli* O78 strain were comparable to the values (9.76 h and 1.26) obtained for enrofloxacin against *Pasteurella multocida* in buffalo calves [1] and the values (9.70 h and 1.40) obtained for marbofloxacin against *E. coli* [34]. According to previous reports, the values of $AUC_{0\text{-}24h}$/MPC of 9 to 12 h could prevent occurrence of resistant mutants for marbofloxacin against *E. coli* [35], which means average plasma concentration being 37.5 ~ 50% of MPC value can achieve a efficacy of preventing resistant mutants based on the dimensional perspective of AUC/MIC theory [36]. In order to cure diseased animals and control selection and development of drug resistance, the drug concentration in serum should exceed the MPC value as long as possible [7]. In this study, the value of T > MPC for sarafloxacin was 1.85 h, which was short due to high MPC. Similarly, $AUC_{0\text{-}24h}$/MPC and C_{max}/MPC from this study were lower than the values reported in literature for preventing the selection of resistant mutants. Therefore, the AUC/MPC of 8.37 h of sarafloxacin may be insufficient for preventing resistant mutant in the current work. Further study is needed to better understand the PK/PD characteristic for sarafloxacin, considering the interaction of drugs, pathogens and animal species.

Conclusions

To our knowledge, it is the first report about the PK/PD modeling study for sarafloxacin in Muscovy ducks targeting avian pathogenic *E. coli* O78 strain. Ex vivo PK/PD modeling and the MPC theory were used to optimize reasonable dosage regimens. Our findings suggested that a single dose of 10 mg/kg BW administered orally is insufficient to treat infection caused by *E. coli* O78 with an MIC of 0.125 or higher. In addition, a higher dose of sarafloxacin is needed to minimize occurrence of antimicrobial resistance with consideration of MPC theory.

Abbreviations
i.v.: Intravenous; LOD: Limit of detection; LOQ: Limit of quantification; MBC: Minimal bactericidal concentration; MIC: Minimal inhibitory concentration; MPC: Mutant prevention concentration; p.o.: Per os; PK/PD: Pharmacokinetics and pharmacodynemics

Acknowledgements
None.

Funding
This study was supported by Program for Changjiang Scholars and Innovative Research Team in University of Ministry of Education of China (Grant No. IRT13063) and the National Key Research and Development Program of China (2016YFD0501310).

Authors' contributions
YL, YZ and WS designed and conducted the experiment. JS and XL ran the simulations and analyzed the resulting data. YY drafted the manuscript. All authors read, revised, and approved the final manuscript.

Competing interests
The authors declare that they have no competing interests.

Consent for publication
Not applicable.

Author details
[1]National Risk Assessment Laboratory for Antimicrobial Resistance of Animal Original Bacteria, South China Agricultural University, Guangzhou 510642, China. [2]Guangdong Provincial Key Laboratory of Veterinary Pharmaceutics Development and Safety Evaluation, South China Agricultural University, Guangzhou 510642, China. [3]Laboratory of Veterinary Pharmacology, College of Veterinary Medicine, South China Agricultural University, Guangzhou, Guangdong 510642, China. [4]College of Veterinary Medicine, National Reference Laboratory of Veterinary Drug Residues, South China Agricultural University, Guangzhou 510642, China.

References

1. Balaje RM, Sidhu PK, Kaur G, Rampal S. Mutant prevention concentration and PK-PD relationships of enrofloxacin for Pasteurella multocida in buffalo calves. Res Vet Sci. 2013;95(3):1114–24.
2. Drlica K. The mutant selection window and antimicrobial resistance. J Antimicrob Chemother. 2003;52(1):11–7.
3. Craig WA. Pharmacokinetic/pharmacodynamic parameters: rationale for antibacterial dosing of mice and men. Clin Infect Dis. 1998;26(1):1–10. quiz 11-12.
4. Drusano GL. Prevention of resistance: a goal for dose selection for antimicrobial agents. Clin Infect Dis. 2003;36 Suppl 1:S42–50.
5. Toutain PL, del Castillo JR, Bousquet-Melou A. The pharmacokinetic-pharmacodynamic approach to a rational dosage regimen for antibiotics. Res Vet Sci. 2002;73(2):105–14.
6. Liang B, Bai N, Cai Y, Wang R, Drlica K, Zhao X. Mutant prevention concentration-based pharmacokinetic/pharmacodynamic indices as dosing targets for suppressing the enrichment of levofloxacin-resistant subpopulations of Staphylococcus aureus. Antimicrob Agents Chemother. 2011;55(5):2409–12.
7. Xu L, Wang H, Yang X, Lu L. Integrated pharmacokinetics/pharmacodynamics parameters-based dosing guidelines of enrofloxacin in grass carp Ctenopharyngodon idella to minimize selection of drug resistance. BMC Vet Res. 2013;9:126.
8. Zeng T, Jiang X, Li J, Wang D, Li G, Lu L, Wang G. Comparative proteomic analysis of the hepatic response to heat stress in Muscovy and Pekin ducks: insight into thermal tolerance related to energy metabolism. PLoS One. 2013;8(10):e76917.
9. Zhuang QY, Wang SC, Li JP, Liu D, Liu S, Jiang WM, Chen JM. A clinical survey of common avian infectious diseases in China. Avian Dis. 2014;58(2):297–302.
10. La Ragione RM, Sayers AR, Woodward MJ. The role of fimbriae and flagella in the colonization, invasion and persistence of Escherichia coli O78 : K80 in the day-old-chick model. Epidemiol Infect. 2000;124(3):351–363.
11. Dho-Moulin M, Fairbrother JM. Avian pathogenic Escherichia coli (APEC). Vet Res. 1999;30(2-3):299–316.
12. Ewers C, Janssen T, Wieler LH. Avian pathogenic Escherichia coli (APEC). Berl Munch Tierarztl Wochenschr. 2003;116(9-10):381–95.
13. Lutful Kabir SM. Avian colibacillosis and salmonellosis: a closer look at epidemiology, pathogenesis, diagnosis, control and public health concerns. Int J Environ Res Public Health. 2010;7(1):89–114.
14. Jones RN, Erwin ME. In vitro susceptibility testing and quality control parameters for sarafloxacin (a-56620): a fluoroquinolone used for treatment and control of colibacillosis in poultry. Quality control study group. Diagn Microbiol Infect Dis. 1998;32(1):55–64.
15. Ding HZ, Zeng ZL, Fung KF, Chen ZL, Qiao GL. Pharmacokinetics of sarafloxacin in pigs and broilers following intravenous, intramuscular, and oral single-dose applications. J Vet Pharmacol Ther. 2001;24(5):303–8.
16. Aliabadi FS, Lees P. Pharmacokinetics and pharmacokinetic/pharmacodynamic integration of marbofloxacin in calf serum, exudate and transudate. J Vet Pharmacol Ther. 2002;25(3):161–74.
17. Parshikov IA, Freeman JP, Lay Jr JO, Moody JD, Williams AJ, Beger RD, Sutherland JB. Metabolism of the veterinary fluoroquinolone sarafloxacin by the fungus Mucor ramannianus. J Ind Microbiol Biotechnol. 2001;26(3):140–4.
18. Haritova AM, Rusenova NV, Parvanov PR, Lashev LD, Fink-Gremmels J. Pharmacokinetic-pharmacodynamic modelling of danofloxacin in turkeys. Vet Res Commun. 2006;30(7):775–89.
19. Walker RD. The use of fluoroquinolones for companion animal antimicrobial therapy. Aust Vet J. 2000;78(2):84–90.
20. Products TEAftEoM, Unit VME: Committee for veterinary medicinal products saraflocaxin (Salmonidae) Summary Report (2). 1998, EMEA/MRL/349/98-FINAL February 1998.
21. The European Agency for the Evaluation of Medicinal Products Veterinary Medicines and Inspections. http://www.ema.europa.eu/docs/en_GB/document_library/EPAR_-_Scientific_Discussion/veterinary/000031/WC500062807.pdf. Accessed 14 Dec 2008.
22. Ho SP, Cheng CF, Wang WS. Pharmacokinetic and depletion studies of sarafloxacin after oral administration to eel (Anguilla anguilla). J Vet Med Sci. 1999;61(5):459–63.
23. Institute of Laboratory Animal Research CoLS, Council. NR. Guide for the care and use of laboratory animals. Washington, DC: National Academy Press; 1996.
24. Illambas J, Potter T, Cheng Z, Rycroft A, Fishwick J, Lees P. Pharmacodynamics of marbofloxacin for calf pneumonia pathogens. Res Vet Sci. 2013;94(3):675–81.
25. CLSI: Performance Standards for Antimicrobial Disk and Dilution Susceptibility Tests for Bacterial Isolated from Animals; Approved Standard-Fourth Edition and Supplement, VET01A4E and VET01S2E PA: Clinical and Laboratory Standards Institute 2013
26. Marcusson LL, Olofsson SK, Komp Lindgren P, Cars O, Hughes D. Mutant prevention concentrations of ciprofloxacin for urinary tract infection isolates of Escherichia coli. J Antimicrob Chemother. 2005;55(6):938–43.
27. Elias G, Lee JS, Hwang MH, Park YS, Cho KH, Kim YH, Park SC. Pharmacokinetics and pharmacokinetic/pharmacodynamic integration of orbifloxacin in Korean Hanwoo cattle. J Vet Pharmacol Ther. 2009;32(3):219–28.
28. Gebru E, Lee JS, Chang ZQ, Hwang MH, Cheng H, Park SC. Integration of pharmacokinetic and pharmacodynamic indices of orbifloxacin in beagle dogs after a single intravenous and intramuscular administration. Antimicrob Agents Chemother. 2009;53(7):3024–9.

29. Linde HJ, Lehn N. Mutant prevention concentration of nalidixic acid, ciprofloxacin, clinafloxacin, levofloxacin, norfloxacin, ofloxacin, sparfloxacin or trovafloxacin for Escherichia coli under different growth conditions. J Antimicrob Chemother. 2004;53(2):252–7.
30. Yuan L, Wang R, Sun L, Zhu L, Luo X, Sun J, Fang B, Liu Y. Pharmacokinetics of marbofloxacin in Muscovy ducks (Cairina moschata). J Vet Pharmacol Ther. 2011;34(1):82–5.
31. Goudah A, Hasabelnaby S. Pharmacokinetics, plasma protein binding and bioavailability of moxifloxacin in Muscovy ducks after different routes of administration. Res Vet Sci. 2010;88(3):507–11.
32. Lees P, Aliabadi FS. Rationalising dosage regimens of antimicrobial drugs: a pharmacological perspective. J Med Microbiol. 2000;49(11):943–5.
33. Papich MG. Pharmacokinetic-pharmacodynamic (PK-PD) modeling and the rational selection of dosage regimes for the prudent use of antimicrobial drugs. Vet Microbiol. 2014;171(3-4):480–6.
34. Gebru E, Choi MJ, Lee SJ, Damte D, Park SC. Mutant-prevention concentration and mechanism of resistance in clinical isolates and enrofloxacin/marbofloxacin-selected mutants of Escherichia coli of canine origin. J Med Microbiol. 2011;60(Pt 10):1512–22.
35. Ferran A, Dupouy V, Toutain PL, Bousquet-Melou A. Influence of inoculum size on the selection of resistant mutants of Escherichia coli in relation to mutant prevention concentrations of marbofloxacin. Antimicrob Agents Chemother. 2007;51(11):4163–6.
36. Toutain PL, Bousquet-Melou A, Martinez M. AUC/MIC: a PK/PD index for antibiotics with a time dimension or simply a dimensionless scoring factor? J Antimicrob Chemother. 2007;60(6):1185–8.

Iron-regulated gene *ireA* in avian pathogenic *Escherichia coli* participates in adhesion and stress-resistance

Yaxin Li, Jianjun Dai, Xiangkai Zhuge, Haojin Wang, Lin Hu, Jianluan Ren, Ling Chen, Dezhi Li and Fang Tang*

Abstract

Background: Avian pathogenic *Escherichia coli* (APEC) causes avian colibacillosis, which results in economic and welfare costs in the poultry industry worldwide. The pathogenesis of avian pathogenic *E. coli* strains is not well defined. Here, the function of an outer membrane protein encoded by the *ireA* gene of avian pathogenic *E. coli* strain DE205B was investigated.

Results: The *ireA* gene was distributed in 32.9 % (46/140) of tested *E. coli* strains, with high percentages in the phylogenetic ECOR groups B2 (58.8 %, 10/17) and D (55.9 %, 19/34). The gene expression level of *ireA* of APEC strain DE205B in high Fe M9 media was 1.8 times higher ($P < 0.05$) than that in low Fe M9 media. An *ireA* deletion mutant and complementary strain were constructed. Compared with the wild-type strain DE205B, the expression of most ferric uptake genes in the *ireA* deletion mutant were significantly upregulated ($P < 0.05$). The adhesion ability of the *ireA* deletion mutant to DF-1 cells was significantly decreased. The survival rate of *ireA* deletion mutant was reduced 21.17 % ($P < 0.01$), 25.42 ($P < 0.05$) and 70.0 % ($P < 0.01$) under alkali, high osmolarity, and low temperature (4 °C) conditions, respectively, compared with the wild-type strain.

Conclusions: The results suggested that the protein encoded by the iron-regulated gene *ireA* has roles in adhesion and stress resistance in avian pathogenic *E. coli*.

Keywords: APEC, *IreA*, Virulence, Adhesion, Stress resistance

Background

Avian pathogenic *Escherichia coli* (APEC), a subgroup of extra-intestinal pathogenic *E. coli* (ExPEC) causes avian colibacillosis and imposes economic losses on the poultry industry worldwide [1]. However, the pathogenesis of APEC is poorly understood. Many virulence genes have been studied to identify virulence factors in APEC, including those involved in adhesion, iron-regulation, toxin/cytotoxin production and serum resistance [2]. Iron is an essential element involved in important biological processes [3]. Biological activities in cells, such as peroxide reduction, nucleotide biosynthesis and electron transport, are facilitated by iron ions [4]. Extra-intestinal sites have low iron contents; therefore, ExPEC strains struggle to take up iron from the host during infection [5]. During natural infection, the initiation, progression and transmission of most bacterial infections depend on the ability of the invading pathogen to acquire iron from the complicated environment [6]. During iron acquisition, the cell must produce transmembrane receptors for siderophores that chelate iron ions [7]. There are various receptors that chelate iron ions encoded by bacterial genes, such as *chuA*, the *SitABCD* system, *iron*, *iha*, *iutA*, and *ireA*. Outer membrane protein ChuA participates in heme acquisition in enterohemorrhagic *E. coli* and uropathogenic *E. coli* (UPEC) strains, and is important for the pathogenicity of APEC [8, 9]. The *SitABCD* system, identified in the APEC strain MT512 by comparative genomic analysis, was reported to be associated with the pathogenicity of APEC [9, 10].

IreA was suggested to be involved in Fe acquisition and to act as an iron-regulated virulence gene in the blood- or urine-derived ExPEC *E. coli* isolated from

* Correspondence: tangfang@njau.edu.cn
Key Laboratory Animal Bacteriology, Ministry of Agriculture, College of veterinary medicine, Nanjing Agricultural University, No.1 Weigang, Nanjing 210095, Jiangsu province, People's Republic of China

humans [11]; however, its exact role in APEC strains remains unknown. Herein, an *ireA* deletion mutant was constructed to study the *ireA* gene function in the APEC strain DE205B.

Results

Prevalence of the *ireA* gene among *E. coli* Strains

As shown in Table 1, *ireA* was present in 32.9 % (46/140) of *E. coli* strains, with 19.0 % (12/63) in phylogenetic ECOR group A, 19.2 % (5/26) in B1, 58.8 % (10/17) in B2 and 55.9 % (19/34) in group D (Additional file 1: Table S1). Thus, the *ireA* gene was significantly more frequently distributed in the B2 and D groups than in the A and B1 groups.

Expression of the *ireA* gene

The *ireA* gene expression was tested by Immunoblotting. Western blotting was performed with anti-His serum, showing expected fusion protein bands for *ireA* (39 kDa) from strains DE205B. However, only fusion his protein (18 kDa) was detected from the blank plasmid control (Fig. 1). These results indicated that *ireA* was expressed under laboratory conditions.

Gene expression of *ireA* in M9 media with different iron content

The relative gene expression of *ireA* in low Fe M9 media was 1.8 times higher than that in high Fe M9 media ($P < 0.01$) (Fig. 2).

Growth curve

The CFU of the wild-type strain DE205B, mutant strain DE205BΔ*ireA* and the complementary strain DE205BCΔ*ireA* was monitored for 12 h. There was no significant difference between the growth curves of the wild-type and mutant strains (Fig. 3), which indicated that deletion of *ireA* had no effects on the growth of DE205B.

Expression variations of Ferric uptake system and adherence genes

The expressions of *fepC, feoB, chuT, fyuA, irp1, irp2, chuA* and *fepA* were detected in the mutant and compared with their expressions in the wild-type strain DE205B. Most of the ferric uptake genes in the mutant strain DE205BΔ*ireA*, except *irp1, irp2* and *chuA*, were significantly upregulated ($P < 0.05$) (Fig. 4). *Irp1, irp2* and *chuA* were non-significantly upregulated. Furthermore, the expressions of the eight ferric uptake genes in the complementary strain DE205BCΔ*ireA* were restored to wild-type levels.

The expression of adherence genes *yfcO, yfcQ, aufG, fmlD, fmlE, yadN* and *fimH* showed no significant difference between the wild-type strain DE205B and the *ireA* mutant strain (Fig. 5).

Table 1 Distribution of the *ireA* gene in *Escherichia coli* strains

ECOR group	Strain counts	Strain counts positive for *ireA*	Percentage
A	63	12	19.0 %
B1	26	5	19.2 %
B2	17	10	58.8 %
D	34	19	55.9 %
Total	140	46	32.9 %

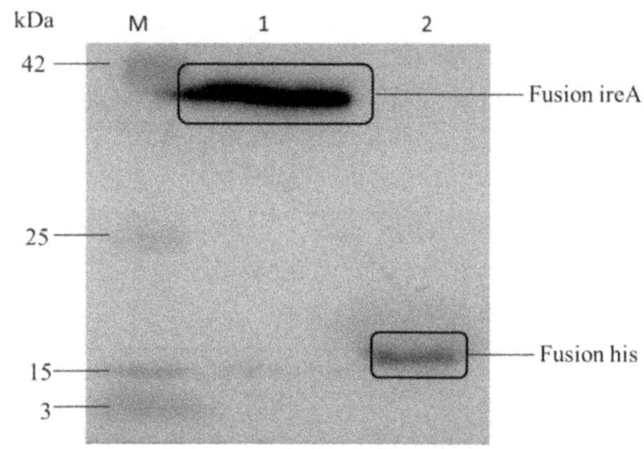

Fig. 1 Expression of *ireA* by western blotting. Expression of fusion *ireA* protein was detected by immunoblotting. Fusion *ireA* was detected in pET32a(+), while there is only his protein was detected in the blank plasmid. Lane M, protein marker; lane 1, fusion *ireA*; lane 2, fusion his

Adherence assays

The number of mutant DE205BΔ*ireA* bacteria adhering to DF-1 cells was significantly decreased compared with

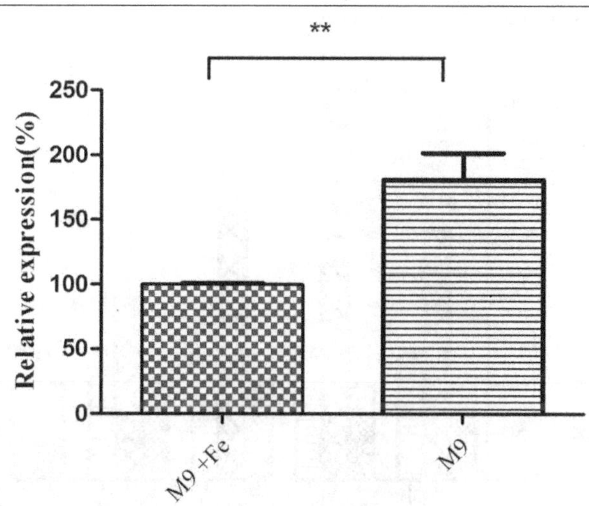

Fig. 2 Expression of *ireA* in M9 media. The first and second columns represent the relative gene expressions of *ireA* in M9 media with low and high Fe content, respectively. The gene expression levels showed significant differences in the two kinds of media ($P < 0.01$)

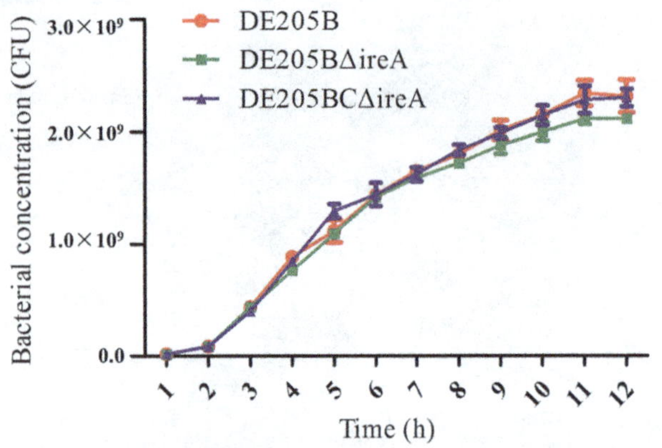

Fig. 3 Growth curve of different strains. Growth curves of the wild-type strain DE205B, mutant strain DE205BΔ*ireA* and complementary strain DE205BCΔ*ireA*. Bacterial growth was estimated by plate counting as Colony Forming Units (CFU)

the number of DE205B wild-type adherent cells ($P < 0.05$) (Fig. 6). The adhesion to DF-1 cells of complementary strain DE205BCΔ*ireA* was partly restored to wild-type levels.

Animal infection

The LD_{50} of the wild-type, deletion mutant and complementary strains were 1.74×10^5, 2.45×10^5, and 3.16×10^5, respectively (Table 2). The results showed that there was no significant difference between the LD_{50} of the wild-type and deletion mutant strains, indicating that the deletion of *ireA* gene has no obvious effect on the virulence of DE205B toward ducks.

Determination of resistance to environmental stress

Compared with the wild-type strain, the survival rate of the *ireA* deletion mutant was reduced by 21.17 % ($P < 0.01$) and 25.42 % ($P < 0.05$) under alkali and high osmolarity conditions, respectively (Fig. 7). The resistance to alkali and high osmolarity conditions of the complementary strain DE205BCΔ*ireA* was almost restored to wild-type levels. For the temperature challenge, compared to the wild type strain, the *ireA* deletion mutant was reduced 70.0 % ($P < 0.01$) under the low (4 °C) temperature (Fig. 8). The resistance to low temperature of the complementary strain DE205BCΔ*ireA*was partly restored. The results showed that presence of the *ireA* gene increased the stress-resistance of APEC strain DE205B.

Discussion

The *ireA* gene is an iron-regulated gene and is involved in iron acquisition in human pathogenic *E. coli* isolates and our study proved this protein functions in APEC. Additionally, we identified two new functions of *ireA* using the deletion mutant. In the present study, *ireA* was demonstrated to contribute to the adhesion to DF-1 cells. Moreover, the expressions of several adhesion genes were tested and the results showed no significant differences between wild-type and mutant strain, indicating that the *ireA* gene indeed plays a role in adhesion. Tarr et al., identified adhesin Iha from an O157:H7 strain of *E. coli* [12]. This adhesin shared high similarities with several identified or putative siderophore receptors. Siderophore receptor IrgA was reported to contribute to growth in the rabbit ileal loop model *in vivo* and to enhance virulence in an infant mouse model, suggesting a possible role in colonization [13, 14]. Here, we proved that iron-regulated gene *ireA* plays a role in the adhesion of APEC strains. The *ireA* gene also increased stress-resistance under alkali and high osmolarity conditions, as well as underlow temperature. Thus, the

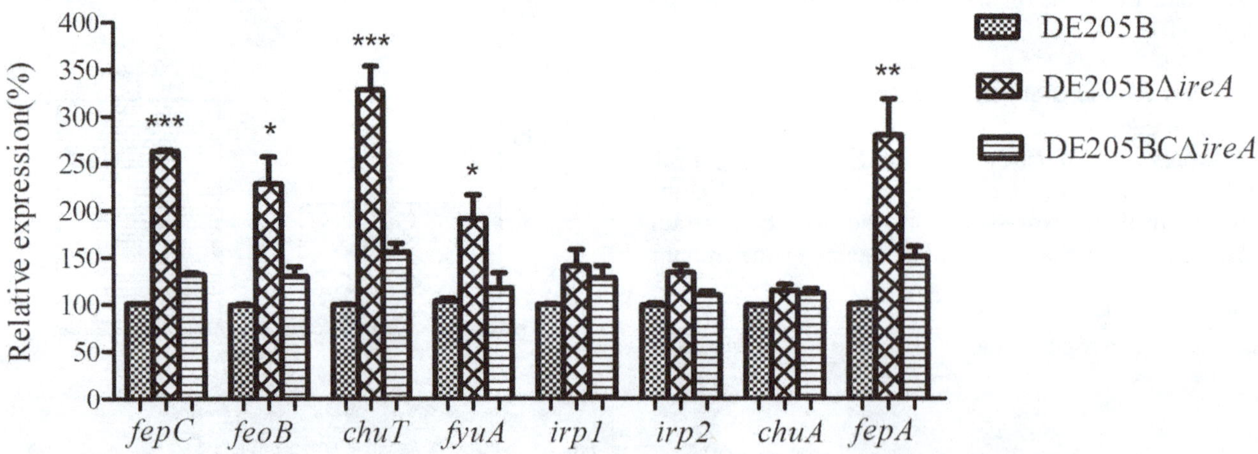

Fig. 4 Expressions of Fe acquisition genes. Expressions of Fe acquisition genes of the wild-type strain DE205B, mutant strain DE205BΔ*ireA* and complementary strain DE205BCΔ*ireA* were tested by qPCR. The relative expression levels in the different mutant strains were calculated using the $2^{-\Delta\Delta Ct}$ method

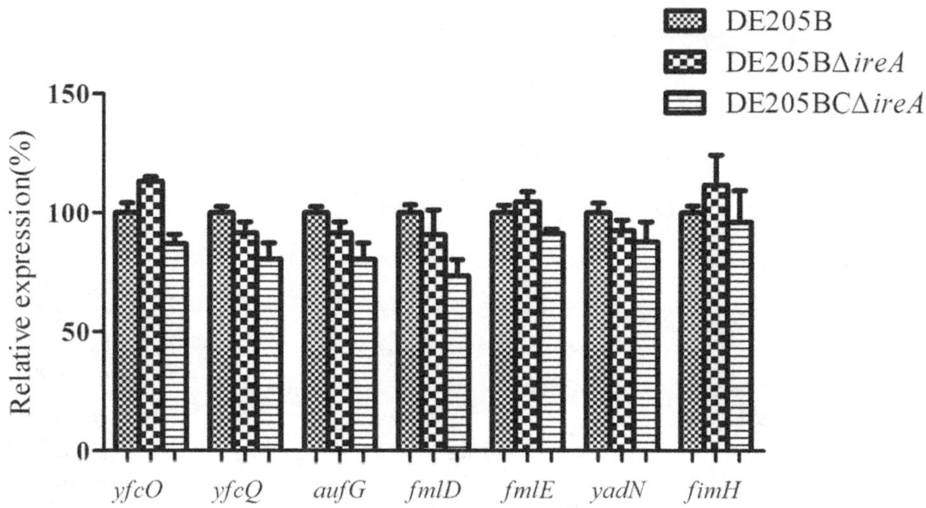

Fig. 5 Expressions of adhesion genes. Expressions of adhesion genes, including *yfcO, yfcQ, aufG, fmlD, fmlE, yadN* and *fimH*, of the wild-type strain DE205B, mutant strain DE205BΔ*ireA* and complementary strain DE205BCΔ*ireA* were tested by qPCR. The relative expression levels in the different mutant strains were calculated using the $2^{-\Delta\Delta Ct}$ method

redundancy of siderophore receptors might reflect their multifunctional roles.

E. coli strains were reported to be classified into four main phylogenetic groups (A, B1, B2, and D) [15]. Virulent ExPEC strains mainly belong to phylogroup B2 and D, whereas most commensal strains belong to phylogroup A [16]. The *ireA* gene was distributed more frequently in the B2 (58.8 %) and D (55.9 %) groups than in the A (19 %) and B1 (19.2 %) groups, indicating that *ireA* might be associated with the virulence of the APEC strain DE205B. Thus, the result correlated with that Russo's report: *ireA* was detected in 13 (26 %) of 50 random clinical isolates from patients and in none (0 %) of 14 fecal isolates, which presumably represented commensal strains [11]. Taken together, these results indicated that *ireA* might be a virulence gene in both human and avian ExPEC *E. coli* strains.

The expression level of *ireA* in DE205B was decreased in high Fe M9 media compared with that in low Fe media, indicating that *ireA* is involved in iron-regulation in this APEC strain. This result agreed with the report of Russo et al., who found that *ireA* was a iron-regulated virulence gene in the blood- or urine-derived isolates of ExPEC *E. coli* [11]. Most ferric uptake genes, such as *fepC, feoB, chuT, fyuA* and *fepA* were upregulated in the *ireA* deletion mutant strain. This might represent a compensatory function for *ireA* gene deletion. Fe acquisition is important for many microorganisms, especially for pathogens that grow in the host, which attempts to limit Fe availability. It is thought that pathogens harbor

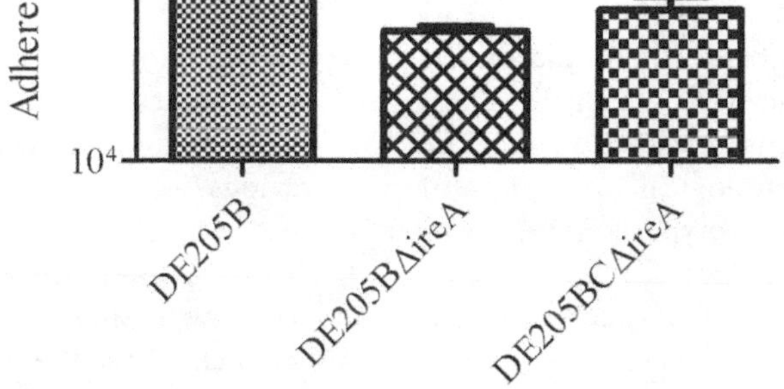

Fig. 6 Adherence assays. The adhesion abilities of the wild-type strain DE205B, mutant strain DE205BΔ*ireA* and complementary strain DE205BCΔ*ireA* to DF-1 cells were tested. The numbers of adherent cells were calculated by plate counting. The number of DE205BΔ*ireA* mutant bacteria adhering to DF-1 cells was significant decreased compared with the number of DE205B wild-type bacteria ($P < 0.05$)

Table 2 LD_{50} of wild-type and mutant strains

Challenge dose (CFU/ml)	Duck mortality		
	DE205B	DE205BΔ*ireA*	DE205BCΔ*ireA*
10^8	7/7	7/7	7/7
10^7	7/7	7/7	7/7
10^6	6/7	6/7	6/7
10^5	3/7	2/7	1/7
LD_{50}	1.74×10^5	2.45×10^5	3.16×10^5

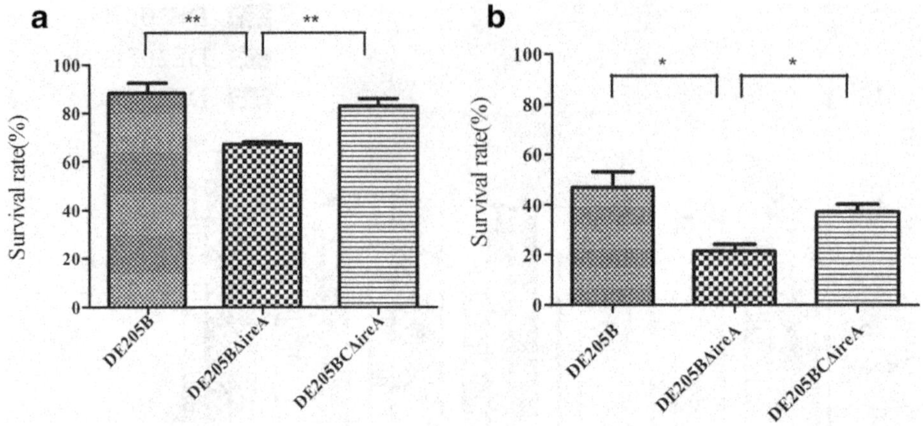

Fig. 7 Resistance to alkaline and high osmolarity. The resistance to alkali (**a**) and high osmolarity (**b**) of wild-type strain DE205B, mutant strain DE205BΔ*ireA* and complementary strain DE205BCΔ*ireA* was tested by exposing the strains to alkaline and high osmolarity conditions and calculating their survival rates. Compared with the wild-type strain, the survival rate of the *ireA* deletion mutant was reduced 21.17 % ($P < 0.01$) and 25.42 ($P < 0.05$) under alkaline and high osmolarity conditions, respectively

multiple Fe acquisition systems to ensure that Fe is gained from the host cells to provide a selective advantage. Alternatively, certain siderophores, and their cognate receptors, might be more active in certain environments, such as inside or outside the gastrointestinal tract [17, 18]. Moreover, multiple systems might represent 'alternatives' that protect against the disruption of one system caused by genomic rearrangements or mutations.

In the duck infection experiments, the LD_{50} showed no significant difference between the wild-type DE205B and the *ireA* deletion mutant strain. Thus, it seemed that *ireA* deletion had no obvious effect on the virulence of DE205B. However, DE205B has several Fe acquisition systems. We showed that most of the other Fe acquisition genes were upregulated in the *ireA* gene deletion mutant. Thus, the *ireA* gene might indeed contribute to the virulence of the APEC strain DE205B, while other Fe acquisition genes displayed compensatory functions when the *ireA* gene was deleted.

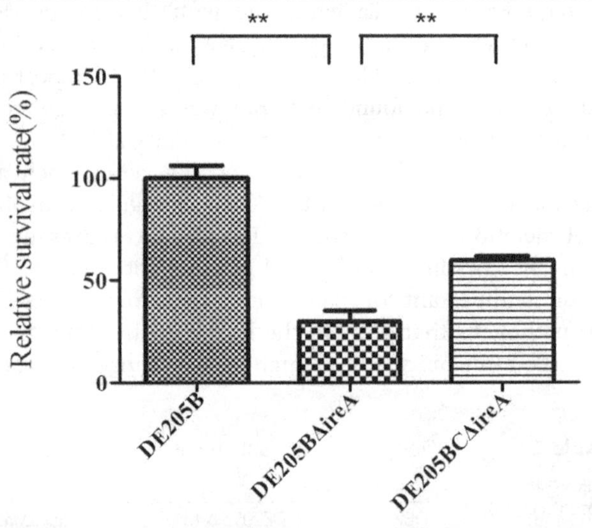

Fig. 8 Challenge under the low temperature of different strains. Each bacterial suspension with concentration of 10^7 CFU/ml (DE205B, DE205BΔ*ireA* or DE205BCΔ*ireA*) were incubated at 4 °C for 7days. The survival rates of wild-type and mutant strains were calculated by plate counting and compared using GraphPad Prism 5. The *ireA* deletion mutant was reduced 70.0 % ($P < 0.01$) under the low (4 °C) temperature compared to that of the wild type strain

Conclusions

In summary, the *ireA* gene was mainly distributed in the more virulent phylogenetic ECOR group B and D. Compared with the wild-type strain, the adhesion and resistance to environmental stress of the *ireA* deletion mutant were significant decreased. This indicated that *ireA* is a Fe iron-regulated gene that aids adhesion and stress-resistance in the APEC strain DE205B.

Methods

Bacterial strains, plasmids and growth conditions

The APEC strain DE205B, which was characterized previously, was isolated from the brain of a duck with neurological symptoms in our previous work [19–22]. Its serotype is O2:K1, which is one of the predominant serotypes of APEC [9, 23]. All *E. coli* strains were grown in Luria-Bertani (LB) medium at 37 °C with shaking or on LB plates with 2 % agar. When necessary, the LB medium was supplemented with appropriate antibiotics: ampicillin (Amp; 100 μg/mL) and kanamycin (Kan; 50 μg/mL), unless otherwise specified. Information on the main strains and plasmids used in this study are listed in Table 3. M9 minimal medium was used to assess the expression of *ireA*, which was prepared as

Table 3 Bacterial strains and plasmids used in the present study

Strain or plasmid	Characteristics	Reference
Strain		
DE205B	O2:K1, NalR	[16, 19]
DE205BΔ*ireA*	*ireA* deletion mutant strain	This study
DE205BCΔ*ireA*	*ireA* complementary strain	This study
Plasmid		
pKD46	Amp, express λ red recombinase	[29]
pKD4	kan, template plasmid	[29]
pSTV28	Cm, expression using lac promotor	TAKARA
pCP20	Cm, Amp, yeast Flp recombinase gene, FLP	[29]

follows: an aliquot was mixed with200 ml of 5 × M9 salt solution (containing$Na_2PO_4 \cdot 7\ H_2O$, 12.8 g; KH_2PO_4, 3.0 g; NaCl, 0.5 g; NH_4Cl, 1.0 g;),2 ml of 1 M $MgSO_4$, 20 ml of 20 % glucose solution, 0.1 ml of1 M $CaCl_2$, and then dissolved in1000 ml double distilled water andfiltrated through a 0.22-μm membrane.

Prevalence of *ireA* among *E. coli* Strains

The distribution of *ireA* among 140 *E. coli* strains (Additional file 1: Table S1) maintained in our laboratory was tested using PCR. The PCR primers were designed using Primer Premier 5. The specific primers *ireA*-F and *ireA*-R are listed in Table 4. The PCR conditions were: 5 min at 95 °C for initial denaturing; 30 cycles of 1 min at 95 °C, 30 s at 50 °C and 1 min at 72 °C; followed by 10 min at 72 °C for extension. The DNA of DE205B and ddH_2O were used as positive and negative templates, respectively. The PCR products were electrophoresed through 1 % agarose gels. Phylogenetic *E. coli* reference (ECOR) groups of single isolates of the 140 *E. coli* strains were determined using triplex PCR, as described previously [16, 24].

Expression of the *ireA* gene

The expression of the *ireA* gene was tested by fusion expression and western blotting as previously reported [25, 26]. The fusion fragment of *ireA* (including the *ireA* promoter and 579bp of *ireA* sequence) and His tag were inserted into plasmid pET32a(+). The fusion PCR primers P1 and P2 were listed in Table 4. Plasmid pET32a(+) without the fusion fragment was used as a blank control. For immunoblotting, protein samples were subjected to sodium dodecylsulfate polyacrylamide gel electrophoresis (SDS-PAGE) and transferred to polyvinylidene fluoride membranes (Amersham Pharmacia Biotech, Piscataway, NJ, USA), as described previously [27]. Anti-His serum was the primary antibody, horseradish peroxidase-conjugated goat anti-mouse IgG was the secondary antibody and 3,3′-diaminobenzidine was used as the substrate.

Regulation of *ireA* expression in M9 media

M9 minimal medium was used to assess the expression of *ireA*.M9 medium or M9 medium with Fe (0.1 mM $Fe(NO_3)_3$) were used as low and high Fe content media, respectively. DE205B was cultured in both M9 media to the mid-log phase and the expression of *ireA* was detected by quantitative real-time reverse transcription PCR(qRT-PCR). The real –time PCR primers were designed by PrimerQuest Tool IDT (http://sg.idtdna.com/primerquest/Home/Index). Briefly, total RNA was extracted from 1 ml of bacteria culture using the Trizol RNA isolation protocol (Invitrogen, Shanghai, China) and cDNA was amplified by reverse transcription according to the instructions of the primeScript RT reagent Kit (Takara). Quantitative real-time PCR (qPCR) was carried out using the ABI Prism 7300 and Sequence Detection System software version 1.4 (Applied Biosystems, Foster City, CA, USA), according to the instructions of the SYBR Premix Ex Taq (Takara, Dalian, China). QPCR primers for *ireA* (Q*ireA*-F and Q*ireA*-R) are listed in Table 4. *DnaE* was used as a reference gene. Assays were performed three times. The relative expressions of *ireA* in different media were calculated using the $2^{-\Delta\Delta Ct}$ method [28]. Statistical analysis was performed using an unpaired *t* test in Graphpad Prism 5.0.

Construction of the *ireA* deletion mutant and complementary strain

An *ireA* knockout strain of DE205B was constructed using the lambda red recombinase system described by Datsenko and Wanner [29]. The specific primers *ireA*Mu-F and *ireA*Mu-R were designed to amplify the target gene *ireA*. The kanamycin resistance gene, which contained sequences homologous to the 5′ and 3′ ends of the target sequence, was amplified using plasmid pKD4 as a template. The PCR products were then transformed by electroporation into DE205B containing the lambda red recombinase expression plasmid pKD46. The transformed bacterial cells were first incubated at 30 °C for 2 h in super optimal broth with catabolite repression (SOC) broth, and then grown on LB agar containing kanamycin at 37 °C. Mutants were confirmed by PCR and sequenced using primers k1 and k2 (Table 4) in combination with primers *ireA*-1 and *ireA*-2 (Table 4) flanking the *ireA* region. To remove the kanamycin resistance gene, plasmid pCP20 was transformed into the mutant and a kanamycin sensitive mutant strain was selected. Finally, the *ireA* deletion mutant strain without kanamycin resistance was named as DE205Bδ*ireA* (Additional file 2: Figure S1).

To construct the complementary strain, the *ireA* gene, including its putative promoters, was amplified using primers *ireA*Co-F and *ireA*Co-R (Table 4). The following amplification program were used: 5 min at 95 °C for

Table 4 Primers used in the present study

Primers	Primer sequence (5′–3′)	Gene	Reference
ireA-F	AGATACGCTTGTTGTTAC	*ireA*	This study
ireA-R	CATTCCATGCTGCTAC		
ireAMu-F	GTAAATTCCCTCTTTGCTAACGCAAATCATTATC ATTACGCCTTTGGCAAAGGGAAATTTGTGTAGG CTGGAGCTGCTTCGA	Upstream region of *ireA*	This study
ireAMu-R	CATTACTGATTACTACACTGGTACCTGAGGCTC ACGGCCTCAGGTTGTCTTTATATACTCCATATGA ATATCCTCCTTAG	Downstream region of *ireA*	
ireA-1	TACTCCCCATCCCCGGGCAA	*ireA*	This study
ireA-2	GGGGGCAGCAATATCCGGTG		
k1	CAGTCATAGCCGAATAGCCT	*kanR*	[27]
k2	CGGTGCCCTGAATGAACTGC		
ireACo-F	TACGGATCCCTGAACAATAGCGAT	*ireA*	This study
ireACo-R	GCTAAGCTTTTACAACCTGGAAAC		
QireA-F	AAACATGGGATGGCGTACTT	*ireA*	This study
QireA-R	AATCAATGGGCCTGACAGATAG		
QFeoB-F	GCACTCTTTGTGCATGGTATTC	*FeoB*	This study
QFeoB-R	TGGCAGCACGGTGTTAAT		
QfepA-F	CAATGCGCCAGAACATAAAGAG	*fepA*	This study
QfepA-R	TGTCGAGGTTGCCATACAAG		
QfepC-F	TCGTTACGCCAGCCATTT	*fepC*	This study
QfepC-R	TGCAGCGCAGACCATAAA		
QfyuA-F	ATGCCTATGTGGGATGGAATG	*fyuA*	This study
QfyuA-R	CCAGTCATCGGTGGTGTATTT		
Qirp1-F	GGCGAACCCTGCTATGTATT	*irp1*	This study
Qirp1-R	GTCCATGCAGTACCAGCTAAA		
Qirp2-F	GCGGCTGATTACCAACAATTAC	*irp2*	This study
Qirp2-R	CTGGATCAGGTTGCTCTCTTC		
QChuA-F	TAGGCCACATCAAGGCTAAAC	*ChuA*	This study
QChuA-R	CGGCGACAACTATGTCGTATAA		
QdnaE-F	ATGTCGGAGGCGTAAGGCT	*dnaE*	This study
QdnaE-R	TCCAGGGCGTCAGTAAACAA		
P1	TTGCCGGAATTCTCAGGGGGCCA GTCTACTGAATGAG	fusion *ireA*	This study
P2	ACCGTCGTCGACTTAGTGATGATGATGAT GATGAGAACCATACAGGGAAGACATAGGG		
QyfcO-F	TGCATAACTCGTCATGTCCTGTCTCCGTTG	*yfcO*	This study
QyfcO-R	AGCGTTTTCTCAATCGTTCCGCCCGTC		
QyfcQ-F	CCTGCATTTCTACGGCAATTTAC	*yfcQ*	This study
QyfcQ-R	CGGTCACCATCAGGTCTTTAC		
QaufG-F	TGCTCTGGCAACATCAGTAG	*aufG*	This study
QaufG-R	ACTAACAGGTAAAGTCAGGAAAGT		
QfmlD-F	CAGGCTCCCTACAGTCATATAAAG	*fmlD*	This study
QfmlD-R	TCGGTGTCTTATCACCAATATCC		
QfmlE-F	CAGTGCCAGACAATTTCCAAC	*fmlE*	This study
QfmlE-R	CCGTTAAATGCAACCTGAACTC		

Table 4 Primers used in the present study *(Continued)*

QyadN-F	CCACTGTTAATGGCGGTGTA	*yadN*	This study
QyadN-R	TTTAGCCAGGCGAGAAGAAC		
QfimH-F	CTTATGGCGGCGTGTTATCT	*fimH*	This study
QfimH-R	CGGCTTATCCGTTCTCGAATTA		

initial denaturing; 35 cycles of 30 s at 95 °C, 30 s at 55 °C and 2.5 min at 72 °C; 10 min at 72 °C for extension. The PCR product of *ireA* gene was purified and subcloned into plasmid pSTV-28. The complementary strain DE205BCΔ*ireA* was generated by transforming vector pSTV-28-*ireA* into the deletion mutant (Additional file 3: Figure S2).

Growth curve

The growths of the DE205B wild-type and mutant strains were compared in LB medium at 37 °C over a course of 12 h, starting at 10^7 CFU/ml. Bacterial growth was estimated by plate counting as Colony Forming Units (CFU). Assays were performed three times.

The expression of the Ferric uptake system and adherence genes

The effect of *ireA* deletion on the regulation of the ferric uptake system, including *fepC, feoB, chuT, fyuA, irp1, irp2, chuA* and *fepA* was detected using qRT- PCR. Seveal adherence genes, including *yfcO, yfcQ, aufG, fmlD, fmlE, yadN* and *fimH* were also selected to test their expression levels. The wild-type DE205B and the *ireA* deletion mutant were cultured in LB to mid-log phase and total RNA was extracted from 1 ml of bacterial culture using the Trizol RNA isolation protocol (Gibco BRL, USA, cat. no.15596-026). cDNA was reverse transcribed and real-time PCR was carried out as described above. The qRT-PCR primers for the ferric uptake system and adherence genes are listed in Table 4. The real-time PCR primers were designed unsing PrimerQuest Tool IDT (http://sg.idtdna.com/primerquest/Home/Index). The relative expression levels of the genes were calculated using the $2^{-\Delta\Delta Ct}$ method [28]. Assays were performed three times, and the statistical analysis was performed using an unpaired *t* test in Graphpad Prism 5.0. On the figures, error bars indicate the standard deviation.

Adherence assays

The adherence assay was performed as described previously [24]. Briefly, chicken embryo fibroblast (CEF) DF-1 cells were seeded at approximately 1×10^5 cells per well in 24-well tissue culture trays (TPP, Shanghai, China) and grown in Dulbecco's modified Eagle medium (DMEM) with 10 % fetal bovine serum at 37 °C in a 5 % CO_2 humidified atmosphere without antibiotics. DF-1 cells were washed once with DMEM and then inoculated with 500 ul of 2×10^7 CFU/ml bacteria per well for 2 h at 37 °C in the presence of 5 % CO_2. The cells were washed, lysed with ddH_2O, and the number of bacterial cells was calculated by plate counting. In all assays, wells only containing DF-1 cells were used as negative controls. The adherence assays were conducted three times. The statistical analysis was performed using an unpaired *t* test in Graphpad Prism 5.0.

Animal infections

Animal infections were performed as described previously [19, 20]. We purchased 7-day-old ducklings and young duck feeds from Anhui Poultry Farm (Anhui, China). Bacterial strains were cultured to the exponential phase, harvested, washed three times in PBS and then adjusted to the appropriate doses. Twenty-five 7-day-old ducks were inoculated intramuscularly 0.2 ml of each bacterial suspension (DE205B, DE205BΔ*ireA* or DE205BCΔ*ireA*) at four concentrations (5×10^8 CFU/ml, 5×10^7 CFU/ml, 5×10^6 CFU/ml, and 5×10^5 CFU/ml). Assays were performed three times. Seven ducks were used for each dose. Seven ducks were injected with PBS as a negative control. Death of the ducks was monitored for 7 days post infection. We calculated the LD_{50} of each strain using the method described by Spearman-Karber [30].

Determination of resistance to environmental stress

Resistance to environmental stress was tested for the wild-type and the mutant strain, as described by La Ragione et al. [31]. Bacteria were cultured in LB broth overnight and harvested by centrifugation. The cells were resuspended in PBS and adjusted to 10^7 CFU/ml in PBS. For alkali challenge, 100 μl of adjusted cells were mixed with 100 μl Tris buffer (1 M, pH10.0) and 800 μl ddH_2O (final concentration, 100 mM, pH10.0) and incubated at 37 °C for 30 min. For high osmolarity endurance, cells were mixed with an equal volume of 4.8 M NaCl (final concentration, 2.4 M) and incubated at 37 °C for 1 h. Bacteria were exposed to PBS (pH 7.0) as a control.

Temperature challenge was performed as previously described with modifications [32], each bacterial suspension, at a concentration of 10^7 CFU/ml (DE205B, DE205BΔ*ireA* or DE205BCΔ*ireA*) was incubated at 4 °C for 7days. Assays were performed three times. The survival rates of wild-type and mutant strains were calculated by plate counting and compared using GraphPad Prism 5.

Additional files

Additional file 1: Table S1. Detailed information about the distribution of the *ireA* gene in APEC strains.

Additional file 2: Figure S1. Technical routes of construction of the *ireA* deletion mutant.

Additional file 3: Figure S2. Technical routes of construction of the *ireA* complementary strain.

Acknowledgements
Authors are grateful to all of the staff at Key Laboratory Animal Bacteriology of Nanjing Agricultural University for helping conduct the experiments.

Funding
This work was supported by grants from the National Basic Research Program of China (2015CB554203), the Fund of Priority Academic Program Development of Jiangsu Higher Education Institutions (PAPD), the Fundamental Research Funds for the Central Universities (KYZ201326), the Youth Foundation of the National Natural Science Foundation of China (No.31402213), the Natural Science Foundation of Jiangsu Province, China (No. BK20140686).

Authors' contributions
YL carried out the gene deletion and adhesion assays, as well as expression of *ireA* gene, JD carried out the tests of resistance to environmental stress, XZ, HW and LH carried out the animal infections, JR, LC, DL carried out the qPCR and gene prevelance tests. FT responsible for the growth curve, whole exprements design and draft of the manuscript. All authors read and approved the final manuscript.

Competing interests
The authors declare that they have no competing interests.

Consent to publish
Not applicable.

References
1. Dziva F, Hauser H, Connor TR, van Diemen PM, Prescott G, Langridge GC, Eckert S, Chaudhuri RR, Ewers C, Mellata M, et al. Sequencing and functional annotation of avian pathogenic Escherichia coli serogroup O78 strains reveal the evolution of E. coli lineages pathogenic for poultry via distinct mechanisms. Infect Immun. 2013;81(3):838–49.
2. Dissanayake DR, Octavia S, Lan R. Population structure and virulence content of avian pathogenic Escherichia coli isolated from outbreaks in Sri Lanka. Vet Microbiol. 2014;168(2–4):403–12.
3. Garenaux A, Houle S, Folch B, Dallaire G, Truesdell M, Lepine F, Doucet N, Dozois CM. Avian lipocalin expression in chickens following Escherichia coli infection and inhibition of avian pathogenic Escherichia coli growth by Ex-FABP. Vet Immunol Immunopathol. 2013;152(1–2):156–67.
4. Heinemann IU, Jahn M, Jahn D. The biochemistry of heme biosynthesis. Arch Biochem Biophys. 2008;474(2):238–51.
5. Gao Q, Wang X, Xu H, Xu Y, Ling J, Zhang D, Gao S, Liu X. Roles of iron acquisition systems in virulence of extraintestinal pathogenic Escherichia coli: salmochelin and aerobactin contribute more to virulence than heme in a chicken infection model. BMC Microbiol. 2012;12:143.
6. Kouse AB, Righetti F, Kortmann J, Narberhaus F, Murphy ER. RNA-mediated thermoregulation of iron-acquisition genes in Shigella dysenteriae and pathogenic Escherichia coli. PLoS One. 2013;8(5):e63781.
7. Pilarczyk-Zurek M, Chmielarczyk A, Gosiewski T, Tomusiak A, Adamski P, Zwolinska-Wcislo M, Mach T, Heczko PB, Strus M. Possible role of Escherichia coli in propagation and perpetuation of chronic inflammation in ulcerative colitis. BMC Gastroenterol. 2013;13:61.
8. Nagy G, Dobrindt U, Kupfer M, Emody L, Karch H, Hacker J. Expression of hemin receptor molecule ChuA is influenced by RfaH in uropathogenic Escherichia coli strain 536. Infect Immun. 2001;69(3):1924–8.
9. Li G, Laturnus C, Ewers C, Wieler LH. Identification of genes required for avian Escherichia coli septicemia by signature-tagged mutagenesis. Infect Immun. 2005;73(5):2818–27.
10. Schouler C, Koffmann F, Amory C, Leroy-Setrin S, Moulin-Schouleur M. Genomic subtraction for the identification of putative new virulence factors of an avian pathogenic Escherichia coli strain of O2 serogroup. Microbiology. 2004;150(Pt 9):2973–84.
11. Russo TA, Carlino UB, Johnson JR. Identification of a new iron-regulated virulence gene, ireA, in an extraintestinal pathogenic isolate of Escherichia coli. Infect Immun. 2001;69(10):6209–16.
12. Tarr PI, Bilge SS, Vary Jr JC, Jelacic S, Habeeb RL, Ward TR, Baylor MR, Besser TE. Iha: a novel Escherichia coli O157:H7 adherence-conferring molecule encoded on a recently acquired chromosomal island of conserved structure. Infect Immun. 2000;68(3):1400–7.
13. Goldberg MB, DiRita VJ, Calderwood SB. Identification of an iron-regulated virulence determinant in Vibrio cholerae, using TnphoA mutagenesis. Infect Immun. 1990;58(1):55–60.
14. Tashima KT, Carroll PA, Rogers MB, Calderwood SB. Relative importance of three iron-regulated outer membrane proteins for in vivo growth of Vibrio cholerae. Infect Immun. 1996;64(5):1756–61.
15. Herzer PJ, Inouye S, Inouye M, Whittam TS. Phylogenetic distribution of branched RNA-linked multicopy single-stranded DNA among natural isolates of Escherichia coli. J Bacteriol. 1990;172(11):6175–81.
16. Clermont O, Bonacorsi S, Bingen E. Rapid and simple determination of the Escherichia coli phylogenetic group. Appl Environ Microbiol. 2000;66(10): 4555–8.
17. Bearden SW, Perry RD. The Yfe system of Yersinia pestis transports iron and manganese and is required for full virulence of plague. Mol Microbiol. 1999; 32(2):403–14.
18. Tsolis RM, Baumler AJ, Heffron F, Stojiljkovic I. Contribution of TonB- and Feo-mediated iron uptake to growth of Salmonella typhimurium in the mouse. Infect Immun. 1996;64(11):4549–56.
19. Wang S, Niu C, Shi Z, Xia Y, Yaqoob M, Dai J, Lu C. Effects of ibeA deletion on virulence and biofilm formation of avian pathogenic Escherichia coli. Infect Immun. 2011;79(1):279–87.
20. Wang S, Xia Y, Dai J, Shi Z, Kou Y, Li H, Bao Y, Lu C. Novel roles for autotransporter adhesin AatA of avian pathogenic Escherichia coli: colonization during infection and cell aggregation. FEMS Immunol Med Microbiol. 2011;63(3):328–38.
21. Zhuge X, Wang S, Fan H, Pan Z, Ren J, Yi L, Meng Q, Yang X, Lu C, Dai J. Characterization and functional analysis of AatB, a novel autotransporter adhesin and virulence factor of avian pathogenic Escherichia coli. Infect Immun. 2013;81(7):2437–47.
22. Wang S, Shi Z, Xia Y, Li H, Kou Y, Bao Y, Dai J, Lu C. IbeB is involved in the invasion and pathogenicity of avian pathogenic Escherichia coli. Vet Microbiol. 2012;159(3–4):411–9.
23. Blanco JE, Blanco M, Mora A, Jansen WH, Garcia V, Vazquez ML, Blanco J. Serotypes of Escherichia coli isolated from septicaemic chickens in Galicia (northwest Spain). Vet Microbiol. 1998;61(3):229–35.
24. Dai J, Wang S, Guerlebeck D, Laturnus C, Guenther S, Shi Z, Lu C, Ewers C. Suppression subtractive hybridization identifies an autotransporter adhesin gene of E. coli IMT5155 specifically associated with avian pathogenic Escherichia coli (APEC). BMC Microbiol. 2010;10:236.
25. Urban JH, Vogel J. Translational control and target recognition by Escherichia coli small RNAs in vivo. Nucleic Acids Res. 2007;35(3):1018–37.
26. Wu Z, Wu C, Shao J, Zhu Z, Wang W, Zhang W, Tang M, Pei N, Fan H, Li J, et al. The Streptococcus suis transcriptional landscape reveals adaptation mechanisms in pig blood and cerebrospinal fluid. RNA. 2014; 20(6):882–98.

27. Wang S, Bao Y, Meng Q, Xia Y, Zhao Y, Wang Y, Tang F, ZhuGe X, Yu S, Han X, et al. IbeR facilitates stress-resistance, invasion and pathogenicity of avian pathogenic Escherichia coli. PLoS One. 2015;10(3):e0119698.
28. Ali-Benali MA, Alary R, Joudrier P, Gautier MF. Comparative expression of five Lea Genes during wheat seed development and in response to abiotic stresses by real-time quantitative RT-PCR. Biochim Biophys Acta. 2005; 1730(1):56–65.
29. Datsenko KA, Wanner BL. One-step inactivation of chromosomal genes in Escherichia coli K-12 using PCR products. Proc Natl Acad Sci U S A. 2000; 97(12):6640–5.
30. Fung KP, Wong TW. Estimation of quantal dose response of drugs by the Spearman-Karber method: a computer program written in BASIC. J Singapore Paediatr Soc. 1989;31(3–4):129–32.
31. La Ragione RM, Sayers AR, Woodward MJ. The role of fimbriae and flagella in the colonization, invasion and persistence of Escherichia coli O78:K80 in the day-old-chick model. Epidemiol Infect. 2000;124(3):351–63.
32. McLeod A, Mage I, Heir E, Axelsson L, Holck AL. Effect of relevant environmental stresses on survival of enterohemorrhagic Escherichia coli in dry-fermented sausage. Int J Food Microbiol. 2016;229:15–23.

12

Characterization and susceptibility of streptococci and enterococci isolated from Nile tilapia (*Oreochromis niloticus*) showing septicaemia in aquaculture and wild sites in Egypt

Kamelia M. Osman[1*], Khalid S. Al-Maary[2], Aymen S. Mubarak[2], Turki M. Dawoud[2], Ihab M. I. Moussa[2], Mai D. S. Ibrahim[3], Ashgan M. Hessain[4], Ahmed Orabi[1] and Nehal M. Fawzy[5]

Abstract

Background: The present investigation was an endeavor into the elucidation of the disease-causing pathogen of streptococcosis in Nile tilapia (*Oreochromis niloticus*) in Egypt affecting adult fish cultured and wild fish in the Nile river. Fish were obtained from commercial fishermen, collected as part of their routine fishing activities. The researchers observed the routine fishing process and selected fish for use in the study, at the point of purchase from the fisherman.

Results: Diseased fish showed exophthalmia with accumulation of purulent and haemorrhagic fluid around eyes, and ventral petechial haemorrhages. The Post mortem examination revealed, abdominal fat haemorrhage, pericarditis and enlargement of the liver, spleen and kidney. Gram-stained smears revealed the presence of Gram-positive cocci, β-hemolytic, oxidase and catalase negative. Analysis of the 16S rRNA gene confirmed that the 17 tilapia isolates studied were 6/17 *Enterococcus faecalis,* 2/17 *Enterococcus gallinarum,* 3/17 *Streptococcus pluranimalium,* 2/17 *Aerococcus viridans,* 1/17 isolate of each *Streptococcus dysgalactiae, Streptococcus anginosus, Lactococcus garvieae* and *Granulicetella elegans/Leuconostoc mesenteroides cremoris*. It should be noted that there was no mixed infection. Multiple resistance was observed and the most frequent antibiotic combination was penicillin, ampicillin, vancomycin, chloramphenicol, rifampicin, ofloxacin, clindamycin, erythromycin and tetracycline representing eight classes.

Conclusions: Consequently, we concluded that *Streptococcus* species are an emerging pathogen for Nile tilapia aquaculture in Egypt and to be considered as a new candidate in the warm water fish diseases in Egypt with special reference to *L. garvieae, S. dysgalactiae* in addition to *L. mesenteroides cremoris* which was not reported before from tilapia and taking into consideration their zoonotic implications for public health.

Keywords: *Streptococcus* species, Tilapia (*Oreochromis* spp.), Lancefield C, *L. Garvieae, S. Dysgalactiae, L. Mesenteroides cremoris*, Antibiotic resistance

* Correspondence: kamelia-osman@hotmail.com
[1]Department of Microbiology, Faculty of Veterinary Medicine, Cairo University, Giza, Egypt
Full list of author information is available at the end of the article

Background

The common name Nile tilapia (*Oreochromis niloticus*) is a species of Tilapia (*Oreochromis* sp.) which in turn is the regular name for about a hundred species of cichlid fish from the tilapiine cichlid lineage [1]. They are freshwater fish species, local to Africa and Middle East areas [2], and the third biggest group of bony fish. Delineations from Egyptian tombs underscored that Nile tilapia have been developed for more than 4000 years [3]. By the second half from the twentieth century, tilapia were brought into a myriad of tropical, sub-tropical and mild locales of the globe [4] becoming a standout asset amongst the most refined fish species adding to the global nourishment in the fish industry [5] where the sustenance of more than half a billion people in the Third World are supported by fisheries and aquaculture [6]. The market price of farmed tilapia boosted up from 154 million USD in 1984 to 4000 million USD in 2010 [7]. China, with a production capacity of 806,000 MT represents almost 50% of the total global production positioned itself as the largest Nile tilapia producer, with Egypt to follow with 200,000 MT, the Philippines with 111,000 MT, Thailand with 97,000 MT and Indonesia with 72,000 MT. Five other countries come next in their capacity for Nile tilapia production, The Lao People's Democratic Republic, Costa Rica, Ecuador, Colombia and Honduras [8]. Also, although significant quantities of tilapia are also produced annually by Cuba, Israel, Malaysia, the USA, Viet Nam and Zimbabwe, yet it should be noted that, their production is reported to FAO as 'tilapias nei' (which may include other tilapia species) and 'freshwater fishes nei' [8].

Streptococcosis is a worldwide threat and epidemiological studies revealed 500 streptococcal isolates in more than 50 sites in 13 countries (http://www.thefishsite.com/articles/190/streptococcus-in-tilapia/#sthash.G4T0XzsI.dpuf). Streptococcosis, also known as 'pop-eye', is contagious with high mortality and has assumed its importance due to being the most crushing threat as it can bring about huge number of deaths of large size fish causing heavy commercial losses in Australia, Israel, Italy, Japan, Korea, South Africa, Colombia, Indonesia and USA [9, 10]. The global commercial losses estimated to reach 250 million USD in 2008 [11]. Within 3 to 7 days, acute *Streptococcus* infections in fish induce >50% mortality rates [12] while chronic infections the mortalities could extend to several weeks, with a daily death of one or two of the fish. In most cases, the clinical symptoms of *Streptococcus* infection, with no species differences (http://www.thefishsite.com/articles/190/streptococcus-in-tilapia/#sthash.G4T0XzsI.dpuf), is usually in the form of lethargic, erratic swimming (spiraling or spinning swimming), dark skin pigmentation, exophthalmia with opacity and haemorrhage in the eye, abdominal distension, diffused haemorrhage in the operculum, around the mouth, anus and base of the fins and enlarged blackened spleen [8, 10, 13–15].

Streptococcosis is not limited to geographic boundaries or/and host range causing a global flare-up in aquaculture farms [16]. A diversity of fish species are susceptible to infection, including sturgeon, various ornamental fish, including rainbow sharks, red-tailed black sharks, rosey barbs, danios, some cichlids including Venustus (*Nimbochromis* ("Haplochromis") *venustus*) and *Pelvicachromis* sp. and several species of tetras, coho salmon, yellowtail (*Seriola quinqueradiata*), Jacopever *(Sebastes schlegeli*), salmonids, Japanese eel (*Anguilla japonica*), ayu and tilapia (*Oreochromis* spp.), striped bass (*Morone saxatilis*), Atlantic croaker (*Micropogon undulatus),* blue fish (*Pomatomus saltatrix*), channel cat fish, golden shiner (*Notemigonous chrysoleuca*), hardhead (sea) cat fish (*Arius felis*), menhaden (*Brevoortia patronus*), pin fish (*Lagodon rhomboides*), sea trout (*Cynoscion regalis*), silver trout (*Cynoscion nothus*), spot (*Leiostomus xanthurus*), stingray (*Dasyatis* sp.), striped bass (*Morone saxatilis*), striped mullet (*Mugil cephalus*) and turbot (*Scophthalmus maximus*) [17, 18].

The most relevant *Streptococcus* species that cause disease in the tilapia farming globally are *S. iniae, S. agalactiae, S. dysgalactiae* and *Lactococcus garviae* [19, 20]. Since the first description of a streptococcal infection in rainbow trout (*Oncorhynchus mykiss*) [21], the diversity and the inherent characteristics of the bacterial species incriminated with streptococcosis was debatable [9, 17]. High and low temperatures affect the virulence agents at which streptococcosis is induced [22]. Warm water streptococcosis implicates species such as *L. garvieae* (synonym *E. seriolicida*), *S. iniae* (synonym *S. shiloi*), *S. agalactieae* (synonym *S. difficilis*) or *S. parauberis* inducing mortalities at temperatures above 15 °C. Differently, *Vagococcus salmoninarum* or *L. piscium* and *S. phocae* are incriminated in cold water streptococcosis at temperatures below 15 °C. The ability of *S. phocae* to cause cold water streptococcosis was evident when researchers were able to isolate it from marine mammals inhabiting cold waters, including Cape fur seal (*Arctocephalus pusillus pusillus*), ringed seal (*Phoca hispida*) and harbor porpoise (*Phocoena phocoena*) and gray seal (*Halichoerus grypus*), harbor seal (*Phoca vitulina*) and cetaceans [9, 10]. Pathogenic fish *Streptococcus* species have been associated with *S. agalactiae, S. difficilis, S. dysgalactiae, S. equi, S. equisimilis, S.* (= *E.*) *faecium, S. ictaluri, S. iniae, S. milleri, S. parauberis, S. phocae, S. pyogenes* and *S. zooepidemicus.* In addition, *E. faecalis* NCTC 775 T, *E. faecium* NCTC 7171 T, *L. lactis* NCFB 604, *S. mutans* NCFB 2062 provoke streptococcosis in Atlantic salmon and rainbow trout [9, 17].

Zoonotically, streptococcicosis is of great significance to delineate the infectious etiology of streptococcosis in Nile tilapia as a potential cause of disease in humans [16, 17] which caused a significant increase in the use of antibiotics in aquaculture. The present investigation was an endeavor into the elucidation of the disease-causing pathogen of streptococcosis in Nile tilapia (*O. niloticus*) in Egypt affecting adult fish cultured and wild fish in the Nile river by studying the phenotypic, antibiotic resistance and molecular characterization of the streptococcal strains isolated from Nile tilapia demonstrating septicemia.

Methods

Fish sampling

Fish were obtained from commercial fishermen, collected as part of their routine fishing activities. The researchers observed the routine fishing process and selected fish for use in the study, at the point of purchase from the fisherman the fish were deceased and as such no ethical approval was required for this study. A total number of 80 Nile tilapia were collected as freshly dead or moribund fish (Fig. 1a-d) presenting at least one or more of the clinical signs of septicaemia (eye lesions: in the form of unilateral or bilateral eye redness/opacity, skin lesions: detached scales, extensive skin congestion, ulcers, hemorrhage, or dark discoloration in the form of strips, fins: congestion at the base of fins, or even hemorrhages, abdomen: slightly distended in some cases, anal opening: congested protruded anal opening) were collected from different locations in Egypt (River Nile in Giza, Kafr Elzayat, Bani-sweif and a breeding farm at El-Tal El-Kebir) during the period 2013–2014. Selection of locations and farms from which the diseased fish were collected depended on their availability at time sampling, accessibility and proximity. After collection, the sampled fish were placed in expanded polystyrene boxes, covered with a plastic film, transported refrigerated to the laboratory and processed for microbiological analysis within 3 h in order to detect *Streptococcus* spp.. Septicaemic fish samples were submitted to the Fish Disease Department, Animal Health Research Institute, Dokki, Egypt.

Isolation and phenotypic characterization of bacteria

The swabs from the fish matrix that were collected (liver, kidney, brain, spleen and ascitic fluid) were immediately streaked onto Columbia agar supplemented with 5% defibrinated sheep blood (CBA) (Oxoid Ltd., Basingstone, England) plates and incubated at 30 °C for 24 h in 5% CO2 atmosphere. Suspected colonies were picked, purified and subjected to phenotypic differential analysis by conventional procedures by their morphological, physiological and biochemical plate and tube tests and in addition to the Gram-positive identification (GPI) cards of the Vitek 2 system (bioMérieux, France) which was

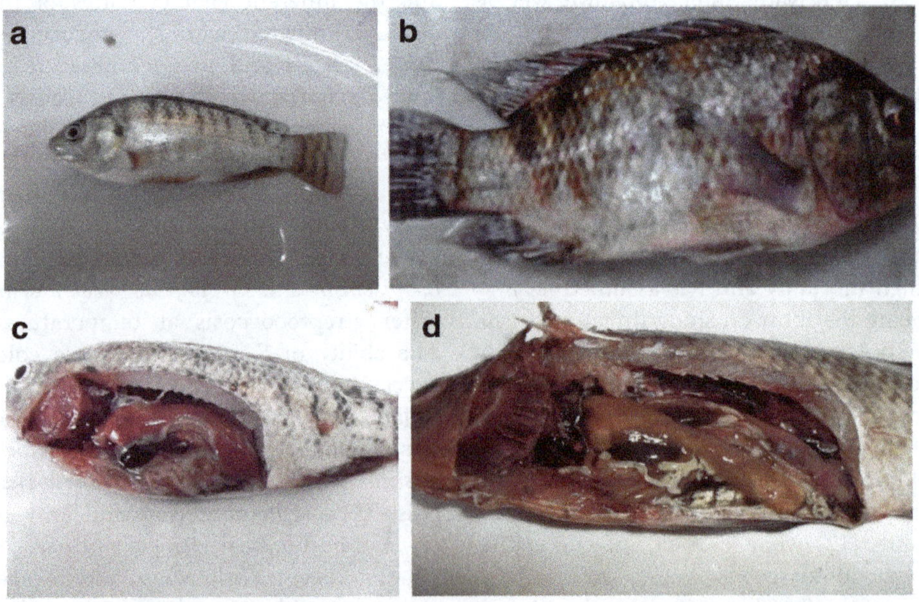

Fig. 1 **a** Body shape of Tilapia fish laterally compressed to oval. Lateral line interrupted with cycloid scales. Caudal fin has distinct vertical stripes and strong body vertical bands. Healthy transparently clear and spherical eye lenses. Normal glistening skin with no pathological lesions observed. **b** Tilapia fish showing externally eye redness, hemorrhage and ulcers on different parts of the body, hemorrhagic dorsal and tail fins, extensively detached scales and distended abdomen with signs of bleeding beneath the skin appearing as small dots the size of a pinprick or as a patch. **c** Shows normal appearance of Tilapia fish with normal liver, kidney, gall bladder and intestines with bright red gills. **d** Tilapia fish postmortum internal findings revealed tipical signs of septicemia in which severely congested gill, kidney, spleen, intestine and heart, dark gall bladder, in addition to hemorrhagic ascites, friable pale liver, muscle redness, and parts of the intestine were devoid of food

used following the manufacturer's instructions. The ability of the strains to grow at 10 and 45 °C was tested in Brain-heart infusion medium over a period of 10 days.

Preparation of genomic DNA and genetic characterization

The suspected *Streptococcus* isolates were cultured in Todd Hewitt Broth at 25 C for 24 h, and genomic DNA was extracted using the Qiagen Genomic-tip 500/G kit (Qiagen, Hilden, Germany) according to the manufacturer's instructions. DNA concentration was estimated spectrophotometrically before use. The extracted DNA was used in the process of amplification of the 16S rRNA gene of the *Streptococcus* species -specific isolates with a pair of specific primers for each species using polymerase chain reaction (PCR) as outlined in Table 1. Seven µl of the amplified products was electrophoresed using 1.0% (*w*/*v*) agarose gel in 1× TBE electrophoresis buffer (0.1 mM Tris/HCI, 0.1 mM boric acid, 0.002 mM EDTA, pH 8.3). The gel was stained with GelRed Nucleic Acid Gel Stain. A negative control (no template DNA) and positive controls consisting of *E. gallinarum* ATCC 49673, *E. faecalis* ATCC 19433, *L. garvieae* ATCC 43921, *S. pluranimalium* ATCC 700864^{T}, *A. viridans* ATCC 11536 T (accession no. M58797), *S. anginosus* ATCC33397 were included in each run.

Serological assays

The Lancefield streptococcal group of the isolated strains was identified using the Oxoid Streptococcal Grouping Kit DR0585 (Oxoid Ltd., Basingstone, England) following the manufacturer's instructions.

Antimicrobial susceptibility testing

The resistance of the isolated strains to antibiotics was assayed by the disc diffusion method [18, 29–31]. *E. faecalis* ATCC 29212, *Escherichia coli* ATCC 25922 and *Aeromonas salmonicida* subsp. *salmonicida* ATCC 33658, *Pseudomonas aeruginosa* ATCC 27853 were used as Quality control strains for disk diffusion susceptibility testing of aquatic bacterial isolates [32]. The upcoming antibiotic discs (Oxoid, Ltd., Basingstoke, England) selected for testing are the most frequently used and prescribed in Egypt which are inhibitors of protein synthesis: phenicols (chloramphenicol), tetracyclines (tetracycline) and macrolides (erythromycin) for both *Enterococcus* and *Streptococcus* species, while aminoglycosides (gentamicin, streptomycin and amikacin) only for *Enterococcus* species; cell wall synthesis: penicillins (penicillin, ampicillin, amoxicillin-clavulonic acid and pipercillin-tazobactum) and glycopeptides (vancomycin) for both *Enterococcus* and *Streptococcus* species and polymyxins (colistin) for *Enterococcus* species; nucleic acid synthesis: ansamycins (rifampicin) and nitrofurantoins (nitrofurantoin) were used for both *Enterococcus* and *Streptococcus* species, fluoroquinolones (ciprofloxacin for *Enterococcus* species and ofloxacin for *Streptococcus* species), quinolones (nalidixic acid for *Enterococcus* species) and lincosamides (clindamycin) for *Streptococcus* species.

Statistical analysis

The experimental data obtained was subjected to multiple linear regressions using Microsoft Excel 2007 to evaluate the statistical analysis between the percentage of antimicrobial resistance (y- range) and actual concentration (x- axis) for all antibiotics to enable us to plot percent inhibition versus drug concentration for each strain.

Table 1 Oligonucleotide primers sequences and size of the PCR-targeted products

Microorganism	Target Gene	Bp fragment	Primer sequence (5′ - 3′)	Annealing Temp (°C)	References
E. faecalis / E. gallinarum	16S rRNA (Genus -specific primers)	112 bp	F- TAC TGA CAA ACC ATT CAT GAT G R- AAC TTC GTC ACC AAC GCG AAC	59 (*E. faecalis*) 50 (*E. gallinarum*)	[23]
E. faecalis	*ddl*$_{E. fecalis}$ (Species-specific primers)	941 bp	F- ATC AAG TAC AGT TAG TCT R- ACG ATT CAA AGC TAA CTG	55	[24]
L. garvieae	16S rRNA (species-specific primers)	1100 bp	F- CAT AAC AAT GAG AAT CGC R- GCA CCC TCG CGG GTTG	58	[25]
S. pluranimalium	16S rRNA (species-specific primers)	1500 bp	F- AGA GTT TGA TCC TGG CTC AG R- ACG GCT ACC TTG TTA CGA CTT	52	[26]
A. viridans	16S rRNA gene (species-specific primers)	540 bp	F- GTG CTT GCA CTT CTG ACG TTA GC R- TGA GCC GTG GGC TTT CAC AT	55	[27]
S. anginosus	MIL (*pbp2b*) (Anginosus Group specific)	275 bp	F- TGC TGC AAC GGT AGC TAA TGG R- GAA AGG TTT CTG CTG TCC CTG	58	[28]
	16srRNA (Species-specific primers)	105 bp	F- GCG TAG GTA ACC TGC CTA TTA GA R- CGC AGG TCC ATC TAC TAGC	58	

Results

Biochemical and molecular characterization

The microbiological cultures on CBA from the swabs taken from the internal organs (kidney, spleen and brain) and ascitic fluid revealed the presence of pinpoint white colonies (0.5 mm Ø) in pure culture or as major colony type. The Gram-stained smears that were taken from the presumptive *Streptococcus* colonies revealed Gram-positive chain forming cocci (0.6–0.9 μm Ø) small or medium sized in diploids, short chain, chain in the form of Y / V-shape, or in long chain, β-haemolytic, catalase and aesculin hydrolysis test negative, ability to grow at 25 and 37 °C and at pH 9.6 in the absence of 6.5% NaCl or 40% bile salts. Table 2 illustrates the effect of incubation temperature and NaCl 6.5% and bile salts on the growth of different isolates their role in identification of different types of isolates. The seventeen isolates were identified using Vitek 2 compact through the biochemical characterization of different isolates.

None of our 16 isolates could be serologically typed to any Lancefield group and in the Vitek 2 inconclusive results were obtained. The only result obtained was with the *S. dysgalactiae* subspecies *equisimilis* (one isolate) which was grouped in the C group.

Analysis of the 16S rRNA gene confirmed that the 17 tilapia isolates studied were 6/17 *E. faecalis,* 2/17 *E. gallinarum,* 3/17 *S. pluranimalium,* 2/17 *A. viridans,* 1/17 isolate of each *S. dysgalactiae, S. anginosus, L. garvieae* and *Granulicatella elegans.*

Prevalence and identification of *Enterococcus, Lactococcus* and *Streptococcus* species isolated from diseased fish

Overall, 17 *Streptococcus* species were collected and the *Streptococcus* spp. occurred in 8/80 (10%) liver samples, 4/80 (5%) spleen samples, in 3/80 (3.8%) kidney samples and 1/80 (1.3%) brain and ascitic fluid samples each. The logistic regression showed that the recovery of *Streptococcus* spp. was significantly affected by fish matrix ($P < 0.001$). The test of independence showed a significant association between the recovery of *Streptococcus* spp. from a given matrix and the location (Table 3).

The rate of bacteria isolated from the diseased tilapia fish, were isolated in a rate of 21.25%. *E. faecalis* showed the highest number of isolates (6 isolates) in a rate of 7.5%, followed by *S. pluranimalium* (3.75) (Table 3). *E. faecalis* was the most predominant isolate (6/80; 1.9%) and the liver was the most prominent site for the infection with *E. faecalis* (3.75%). Also, *E. faecalis* was the sole isolate from the ascitic fluid (1.25%). *S. pluranimalium* was the second predominant isolate (0.93%) being also predominantly localized in the liver (2.5%) and spleen (1.3%). Similarly, *E. gallinarum* was isolated at a rate of 1.3% from the liver and kidney. *S. dysgalactiae* subspecies *equisimilis* was only isolated from the brain (1.25%).

Antimicrobial susceptibility

The susceptibility of 17 *Streptococcus* strains was assessed against 18 different antibiotics (Fig. 2). Highest resistant to Tetracycline 94.1% (16/17) the lowest resistance was observed for Nitrofurantoin, Streptomycin, Gentamicin and Trimethoprim/Sulphamethaxozol 5.9% (1/17 each). The 17 isolates showed total susceptibility to Amoxicillin/Clavulanic acid, Piperacillin/Tazobactam, Nalidixic acid, Colistin and Amikacin. There was no significant relationship between the percentage of antimicrobial resistance (y- range) and actual concentration (x- axis) for all combined antibiotics and consequently no regression line could be drawn (Table 4).

Multiple resistance was observed in 16/17 strains (94.1%). In strains with multiple resistance, the most frequent antibiotic combination was penicillin, ampicillin, vancomycin, chloramphenicol, rifampicin, ofloxacin,

Table 2 Differential diagnosis between different bacterial species using growth conditions

Isolate	Growth at		Growth on 6.5% NaCl BHI agar			Growth at 40% Bile Salt BHI agar
	10 C	45 C	After 24 h	After 48 h	After 72 h	After 7 days
Aerococcus viridans	After 48 h (very faint) but good after 72 h	+	No growth	Very weak growth	Weak growth	No growth
E. faecalis	after 48 h	+	Very weak growth	Good growth	Very good growth	No growth
Lactococcus garvieae	after 48 h (very faint) but good after 72 h	+	No growth	Very weak growth	Very good growth	No growth
S. pluranimalium	After 48 h	+	very weak growth	Very weak growth	Very good growth	No growth
E. gallinarum	After 48 h (very faint) but good after 72 h	_	No growth	No growth	No growth	No growth
S. dysgalactiae subspecies *equisimilis*	No growth	+	No growth	No growth	No growth	No growth
S. anginosus	No growth	No growth	No growth	No growth	No growth	No growth

Table 3 Prevalence and Types of *Enterococcus, Lactococcus* and *Streptococcus* species isolated from diseased fish organs using 16 s rRNA

Matrix	Total No.	Species																	
		E. faecalis		*S. pluranimalium*		*A. viridans*		*E. gallinarum*		*S. anginosus*		*L. garvieae*		*S. dysgalactiae equisimilis*		*Granulicetella elegans / Leuconostoc mesenteroides cremoris*		Total	
		n	%	n	%	n	%	n	%	n	%	n	%	n	%	n	%	n	%
Liver	80	3	3.8	2	2.5	1	1.3	1	1.3	1	1.3	1	1.3	0	0	0	0	8	10.0
Kidney	80	1	1.3	0	0	1	1.3	1	1.3	0	0	0	0	0	0	0	0	3	3.8
Brain	80	0	0	0	0	0	0	0	0	0	0	0	0	1	1.3	0	0	1	1.3
Spleen	80	1	1.3	1	1.3	0	0	1	1.3	0	0	0	0	0	0	1	1.3	4	5
Ascitic fluid	3	1	33.3	0	0	0	0	0	0	0	0	0	0	0	0	0	0	1	33.3
Total	323	6	1.9	3	0.9	2	0.6	2	0.9	1	0.3	1	0.3	1	0.3	1	0.3	17	5.3

n, number of isolates

clindamycin, erythromycin and tetracycline (7/17, 41.2%) representing eight classes (Table 5).

Discussion

In this work, a collection of 17 strains of *Streptococcus* species isolated from diseased tilapia were biochemically, serologically and genetically characterized and data on their prevalence of the disease in Egypt. In contrast to other results [18], 16 of our isolates could not be serologically typed to any Lancefield group and in the Vitek 2 inconclusive results were obtained, a phenomenon which was also previously observed by Figueiredo et al. [33]. On the other hand, our sole isolate of *S. dysgalactiae* subspecies *equisimilis* which was grouped in the C group was also identified in Japan by Nomoto et al. [34, 35] and Abdelsalam et al. [36], in the amberjack (*Seriola dumerili*) and yellowtail (*Seriola quinqueradiata*) and in Amur sturgeon (*Acipenser schrenckii*) in China [37] and in Nile tilapia (*Oreochromis niloticus* (L.) in Brazil [20].

Our detection of *Streptococcus* species in the three organ tissues (liver, spleen and kidney) implicates them as the target organs of the organism [38–40]. Fish pathogenic strains have been described, as either an α- or ß-haemolytic or as non-haemolytic [41]. Superficially, this data could surmise heterogeneity amid the pathogens,

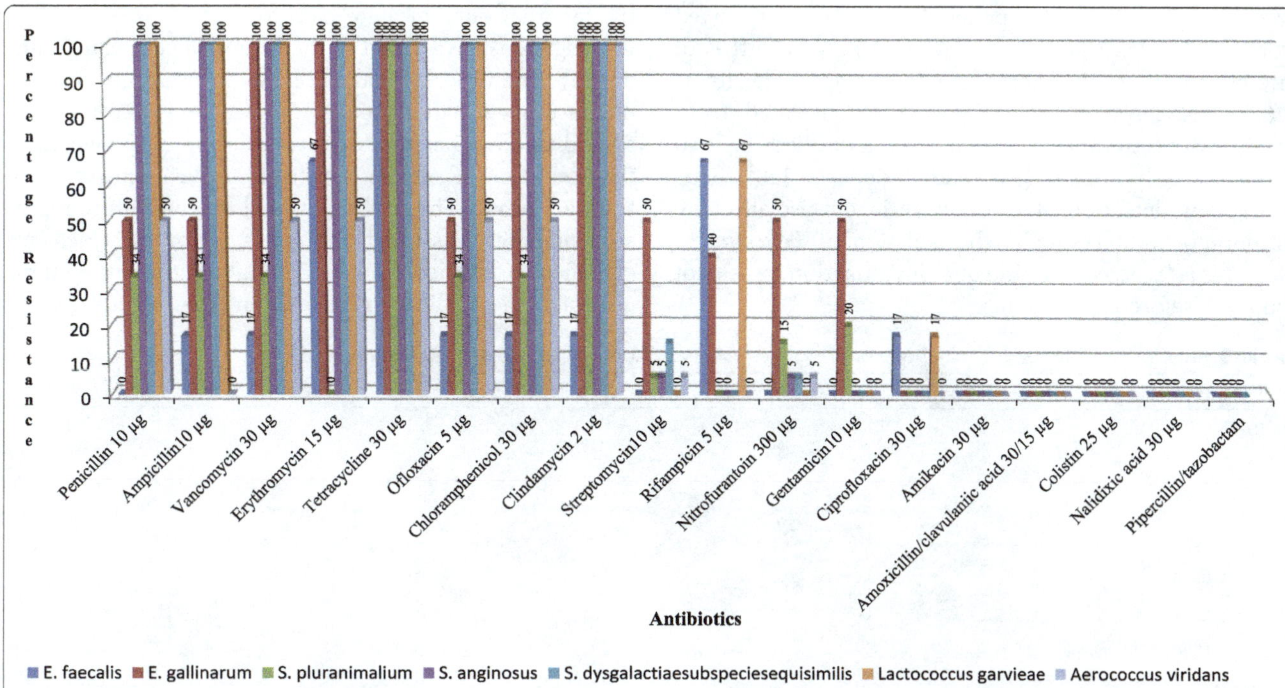

Fig. 2 Percentage resistance of the seven species of streptococci isolated from Nile tilapia (*Oreochromis niloticus*) to the 18 antibiotics tested

Table 4 Statistical analysis between the percentage of antimicrobial resistance (y- range) and actiual concentration (x- axis) of antibiotics for the isolated seven strains

	E. faecalis	*E. gallinarum*	*S. pluranimalium*	*S. anginosus*	*S. dysgalactiae subspecies equisimilis*	*L. garvieae*	*A. viridans*
E. faecalis	1						
E. gallinarum	0.534252	1					
S. pluranimalium	0.434469	0.696294	1				
S. anginosus	0.458603	0.7774	0.693549	1			
S. dysgalactiae subspecies equisimilis	0.455604	0.783461	0.692309	0.999059	1		
L. garvieae	0.593849	0.767848	0.650752	0.953986	0.950886	1	
A. viridans	0.555896	0.785501	0.873946	0.824254	0.823841	0.784558	1

inspite of the fact that some confirmed ranks such as *S. agalactiae*, incorporates both α– and ß-haemolytic strains. It should be noted that, many features are common within the predominance of fish pathogens [9]. Yet, this does not exclude some discrepancies reported in isolates recovered from the Transvaal in South Africa [42] and other isolates from Japan [43–45]. Such discrepancies could be due to the dissimilarity and absence of a standardized test protocols and/or point to heterogeneity in the species composition of the organisms.

The development and application of molecular methodology has been of great benefit and advantage through facilitating identification precision, classification of streptococci [17] and time-saving. Thus, our use of the PCR in the species -specific analysis of the 16S rRNA gene was of great assistance in the present investigation and unequivocally demonstrated that all of them belonged to the *Streptococcus* species. To a certain degree, geographical discrepancies have been reported from South Africa [42], Japan [46] and Italy [47]. It is of interest to reveal that according to the available literature, *L. garvieae* although being rarely isolated from tilapia with streptococcosis, it was identified in two countries only, Brazil [19] and Indonesia [10]. This makes our detection of *L. garvieae* in our isolates, the third report. Interestingly, the isolation of *Leuconostoc mesenteroides cremoris* in our investigation was not reported before from tilapia.

Aquaculture is a developing field where antibiotics are intensely used, either specifically to the water or in fish sustenance, as prophylactics to control infections, which has brought about the blooming of AR genes in the aquatic environment [48]. The measure of AMR in aquaculture is under dispute as there is an absence of consent on a standard indicator organism. Ratably, the utilization of antimicrobials in aquaculture seems, by all accounts, to be of substantially more prominent greatness when compared with terrestrial animals. A shortage of solid ratable and subjective information on antimicrobial use (AMU) in different animal production systems over the area is a noteworthy hole in the exploration. Subjective and ratable accessible information (for the most part AMU recurrence of particular antimicrobials) from particular examinations recommends a high assorted variety of antimicrobials utilized both as development promoters (AGPs), and in addition for prophylactic and treatment purposes, despite the fact that outcomes are hard to look at crosswise over investigations. As a result of the extensive contrasts in underway frameworks, sampling and assay techniques, phenotypic evaluations of AMR pervasiveness in this audit should be deciphered with extraordinary care. Generally, the collection of samples are liable to have an expansive testing mistake. The antibiotics used in aquaculture represent different classes of antibiotics, some of which are classified as "Highest Priority Critically Important Antimicrobials" in medical treatment in the WHO list of

Table 5 Antibiotic resistance combinations profile of the 17 *Streptococcus* species isolated from Nile tilapia

Antibiotic resistance combination profile	number of isolates/17	% of isolates	number of antibiotics	Number of classes
P, Am	1	5.9	2	1
P, Am,VA	1	5.9	3	2
P, Am,VA, C	2	43	4	3
P, Am,VA, C, RD	1	5.9	5	4
P, Am,VA, C, RD, OFX	1	1.9	6	5
P, Am,VA, C, RD, OFX, DA	1	5.9	7	6
P, Am,VA, C, RD, OFX, DA, E	3	17.6	8	7
P, Am,VA, C, RD, OFX, DA, E, TE	7	41.2	9	8

P penicillin, *Am* ampicillin, *Va* vancomycin, *C* chloramphenicol, *RD* rifampicin, *OFX* ofloxacin, *DA* clindamycin, *E* erythromycin, *TE* tetracycline

Critically important antimicrobials for human medicine (CIA list) such as fluoroquinolones, 3rd and 4th Generation cephalosporins, Macrolides and ketolides and Glycopeptides [49]. Fortunately, the isolated strains in the present investigation were not resistant to any of the CIA list with the exception of erythromycin. Globally, the use of antimicrobial agents is regulated differently from country to country, being either very strict or under-regulated. Possible hazards associated with drug abuse in fish farming are the presence of residues in food and the development of antibiotic resistance in the bacterial population. In agreement, to our surprise numerous multi-ABR- bacteria (49%) were observed among our isolates, irrespective of their traditional resistance to beta lactam antibiotics [50, 51]. It was theorized that, resistance to these antibiotics could be a result of their overuse or/and misuse in the aquaculture industry, could arise from gene mutations or by acquisition of transferable genetic elements such as integrons [50, 52]. The property of horizontal spread of resistance genes was incriminated to be responsible for the recorded levels of multi-resistance. Notwithstanding AMU in aquaculture, the basic routine with regards to releasing fertilizer from earthbound creatures into water frameworks leaves the aquatic environments especially powerless against the improvement of AMR.

Conclusion

Worldwide death of fish caused by streptococcal infection remains an extortionate issue for growers of Nile tilapia and other warmwater fish, yet can be handled effectively with a cohesive, supportable scheme incriminating vaccines and new-generation antibiotics developed specifically for aquaculture. Strains of *Streptococcus* associated with infection in humans can cause people handling affected whole raw fish, primarily tilapia, to become at risk of developing neonatal meningitis and sepsis (early-onset and late-onset disease), cellulitis, subdural empyema, endocarditis or arthritis following a puncture wound [53–55]. Substantially, our results highlight the necessity to encourage conscientious fish producers, efficient husbandry performances and judicious practise of antibiotics in aquaculture. It should be emphasized that, *S. dysgalactiae* has emerged as a causative agent in fish disease, with a highly medical significance in mammalian and human health as alpha-hemolytic Lancefield group C *S. dysgalactiae* of fish origin, was implicated in ascending upper limb cellulitis in humans [56].

Abbreviations

AGPs: Antimicrobial growth promoters; AMU: Antimicrobial usage; CBA: Columbia blood agar; CIA: Central Intelligence Agency; FAO: Food and Agriculture Organization; GPI: Gram-positive identification; MT: Metric tons; USD: United States Dollar; WHO: World Health Organization

Acknowledgements

The authors extend their appreciation to the Deanship of Scientific Research at King Saud University for funding the work through the research group project No.: RGP-162.

Funding

The work was funded through the research group project No.: RGP-162.

Authors' contributions

KO developed the concept, designed experiments, collected, and analyzed data and prepared the manuscript; KAM, IM, MI and AH contributed their scientific advice during the work and manuscript revision; AO and NF performed the experiments. All authors discussed the results and implications and commented on the manuscript at all stages. All authors read and approved the final manuscript.

Consent for publication

Not applicable.

Competing interests

The authors declare that they have no competing interests.

Author details

[1]Department of Microbiology, Faculty of Veterinary Medicine, Cairo University, Giza, Egypt. [2]Department of Botany and Microbiology, College of Science, King Saud University, Riyadh, Kingdom of Saudi Arabia. [3]Department of Public Health, College of Applied Medical Science, King Khalid University, Abha, Kingdom of Saudi Arabia. [4]Department of Health Science, College of Applied Studies and Community Service, King Saud University, Riyadh, Kingdom of Saudi Arabia. [5]Department of Fish Diseases and Management, Animal Health Research Institute, Dokki, Giza, Egypt.

References

1. Jamie Allen's. Family tree & ancient genealogical allegations version 77, 2016. The PEDIGREE of Nile tilapia.
2. Trewaves E. Tilapia fishes of the genera Sarotherodon. British Museum (Natural History): Oreochromis. Danakilia; 1983.
3. Balarin JD, Hatton JP. Tilapia: A guide to their biology and culture in Africa. Stirling, UK: University of Stirling; 1979.
4. Pillay TVR. Aquaculture principles and practices. Fishing news books. Oxford, UK: Blackwell Science; 1990.
5. FAO. Food and Agriculture Organization of the United Nations. Fishstat plus. FAO. Rome 2004.
6. Babylon Software Ltd. Babylon's 10 online Dictionary & Translation, Copyright © 2014–2016.
7. Food FAO. Agriculture Organization of the United Nations. Yearbook 2010, fishery and aquaculture statistics. Rome. 2012;
8. FAO. Fisheries and Aquaculture Department. About us - Fisheries and Aquaculture Department. In: FAO Fisheries and Aquaculture Department [online]. Rome. Updated. [Cited 15 September 2016]. http://www.fao.org/fishery/about/en
9. Austin B, Austin DA. Bacterial fish pathogens: disease of farmed and wild fish, fifth edition ISBN 978-94-007-4883-5 ISBN 978-94-007-4884-2 (eBook) springer Dordrecht Heidelberg new York London Library of Congress control number: 2012946925 © springer science+business media Dordrecht 2012.

10. Anshary H, Kurniawan RA, Sriwulan S, Ramli R, Baxa DV. Isolation and molecular identification of the etiological agents of streptococcosis in Nile tilapia (*Oreochromis niloticus*) cultured in net cages in Lake Sentani, Papua, Indonesia. Springer Plus. 2014;3:627. doi:10.1186/2193-1801-3-627.
11. Klesius PH, Shoemaker CA, Evans JJ. *Streptococcus*: a worldwide fish health problem. 8th international symposium on tilapia in aquaculture. Cairo. 2008: 83–107.
12. Yanong RPE, Francis-Floyd R. Streptococcal Infections of Fish. This document is Circular 57, one of a series of the Fisheries and Aquatic Sciences Department, Florida Cooperative Extension Service, Institute of Food and Agricultural Sciences, University of Florida. Original publication date April 2002. Revised August 2006. Reviewed June 2013. Visit the EDIS website at http://edis.ifas.ufl.edu 2013.
13. Siti-Zahrah A, Padilah B, Azila A, Rimatulhana R, Shahidan R. Multiple streptococcal species infection in cage-cultured red tilapia but showing similar clinical signs, pp. 313–320. In: Bondad-Reantaso MG, Mohan CV, Crumlish M, Subasinghe RP, editors. Diseases in Asian Aquaculture VI. Manila, Philippines: Fish Health Section, Asian Fisheries Society; 2008. p. 505.
14. Amal MNA, Zamri-Saad M. Streptococcosis in tilapia (*Oreochromis niloticus*): a review. Pertanika J Trop Agric Sci. 2011;34:195–206.
15. Li YW, Liu L, Huang PR, Fang W, Luo ZP, Peng HL, et al. X chronic streptococcosis in Nile tilapia, *Oreochromis niloticus* (L.), caused by *Streptococcus agalactiae*. J Fish Dis. 2014;37:757–63. doi:10.1111/jfd.12146.
16. Sudheesh, P. S., Al-Ghabshi, A., Al-Mazrooei, N., and Al-Habsi, S. (2012). Comparative Pathogenomics of bacteria causing infectious diseases in fish. Inter J Evol biol. 2012;2012:457264. doi:https://doi.org/10.1155/2012/457264.
17. Toranzo AE, Magarin B, Romalde JL. A review of the main bacterial fish diseases in mariculture systems. Aquaculture. 2005;246:37–61. doi:10.1016/j.aquaculture.2005.01.002
18. Romalde JL, Ravelo C, Valdes I, Magariños B, de la Fuente E, Martín CS, et al. *Streptococcus phocae*, an emerging pathogen for salmonid culture. Vet Microbiol. 2008;130:198–207. doi:10.1016/j.vetmic.2007.12.021.
19. Evans JJ, Klesius PH, Shoemaker CA. First isolation and characterization of *Lactococcus garvieae* from Brazilian Nile tilapia, *Oreochromis niloticus* (L.) and pintado, *Pseudoplathystoma corruscans* (Spix & Agassiz). J Fish Dis. 2009;32: 943–51. doi:10.1111/j.1365-2761.2009.01075.x.
20. Netto LN, Leal CA, Figueiredo HC. *Streptococcus dysgalactiae* as an agent of septicaemia in Nile tilapia, *Oreochromis niloticus* (L.). J Fish Dis. 2011;4:251–4. doi:10.1111/j.1365-2761.2010.01220.x.
21. Hoshina T, Sano T, Morimoto Y. A *Streptococcus* pathogenic for fish. J Tokyo Univ Fisher. 1958;44:57–8.
22. Ghittino C. La estreptococosis en los peces. Aquatic 2, art. 1999;605. Available at URL http://aquatic.unizar.es/n2/art605/lact_rev.htm.
23. Karsidani SH, Soltani M, Nikbakhat-Brojeni G, Ghasemi M, Skall H. Molecular epidemiology of zoonotic streptococcosis/lactococcosis in rainbow trout (*Oncorhynchus mykiss*) aquaculture in Iran. Iran J Microbiol. 2010;2:198–209.
24. Biavasco F, Foglia G, Paoletti C, Zandri G, Magi G, Guaglianone E, et al. VanA-type enterococci from humans, animals, and food: species distribution, population structure, Tn*1546* typing and location, and virulence determinants. Appl Environ Microbiol. 2007;73:3307–19. doi:10.1128/AEM.02239-06.
25. Fadaeifard F, Momtaz H, Rahimi E, Mirzakhani A. Detection of *Streptococcus iniae* and *Lactococcus garvieae* by multiplex polymerase chain reaction (PCR) in some rainbow trout farms of Iran. Afr J Biotechnol. 2012;11:260–3. doi: 10.5897/AJB11.2651.
26. Wan L, Chen SJ, Wang CD, Li DS, Zheng Z, Wang CD, et al. Identification and genotypic analysis of *Streptococcus* spp. isolated from Giant pandas in China by PCR-based methods. Afr J Microbiol Res. 2012;6:1380–6. doi:10.5897/AJMR11.805.
27. Martin V, Vela AI, Gilbert M, Cebolla J, Goyache J, Domínguez L, et al. Characterization of *Aerococcus viridans* isolates from swine clinical specimens. J Clin Microbiol. 2007;45:3053–7. doi:10.1128/JCM.00156-07.
28. Takao A, Nagamune H, Maeda N. Identification of the anginosus group within the genus *Streptococcus* using polymerase chain reaction. FEMS Microbiol Lett 2004;233:83–89. doi:10.1016/j.femsle.2004.01.042.
29. Channaiah LH, Subramanyam B, McKinney LJ, Zurek L. Stored-product insects carryantibiotic-resistant and potentially virulent enterococci. FEMS Microbiol Ecol. 2010;74:464–71. doi:10.1111/j.1574-6941.2010.00949.x.
30. CLSI. The Clinical and Laboratory Standards Institute. Methods for Antimicrobial Disk Susceptibility Testing of Bacteria Isolated From Aquatic Animals. In: Approved guideline (VET03-a). Pennsylvania, USA: Wayne; 2014.
31. Iweriebor BC, Gaqavu S, Obi LC, Nwodo UU, Okoh AI. Antibiotic susceptibilities of *Enterococcus* species isolated from hospital and domestic wastewater effluents in Alice, eastern Cape Province of South Africa. Int J Environ Res Public Health. 2015;12:4231–46. doi:10.3390/ijerph120404231.
32. Miller RA, Walker RD, Baya A, Clemens K, Coles M, Hawke JP, et al. Antimicrobial susceptibility testing of aquatic bacteria: quality control disk diffusion ranges for *Escherichia coli* ATCC 25922 and *Aeromonas salmonicida* subsp. *salmonicida* ATCC 33658 at 22 and 28°C. J Clin Microbiol. 2003;41: 4318–23. doi:10.1128/JCM.41.9.4318-4323.2003.
33. Figueiredo HCP, Netto LN, Leal CAG, Pereira Ulisses P, Mian Glaúcia F. *Streptococcus iniae* outbreaks in Brazilian Nile tilapia (*Oreochromis niloticus* L.) farms. Braz J Microbiol. 2012;43:576–80. doi:10.1590/S1517-83822012000200019.
34. Nomoto R, Munasinghe LI, Jin DH, Shimahara Y, Yasuda H, Nakamura A, et al. Lancefield group C *Streptococcus dysgalactiae* infection responsible for fish mortalities in Japan. J Fish Dis. 2004;27:679–86. doi:10.1111/j.1365-2761.2004.00591.x.
35. Nomoto R, Unose N, Shimahara Y, Nakamura A, Hirae T, Maebuchi K, et al. Characterization of Lancefield group C *Streptococcus dysgalactiae* isolated from farmed fish. J Fish Dis. 2006;29:673–82. doi:10.1111/j.1365-2761.2006.00763.x.
36. Abdelsalam M, Chen SC, Yoshida T. Phenotypic and genetic characterizations of *Streptococcus dysgalactiae* strains isolated from fish collected in Japan and other Asian countries. FEMS Microbiol Lett. 2010;302: 32–8. doi:10.1111/j.1574-6968.2009.01828.x.
37. Yang W, Li A. Isolation and characterization of *Streptococcus dysgalactiae* from diseased *Acipenser schrenckii*. Aquaculture. 2009;294:14–7. doi:10.1016/j.aquaculture.2009.05.018.
38. Eldar A, Bejerano Y, Livoff A, Horovitcz A, Bercovier H. Experimental streptococcal meningo-encephalitis in cultured fish. Vet Microbiol. 1995;43: 33–40. doi:10.1016/0378-1135(94)00052-X.
39. Lahav D, Eyngor M, Hurvitz A, Ghittino C, Lublin A, Eldar A. *Streptococcus iniae* type 11 infections in rainbow trout *Oncorhynchus mykiss*. Dis Aquatic Org. 2004;62:177–80. doi:10.3354/dao062177.
40. Abuseliana AF, Daud HHM, Abdul Aziz S, Bejo SK, Alsaid M. Pathogenicity of *Streptococcus agalactiae* isolated from a fish in Selangor to juvenile red tilapia (*Oreochromis* sp.). J Anim Vet Adv. 2011;10:914–9. doi:10.3923/javaa.2011.914.919.
41. Murray PR, Baron EJ, Jorgensen JJ, et al. *Streptococcous* general methods in: manual of ClinicalMicrobiology, 2003; 8th ed. Section 1, ASM press: Washington, DC.
42. Boomker J, Imes GD Jr, Cameron CM, Naude TW, Schoonbee HJ. Trout mortalities as a result of a Streptococii infection. Onderstepoort J Vet Res. 1979;46:71–7.
43. Minami T, Nakamura M, Ikeda Y, Ozak HA. Beta-hemolitic *Streptococcus* isolated from cultured yellowtail. Fish Pathol. 1979;14:15–9. doi:10.3147/jsfp.14.33
44. Kitao T, Aoki T, Sakoh R. Epizootic caused by b-haemolytic *Streptococcus* species in cultured freshwater fish. Fish Pathol. 1981;15:301–7.
45. Ugajin M. Studies on *Streptococcus* sp as a causative agent of an epizootic among the cultured ayu (*Plecoglossus altivelis*) in Tochigi prefecture, Japan, 1980. Fish Pathol. 1981;16:119–27. doi:10.3147/jsfp.16.119
46. Kusuda R, Komatsu I, Kawai K. *Streptococcus* sp. isolated from an epizootic of cultured eels. Nippon Suisan Gakkaishi. 1978;44:295.
47. Ghittino C, Prearo M. Report of streptococcosis in rainbow trout (*Oncorhynchus mykiss*) in Italy: preliminary note. Boll Soc Ital Patalog Ittica. 1992;8:4–11.
48. Heuer OE, Kruse H, Grave K, Collignon P, Karunasagar I, Angulo FJ. Human health consequences of use of antimicrobial agents in aquaculture. Clin Infect Dis. 2009;49:1248–53. doi:10.1086/605667.
49. WHO. The World Health Organization. WHO fact sheets on food safety: Highest Priority Critically Important Antimicrobials, 2016.
50. Defoirdt T, Sorgeloos P, Bossier P. Alternatives to antibiotics for the control of bacterial disease in aquaculture. Curr Opin Microbiol. 2011;14:251–8. doi:10.1016/j.mib.2011.03.004.
51. Di Cesare A, Luna GM, Vignaroli C, Pasquaroli S, Tota S, Paroncini P, et al. Aquaculture can promote the presence and spread of antibiotic-resistant enterococci in marine sediments. PLoS One. 2013;8(4):e62838. doi:10.1371/journal.pone.0062838.
52. Huddleston JR. Horizontal gene transfer in the human gastrointestinal tract: potential spread of antibiotic resistance genes. Infect Drug Resis. 2014;7: 167–76. doi:10.2147/IDR.S48820.

53. MMWR. Invasive infection with *Streptococcus iniae*, Ontario, 1995–1996. Morb Mort Weekly Rep. 1996;45:650–3. available on-line from the Centers for Disease Control's website at www.cdc.gov/mmwr
54. Weinstein MR, Litt M, Kertesz DA, Wyper P, Rose D, Coulter M, et al. Invasive infections due to a fish pathogen, *Streptococcus iniae* study group. New Eng J Med. 1997;337:589–94. doi:10.1056/NEJM199708283370902.
55. Aryasinghe L, Sabbar S, Kazim Y, Awan LM, Khan HK. Streptococcus *pluranimalium*: a novel human pathogen? Inter J Surg Case Rep. 2014;5: 1242–6. doi:10.1016/j.ijscr.2014.11.029.
56. Koh TH, Sng LH, Yuen SM, Thomas CK, Tan PL, Tan SH, et al. Streptococcal cellulitis following preparation of fresh raw seafood. Zoonoses Public Health. 2009;56:206–8. doi:10.1111/j.1863-2378.2008.01213.x.

13

Antimicrobial resistance and genomic rep-PCR fingerprints of *Pseudomonas aeruginosa* strains from animals on the background of the global population structure

Isa Serrano[1], Daniel De Vos[2], José Pedro Santos[1], Florence Bilocq[2], Alexandre Leitão[1], Luis Tavares[1], Jean-Paul Pirnay[2] and Manuela Oliveira[1*]

Abstract

Background: *Pseudomonas aeruginosa* is an important human opportunistic pathogen responsible for fatal nosocomial infections worldwide, and has emerged as a relevant animal pathogen. Treatment options are dramatically decreasing, due to antimicrobial resistance and the microorganism's large versatile genome.

Antimicrobial resistance profiles, serotype frequency and genomic profile of unrelated *P. aeruginosa* isolates of veterinary origin ($n = 73$), including domesticated, farm, zoo and wild animals mainly from Portugal were studied. The genomic profile, determined by DiversiLab system (Rep-PCR-based technique), was compared with the *P. aeruginosa* global population structure to evaluate their relatedness.

Results: Around 40% of the isolates expressed serotypes O6 (20.5%) and O1 (17.8%). A total of 46.6% of isolates was susceptible to all antimicrobials tested. Isolates obtained from most animals were non-multidrug resistant (86.3%), whereas 11% were multidrug resistant, MDR (non-susceptible to at least one agent in ≥ three antimicrobial categories), and 2.7% extensively drug resistant, XDR (non-susceptible to at least one agent in all but two or fewer antimicrobial categories). Resistance percentages were as follows: amikacin (0.0%), aztreonam (41.1%), cefepime (9.6%), ceftazidime (2.7%), ciprofloxacin (15.1%), colistin (0.0%), gentamicin (12.3%), imipenem (1.4%), meropenem (1.4%), piperacillin + tazobactam (12.3%), ticarcillin (16.4%), ticarcillin + clavulanic acid (17.8%), and tobramycin (1.4%).

Animal isolates form a population with a non-clonal epidemic structure indistinguishable from the global *P. aeruginosa* population structure, where no specific 'animal clonal lineage' was detected.

Conclusions: Serotypes O6 and O1 were the most frequent. Serotype frequency and antimicrobial resistance patterns found in *P. aeruginosa* from animals were as expected for this species. This study confirms earlier results that *P. aeruginosa* has a non-clonal population structure, and shows that *P. aeruginosa* population from animals is homogeneously scattered and indistinguishable from the global population structure.

Keywords: Animal origin, Antimicrobials, Environment, MDR, Non-clonal, Population, Pseudomonas aeruginosa, Rep-PCR, Serotype, XDR

* Correspondence: moliveira@fmv.ulisboa.pt
[1]CIISA/Faculty of Veterinary Medicine, University of Lisbon, Lisbon, Portugal
Full list of author information is available at the end of the article

Background

Pseudomonas aeruginosa is an infectious bacterial species, with a world-wide dispersion, capable to infect and promote disease in different tissues [1], and responsible for remarkable morbidity and mortality rates in humans [2].

P. aeruginosa is a ubiquitous bacterial species, with an exceptional capacity to adapt to different aquatic and terrestrial ecological niches [3, 4]. Its high adaptability is in part explainable by its metabolic versatility [4–6]. This opportunistic bacterium migrates from its natural environment, colonizing and infecting a wide range of organisms [5, 6], including plants [7] and different animals, such as fruit flies [8], waxmoth [9], zebrafish [10] and mammals [11, 12].

In veterinary medicine, *P. aeruginosa* is responsible for a large variety of infections such as ocular infections [13], mastitis [14, 15], discospondylitis [16], otitis [17, 18], pyoderma [19], ulcerative keratitis [20], urinary tract infections [21] and incision, joint, invasive device and wound infections [22]. The most imminent problems are otitis externa in dogs, mastitis in cattle, dermatitis in rabbits and fleece rot in sheep. However, the importance of animal infections caused by *P. aeruginosa* has been disregarded due to the low detection of animal clinical cases [23].

Overall, infections caused by *P. aeruginosa* are hard to treat because this bacterium shows intrinsic and acquired resistance to different antimicrobial compounds [6]. It has been argued that the presence of specific outer membrane proteins involved in efflux transport systems or affecting cell permeability may explain the intrinsic resistance of *P. aeruginosa* to antimicrobials [24–26]. *P. aeruginosa* strains are also able to express a wide variety of acquired resistance mechanisms, including the production of β-lactamases and carbapenemases [14], mainly due to mutations in chromosomal resistance genes or acquisition of resistance genes from other bacteria through plasmids [18]. Moreover, resistance transmission from humans to animals has been acknowledged [27, 28].

Different studies have been consensual about the fact that *P. aeruginosa* clinical isolates are indistinguishable from the ones from the environment, either genotypically, chemotaxonomically, or functionally [5, 29, 30]. In order to understand the global population structure, clinical and environmental isolates collected around the world were recently analyzed [4, 5]. Authors concluded that *P. aeruginosa* has an epidemic population structure, which is non-clonal. There are no specific *P. aeruginosa* clones related with specific diseases, habitat or animal species [5, 23].

The objective of this study was to characterize the antimicrobial resistance patterns, serotype frequency, and genomic profile of a collection of *P. aeruginosa* isolates from a wide variety of animal species with different kinds of infections, from different geographic regions of Portugal. A rapid and accurate genotyping method based on Rep-PCR, the DiversiLab system, was used and the genomic profile was then compared with the *P. aeruginosa* global population structure to evaluate their relatedness.

Methods

P. aeruginosa isolates

In this study, a total of 73 *P. aeruginosa* isolates were used, belonging to a collection of animal isolates from the Faculty of Veterinary Medicine, Technical University of Lisbon (Additional file 1: Table S1). Isolates were collected from 2003–2012 in different geographic regions of Portugal, except for one sea turtle isolate sampled in Principe Island in the Gulf of Guinea. Our batch included 50 isolates from pets [dog ($n = 39$), cat ($n = 5$), parrot ($n = 4$), turtle ($n = 2$)], 15 from farm animals [horse ($n = 6$), cow ($n = 5$), sheep ($n = 2$), pig ($n = 1$), goat ($n = 1$)], 7 from zoo animals [seal ($n = 1$), dolphin ($n = 2$), kangaroo ($n = 2$), tamarind ($n = 2$)] and one from a wild free-living sea turtle.

Bacteria were isolated on Columbia blood agar (COS, BioMérieux, Marcy-l'Etoile, France), identified through their morphologic characteristics and biochemical profile (API 20 NE, BioMérieux, Marcy-l'Etoile, France) and kept frozen at -80 °C until further processing. *P. aeruginosa* control strain ATCC 27853 was used in this study.

Molecular identification

Species identification of the isolates was confirmed using a previously described PCR assay targeting the *P. aeruginosa* species-specific *oprI* and *oprL* genes [24].

Serotyping

Isolates were grown overnight on Luria-Bertani agar medium (Gibco-BRL-Life Technologies, Brussels, Belgium) at 37 °C, after which were serotyped by slide agglutination according to the International Antigenic Typing Scheme (IATS) for *P. aeruginosa* [31], using a panel of 16 type O monovalent antisera (Bio-Rad, Temse, Belgium). Four antisera pools, each containing four antisera, were also used: pool A (O1, O3, O4, O6); pool E (O2, O5, O15, O16); pool C (O9, O10, O13, O14); and pool F (O7, O8, O11, O12).

Antimicrobial resistance

Antimicrobial resistance studies were performed by using the Vitek 2 system (BioMerieux, Marcy-l'Etoile, France) in accordance with the manufacturer's instructions. *P. aeruginosa* ATCC 27853 was included as control strain. The following antimicrobials were tested: amikacin, aztreonam, cefepime, ceftazidime, ciprofloxacin, colistin, gentamicin, imipenem, meropenem, piperacillin

+ tazobactam, ticarcillin, ticarcillin + clavulanic acid, and tobramycin. Antimicrobial resistance phenotypes, represented by the minimum inhibitory concentrations (MICs) were interpreted according to CLSI guidelines: CLSI, Performance Standards for Antimicrobial Disk and Dilution Susceptibility Tests for Bacteria Isolated From Animals [32]. The breakpoints of aztreonam, cefepime, ceftazidime, ciprofloxacin, colistin, meropenem, piperacillin + tazobactam, and tobramycin were not defined at the above CLSI, so their MICs were interpreted using: CLSI Performance Standards for Antimicrobial Susceptibility Testing [33].

Rep-PCR genotyping

DiversiLab system (rep-PCR) was used for isolates genotyping. *P. aeruginosa* DNA was extracted using the UltraCleanTM Microbial DNA Isolation Kit (Mo Bio Laboratories Inc., Solana Beach, CA) according to the manufacturer's instructions. DNA quantification was measured using a NanoDrop ND-1000 spectrophotometer (NanoDrop Technologies, Wilmington, DE, USA). Then, rep-PCR was performed using PTC 200 thermocycler and *Pseudomonas* fingerprinting kit (Bacterial Barcodes, bioMe´rieux, Athens, GA, USA) in a total reaction volume of 25 μl. The reaction mixture consisted of 18 μl of rep-PCR MM1, 2.5 μl of Gene Amp 10X, 2 μl of primer Mix, 0.5 μl of AmpliTaq DNA polymerase (Applied Biosystems, Foster City, CA, USA) and 2 μl of genomic DNA (25–50 ng/ml). Thermal conditions were as follows: initial denaturation step at 94 °C for 2 min, 35 cycles including denaturation at 94 °C for 30 s, annealing at 50 °C for 30 s and extension at 70 °C for 90 s, followed by a final extension step at 70 °C for 3 min.

PCR products were analyzed using the Agilent 2100 BioAnalyzer (Agilent Technologies, Santa Clara, CA, USA). Then, the amplified fragments (sizes from 100–1000 bp) were electrophoretically separated using a microfiluidic labchip. In order to monitor reproducibility, the *P. aeruginosa* ATCC 27853 reference strain was used as a control in each PCR reaction and in each chip. Electropherograms were downloaded and automatically analyzed by the DiversiLab software (version 3.4) (BioMerieux, Brussels, Belgium). All fingerprint patterns were normalized, then, the Pearson correlation coefficient was used in order to calculate the distance matrices among all samples. Based on UPGMA and multidimensional scaling, the DiversiLab software created a customized report presenting a dendrogram, electropherograms, virtual gel images and scatter plots. Relatedness among isolates was deduced as previously described [34]: isolates showing similarity levels above 95% were considered as linked, while isolates with similarity levels below 95% were considered as different. Closely related isolates differing by a maximum of two band classes were collapsed into one node.

Results

Molecular identification and serotype distribution

Both target genes used in rep-PCR (*oprI* and *oprL*) were detected in all 73 *P. aeruginosa* isolates tested, confirming their identification as *Pseudomonas aeruginosa*. Isolates were serotyped, being observed that most isolates belonged to serotypes O6 (20.5%), O1 (17.8%), O11 (9.6%), O3 (5.5%) and O9 (5.5%) (Table 1). Isolates belonging to serotypes O4, O10, O15 and O12 were also detected, but at a lower percentage. PA isolates (strains that polyagglutinate in pools E (O2 + O5 + O15 + O16) and F (O7, O8, O11, O12), but not in the individual antisera) were 12.3%. Nine isolates (12.3%) were classified as NT/NA: NT (Non Typeable strains which are polyagglutinating), NA (strains that do Not Agglutinate in any pool or individual antiserum) (Table 1).

Antimicrobial resistance

A total of 46,6% of isolates was susceptible to all antimicrobials tested. Table 2 summarizes the frequency of resistant isolates for all antimicrobials tested, where intermediate isolates are also classified as resistant (low-level resistance). Resistance to aztreonam (41.1%) was the highest. Resistance to ciprofloxacin (15.1%), piperacillin + tazobactam (12.3%), ticarcillin (16.4%) and ticarcillin + clavulanic acid (17.2%), was between 10% and 20%. Resistance was lowest for cefepime (9.6%), ceftazidime (2.7%), imipenem (1.4%), gentamicin (12.3%), meropenem (1.4%), and tobramycin (1.4%). All isolates were susceptible to amikacin and to colistin (Table 2).

The number of isolates with high-level resistance is higher than the number of isolates with low-level resistance (intermediate) (Table 2).

Table 1 Serotype percentage of *P. aeruginosa* animal isolates (*n* = 73)

Serotype	Number	Percentage
O6	**15**	**20.5**
O1	**13**	**17.8**
PA	**9**	**12.3**
NT/NA	**9**	**12.3**
O11	**7**	**9.6**
O3	**4**	**5.5**
O9	**4**	**5.5**
O4	3	4.1
O10	3	4.1
O15	3	4.1
O12	2	2.7

Serotypes with a percentage of more than 5% are expressed in boldface
NT, Non Typeable strains which are polyagglutinating; PA, strains that PolyAgglutinate in pools E (O2 + O5 + O15 + O16) and F (O7, O8, O11, O12), but not in the individual antisera; NA, strains that do Not Agglutinate in any pool or individual antiserum

Table 2 Antimicrobial resistance of *P. aeruginosa* isolates ($n = 73$)

Antimicrobials	MIC breakpoint (µg/mL)	Resistance % (n)		
		High[a]	Low[b]	Total
Amikacin	≤16 - ≥64	0.0	0.0	0.0
Aztreonam	≤8 - ≥32	15.1 (11)	26.0 (19)	41.1 (30)
Cefepime	≤8 - ≥32	0.0	9.6 (7)	9.6 (7)
Ceftazidime	≤8 - ≥32	0.0	2.7 (2)	2.7 (2)
Ciprofloxacin	≤1 - ≥4	15.1 (11)	0.0	15.1 (11)
Colistin	≤2 - ≥8	0.0	0.0	0.0
Gentamicin	≤4 - ≥16	2.7 (2)	9.6 (7)	12.3 (9)
Imipenem	≤4 - ≥16	1.4 (1)	0.0	1.4 (1)
Meropenem	≤2 - ≥8	1.4 (1)	0.0	1.4 (1)
Piperacillin + tazobactam	≤16/4 - ≥128/4	1.4 (1)	11.0 (8)	12.3 (9)
Ticarcillin	≤64 - ≥128	16.4 (12)	0.0	16.4 (12)
Ticarcillin + clavulanic acid	≤64/2 - ≥128/2	17.8 (13)	0.0	17.8 (13)
Tobramycin	≤4 - ≥16	1.4 (1)	0.0	1.4 (1)

[a]High, high-level resistant; [b]Low, low-level resistant (Intermediate)

The distribution of antimicrobial resistance per serotype was as follows: serotype O1 isolates were resistant to aztreonam (46.2%), cefepime (7.7%), ciprofloxacin (7.7%), gentamicin (7.7%), piperacillin + tazobactam (15.4%), ticarcillin (15.4%), and ticarcillin + clavulanic acid (15.4%); serotype O6 isolates were resistant to aztreonam (26.7%), ciprofloxacin (20.0%), gentamicin (6.7%), ticarcillin (13.3%), and ticarcillin + clavulanic acid (13.3%). These two serotypes, representing 38% of animal isolates, are in accordance to the total results, except the fact that serotype O6 was fully susceptible to the two cephalosporins tested, whereas the total resistance for cephalosporins was 2.7% (ceftazidime) and 9.6% (cefepime).

Multidrug resistant (MDR) isolates are non-susceptible to at least one agent in ≥ three antimicrobial categories, and extensively drug resistant (XDR) isolates non-susceptible to at least one agent in all but two or fewer antimicrobial categories [35]. According to Magiorakos AP et al., 2012 [33], ticarcillin is not used to define MDR and XDR isolates, thus it was not used to define MDR and XDR isolates in this study. Isolates obtained from most animals were non-multidrug resistant (nor MDR, nor XDR) (86.3%). Only 2.7% of the isolates were XDR and 11.0% were MDR.

MDR was found in isolates belonging to serotypes O1, O6, O11, O15, and to PA and NT isolates. MDR profiles observed were as follows: aztreonam / ciprofloxacin / ticarcillin + clavulanic acid (3/8) aztreonam / cefepime / ticarcillin + clavulanic acid / piperacillin + tazobactam (1/8), aztreonam / ceftazidime / ticarcillin + clavulanic acid / piperacillin + tazobactam (1/8), aztreonam / ciprofloxacin / gentamicin / ticarcillin + clavulanic acid (1/8), aztreonam / cefepime / gentamicin / ticarcillin + clavulanic acid / piperacillin + tazobactam (1/8), aztreonam / cefepime / ciprofloxacin / ticarcillin + clavulanic acid / piperacillin + tazobactam (1/8).

The two XDR isolates were obtained only from dogs. One isolate expressed serotype O12 and was susceptible to only one antimicrobial category (polymyxin) and non-susceptible to at least one agent in all other antimicrobial categories (including aminoglycosides, as it was non-susceptible to gentamicin). The other XDR isolate, was a PA isolate fully susceptible to two antimicrobial categories (carbapenems and polymyxin) and non-susceptible to at least one agent in all other antimicrobial categories (including cephalosporins, as it was non-susceptible to cefepime, and aminoglycosides, as it was non-susceptible to gentamicin).

Genotyping

Fully automated rep-PCR (DiversiLab system) was used as a rapid method to genetically analyze the population structure of *P. aeruginosa*. The total genome profile was determined by rep-PCR and combined with former data from clinical (animal and human) and environmental *P. aeruginosa* isolates collected across the world, previously studied through a polyphasic approach consisting of three outer membrane (lipo)protein gene sequences (*oprI*, *oprL* and *oprD*), amplified fragment length polymorphism, serotype and pyoverdine type [4].

Genotyping with rep-PCR did not show any animal specific cluster, as showed in Fig 1. The dendrogram included a total of 151 *P. aeruginosa* isolates: 73 from this study, and 5 isolates which were not fully characterized from animals collected in Portugal (these 78 are delineated in blue), and 73 *P. aeruginosa* isolates from clinic (animal and human) and environmental samples from a previous study [4]. Considering a similarity of ≥80% clusters obtained included isolates from all origins: animal, human and environmental (Fig. 1). In fact, all animal isolates from this study, including the 78 animal clinical isolates collected from 2003–2012 in Portugal and the one sea turtle isolate sampled in the Gulf of Guinea, were homogeneously scattered in the global *P. aeruginosa* population structure previously depicted by Pirnay et al., (2002) [4].

Discussion

Rep-PCR is a rapid method for bacterial genome fingerprinting, based on highly conserved repetitive sequence elements [repetitive extragenic palindromic (REP) sequence] within bacterial genomes, which are amplified by PCR, allowing the analyses of strain-specific patterns [36]. DiversiLab system used in our study is more

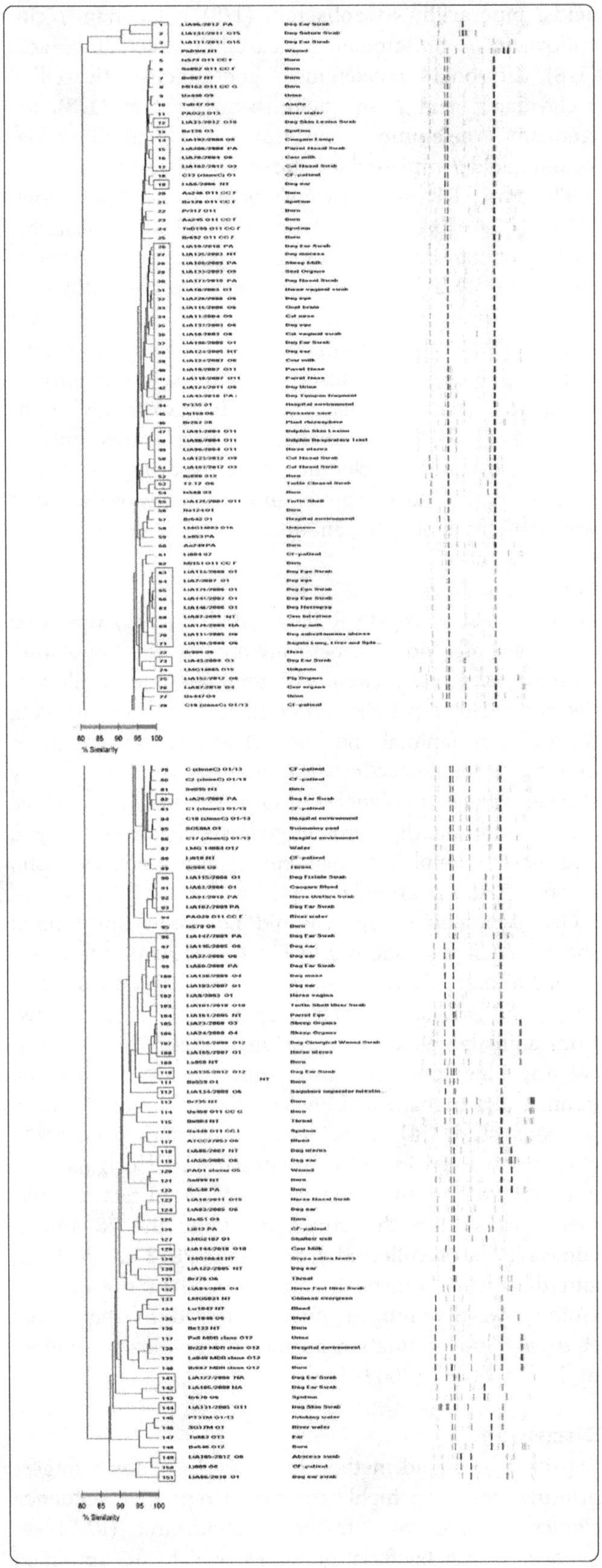

Fig. 1 Normalized rep-PCR patterns and dendrogram for a total of 151 *P. aeruginosa* isolates: 73 *P. aeruginosa* isolates of this study plus 5 animal isolates not fully characterized (all delineated in blue), and 73 *P. aeruginosa* isolates from clinic (animal and human) and environmental origin from a previous study [4]. DiversiLab dendrogram based on UPGMA and Pearson correlation coefficient. Percentages of similarity are shown below the dendrogram

reproducible than standard rep-PCR method, as the analysis is fully automated [37].

Multilocus sequence typing (MLST) is a strain-typing system that focuses exclusively on seven conserved housekeeping genes. The analysis of these genes, less likely to undergo horizontal gene transfer because of selective neutrality, provides a more accurate imprint of the recombination effect [5, 38]. The combination of alleles at the seven loci provided an allelic profile, or sequence type (ST). The relatedness between isolates is determined through a dendrogram from the matrix of pairwise differences between STs [39]. These data can be used in different aspects of evolutionary biology, whether to understand the evolution of genetic lineages or to estimate the relative contribution of recombination and single mutations in bacterial species [40]. MLST is therefore suitable for phylogenetic analysis enabling to track the global clonal history of the species with high accuracy [38]. Another advantage of MLST is that sequence data are portable between laboratories enabling to compare data from different geographic areas [40].

Although MLST is highly informative, the genetic variation indexed by MLST accumulates slowly, being more useful for long term epidemiological studies [39]. It has a limited resolution when applied to closely related stains [37]. On the other hand, DiversiLab is efficient to detect subtle genomic differences when applied to very closely related strains, being more useful for short term studies and outbreaks investigation [37].

Although we did not perform MLST, DiversiLab system results allow concluding that all animal isolates from this study were homogeneously scattered in the global *P. aeruginosa* population structure (Fig. 1), confirming earlier results that *P. aeruginosa* has a non-clonal population structure [4].

Our results are in accordance with the previous study by Pirnay et al., (2002) [4], in which a total of 73 *P. aeruginosa* clinical and environmental isolates collected worldwide presented predominantly the following serotypes: O1 (12.3%), O6 (10.9%), O11 (15.1%). The only exception was for serotype O12, which was less frequent in our study (2.7% versus 9.6%) (Table 1) [4]. Our results also agree with a recent study [41], regarding *P. aeruginosa* isolates from nosocomial pneumonia cases from several hospitals located in different countries. In both studies, frequency of serotypes O6, O11, O1, O4, O12 and O15 was similar, as also observed for not typeable isolates. By the contrary, different results were observed regarding serotype O10 (4.1% versus 9.8%), and we were not able to detect serotypes O2, O7 and O8 (Table 1).

P. aeruginosa is generally resistant against a wide spectrum of antimicrobial agents. Hence, only a few agents, including some extended-spectrum β-lactams, aminoglycosides, and fluoroquinolones are still effective [42, 43]. Resistance patterns were typical for this species. Near 50% of isolates was susceptible to all antimicrobials tested (46.6%). As expected, the aminoglycosides, carbapenems, cephalosporins, and polymyxin studied had also low resistance levels, maximum 12.3% (Table 2), thus amikacin, cefepime, ceftazidime, colistin, gentamicin, imipenem, meropenem, and tobramycin are generally effective in animals. Of notice that carbapenems are critically important antimicrobials and should be reserved for human use. The latest European Medicines Agency report, published in October 2015, shows that sales of antimicrobials for use in animals in Europe fell by approximately 8% between 2011 and 2013. However, there are notably differences between countries: 11 countries have decreased the sales of veterinary antimicrobial agents, whereas 6 countries including Portugal increased [44]. The greater percentages of sales for food-producing animals, including horses, in mg per population correction unit (mg/PCU), of the various veterinary antimicrobial classes, in Portugal, in 2013, were tetracyclines (39.2), penicillins (16.9), macrolides (12.4), polymyxins (10.1) [44].

There was a high resistance rate among animal isolates tested against monobactam aztreonam (41.1%). Resistance rates of penicillins [ticarcillin (16.4%), ticarcillin + clavulanic acid (17.8%), piperacillin + tazobactam (12.3%)] and the fluoroquinolone ciprofloxacin (15.1%) were inferior to 20% (Table 2).

The higher resistance rates among those critical antimicrobials should most probably result from intrinsic antimicrobial resistance traits of *P. aeruginosa*, such as low cell wall permeability, and its capacity to express acquired resistance mechanisms [14], and to a lesser degree to veterinary medicine antimicrobial consumption. It should be addressed that probably this collection of strains from animals are probably more resistant than in general, since often specimens are collected from chronic cases.

Near 14% of isolates were MDR and XDR (13.7%), pointing to the importance of the transmission of antimicrobial resistance genes in *P. aeruginosa* from animals. The antimicrobial resistance is a priority to FAO/OIE/WHO under the concept "One Health". Is crucial to include an international perspective in any politics about antimicrobial resistance. To decrease antimicrobial resistance in veterinary isolates, it is important to continue to implement responsible-use campaigns, to raise awareness of the threat of antimicrobial resistance, and to restrict its use and targets [44]. In the future, a safe and gradual implementation of alternatives to antimicrobials will be crucial to face antimicrobial resistance [45].

Interestingly, the XDR isolate only susceptible to amikacin, colistin, and tobramycin, was isolated from a dog with an infected surgical wound and was serotyped as O12 which is a serotype associated with human XDR clonal-cluster [5, 46]. Based on this observation, can one can speculate the possibility of resistance transmission from humans to animals [27, 28].

Conclusions

The reported data shows that serotype frequency and the resistance patterns of *P. aeruginosa* collected from animals were typical for this species. The intrinsic resistance mechanism of *P. aeruginosa* should explain the presence of multidrug profiles and the high resistance rates observed in some critical antimicrobials. This study confirms earlier results that *P. aeruginosa* has a non-clonal population structure, and demonstrates the similarity between environmental and clinical isolates from animals and humans. They are all part of the global *P. aeruginosa* population and form a non-clonal epidemic structure. No specific 'animal clonal lineage' could be detected.

Acknowledgments

The authors want to thank to the Interdisciplinary Research Center for Animal Health (CIISA), Faculty of Veterinary Medicine, University of Lisbon (FMV/UL), Portugal, Fundação para a Ciência e a Tecnologia (FCT), Portugal (Project UID/CVT/00276/2013), and to the Laboratory for Molecular and Cellular Technology, Queen Astrid Military Hospital, Brussels, Belgium, for supporting this work.

Funding

Fundação para a Ciência e a Tecnologia (FCT), Portugal (Project UID/CVT/00276/2013); Interdisciplinary Research Center for Animal Health (CIISA), Faculty of Veterinary Medicine, University of Lisbon (FMV/UL), Portugal; Laboratory for Molecular and Cellular Technology, Queen Astrid Military Hospital, Brussels, Belgium.

Authors' contributions

IS Analyzed the data and wrote the manuscript. MO conceived the study and participated in its coordination, helped to draft the manuscript. JPS carried out the phenotypic assays and the molecular genetic studies. FB carried out the phenotypic assays and the molecular genetic studies. AL helped to draft the manuscript. LT participated in the study design and coordination. JPP participated in results analysis and helped to draft the manuscript. DdV conceived the study and participated in its coordination, helped to draft the manuscript. All authors read and approved the final manuscript.

Competing interests
The authors declare that they have no competing interests.

Consent for publication
Not applicable.

Author details
[1]CIISA/Faculty of Veterinary Medicine, University of Lisbon, Lisbon, Portugal. [2]Laboratory for Molecular and Cellular Technology, Queen Astrid Military Hospital, Brussels, Belgium.

References

1. Lyczak JB, Cannon CL, Pier GB. Establishment of Pseudomonas aeruginosa infection: lessons from a versatile opportunist. Microbes Infect. 2000;2(9): 1051–60.
2. Talbot GH, Bradley J, Edwards Jr JE, Gilbert D, Scheld M, Bartlett JG. Bad bugs need drugs: an update on the development pipeline from the Antimicrobial Availability Task Force of the Infectious Diseases Society of America. Clin Infect Dis. 2006;42(5):657–68.
3. Goldberg JB. Pseudomonas: global bacteria. Trends Microbiol. 2000;8(2):55–7.
4. Pirnay JP, De Vos D, Cochez C, Bilocq F, Vanderkelen A, Zizi M, Ghysels B, Cornelis P. Pseudomonas aeruginosa displays an epidemic population structure. Environ Microbiol. 2002;4(12):898–911.
5. Pirnay JP, Bilocq F, Pot B, Cornelis P, Zizi M, Van Eldere J, Deschaght P, Vaneechoutte M, Jennes S, Pitt T, et al. Pseudomonas aeruginosa population structure revisited. PloS One. 2009;4(11), e7740.
6. Silby MW, Winstanley C, Godfrey SA, Levy SB, Jackson RW. Pseudomonas genomes: diverse and adaptable. FEMS Microbiol Rev. 2011;35(4):652–80.
7. Rahme LG, Ausubel FM, Cao H, Drenkard E, Goumnerov BC, Lau GW, Mahajan-Miklos S, Plotnikova J, Tan MW, Tsongalis J, et al. Plants and animals share functionally common bacterial virulence factors. Proc Natl Acad Sci USA. 2000;97(16):8815–21.
8. Apidianakis Y, Rahme LG. Drosophila melanogaster as a model host for studying Pseudomonas aeruginosa infection. Nat Protoc. 2009;4(9):1285–94.
9. Miyata S, Casey M, Frank DW, Ausubel FM, Drenkard E. Use of the Galleria mellonella caterpillar as a model host to study the role of the type III secretion system in Pseudomonas aeruginosa pathogenesis. Infect Immun. 2003;71(5):2404–13.
10. Clatworthy AE, Lee JS, Leibman M, Kostun Z, Davidson AJ, Hung DT. Pseudomonas aeruginosa infection of zebrafish involves both host and pathogen determinants. Infect Immun. 2009;77(4):1293–303.
11. Potvin E, Lehoux DE, Kukavica-Ibrulj I, Richard KL, Sanschagrin F, Lau GW, Levesque RC. In vivo functional genomics of Pseudomonas aeruginosa for high-throughput screening of new virulence factors and antibacterial targets. Environ Microbiol. 2003;5(12):1294–308.
12. Snouwaert JN, Brigman KK, Latour AM, Malouf NN, Boucher RC, Smithies O, Koller BH. An animal model for cystic fibrosis made by gene targeting. Science. 1992;257(5073):1083–8.
13. Ledbetter EC, Mun JJ, Kowbel D, Fleiszig SM. Pathogenic phenotype and genotype of Pseudomonas aeruginosa isolates from spontaneous canine ocular infections. Invest Ophthalmol Vis Sci. 2009;50(2):729–36.
14. Nam HM, Lim SK, Kang HM, Kim JM, Moon JS, Jang KC, Kim JM, Joo YS, Jung SC. Prevalence and antimicrobial susceptibility of gram-negative bacteria isolated from bovine mastitis between 2003 and 2008 in Korea. J Dairy Sci. 2009;92(5):2020–6.
15. Sela S, Hammer-Muntz O, Krifucks O, Pinto R, Weisblit L, Leitner G. Phenotypic and genotypic characterization of Pseudomonas aeruginosa strains isolated from mastitis outbreaks in dairy herds. J Dairy Res. 2007; 74(4):425–9.
16. Sura R, Creden A, Van Kruiningen HJ. Pseudomonas-associated discospondylitis in a two-month-old llama. J Vet Diagn Invest. 2008;20(3):349–52.
17. McKay L, Rose CD, Matousek JL, Schmeitzel LS, Gibson NM, Gaskin JM. Antimicrobial testing of selected fluoroquinolones against Pseudomonas aeruginosa isolated from canine otitis. J Am Anim Hosp Assoc. 2007;43(6):307–12.
18. Rubin J, Walker RD, Blickenstaff K, Bodeis-Jones S, Zhao S. Antimicrobial resistance and genetic characterization of fluoroquinolone resistance of Pseudomonas aeruginosa isolated from canine infections. Vet Microbiol. 2008;131(1-2):164–72.
19. Hillier A, Alcorn JR, Cole LK, Kowalski JJ. Pyoderma caused by Pseudomonas aeruginosa infection in dogs: 20 cases. Vet Dermatol. 2006;17(6):432–9.
20. Lin CT, Petersen-Jones SM. Antibiotic susceptibility of bacteria isolated from cats with ulcerative keratitis in Taiwan. J Small Anim Pract. 2008;49(2):80–3.
21. Werckenthin C, Alesik E, Grobbel M, Lubke-Becker A, Schwarz S, Wieler LH, Wallmann J. Antimicrobial susceptibility of Pseudomonas aeruginosa from dogs and cats as well as Arcanobacterium pyogenes from cattle and swine as determined in the BfT-GermVet monitoring program 2004-2006. Berl Munch Tierarztl Wochenschr. 2007;120(9-10):412–22.
22. Weese JS. A review of multidrug resistant surgical site infections. Vet Comp Orthop Traumatol. 2008;21(1):1–7.
23. Haenni M, Hocquet D, Ponsin C, Cholley P, Guyeux C, Madec JY, Bertrand X. Population structure and antimicrobial susceptibility of Pseudomonas aeruginosa from animal infections in France. BMC Vet Res. 2015;11:9.
24. De Vos D, Lim Jr A, Pirnay JP, Struelens M, Vandenvelde C, Duinslaeger L, Vanderkelen A, Cornelis P. Direct detection and identification of Pseudomonas aeruginosa in clinical samples such as skin biopsy specimens and expectorations by multiplex PCR based on two outer membrane lipoprotein genes, oprI and oprL. J Clin Microbiol. 1997;35(6):1295–9.
25. Masuda N, Sakagawa E, Ohya S. Outer membrane proteins responsible for multiple drug resistance in Pseudomonas aeruginosa. Antimicrob Agents Chemother. 1995;39(3):645–9.
26. Nikaido H. Prevention of drug access to bacterial targets: permeability barriers and active efflux. Science. 1994;264(5157):382–8.
27. Mohan K, Fothergill JL, Storrar J, Ledson MJ, Winstanley C, Walshaw MJ. Transmission of Pseudomonas aeruginosa epidemic strain from a patient with cystic fibrosis to a pet cat. Thorax. 2008;63(9):839–40.
28. Wang Y, Wang X, Schwarz S, Zhang R, Lei L, Liu X, Lin D, Shen J. IMP-45-producing multidrug-resistant Pseudomonas aeruginosa of canine origin. J Antimicrob Chemother. 2014;69(9):2579–81.
29. Alonso A, Rojo F, Martinez JL. Environmental and clinical isolates of Pseudomonas aeruginosa show pathogenic and biodegradative properties irrespective of their origin. Environ Microbiol. 1999;1(5):421–30.
30. Romling U, Wingender J, Muller H, Tummler B. A major Pseudomonas aeruginosa clone common to patients and aquatic habitats. Appl Environ Microbiol. 1994;60(6):1734–8.
31. Liu PV, Wang S. Three new major somatic antigens of Pseudomonas aeruginosa. J Clin Microbiol. 1990;28(5):922–5.
32. CLSI. Performance Standards for Antimicrobial Disk and Dilution Susceptibility Tests for Bacteria Isolated from Animals, CLSI supplement VET01S. 3rd ed. Wayne: Clinical and Laboratory Standards Institute; 2015.
33. CLSI. Performance Standards for Antimicrobial Susceptibility Testing, CLSI supplement M100-S25. Wayne: Clinical and Laboratory Standards Institute; 2015.
34. Doleans-Jordheim A, Cournoyer B, Bergeron E, Croize J, Salord H, Andre J, Mazoyer MA, Renaud FN, Freney J. Reliability of Pseudomonas aeruginosa semi-automated rep-PCR genotyping in various epidemiological situations. Eur J Clin Microbiol Infect Dis. 2009;28(9):1105–11.
35. Magiorakos AP, Srinivasan A, Carey RB, Carmeli Y, Falagas ME, Giske CG, Harbarth S, Hindler JF, Kahlmeter G, Olsson-Liljequist B, et al. Multidrug-resistant, extensively drug-resistant and pandrug-resistant bacteria: an international expert proposal for interim standard definitions for acquired resistance. Clin Microbiol Infect. 2012;18(3):268–81.
36. Olive DM, Bean P. Principles and applications of methods for DNA-based typing of microbial organisms. J Clin Microbiol. 1999;37(6):1661–9.
37. Maatallah M, Bakhrouf A, Habeeb MA, Turlej-Rogacka A, Iversen A, Pourcel C, Sioud O, Giske CG. Four genotyping schemes for phylogenetic analysis of Pseudomonas aeruginosa: comparison of their congruence with multi-locus sequence typing. PLoS One. 2013;8(12), e82069.
38. Khan NH, Ahsan M, Yoshizawa S, Hosoya S, Yokota A, Kogure K. Multilocus sequence typing and phylogenetic analyses of Pseudomonas aeruginosa Isolates from the ocean. Appl Environ Microbiol. 2008;74(20):6194–205.
39. Enright MC, Spratt BG. A multilocus sequence typing scheme for Streptococcus pneumoniae: identification of clones associated with serious invasive disease. Microbiology. 1998;144(Pt 11):3049–60.
40. Spratt BG. Multilocus sequence typing: molecular typing of bacterial pathogens in an era of rapid DNA sequencing and the internet. Curr Opin Microbiol. 1999; 2(3):312–6.

41. Lu Q, Eggimann P, Luyt CE, Wolff M, Tamm M, Francois B, Mercier E, Garbino J, Laterre PF, Koch H, et al. Pseudomonas aeruginosa serotypes in nosocomial pneumonia: prevalence and clinical outcomes. Crit Care (London, England). 2014;18(1):R17.
42. Harada K, Arima S, Niina A, Kataoka Y, Takahashi T. Characterization of Pseudomonas aeruginosa isolates from dogs and cats in Japan: current status of antimicrobial resistance and prevailing resistance mechanisms. Microbiol Immunol. 2012;56(2):123–7.
43. Lister PD, Wolter DJ, Hanson ND. Antibacterial-resistant Pseudomonas aeruginosa: clinical impact and complex regulation of chromosomally encoded resistance mechanisms. Clin Microbiol Rev. 2009;22(4):582–610.
44. EMA - European Medicines Agency. Sales of veterinary antimicrobial agents in 26 EU/EEA countries in 2013 (EMA/387934/2015). In: European Surveillance of Veterinary Antimicrobial Consumption; 2015.
45. Oliveira M, Serrano I (eds.). Frontiers in antimicrobial agents - The challenges of antimicrobial resistance in the development of new therapeutics. Sharjah: Bentham Science Publishers; 2016.
46. Pirnay JP, De Vos D, Cochez C, Bilocq F, Pirson J, Struelens M, Duinslaeger L, Cornelis P, Zizi M, Vanderkelen A. Molecular epidemiology of Pseudomonas aeruginosa colonization in a burn unit: persistence of a multidrug-resistant clone and a silver sulfadiazine-resistant clone. J Clin Microbiol. 2003;41(3): 1192–202.

Neoplastic diseases in the domestic ferret (*Mustela putorius furo*) in Italy: classification and tissue distribution of 856 cases (2000–2010)

Giancarlo Avallone[1], Annalisa Forlani[2], Marco Tecilla[3*], Elena Riccardi[2], Sara Belluco[4], Sara Francesca Santagostino[5], Guido Grilli[3], Kiumars Khadivi[6] and Paola Roccabianca[3]

Abstract

Background: The aim of this study was to describe the prevalence and tissue distribution of neoplasms in Italian ferrets, compared to the epidemiological data previously reported in USA and Japan.

Methods: Signalment and diagnoses of pathological submissions received between 2000 and 2010 were searched; cases with the diagnosis of neoplasm were selected and original sections reviewed to confirm the diagnosis.

Results: Nine-hundred and ten samples were retrieved, 690 of which included at least one tumour for a total of 856 tumours. Ferrets with multiple neoplasms were 134 (19.4%). Median age was 5 years, and F/M ratio was 0.99. Endocrine neoplasms were the most common. Other frequent tumours were cutaneous mast cell tumours, sebaceous tumours, and lymphomas. Cutaneous squamous cell carcinomas (SCC) were consistently associated with sebaceous tumours. Twenty-four abdominal spindle cell tumours with an undefined origin were observed. Lymphomas and islet cell tumours had a lower incidence compared with previous extra-European studies.

Discussion: Epidemiological information on ferret tumours derives from extra-European countries, mostly USA and Japan. In these countries similar distributions with minor discrepancies have been reported. Compared to previous reports, adrenal tumours were more frequent than pancreatic islet cell neoplasms, and a higher number of mesenchymal neoplasms arising from the adrenal capsule was noted. An unusual association between SCC and sebaceous gland neoplasms and a high number of intrabdominal spindle cell neoplasms with unclear primary origin were noted and grants further investigation.

Conclusions: The tissue distribution of tumours recorded in this study paralleled previous findings in ferrets from USA and Japan. Some differences have been noted in the frequency of lymphoma, adrenal mesenchymal tumours and cutaneous tumours. Some tumours that are among the most common in other species seem to be uncommon in ferrets and are characterized by distinctive predilection sites.

Keywords: Ferret, Tumours, Neoplastic diseases

* Correspondence: marco.tecilla@unimi.it; marco.tecilla@gmail.com
[3]Department of Veterinary Medicine, University of Milan, Via Celoria 10, 20100 Milan, Italy
Full list of author information is available at the end of the article

Background

The ferret (*Mustela putorius furo*) is a popular non-conventional companion animal for which a prevalence of neoplastic diseases ranging from 5.2 to 12% has been described [1–4].

Tumours of the endocrine system are the most common neoplasms in ferrets with a majority of pancreatic islet and adrenal tumours [1–4]. Pancreatic islet beta cell tumours represent the most frequent neoplasm and almost the totality of primary pancreatic neoplasms in ferrets [1–5]. Genetic and nutritional components have been postulated to predispose ferrets to the onset of this tumour type in the United States [5]. Adrenal tumours have been reported as the second most frequent endocrine disease both in the United States and Japan [1–4]. The pathogenesis leading to adrenal gland disease is still debated; however, early gonadectomy combined with an artificially prolonged photoperiod experienced by indoor pet ferrets, along with a possible genetic component, seem to predispose to adrenal tumours [6].

The second most common affected systems are the hemolymphatic and the integumentary system, with similar frequencies [1–4]. Hemolymphatic neoplasms have a slightly higher frequency in ferrets from North America [1], while the contrary occurs for integumentary neoplasms in ferrets from Japan [3]. The epidemiological similarities of neoplastic disease between Japanese and U.S. ferrets could be explained by the fact that most Japanese pet ferrets are imported from North America, and their husbandry, including diet, is comparable [3].

To the best of our knowledge, there are no epidemiologic reports with reference to domestic ferret neoplastic diseases in Europe and, specifically, in Italy. This represents an 11-year retrospective study investigating tumour types and their prevalence in ferrets from Northern Italy.

Methods

The electronic archives of the exotic and non-conventional companion animal diagnostic service were searched from its establishment in 2000 till 2010 covering a 11-year period. Records of histopathological samples from ferrets (biopsies and necropsies) including at least one neoplastic lesion were retrieved, and data regarding gender, age, breed, site of the lesions and histological diagnoses were collected. In Italy, early gonadectomy is frequent in ferrets; however the neutering status was inconsistently included, therefore, gender was categorized into male (61 ferrets), female (76 ferrets), neutered males (252 ferrets), neutered females (238 ferrets) and unknown (59 ferrets).

Tumour types were classified according to the published references or the pertinent fascicles of the World Health Organization "International Histological Classification of Tumours of Domestic Animals" [7].

Neoplasms were grouped by affected organ system (e.g. skin and subcutis, gastrointestinal tract, etc.) with the exclusion of lymphoid neoplasms that were grouped independently from the organ or tissue of origin. Cases of neoplastic diseases with low frequency were grouped in a set named "miscellaneous". Neoplasms developing in the same ferret but with different tissue of origin and different malignancy were recorded as independent neoplasms using the same identification number for the ferret. Hyperplastic lesions were excluded. The diagnoses were reviewed independently by 4 board certified pathologists. Differences between the diagnoses were discussed jointly to achieve an agreement.

Results

The number of pathological specimens collected from ferrets during an 11-year period was 910. Of these, 690 samples contained at least one neoplastic lesion. Multiple neoplasms occurred in 134 cases (19.4%): 111 ferrets were diagnosed with two tumours, 16 with three, 5 with four, and 2 with five different tumours. Consequently, a total of 856 tumours was included in this study. The tissue distribution of all neoplasms excluding lymphoid tumours is summarized in Table 1. The tissue distribution of lymphoid neoplasm is summarized in Table 2.

Specifically, of the 856 tumours, 313 adrenal tumours were collected, along with 200 pancreatic, 156 cutaneous and subcutaneous, 74 lymphoid, 26 skeletal, 24 intra-abdominal, 20 hepatic, 15 digestive tract, and 14 genital tumours. Fifteen cases were grouped under the "miscellaneous" category. Age was recorded in 459 cases. The mean age of affected ferrets was 4.5 years, and the median was 5, with a range from 7 months to 10 years. Age distribution in all affected ferrets and in ferrets with adrenocortical, insular and hemolymphatic tumours, is summarized in Fig. 1. Gender was recorded in 641 cases (321 males and 320 females). The F/M ratio was 0.99. Endocrine neoplasms were the most common (57.0%), followed by cutaneous/subcutaneous (18.2%) and lymphoid tumours (8.6%).

Adrenal gland

A total of 313 adrenal tumours were diagnosed in 303 ferrets, accounting for 36.6% of cases. Age ranged from 1 to 10 years (mean 4.4, median 4.5 years). Of the 313 adrenal tumours, 289 were cortical (228 carcinomas and 61 adenomas), eight of which were characterized by myxoid differentiation, while 13 derived from the adrenal medulla (11 pheochromocytomas and two neuroblastomas). Ten cases were mesenchymal, including two leiomyosarcomas, five leiomyomas and three spindle cell sarcomas. One case was diagnosed as undifferentiated malignant neoplasm NOS. Mesenchymal tumours were characterized by connection with adrenal gland capsule

Table 1 tissue distribution and specific diagnosis of tumors in ferrets

Organ system	Differentiation/ site	Diagnosis	N° of cases
Adrenal gland	Cortical	Cortical carcinoma	228
		Cortical adenoma	61
	Medullary	Pheochromocytoma	11
		Neuroblastoma	2
	Other	Leiomyoma	5
		Spindle cell sarcoma	3
		Leiomyosarcoma	2
		Malignant neoplasia NOS	1
Pancreas	Insular	Islet cell tumor	190
	Exocrine	Exocrine adenocarcinoma	6
		Exocrine adenomas	4
Skin and subcutis	Mastocytic	Mast cell tumor	68
	Sebaceous	Sebaceous epithelioma	22
		Sebaceous adenoma	16
	Apocrine	Apocrine adenocarcinoma	10
		Apocrine adenoma	8
	Squamous	Squamous cell carcinoma	9
	Vascular	Hemangioma	8
		Angiosarcoma	1
	Other	Fibroma	3
		Leiomyoma	3
		Basal cell carcinoma	2
		Trichoblastoma	2
		Leiomyosarcoma	1
		Rhabdomyosarcoma	1
		Infundibular keratinizing acanthoma	1
		Lipoma	1
Skeletal system		Chordoma	24
		Osteosarcoma	2
Abdominal cavity		Spindle cell tumor with polygonal cells	22
		Leiomyosarcoma	1
		Hemangioma	1
Liver	Cholangiocellular	Cholangiocellular carcinoma	6
	Vascular	Hemangiosarcoma	4
		Hemangioma	2
	Hepatocellular	Hepatocellular carcinoma	3
		Hepatocellular adenoma	2
	Round cell tumor	Undifferentiated NOS	3
Digestive tract	Oral cavity	Squamous cell carcinoma	3
		Fibromatous epulis	1
		Sarcoma NOS	1

Table 1 tissue distribution and specific diagnosis of tumors in ferrets *(Continued)*

	Stomach	Gastric carcinoma	3
	Intestine	Adenocarcinoma	6
		Leiomyoma	1
Genital system	Ovary	Gonadostromal tumor	3
		Carcinoma	1
	Uterus	Adenocarcinoma	2
		Leiomyoma	1
	Vagina	Papilloma	1
	Testicle	Seminoma	3
		Gonadostromal tumor	2
	Prostate	Adenocarcinoma	1
Miscellaneous	Lymph node	Metastatic neoplasm	4
		Hemangioma	1
	Spleen	RCT NOS	3
		Myelolipoma	1
	Kidney	Sarcoma NOS	1
	Lung	Adenocarcinoma	1
	Mediastinum	Hemangioma	1
	Thoracic cavity	Sarcoma NOS	1
	Salivary gland	Adenoma	1
	Lacrimal gland	Adenoma	1

and compression of adrenal parenchyma. Ten ferrets were affected by two simultaneous neoplasms (six cortical tumours associated with pheochromocytoma, three cortical tumours associated with mesenchymal tumours, and one pheochromocytoma associated with a mesenchymal tumour). The majority of cortical carcinomas were well differentiated and the main criteria for histological malignancy were infiltrative growth in the periadrenal adipose tissue (Fig. 2a and b), invasion of adjacent large vessels and poor demarcation from surrounding tissues [4].

Pancreas

A total of 200 pancreatic tumours were diagnosed in 196 ferrets, accounting for 23.4% of cases. Age ranged from 2 to 8 years (mean 5.3, median 5 years). Of the 200 pancreatic tumours, 190 were islet cell tumours and ten were exocrine [four adenomas (Fig. 2c) and six adenocarcinomas (Fig. 2d)]. Four ferrets were affected by concomitant insular and pancreatic exocrine tumour. The majority of insular tumours were well differentiated.

Skin and subcutis

Excluding lymphoid tumours, a total of 156 cutaneous and subcutaneous tumours were diagnosed in 119

Table 2 Tissue distribution of hemolymphatic tumors in ferrets

Differentiation	Distribution	N° of cases
Lymphoma	Nodal	16
	Splenic	14
	Gastrointestinal	13
	Multicentric	8
	Cutaneous	5
	Hepatic	5
	Hepatosplenic	5
	Pancreatic	1
	Renal	1
	Intra-abdominal NOS	2
Plasma cell tumor	Splenic	2
	Nodal	1
	Multicentric	1

ferrets, accounting for 18.2% of the cases. Age ranged from 1 to 10 years (mean 4.7, median 5 years). Sixty-eight mast cell tumours (Fig. 2e) were diagnosed. Sebaceous gland neoplasms were the second most frequent cutaneous neoplasm and included 22 epitheliomas (three of which were associated with a squamous cell carcinoma and five with squamous metaplasia), 16 adenomas (six of which associated with squamous cell carcinoma and three with squamous metaplasia). A total of nine squamous cell carcinomas (Fig. 2f) were diagnosed, accounting for 5.8% of cutaneous tumours, and were all associated with sebaceous tumours.

Eighteen apocrine gland neoplasms were diagnosed (ten adenocarcinomas and eight adenomas). Three out of ten adenocarcinomas were located in the preputial region. Other tumour types included: eight hemangiomas, three fibromas, three leiomyomas, two trichoblastomas, two basal cell carcinomas, one angiosarcoma, one leiomyosarcoma, one rhabdomyosarcoma, one infundibular keratinizing acanthoma, and one lipoma. In this group, 25 ferrets had multiple neoplasms. Of these, sixteen were diagnosed with two tumours, six with three tumours, and three with four tumours.

Hemolymphatic tumours

Seventy-four tumours affecting the lymphoid tissue were retrieved, accounting for 8.6% of cases. Age ranged from 7 months to 8.5 years (mean 3.4, median 3.5 years). Seventy were lymphomas; the majority were primary nodal (16), 14 splenic, 13 were localized in the gastrointestinal tract (four in the stomach and nine in the intestine), eight were multicentric, five were cutaneous (two of which were epitheliotropic), five hepatic, five hepatosplenic, one pancreatic and one renal. Two cases consisted of an intra-abdominal mass with no connection to recognizable organs or tissues. Four plasma cell tumours were diagnosed: two were splenic, one nodal and one multicentric.

Skeletal system

Twenty-six tumours arising from the skeletal system were retrieved (3% of the caseload). The majority were chordomas (24 cases) and two were osteosarcomas. Age

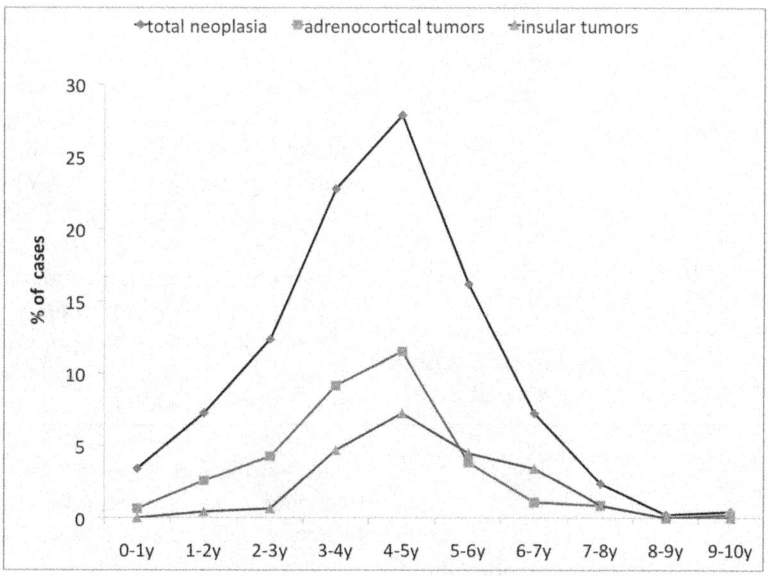

Fig. 1 Histogram representing age distribution for all neoplastic lesions (*line with squares*) and for each of the most represented neoplastic categories: adrenocortical (*line with diamonds*), insular (*line with triangles*) and hemolymphatic (*lines with circles*) tumors in ferrets. The number of cases is expressed as percentage of the total cases for which the age was indicated

ranged from 8 months to 7 years (mean 3.7, median 4 years). All chordomas were located on the tail, whereas the two osteosarcomas arose from the maxilla.

Abdominal cavity

Twenty-four intra-abdominal tumours without connection to any recognizable organ or tissue were diagnosed, accounting for 2.8% of cases. Age ranged from 1 to 8 years (mean 3.4, median 3 years), all ferrets were female. Twenty-two were well demarcated tumours with a diameter ranging from 0.8 to 4 cm, composed mostly of interlacing bundles of spindle cells intermixed with polygonal cells with vacuolated cytoplasm. The remaining two cases were one leiomyosarcoma and one hemangioma respectively.

Liver

Twenty-six tumours were detected in the liver. Excluding lymphoid tumours, 20 hepatic tumours were diagnosed (3% of the caseload), including six cholangiocellular carcinomas, six vascular tumours (four hemangiosarcomas and two hemangiomas), five hepatocellular tumours (three carcinomas and two adenomas), and three undifferentiated RCTs. Age ranged from 2 to 7 years (mean 4.4, median 4 years).

Digestive tract

Thirty tumours were detected in the digestive tract. Excluding lymphoid tumours, a total of 15 tumours (accounting for the 1.75% of the caseload) arising from the digestive tract were diagnosed. Age ranged from 2 to 7 years of age (mean 4.2, median 4 years). Five cases were in the oral cavity (three squamous cell carcinomas, one fibromatous epulis and one sarcoma NOS), seven in the intestine (six adenocarcinomas and one leiomyoma) and three were gastric carcinomas.

Female genital system

Eight tumours, accounting for the 0.9%, were diagnosed. Ovarian neoplasms included three gonadostromal tumours (theca cell tumours) and one cystic papillary adenocarcinoma. Neoplasms arising from the uterus were two adenocarcinomas and one leiomyoma. One single vaginal papilloma was recorded. Age ranged from 1 to 6 years (mean 3.2, median 2.8 years).

Male genital system

Six tumours were diagnosed (accounting for the 0.7% of the cases) and included three seminomas, two gonadostromal tumours (Leydig cell tumour) and one prostatic adenocarcinoma. Age ranged from 3 to 7 years (mean 5, median 5 years).

Miscellanea

Other 14 tumours identified, accounting for the 1.6% of the caseload. The miscellanea tumors included: four cases in which a tumour metastatic to the lymph node was the sole sample submitted (three adenocarcinomas with apocrine differentiation and one undifferentiated neuroendocrine tumour), three splenic round cell tumours NOS, one primary nodal hemangioma, one lacrimal gland adenoma, one salivary gland adenoma, one renal sarcoma, one splenic myelolipoma, one mediastinal hemangioma, one pulmonary adenocarcinoma and one sarcoma arising in the thoracic cavity. Age ranged from 3 to 7 years (mean 5.1, median 5 years).

Discussion

Epidemiological information on tumours in ferrets derives from extra-European countries, mostly USA and Japan [1–4]. In these countries, similar distributions have been reported, with minor discrepancies on the frequency of hemolymphatic and integumentary tumours [1–4]. In our study, the histologic type and tissue distribution of 856 neoplasms from Italian ferrets is reported. A predilection of gender was not observed, and the age of affected ferrets was variable, paralleling the findings of previous reports [1–6].

Additionally, similar to previous reports, endocrine neoplasms represented the majority of tumours in domestic ferrets [1–4]. On the contrary, adrenal tumours were more frequent compared to pancreatic islet cell neoplasms in this report. This discrepancy can be explained partially by the criteria applied in this study to classify islet cell tumours: multiple islet cell tumours in the same sample were regarded as a single case, interpreting the development of multiple identical pancreatic neoplasms in the same animal as the consequence of the same pathological process.

Most adrenal neoplasms were malignant and originated from the cortex, whereas pheochromocytomas were less common, paralleling previous observations [6, 8]. Similar to previous studies [6, 8], no female/male predisposition was highlighted. In fact, early gonadectomy and neutering (commonly performed in Italian ferrets), combined with the artificial prolonged photoperiod experienced by indoor pet ferrets are believed to predispose both genders to the development of adrenocortical tumours.

Interestingly, we observed a higher frequency of mesenchymal neoplasms arising from the adrenal capsule compared with other reports [1–4]. These tumours were characterized by scant amount of residual adrenal tissue and by smooth muscle differentiation in the majority of cases.

Pancreatic islet cells tumours have been well characterized in ferrets over the last 20 years [5], and are reported as the most common neoplasm in middle aged

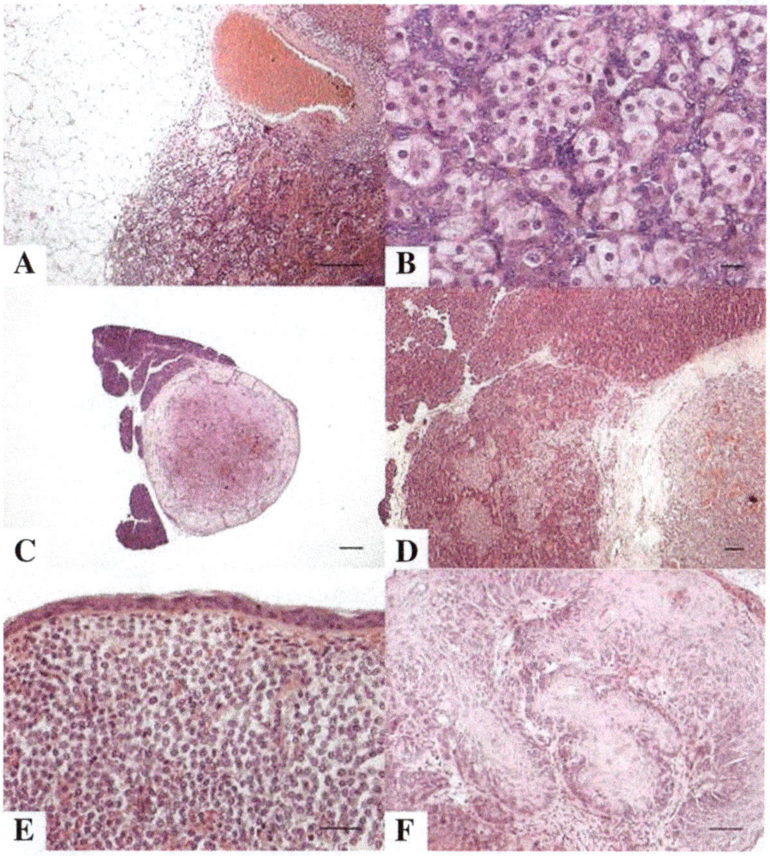

Fig. 2 a Adrenocortical carcinoma, adrenal gland, ferret. Neoplastic cells infiltrate the capsule and adjacent adipose tissue with a mild desmoplasia, and minimal lymphoplasmacytic inflammation. Bar 50 micron, Hematoxylin and eosin stain. **b** Adrenocortical carcinoma, adrenal gland, ferret. Concurrent presence of large polygonal cells of the zona fasciculate characterized by granular cytoplasm and of smaller cells with high nuclear/cytoplasmic ratio. Bar 50 micron, Hematoxylin and eosin stain. **c** Insular adenoma, pancreas, ferret. Typical expansile growth delimited by a thick fibrous capsule. Cells are organized in dense pockets with minimal highly vascularized stroma. Bar 1 mm, Hematoxylin and eosin stain. **d** Insular adenocarcinoma, pancreas, ferret. The tumor is characterized by infiltration of the capsule and adjacent exocrine pancreas by neoplastic cells. Bar 50 micron, Hematoxylin and eosin stain. **e** Squamous cell carcinoma, skin, ferret. Cords of atypical keratinocytes of the spinous layer are proliferating and invading the superficial dermis. Asynchronous keratinocyte maturation and keratin pearls are visible. Bar 50 micron, Hematoxylin and eosin stain. **f** Well differentiated mast cell tumor, haired skin, ferret. The dermis is diffusely obscured and substituted by dense sheets of well-differentiated mast cells. Bar 50 micron, Hematoxylin and eosin stain

to older ferrets [1–5]. On the contrary, islet cell tumours were the second most common neoplasm in our study, with a majority demonstrating an infiltrative growth. Nevertheless, the infiltrative growth has not been demonstrated to be an indication of malignancy in these tumours [2, 4]. A slight prevalence of male ferrets was observed; this statement is in agreement with previous reports [5].

Cutaneous and subcutaneous mast cell tumours were the most frequent skin neoplasms, followed by sebaceous and apocrine gland tumours. This data parallels one study reporting mast cell tumour as one of the most frequent skin tumour of ferrets [9], but is in contrast with several reports in which sebaceous gland tumours as the most frequent cutaneous neoplasm [1–4].

In our caseload, the number of sebaceous epitheliomas was slightly higher than adenomas. Both tumour types were characterized by squamous differentiation, and by areas of SCC development in nine cases. The presence of squamous metaplasia has been previously reported in these tumours that have been defined as “basal cell tumour with sebaceous and squamous differentiation” and interpreted as putatively arising from pluripotential basal cells [10]. The occurrence of SCC within sebaceous tumours has been previously reported in long-standing lesions in ferrets, but valid hypotheses able to explain this association are lacking [2, 4].

The prevalence of vascular cutaneous/subcutaneous neoplasms in our caseload parallels previous reports [3, 10]. On the contrary, cutaneous neoplasms of smooth muscular origin were less common in this study [3, 11].

The lymphoid tissue was the third most commonly involved by neoplastic disease after endocrine tissues and skin/subcutis. Most lymphomas were nodal, followed by lymphoma arising from the spleen and the gastrointestinal tract. The frequency of lymphoma was lower than what previously reported [1–4]. In the United States, lymphoma has been hypothesized to have a viral etiology in ferrets [12–14]. However, the agent has not been identified even if horizontal transmission of lymphoma using cell or cell free inoculation has been demonstrated, supporting this hypothesis [12–14]. The different frequency of lymphoma in our caseload compared with ferrets from the U.S. could be related to a dissimilar distribution of this putative etiological agent. A further hypothesis may derive from the fact that, in veterinary practice, lymphomas are frequently diagnosed by cytology only; thus, the number of lymphomas in our caseload could be underestimated. Similarly to what is reported in literature, hemangiosarcomas occurred more commonly in the liver, hemangiomas mainly in the skin, and rarely in thoracic and abdominal cavity, likely in association with serosal membranes [4, 15].

Skeletal tumours consisted mainly of chordomas, and were located on the tail as previously reported [3, 16]. On the contrary, osteosarcomas were rare and arose in the maxillary region rather than in the appendicular bones.

It is worth mentioning the high number of spindle cells tumours with vacuolated cells evidenced within the abdominal cavity, without connection to identifiable organs or tissues. No reports of these tumours seem to be available [1–4]. The large size of these neoplasms can be explained by the lack of associated clinical signs, leading to a late diagnosis. In these abdominal tumours, the spindle cell component accounted for almost the 90% of the neoplasm, while the vacuolated component was minimal. The morphology of the polygonal neoplastic vacuolated cells strongly resembled adrenal cortical cells, suggesting a possible origin from ectopic adrenal tissue. The documented presence of a spindle cell component within certain adrenal neoplasms likely supports this hypothesis [17, 18], and has been considered both a normal stromal component of the tumours or part of the tumours itself [17, 18].

Conclusions

In conclusion, the frequency and the tissue distribution of tumours recorded in this study paralleled previous findings, with some differences regarding the frequency of lymphoma, adrenal mesenchymal tumours and the type of cutaneous tumours. Some tumours that are among the most common in other species, such as hemangiosarcoma, osteosarcoma and SCC, seem to be uncommon in ferrets and to be characterized by distinctive predilection sites. The unusual association between SCC and sebaceous gland neoplasms and the primary origin of intrabdominal spindle cell neoplasms grants further investigation.

Abbreviations

MCT: Mast cell tumors; NOS: Not otherwise specified; RCT: Round cell tumors; SCC: Squamous cell carcinomas

Acknowledgements

No acknowledgements required.

Funding

The author (s) received no financial support for the research, authorship, and/or publication of this article.

Authors' contributions

GA: study design, selection of cases, reviewing of the histological diagnosis, interpretation of data for the work, literature search, participated in writing. AF: selection of cases, reviewing of the histological diagnosis, execution analysis, interpretation of data for the work, literature search, participated in writing. MT: selection of cases, reviewed the study proposal, participated in writing, image editing. ER: reviewing of the histological diagnosis, editing of the manuscript. SB: reviewing of the histological diagnosis, editing of the manuscript. SF: reviewed the study proposal, selection of cases, participated in writing. GG: reviewed the study proposal, editing of the manuscript. KK: provided some of the cases, editing of the manuscript. PR: study design, selection of cases, reviewing of the histological diagnosis, participated in writing. All authors read and approved the final manuscript.

Competing interests

The authors declare that they have no competing interests.

Consent for publication

Not applicable.

Ethics approval and consent to participate

Material came from submitted surgically excised tumours of privately owned pets representing routine diagnostic biopsy material submitted by private practitioners and was utilized under owner's consent.

The caseload included in the study was collected during a temporal range (2000-2010) when Italian National did not require ethical approval, although the local ethics committee in this particular case did not consider necessary an ethics approval procedure to be necessary seen the retrospective nature of the study and the absence of private information disclosure involved in the study.

Author details

[1]Department of Veterinary Medical Sciences (DIMEVET), University of Bologna, Ozzano dell'Emilia, Italy. [2]IDEXX Laboratories Ltd. Grange House, Sandbeck Way, Wetherby, West Yorkshire LS22 7DN, UK. [3]Department of Veterinary Medicine, University of Milan, Via Celoria 10, 20100 Milan, Italy. [4]Equipe recherche UPSP ICE 2011-03-101: Oncology, and Laboratoire de Pathologie et Morphologie Clinique, Vetagro-sup, France. [5]Laboratory of Comparative Pathology, Memorial Sloan Kettering Cancer Center, 1275 York Av, Box 270, New York, USA. [6]Private practicioner, Milan, Italy.

References

1. Li X, Fox JG, Padrid PA. Neoplastic diseases in ferrets: 574 cases (1968-1997). J Am Vet Med Assoc. 1998;212:1402–6.
2. Quesenberry KE, Carpenter JW, editors. Ferrets, rabbits, and rodents: clinical medicine and surgery. 3rd ed. St. Louis: Elsevier/Saunders; 2012.
3. Miwa Y, Kurosawa A, Ogawa H, Nakayama H, Sasai H, Sasaki N. Neoplasitic diseases in ferrets in Japan: a questionnaire study for 2000 to 2005. J Vet Med Sci Jpn Soc Vet Sci. 2009;71:397–402.
4. Fox JG, Marini RP, editors. Other systemic diseases. biol. dis. ferret. 3rd ed. Ames: Wiley; 2014. p. 421–38.
5. Chen S. Pancreatic endocrinopathies in ferrets. Veterinary Clin. North Am. Exot. Anim. Pract. 2008;11:107–23. vii.

6. Simone-Freilicher E. Adrenal gland disease in ferrets. Veterinary Clin. North Am. Exot. Anim. Pract. 2008;11:125–37.
7. Head KW, Armed Forces Institute of Pathology (U.S.), American Registry of Pathology, WHO Collaborating Center for Worldwide Reference on Comparative Oncology. Histological classification of tumors of domestic animals. Washington, DC: Published by the Armed Forces Institute of Pathology in cooperation with the American Registry of Pathology and the World Health Organization Collaborating Center for Worldwide Reference on Comparative Oncology; 2003.
8. Bielinska M, Kiiveri S, Parviainen H, Mannisto S, Heikinheimo M, Wilson DB. Gonadectomy-induced adrenocortical neoplasia in the domestic ferret (Mustela putorius furo) and laboratory mouse. Vet Pathol. 2006;43:97–117.
9. Parker GA, Picut CA. Histopathologic features and post-surgical sequelae of 57 cutaneous neoplasms in ferrets (Mustela putorius furo L.). Vet Pathol. 1993;30:499–504.
10. Kanfer S, Reavill DR. Cutaneous neoplasia in ferrets, rabbits, and guinea pigs. Veterinary Clin North Am Exot Anim Pract. 2013;16:579–98.
11. Mikaelian I, Garner MM. Solitary dermal leiomyosarcomas in 12 ferrets. J Vet Diagn Investig Off Publ Am Assoc Vet Lab Diagn Inc. 2002;14:262–5.
12. Erdman SE, Reimann KA, Moore FM, Kanki PJ, Yu QC, Fox JG. Transmission of a chronic lymphoproliferative syndrome in ferrets. Lab Investig J Tech Methods Pathol. 1995;72:539–46.
13. Erdman SE, Kanki PJ, Moore FM, Brown SA, Kawasaki TA, Mikule KW, et al. Clusters of lymphoma in ferrets. Cancer Invest. 1996;14:225–30.
14. Batchelder MA, Erdman SE, Li X, Fox JG. A cluster of cases of juvenile mediastinal lymphoma in a ferret colony. Lab Anim Sci. 1996;46:271–4.
15. Cross BM. Hepatic vascular neoplasms in a colony of ferrets. Vet Pathol. 1987;24:94–6.
16. Dunn DG, Harris RK, Meis JM, Sweet DE. A histomorphologic and immunohistochemical study of chordoma in twenty ferrets (Mustela putorius furo). Vet Pathol. 1991;28:467–73.
17. Gliatto JM, Alroy J, Schelling SH, Engler SJ, Dayal Y. A light microscopical, ultrastructural and immunohistochemical study of spindle-cell adrenocortical tumours of ferrets. J Comp Pathol. 1995;113:175–83.
18. Newman SJ, Bergman PJ, Williams B, Scase T, Craft D. Characterization of spindle cell component of ferret (Mustela putorius furo) adrenal cortical neoplasms - correlation to clinical parameters and prognosis. Vet Comp Oncol. 2004;2:113–24.

Transcriptome profiling of *Staphylococci*-infected cow mammary gland parenchyma

Ewa M Kosciuczuk[1,4], Paweł Lisowski[1], Justyna Jarczak[1], Alicja Majewska[2], Magdalena Rzewuska[3], Lech Zwierzchowski[1] and Emilia Bagnicka[1*]

Abstract

Background: Genome-wide gene expression profiling allows for identification of genes involved in the defense response of the host against pathogens. As presented here, transcriptomic analysis and bioinformatics tools were applied in order to identify genes expressed in the mammary gland parenchyma of cows naturally infected with coagulase-positive and coagulase-negative *Staphylococci*.

Results: In cows infected with coagulase-positive *Staphylococci*, being in 1st or 2nd lactation, 1700 differentially expressed genes (DEGs) were identified. However, examination of the 3rd or 4th lactations revealed 2200 DEGs. Gene ontology functional classification showed the molecular functions of the DEGs overrepresented the activity of cytokines, chemokines, and their receptors. In cows infected with coagulase-negative *Staphylococci*, in the 1st or 2nd lactations 418 DEGs, while in the 3rd or 4th lactations, 1200 DEGs were identified that involved in molecular functions such as protein, calcium ion and lipid binding, chemokine activity, and protein homodimerization. Gene network analysis showed DEGs associated with inflammation, cell migration, and immune response to infection, development of cells and tissues, and humoral responses to infections caused by both types of *Staphylococci*.

Conclusion: A coagulase-positive *Staphylococci* infection caused a markedly stronger host response than that of coagulase-negative, resulting in vastly increased DEGs. A significant increase in the expression of the *FOS*, *TNF*, and genes encoding the major histocompatibility complex proteins (MHC) was observed. It suggests these genes play a key role in the synchronization of the immune response of the cow's parenchyma against mastitis-causing bacteria. Moreover, the following genes that belong to several physiological pathways (KEGG pathways) were selected for further studies as candidate genes of mammary gland immune response for use in Marker Assisted Selection (MAS): chemokine signaling pathway (*CCL2, CXCL5, HCK, CCR1*), cell adhesion molecules (CAMs) pathway (*BOLA-DQA2, BOLA-DQA1, F11R, ITGAL, CD86*), antigen processing and presentation pathway (*CD8A, PDIA3, LGMN, IFI30, HSPA1A*), and NOD-like receptor signaling pathway (*TNF, IL8, IL18, NFKBIA*).

Keywords: Dairy cows, Udder parenchyma, Chronic mastitis, Transcriptomics, Gene expression profiling, microarray, qPCR

Background

In cows, disorders of mammary gland function are most often caused by inflammation from a bacterial infection as the main mastitis pathogens [1]. However, inflammation depends on both environmental factors as well as immune system efficiency [2, 3]. Mechanisms of the immune response depend on different populations of cells and their secreted mediators [4–7]. Expression profile analysis of immune system genes in the mammary gland tissues of both healthy animals and those infected by different pathogens may help explain the specific immune response mechanisms. Furthermore, these analyses could indicate the tissue-specific physiological processes and biochemical pathways involved in different types of infections. Moreover, this knowledge could be essential for the therapy and eradication of mastitis [5]. Microarray technology enables the user to measure vast amounts of gene expression data under different physiological circumstances simultaneously, and,

* Correspondence: e.bagnicka@ighz.pl
[1]Department of Animal Improvement, Institute of Genetics and Animal Breeding Polish Academy of Sciences, 36a Postepu str., Jastrzebiec 05-552, Poland
Full list of author information is available at the end of the article

therefore, it allows for the identification of the genes involved in the defense of the host against microbial infection [8]. It also aids in understanding the processes that occur during mastitis [9].

Studies on gene expression profiles in mammary gland tissues and bovine milk leukocytes have been previously performed. Swanson et al. (2009) [10] reported differences in the expression level of several hundred genes in response to an infection by *Streptococcus uberis*, including a large number of genes associated with the immune system. Mitterhuemer et al. [11] studied the influence of *Escherichia coli* on the local (infected quarters) and systemic (neighboring quarters) transcriptome in the mammary glands of dairy cattle. They revealed that local inflammation influenced the expression of genes engaged in the immune response and inflammation, while the systemic response covered the expression of genes involved in antigen processing and presentation, cytokines, protein degradation, and apoptosis. Lützow et al. (2008) [12] identified two main groups of genes (gene clusters) differentially expressed in the mammary gland of cows in response to infection by *Staphylococcus aureus*. The up-regulated genes encoded proteins involved in intracellular signaling, primarily cytokines and chemokines. The genes with lower expression were encoded for extracellular matrix proteins, cellular cytoskeleton proteins, receptors, and intracellular signaling proteins. Moreover, Gilbert et al. [13] found that crude *E. coli* lipopolysaccharide (LPS), the endotoxin of the Gram-negative bacteria, stimulated expression of many more genes than the *S. aureus* infection did. They also stated that LPS induced different mechanisms of leukocyte enrollment.

However, most of these studies were carried out either in vitro on cultured cells derived from mammary gland tissues [10, 13, 14], on experimentally infected animals [10–12], or on milk somatic cells derived from mastitic cows [15]. Moreover, it should be noted that Krappmann et al. [16] proved that mammary gland epithelial cells, obtained from milk somatic cells using magnetic beads, probably did not reflect the metabolic processes proceeding in secretory cells of the mammary gland itself; therefore, they could not substitute the study on the mammary gland biopsies. Other researchers comparing results obtained in vitro and in vivo in different tissues draw similar conclusion in that the in vitro study does not fully reflect the conditions occurring in the living organism [10, 17–19]. Thus, the present study was performed in vivo in animals with recurrent and incurable mammary gland inflammation. The aim of the study was transcriptional profiling and bioinformatics analysis of genes expressed in secretory tissue (parenchyma) derived from dairy cow mammary glands naturally infected with coagulase-positive and coagulase-negative *Staphylococci* in comparison with those of healthy mammary glands.

Results

The microbiological status of the collected mammary gland samples, as well as information on the average lactose content and milk somatic cell count, was presented in detail previously [20]. Briefly, the microbial status showed that 30% of studied samples were free from bacterial pathogens. In the remaining samples, only bacteria from *Staphylococcus* genus were found. The lowest level of somatic cells was found in milk of healthy cows being in 1st or 2nd lactations and the highest in the milk of cows in 3rd or 4th lactations infected with coagulase-positive *Staphylococci*.

Comparison of gene expression profiles in coagulase-positive *Staphylococci*-infected and healthy mammary gland parenchyma

Comparing transcript levels in the secretory epithelial tissue of cows infected with coagulase-positive *Staphylococci* in the 1st or 2nd lactation (group CoPS-1/2) and in healthy cows (H) identified 1700 differentially expressed genes (DEGs), meeting the criteria of log FC > 0.5 and $P < 0.05$. Among these genes, 1360 were up-regulated and 340 were down-regulated in bacteria-infected cows. For these genes, 223 biological processes, 85 molecular functions, and 36 cellular component categories were ascribed (Additional files 1 and 2). In the bacteria-infected udders, DEGs were associated with the immune defense response, immune system processes, response to wounding, amino acid transport, transportation of metabolic oxoacids, and ketone metabolic processes. When genes were classified according to their molecular functions, the DEGs were responsible for the activities of chemokines, cytokines and their receptors, protein binding, transmembrane transporter activity, and nucleotide binding. The cellular component genes included those encoding proteins of major histocompatibility complex (MHC) classes I and II. Ten categories of the most differentially expressed genes representing biological processes, molecular functions, and cellular components are shown in Additional file 3: Figure S1. The charts show the categories hierarchized according to increasing *P* values.

A comparison of the transcriptomes of cows from the CoPS-1/2 and H groups identified the network of genes responsible for the migration of immune cells. In this network, the "nodes" represent key genes up-regulated in the CoPS-1/2 group: *MMP7* (matrix metallopeptidase7), *PLAU* (plasminogen activator, urokinase), *ANXA2* (annexin A2), *COL1A1* (collagen, type I, alpha 1), and *TIMP1* (TIMP metallopeptidase inhibitor 1). In Additional file 3: Figure S2, the "cellular movement, hematological system development and function, immune cell trafficking" network is presented with differentially expressed genes and key genes included in this network.

In cows undergoing the 3rd or 4th lactations (CoPS-3/4), 2200 DEGs were identified, meeting the criteria of logFC > 0.5 and $P < 0.05$. There were 1389 up-regulated and 811 down-regulated genes in CoPS-3/4 as compared to H (Additional files 4 and 5). The DEGs were involved in 285 biological processes, 71 molecular functions, and 49 cellular component categories. The biological processes influenced by DEGs included inflammatory responses stimulus responses, lipid biosynthesis, and neutral lipid metabolic processes. The identified molecular functions primarily represented cytokine and chemokine activity as well as their receptors, peptidase activity, magnesium ion binding and oxidoreductase activity. In the cellular component category, genes encoding MHC (major histocompatibility complex) protein systems were identified. Ten categories of biological processes, molecular functions, and cellular components of the most differentially expressed genes are shown in Additional file 3: Figure S3. Comparison of mammary parenchyma transcriptomes of cows from the CoPS-3/4 and H groups revealed four networks of genes which differ in expression level: (A) network of cell metabolism, (B) network of the organization and function of the cells, (C) network of the inflammatory response, and (D) network of the response to infection and development of cells and tissues. Networks A, B, and C contain, respectively, the node (key) genes up-regulated in the CoPS-3/4 group: *FOS* (*Bos taurus* FBJ murine osteosarcoma viral oncogene homolog), *ILβ* (interleukin-β), and *TNF* (tumour necrosis factor). Additional file 3: Figure S4 shows the identified networks with differentially expressed genes.

Comparison of gene expression profiles in healthy and coagulase-negative *Staphylococci*-infected mammary gland parenchyma

Comparing transcript levels of the mammary gland parenchyma of the CoNS-1/2 group (cows infected with coagulase-negative *Staphylococci*, being in their 1st or 2nd lactations) with the H group identified 418 DEGs, meeting the criteria of logFC > 0.5 and $P < 0.05$. Of these genes, 117 showed increased (up-regulated) and 301 had decreased (down-regulated) expression in animals infected by bacteria. For these genes, 18 biological processes, five molecular functions, and nine cell component categories were identified (Additional files 6 and 7). Biological processes where DEGs were represented included defense response, stress response, antigen presentation, and inflammatory response. In the case of molecular function categories, odorant binding, receptor binding, and RNA binding were highly associated with coagulase-negative *Staphylococci* infection of the mammary secretory tissues. For cellular component categories, DEGs belonged to a group of genes encoding MHC and extracellular matrix proteins. Ten categories of biological processes, molecular functions, and cellular components of the most differentially expressed genes are shown in Additional file 3: Figure S5 according to increasing P value. In the CoNS-1/2 group, a network of genes responsible for intercellular signaling, including *EGR1* (early growth response protein 1) and *TGFB3* (transforming growth factor beta 3) as key genes ("nodes"), that represented intragenic network were identified (Additional file 3: Figure S6).

Gene expression analysis profiles of udder parenchyma of cows in their 3rd or 4th lactations, infected with coagulase-negative *Staphylococci* (CoNS-3/4 group vs. H group), identified 1200 DEGs, meeting the criteria of logFC > 0.5 and $P < 0.05$. Among these, 933 genes were up-regulated and 267 were down-regulated in the group infected with bacteria. These genes were involved in 206 biological processes, 56 molecular functions, and 46 cellular component categories (Additional files 8 and 9). In the case of biological processes, genes with differed expression were those engaged in the defense response, immune response, signal transduction, lipid biosynthesis, and organic acid metabolism. As to the molecular function, these genes were responsible for protein binding, chemokine activity, calcium ion binding, protein homodimerization, and lipid binding. Among the cellular component categories, genes encoding cell surface proteins and MHC I proteins were identified. Ten categories of biological processes, molecular functions, and cellular components of the most differentially expressed genes, categorized by increasing P value, are shown in Additional file 3: Figure S7.

Genes involved in the response to CoNS infection form five gene networks: (A) cell morphology, (B) organization of the cells, (C) cell proliferation, (D) reaction to tissue injury, and (E) humoral response (Additional file 3: Figure S8). In these networks, several "node" genes were distinguished: *UBC* (ubiquitin) for network A, *FOS* for network B, *TNF* for network C, *SOD2* (superoxide dismutase 2) for network D, and *IL2R* (interleukin-2 receptor) and *PTGS2* (prostaglandin endoperoxide synthase-2) for network E.

KEGG biochemical pathway analysis

To determine over-represented biochemical pathways, including genes up-regulated during *Staphylococci* infections, the Kyoto Encyclopedia of Genes and Genomes (KEGG) database was searched (Table 1). In cows from the CoNS-1/2 group several pathways associated with the body's response to the presence of bacteria were identified. For all pathways, the differences between infected and non-infected udders were significant at $P < 0.05$. Importantly, all identified pathways were associated with immunological processes. A comparison of groups CoPS-1/2 vs. H identified 10 pathways, including genes involved in

Table 1 Pathways and number of genes up- or down-regulated in CoPS-1/2, CoPS-3/4, and CoNS-3/4 bovine groups

Pathway	No. of genes		
	CoPS-1/2	CoPS-3/4	CoNS-3/4
Complement and coagulation cascades	22	21	18
Cytokine-cytokine receptor interaction	31	19	22
Chemokine signaling pathway	25	25	18
Antigen processing and presentation	13	19	18
NOD-like receptor signaling pathway	11	15	10
Cell adhesion molecules (CAMs)	16	24	14
Leukocyte trans-endothelial migration	16	22	12
Toll-like receptor signaling pathway	13	14	11
Gap junction	12	–	–
T cell receptor signaling pathway	–	17	–
Natural killer cell mediated cytotoxicity	–	15	–
Immune network for IgA production	12	12	10
Cytosolic DNA-sensing pathway	–	8	–

the immune response. Analysis of CoPS-3/4 vs. H groups identified 12 pathways and CoNS-3/4 vs. H revealed 11 pathways. For all three comparisons, changes in pathways of complement and coagulation cascades, cytokine-cytokine receptor interaction, antigen processing and presentation, leukocyte trans-endothelial migration, nucleotide oligomerization domain (NOD)-like and Toll-like receptors, chemokine signaling and cell adhesion molecules (*CAMs*) were identified.

In pathways associated with the response of the mammary gland secretory tissues to the bacteria, approximately 10 to 30 DEGs were found, making the detected paths highly significant (with *P*-values ranging from 5×10^{-2} to 5×10^{-9}). Figure 1 shows an example diagram of the signaling pathway of a Toll-like receptor together with the selected DEGs comparing the CoPS-3/4 vs. H groups. The figure shows the dependence of the complement cascade and cytokine pathways on the Toll-like receptor pathway. DEGs in the CoPS-3/4 vs. H comparison were involved in metabolic reactions leading to complement and cytokine pathways.

In the CoPS-1/2 group, intestinal immune network for IgA (immunoglobulin A) production, gap junction, and hematopoietic cell lineage pathways were involved in the immune response to infection. In the CoPS-3/4 group, genes associated with the lysosome, T cell receptor signaling pathway, natural killer cell mediated cytotoxicity, and cytosolic DNA-sensing pathways were differentially expressed as compared to the H group.

Identification of functional gene clusters

Bioinformatics analysis of microarray results showed that the identified DEGs were involved in multiple biological processes. Clustering analysis using the DAVID Functional Clustering Module allowed for a more accurate classification and interpretation of results. Several clusters were identified in each of the transcriptomes. Functional clustering showed that identified clusters were primarily associated with immunological processes (Additional file 10). Analysis of samples collected from cows assigned to the groups CoPS-1/2, CoPS-3/4, CoNS-1/2, and CoNS-3/4 showed six, eight, four, and five clusters, respectively. These clusters contained groups of genes associated with the immune response, antigen presentation, MHC proteins, chemotaxis of leukocytes, leukocyte adhesion, activity of chemokines and cytokines, complement activation, humoral response, B-cell activity, and activity of immunoglobulins. Furthermore, in samples taken from the CoPS-3/4 group, a cluster No. 4, consisting of genes associated with metabolism and biosynthesis of lipids and fatty acid was identified. In samples derived from the CoNS-1/2 animals, three additional clusters were identified and were associated with the serine-threonine kinase receptor signaling pathway, transforming growth factor beta (TGF-β), and a cluster of genes related to the organization of cytoskeletal actin.

Validation of selected genes by real-time quantitative PCR (qPCR)

Validation of microarray results was performed to confirm the accuracy of the transcriptomic analysis for each of the four comparisons using individual, unpooled mRNA samples. The relative transcript levels of validated genes were compared between infected and non-infected samples within age groups separately (lactations 1/2 and 3/4). In concordance with the microarray results, the levels of *SAA3* (serum amyloid A3), *CFB* (complement factor B), and *CP* (cytoplasmic polyadenylation) were higher in both CoPS and both CoNS group samples. Moreover, comparisons between CoPS-1/2 and H-1/2 groups and CoPS-3/4 and H-3/4 groups revealed that, in both CoPS groups, *HP* (haptoglobin) and *IL8* (interleukin 8) gene transcripts were higher than in H groups, while the levels of *CA6* (Carbonic anhydrase 6) and *CA4* (Carbonic anhydrase 4) were higher in H-1/2 and H-3/4 groups, respectively. In the CoNS-3/4 group, *HP* gene expression was higher than in H-3/4 group, similar to both CoPS groups. Patterns of gene expression in cow mammary parenchyma, as measured with real-time PCR (qPCR) between particular groups (CoNS and CoPS vs. H) according to lactation status, are shown in Fig. 2.

Discussion

In the present study, hundreds of genes are differentially expressed in the parenchyma derived from infected cows' mammary glands as compared to healthy ones. The

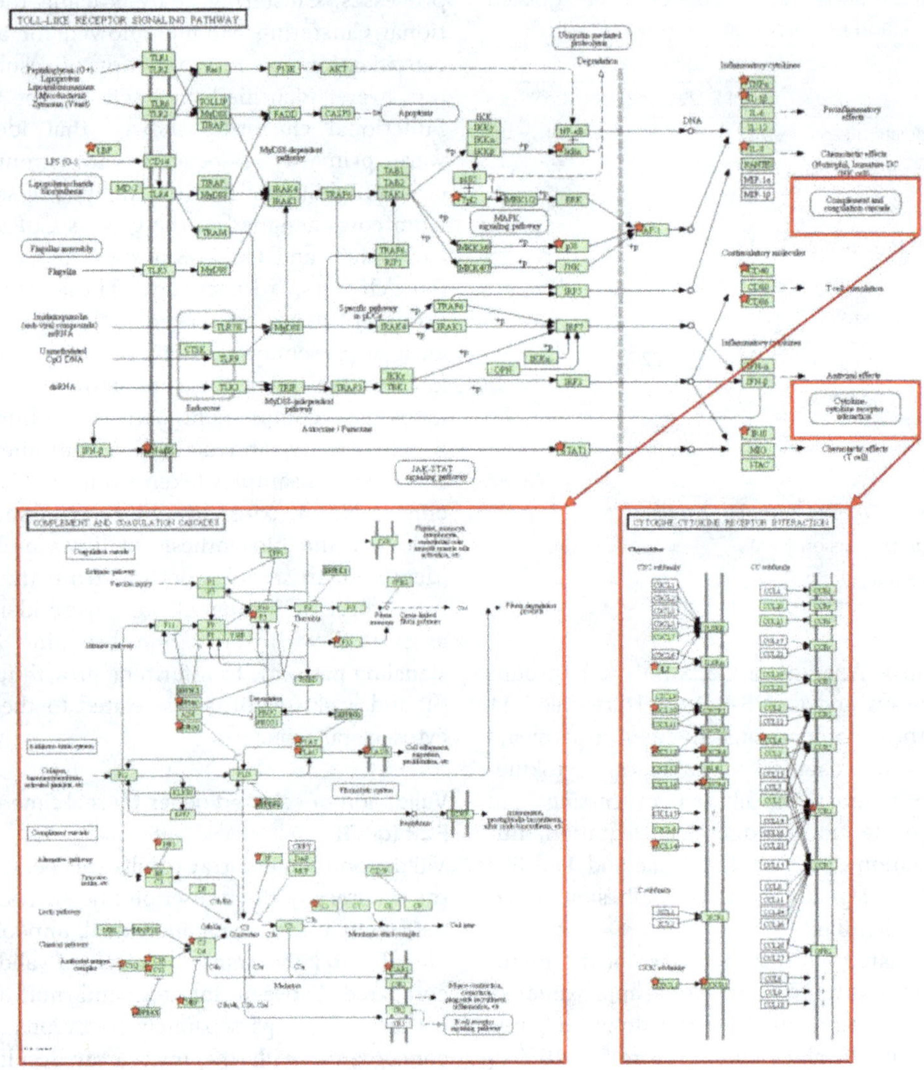

Fig. 1 Gene map of the signaling pathways of the Toll-like receptor, activation of complement and interaction of cytokines (shown only partly) derived from the KEGG database. Genes showing significantly different expression in the CoPS-3/4 vs. H groups are marked with red asterisks. The figure shows the dependence of complement activation and cytokine pathways on the Toll-like receptor pathway (*red arrows*). Differentially expressed genes are located on the paths leading to the complement and cytokine pathways

highest number of DEGs, 2200 genes, was identified in CoPS-3/4 group. The infection caused by coagulase-negative *Staphylococci* (CoNS) influenced a smaller number of genes in this age group – 1200. Cows in lactations 1/2 were also characterized by different gene expression profiles; the numbers of DEGs were 1200 and 418 in the CoPS and CoNS groups, respectively. These results reflected the complex nature of the mammary tissue response to infection with *Staphylococcus* bacteria. The intricacy and complexity of gene expression patterns associated with *S. aureus* infections, both in blood leukocytes and milk somatic cells (MSCs), were emphasized by other researchers [15]. Moreover, the inflammation of mammary glands of other species, such as goat or pig exposed either to *Mycoplasma agalactiae* (goat) or to *E. coli* and *S. aureus* (pig), also resulted in many differentially expressed genes in the early response (until 24 h) to infection [21, 22].

Functional classification of genes

Classifying DEGs according to their ontology, and so grouping them into similar categories in terms of gene function, identified a number of biological processes, molecular functions, and cellular components primarily involved in the immune response. In young cows infected with coagulase-negative *Staphylococci* (CoNS-1/2), increased expression levels of *CFB, CFH,* and *C4BP* were found, encoding complement system factors B and H as well as C4b-binding protein, respectively. In humans, these factors are an important part of the complement

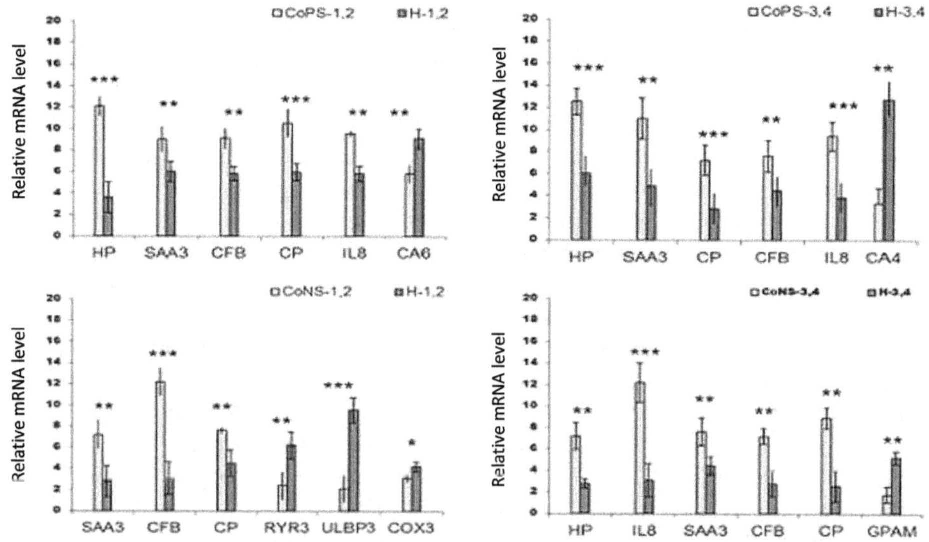

Fig. 2 Validation of microarray analysis using real-time PCR. The relative levels of mRNA expressed are shown as the mean (with standard error – SE) of six animals. Groups differ from each other significantly at $^{*}P < 0.05$, $^{**}P < 0.01$, and $^{***}P < 0.001$

system acting against microbial infections [23] Similar results to ours were obtained by Rinaldi et al. [24] and Whelehan et al. [9]. These authors reported increased expression of acute phase proteins in mammary tissues infected with *E. coli* compared to bacteria free-tissues. Furthermore, the results of Whelehan et al. [9] showed elevated levels of *SAA3* gene transcripts (*SAA3* encodes components of serum amyloid A, belonging to acute phase proteins that act as opsonins) in the udder parenchyma of cows infected with *S. aureus*. In the present study, in CoPS-3/4 and CoNS-3/4 groups, as well as in CoPS-1/2 group, higher expression levels of genes encoding proteins of the canonical pathway of complement activation complex (*C6, C1S, C1QA, C1QB*, and *C4BP*) and the alternative route of the complement system (*CFB* and *CFH*) were observed. This is an interesting observation as the complement system is an example of cooperation between specific and non-specific immune mechanisms [25]. Activation of the complement pathway is important for a rapid response against pathogens, before an organism is able to develop specific mechanisms that operate slowly but more effectively. Numerous studies have reported activation by *S. aureus* of both alternative and classical complement pathways [26, 27], which is consistent with our results showing the activation of genes encoding proteins belonging to both pathways of complement action. Most of these genes, however, belong to the classical complement pathway, which could be due to the recurrent udder inflammation in the examined cows, resulting in production of specific antibodies activating the classical complement pathway. Two pathways of complement activation do not operate completely independently. The C3b component, generated by the classical pathway, can be deposited on the cell surface and thus may further initiate the formation of the alternative pathway. In the CoNS-1/2 group, the immune response to the pathogen relies on the activation of the alternative complement pathway. This may indicate that the organism of a young animal is able to combat infection without the activation of specific immune mechanisms, or that it meets with this certain type of bacteria for the first time.

In CoPS-1/2, CoPS-3/4, and CoNS-3/4 groups, four DEGs were identified with increased expression associated with antigen processing and presentation - *BOLA-DQB*, *BOLA*-DRB3, *BOLA-DQA2*, and *BOLA-DQA1*. These genes and the encoded proteins are critical for the immune system to clear infections [28]. Most studies confirm the paramount importance of class I and class II MHC molecules, which are key in resistance to infection not only in human [29] but also in goat and bovine, including resistance to mastitis [30–32]. Fitzpatrick et al. [33] showed MHC-II up-regulation in the connective tissue derived from *S. uberis* bacteria-infected cow udders. Swanson et al. [10] also reported a higher *HLA-DRA* (in human: HLA class II histocompatibility antigen, DR alpha chain) gene expression in the mammary tissues of cows after intramammary infection with *S. uberis* but not in healthy tissues. Moreover, Brand et al., [30] listed several genes belonging to the major histocompatibility complex (*HLA-DMA, HLA-DMB, HLA-DQA1, HLA-DQB1, HLA-DRA*, and *HLA-DRB1*) as a part of a "dendritic cell maturation" canonical pathway, which was affected by mastitic bacteria. According to Bonnefont et al. [34], the subunits of MHC class II, namely DQA1, DQA2, and DRB1, were also affected by *S. aureus*.

Biochemical pathways

Two biochemical pathways were involved in the bovine immune response to infection with *Staphylococcus* bacteria: the Toll-like receptors pathway and the cytokine receptor interaction pathway. TLRs are membrane receptors that play a key role in the innate immune system, recognizing structurally conserved molecules derived from different microorganisms. Cells of the immune system which recognize the molecular patterns of a pathogen with TLRs, include macrophages and dendritic cells that respond to membrane components of Gram-positive and Gram-negative bacteria [35]. Stimulation of these cells by a pathogen through TLRs induces rapid activation of the innate immune mechanisms, manifested by increased synthesis of pro-inflammatory cytokines and activation of dendritic cells [36]. Toll-like receptors are located on the surface of macrophages, whose activation leads to the synthesis of TNF and IL-8 [12]. In our study, in the signaling pathway of Toll-like receptors, genes such as *TNF, IL-8, CXCL10* (Chemokine Ligand 10 – C-X-C Motif)), and *CD40* (TNF receptor superfamily) have been identified. This observation confirmed the results of other authors who have shown increased expression of *TNF, IL-8, CXCL10,* and *CD40* antigen genes in tissues of cow udders experimentally infected with *E. coli* and *S. aureus* [12, 37]. Moreover, Bonnefont et al. [34] stressed that the components of the chemokine signaling pathway are affected by *S. aureus* infection. The proteins encoded by *TNF, IL-8, CXCL10,* and CD40 genes (the same for both types of infections) are closely related to inflammation and are essential for the activation of neutrophils and their migration to sites of inflammation in the infected mammary gland. On the basis of our study, it can be concluded that bacterial infections by coagulase-positive and coagulase-negative *Staphylococci* evoke similar reactions in the innate immune system. This was also evidenced by the fact that the Toll-like receptors pathway leads to the activation of the next two pathways, which are also shared by both bacterial infections (CoPS and CoNS). One is the complement activation pathway, which involves the genes discussed above in relation to the process of acute inflammation. Another biochemical pathway involved in mammary gland response to bacterial pathogens is the cytokine receptor interaction pathway. In our study, in all groups of cows infected with *Staphylococci* bacteria, a higher level of expression was found for genes encoding chemokine receptors *CXCR4, CXCR6,* and *CX3CR1* (also known as the fractalkine receptor) as compared to the healthy groups of cows. Günther at el. [38], in a study on the secretory epithelial cells of bovine mammary glands infected with *E. coli,* showed an important role of the fractalkine receptor and other CXC receptors in the recruitment and migration of leukocytes to sites of inflammation. Additionally, results of studies on goat and porcine mammary gland epithelial cells also indicated on the influence of the infection on cytokine and chemokine expression levels [21, 22].

Functional gene networks

Comparing CoPS-1/2 cows with controls, we identified a network of differentially expressed genes responsible for the migration of immune cells. In this network, *CD44, PLAU,* and *MMP7* genes can be distinguished, and they are strongly linked to other genes of the determined network. The *CD44* gene encodes a glycoprotein, the hyaluronain receptor, which is an important component of the extracellular matrix [39]. The interaction of CD44 with the glycoprotein hyaluronate (HA) has an important role in the adhesion of leukocytes to the vascular endothelium, as well as their migration to the sites of inflammation [40]. The results of more recent studies showed elevated *CD44* expression in inflammation of the cow mammary gland, particularly in the early stages of the inflammatory response [41]. The increased expression of *CD44* found in our study in a group of younger individuals (1st or 2nd lactations) may be indicative of the acute inflammation and tissue damage.

The *PLAU* gene encodes the urokinase plasminogen activator, which is a part of the fibrinolytic system. PLAU is a protease that converts plasminogen to plasmin by specific cleavage of the plasminogen protein [42]. The results of studies conducted by Lincoln and Leigh [43] and Moyes et al. [44] on a group of dairy cows infected with *S. uberis* also showed induction of the *PLAU* gene. The authors interpreted this result as an indicator of *S. uberis* virulence, causing inflammation of the mammary gland of cows. Plasmin catalyzes the degradation of fibrin and laminin to soluble peptides. Its activity is connected with elevated permeability of the epithelial barrier in the mammary gland during inflammation. The other function of plasmin is activation of MMP precursors [42]. Disintegration of these proteins is carried out either by direct action of plasmin, or indirectly through its activating effect on the MMP precursor cascade [45]. This corresponds to the results of our study, which also demonstrated the activation of the *MMP7* metalloproteinase gene, undergoing higher expression in the cows from the CoPS-1/2 group than in controls. Increased expression of the *MMP7* gene may result in the degradation of the extracellular matrix and the migration of immune cells to sites of inflammation.

In CoNS-3/4 and CoPS-3/4 groups, four and five significant intergenic networks were identified, respectively, which could be ascribed to two common key gene nodes: *TNF* and *FOS.* Furthermore, when comparing CoPS-1/2 cows with healthy ones, the *IL1-β* node (key) gene was identified. It exhibited, inseparably with *TNF,* activity in inflammation [5]. The *TNF, IL1-β,* and *FOS* genes belong to the Toll-like receptor and cytokine receptor interaction signaling pathways, and they were also identified in the CoPS-3/4 experimental group. The *FOS* gene encodes a transcription factor that is a component of the JUN/AP-1 trans-activating complex. In the basic state of a cell, *FOS* has a very low level of expression, but its transcript level increases within several minutes after stimulation by *S. uberis*; therefore, this gene is called "the early response gene" [43, 44]. It is involved in the regulation of cell proliferation, differentiation, and transformation [46]. Lützow et al. [12], after challenging bovine mammary tissues with *S. aureus*, showed increased expression of the *FOS* gene, which is involved in the TLR-2 and TLR-4 signaling pathway. In the studies of *S. uberis* infection, the *FOS* gene was shown to be a component of IL-6 and IL-10 signaling pathways [44].

AP1 has been reported play a crucial role in signaling pathways related to bacterial infections [47]. Functional AP1 sites have been identified in promoters of cytokine (interleukins, interferons) encoding genes [48–50] and other genes participating in the immune response. The C-JUN NH(2)-terminal kinase (JNK) regulates AP1 transcription factor activity and stimulates expression of pro-inflammatory mediators such as TNF [51]. The increased expression of the *FOS* gene found in our study indicated a strong stress caused by infection with coagulase-negative and coagulase-negative *Staphylococci.*

The *IL1B* gene encodes a protein that is a member of the cytokine – interleukin-1β family. This protein is produced by monocytes/macrophages and epithelial cells [5], whereas the *TNF-α* and *TNF-β* genes encode multifunctional pro-inflammatory cytokines that belong to the family of tumor necrosis factors (TNF) [52]. TNF-α plays an important role in the lactating cow's mammary gland by mediating immune inflammatory responses in mastitis [53]. TNF mediates most pro-inflamatory effects that occur upon bacterial infection by promoting NFkB and MAPK activation [47]. Our identification of the proinflammatory cytokine genes as nodal (key) genes indicates their important role in the immune response induced by the two groups of bacteria studied (CoPS and CoNS). These results confirm those found in the literature, as the TNF-β and IL-1 cytokines were previously identified as the most important pro-inflammatory cytokines produced in inflammation. They are also critical in inflammation of the mammary gland of cows caused by *S. aureus* and *E. coli* [12, 54, 55]. As shown by Xiu et al. [56] other cytokines (e.g. Il-8; IL-1-alpha), including chemokines (chemokine ligand 5 – CXCL5; chemokine ligand 5 – C-C motif; chemokine receptor 7 – CXCL7) were upregulated after infection caused by *S. aureus*.

Conclusion

Infection of cow mammary gland parenchyma with coagulase-negative or -positive *Staphylococci* affected genes, which encode proteins showing the same and/or similar molecular functions. Our results provided evidence that coagulase-positive *Staphylococci* caused a much stronger host response than coagulase-negative, resulting in increased number of DEGs as compared with uninfected tissues. Moreover, the response of the udder parenchyma to a *Staphyllococci* infection was stronger in older cows (lactations three or four) than was observed in younger ones (lactations one or two). Gene network analysis predicted DEGs associated with inflammation, cell migration, and the immune response to the infection site, as well as a humoral response in infections caused by both coagulase-positive and coagulase-negative groups of *Staphylococci.*

In both types of infections, caused either by coagulase-positive or coagulase-negative *Staphylococci*, a marked increase was observed in the expression levels of *FOS* and *TNF* genes, and genes encoding the major histocompatibility system proteins *(MHC)-BOLA-DQB, BOLA-DRB3,* or *BOLA-DQA1*. Therefore, we suggest that these particular genes play a key role in immune response synchronization of the cow's udder secretory tissues to mastitis-causing bacteria.

Based on the results of microarray study, the following genes belonging to several physiological pathways (KEGG pathways) were selected for further studies: chemokine signaling pathway (*CCL2, CXCL5, HCK,CCR1*), cell adhesion molecules (CAMs) pathway (*BOLA-DQA2, BOLA-DQA1, F11R, ITGAL, CD86*), antigen processing and presentation pathway (*CD8A, PDIA3, LGMN, IFI30, HSPA1A*), and NOD-like receptor signaling pathway (*TNF, IL8, IL18, NFKBIA*). The listed genes are considered "main genes" involved in mammary gland defense, and these gene polymorphism study has already started to find the associations with resistance to mastitis aiming to include results to MAS in the future. Moreover, epigenetic studies have been conducted in parallel.

Methods

Animals and sample collection

The study was conducted on 30 Holstein-Friesian (HF) dairy cows of the Polish Black and White variety, between the first and fourth lactations. The animals were born and maintained in the Experimental Farm of Institute of Genetics and Animal Breeding in Jastrzębiec, Poland, and they were under constant veterinary supervision. The feeding and maintenance conditions of the animals were previously described [20]. Animals were culled at the third stage of lactation because of reproduction problems (without mastitis) or recurrent and incurable mammary gland infections caused by coagulase-positive or coagulase-negative *Staphylococci.* They were slaughtered in a registered slaughterhouse under constant monitoring conditions by the institutional authorities. The parenchyma samples were taken from deep in the secretory portion of the gland from each quarter immediately after slaughter. The authors were interested in the processes taking place only in parenchyma, therefore, the samples were rinsed in PBS to remove milk and blood from tissue samples and frozen in liquid nitrogen (120 samples total). Milk samples were taken from each quarter two days before slaughter and examined for the presence of bacteria. The exact methodology of the microbiological investigation was previously described [20] and is also shown in Additional file 11.

Tissue samples

The samples were divided into five groups according to the lactation number and health status of the mammary gland, which was established on the basis of previous analysis of the presence of *Staphylococci* infection in quarter milk, somatic cell count (SCC) (IBC_M, Bentley, USA), and lactose content (Fossomatic FT2, FOSS, Denmark). The control group (H) consisted of samples collected from healthy, pathogen-free mammary glands, and one sample was harvested from one cow. Three pathogen-free samples from each of the four lactations were taken for analysis ($N = 12$). The next four groups of samples were divided according to the type of pathogen bacteria and parity (cows with unfinished somatic development, being in the first and second lactations, or cows with complete somatic development, being in the third or fourth lactations). These four groups consisted of samples collected from cows with infections caused by coagulase-negative *Staphylococci*, being in their 1st or 2nd lactations or in the 3rd or 4^{th}lactations (CoNS-1/2 and CoNS-3/4, respectively) and infected with coagulase-positive staphylococci in the 1st/2nd or 3rd/4th lactations (CoPS-1/2 and CoPS-3/4, respectively). Each group consisted of six samples derived from six different animals.

RNA extraction, RNA pooling, sample preparation, and microarray hybridization scheme

The details of total RNA isolation from cow udder secretory tissues were described previously [20]. For each group, three independent RNA pools were obtained by mixing six individual RNA samples from bovine mammary glands, and one mg of pooled RNA was reverse transcribed using the Quick Amp Labeling Kit, Two-Color (Agilent, USA), according to the manufacturer's protocol. For the arrays, combined RNA samples were hybridized in biological duplicates, and two technical replicates were performed for each hybridization. In both biological repetitions, the RNA samples were collected from the same individuals but from different udder quarters with the same health status. The total number of hybridizations was 16 (4 hybridizations for each of the treatment groups: CoPS-1/2, CoPS-3/4, CoNS-1/2, and CoNS-3/4). Hybridizations were performed to compare control RNA derived from healthy individuals, being in the first to fourth lactations (H-1/2/3/4). Established reference, control RNA represents standardized sample of physiologically "healthy" mammary gland RNA for the purpose of analysis and to help streamline and optimize of designed gene expression studies [57]. The broad representation of RNA in designed reference makes the control RNA useful to study of diseased mammary gland transcriptome regardless of the stage of lactation and the age of exanimated animals.

RNA labeling, microarray hybridization, and fluorescent detection

Single strand cRNA was labeled with Cyanine 5-CTP or Cyanine 3-CTP (Agilent, USA). Reaction efficiency and activity were determined by NanoDrop. Hybridization to the Bovine (V2) Gene Expression Microarrays 4 × 44 K (Agilent, USA), washing, and scanning was performed according to the Two-Color Microarray-Based Gene Expression Analysis (Quick Amp Labeling) with Tecan HS Pro Hybridization. Following 17 h of hybridization, arrays were scanned on an Agilent G2565AA scanner. Images were quantified using Agilent Feature Extraction Software (version A.8.5.1.1). Pooling, labeling, and hybridization of RNA sample schemes in the microarray analysis are shown in Additional file 12.

Microarray validation

Real-Time PCR (qPCR) was used to validate the microarray results. Ten genes that belonged to different functional clusters and differed in expression ($p \leq 0.05$) between the control and CoNS-1/2, CoNS-3/4, CoPS-1/2, and CoPS-3/4 were selected for qPCR. These were: *HP, SAA3, CFB, CP, IL8, CA6, CA4, RYR3, ULBP3*, and *GPAM*. The real-time PCR validations were performed in triplicate of individual (unpooled) RNA samples.

Two reference genes were selected as the most stably expressed in the present experimental design, belonging to different functional classes from six housekeeping genes (HKGs) (B-actin – *ACTB*, Glyceraldehyde-3P-dehydrogenase – *GAPDH*, Succinate dehydrogenase complex subunit A – *SDHA*, TATA box-binding protein – *TATABP*, Zeta polypeptide – *YWHAZ*, and Hypoxanthine phosphoribosyltransferase1 – *HPRT1*). The M-values of all putative reference genes were low and ranged between 0.6 and 0.3, and thus all met the criteria for proper references. However, *HPRT1* and *TBP* demonstrated the greatest stability in bovine mammary gland in the present experimental conditions and, therefore, were selected as references. The primer sequences, amplicon length, melting temperature, and GenBank accession numbers of both housekeeping and validated genes are summarized in Additional file 13.

Real-Time PCR amplification was performed with the Light Cycler 480 system (Roche, Germany) using 96-well optical plates with the SYBR Green technique. A PCR mix was prepared in a total volume of 20 µl: 10 µl water, 1 µl forward primer (10 µM), 1 µl reverse primer (10 µM), 2 µl cDNA, and 10 µl SYBR Green I Master Mix (2×) (Roche, Germany). The following amplification program was used: 5 min pre-incubation at 95 °C; 45 cycles amplification with 10 s at 95 °C for denaturation, 15 s at 58-60 °C for annealing, and 20 s at 72 °C for elongation. Negative controls (no cDNA) were run in the same reaction set. A dissociation stage was added to verify the presence of a gene specific peak and the absence of primer-dimer peaks. Real-time products were separated and assessed on 2% agarose gels.

Data normalization methods and selection of differently expressed genes are described in Additional file 14.

Additional files

Additional file 1: Genes with up-regulated expression found in samples derived from cow mammary gland parenchyma infected with coagulase-positive *Staphylococci* in 1stor 2nd lactations (CoPS-1/2) vs. healthy cows (H). (XLS 86 kb)

Additional file 2: Genes with down-regulated expression found in samples derived from cow mammary gland parenchyma infected with coagulase-positive *Staphylococci* in 1st or 2nd lactations (CoPS-1/2) vs. healthy cows (H). (XLS 33 kb)

Additional file 3: Figure S1. Figure S1. Significantly enriched Gene Ontology (GO) categories of genes differentially expressed in mammary secretory tissue between CoPS-1/2 and H cows. **Figure S2.** Gene network graphical representation. Cellular movement, hematological system development and function, and immune cell trafficking in secretory tissue between CoPS-1/2 and H cows. **Figure S3.** Significantly enriched Gene Ontology (GO) categories of genes differentially expressed in mammary secretory tissue between CoPS-3/4 and H cows. **Figure S4.** Gene network graphical representation: (A) Metabolic Disease, (B) Cellular Assembly and Organization, (C) Inflammatory Response, (D) Infectious Disease, Tissue Development in secretory tissue between CoPS-3/4 and H cows. **Figure S5.** Significantly enriched Gene Ontology (GO) categories of genes differentially expressed in mammary secretory tissue between CoNS-1/2 and H cows. **Figure S6.** Gene network graphical representation. Cell-To-Cell Signaling and Interaction in mammary secretory tissue between CoNS-1/2 and H cows. **Figure S7.** Significantly enriched Gene Ontology (GO) categories of genes differentially expressed in mammary secretory tissue between CoNS- 3/4 and H cows. **Figure S8.** Gene network graphical representation: (A) Cell Morphology, (B) Cell Assembly and Organization, (C) Cellular Growth and Proliferation, (D) Organismal Injury and Abnormalities, (E) Humoral Immune Response - in secretory tissue between CoNS-3/4 and H cows.

Additional file 4: Genes with up-regulated expression found in samples derived from cow mammary gland parenchyma infected with coagulase-positive *Staphylococci* in 3rd or 4th lactations (CoPS-3/4).

Additional file 5: Genes with down-regulated expression found in samples derived from cow mammary gland parenchyma infected with coagulase-positive *Staphylococci* in 3rd or 4th lactations (CoPS-3/4).

Additional file 6: Genes with up-regulated expression found in samples derived from cow mammary gland parenchyma infected with coagulase-negative *Staphylococci* in 1st or 2nd lactations (CoNS-1/2).

Additional file 7: Genes with down-regulated expression found in samples derived from cow mammary gland parenchyma infected with coagulase-negative *Staphylococci* in 1st or 2nd lactations (CoNS-1/2).

Additional file 8: Genes with up-regulated expression found in samples derived from cow mammary gland parenchyma infected with coagulase-negative *Staphylococci* in 3rd or 4th lactations (CoNS-3/4).

Additional file 9: Genes with down-regulated expression found in samples derived from cow mammary gland parenchyma infected with coagulase-negative *Staphylococci* in 3rd or 4th lactations (CoNS-3/4).

Additional file 10: Table S1. Gene clusters differing in expression between the CoPS-1/2 (coagulase-positive *Staphyloccoci* in 1st or 2nd lactation) and H (Healthy) groups in the parenchyma of the cow mammary gland. **Table S2.** Gene clusters differing in expression between the CoPS-3/4 (coagulase-positive *Staphyloccoci* in 3rd or 4th lactation) and H (Healthy) groups in the parenchyma of the cow mammary gland. **Table S3.** Gene clusters differing in expression between the CoNS-1/2 (coagulase-negative *Staphyloccoci* in 1st or 2nd lactation) and H (Healthy) groups in the parenchyma of the cow mammary gland. **Table S4.** Gene clusters differing in expression between the CoNS-3/4 (coagulase-positive *Staphyloccoci* in 3rd or 4th lactation) and H (Healthy) groups in the parenchyma of the cowmammary gland.

Additional file 11: Microbiological examination.

Additional file 12: Pooling, labeling, and hybridization of RNA sample schemes used in microarray analysis.

Additional file 13: Table S5. The primer sequences, amplicon length, melting temperature and no. of GenBank access of housekeeping genes examined to use in qPCR analysis. **Table S6.** The primer sequences, amplicon length, melting temperature and No. of GenBank access of validated genes.

Additional file 14: Data normalization and selection of differently expressed genes (DEGs).

Abbreviations

ANXA2: Annexin A2; BoLA: Bovine lymphocyte antigen; BOLA-DQA1: Major histocompatibility complex, class II, DQ alpha, type 1 [*Bos taurus* (cattle)]; BOLA-DQA2: Major histocompatibility complex, class II, DQ alpha 2 [*Bos taurus* (cattle)]; BOLA-DQB: Major histocompatibility complex, class II, DQ beta [*Bos taurus* (cattle)]; BOLA-DRB3: Major histocompatibility complex, class II, DRB3 [*Bos taurus* (cattle)]; C1QA: Complement component 1, q subcomponent, A chain; C1QB: Complement component 1, q subcomponent, B chain; C1S: Complement component 1, s subcomponent; C3B: Complement Component 3b; C4BP: Complement component 4 binding protein; C6: Complement Component 6; CA4: Carbonic anhydrase 4; CA6: Carbonic anhydrase 6; CAMs: Cell adhesion molecules; CCL26: Chemokine (C-C motif) ligand 2; CD40: CD40 molecule; TNF: receptor superfamily; CD44: Cell-surface glycoprotein; CFB: complement factor B; CFH: Complement factor H; COL1A1: Collagen, type I, alpha 1; CoNS-1/2 group: Cows infected with coagulase-negative *Staphylococci*, being in their 1st and 2nd lactations; CoNS-3/4: Cows infected with coagulase-negative staphylococci, being in their 3rd and 4th lactation; CoPS-1/2 group: Cows infected with coagulase-positive *Staphylococci*, in 1st or 2nd lactation; CoPS-3/4 group: Cows infected with coagulase-positive Staphylococci, in 3rd or 4th lactation; COX3: Cytochrome c oxidase subunit 3; CP: Cytoplasmic polyadenylation; CX3CR1: Fractalkine receptor; CXCL10: Chemokine (C-X-C Motif) Ligand 10; CXCR4: C-X-C chemokine receptor type 4 also known as fusin or CD184; CXCR6: C-X-C chemokine receptor type 6; DEGs: Differentially expressed genes; EGR1: Early growth response protein 1; FOS: *Bos taurus* FBJ murine osteosarcoma viral oncogene homolog; FST: Follistatin; GPAM: Glycerol-3-phosphate acyltransferase; GPD1: Glycerolphosphate Dehydrogenase 1; H: Healthy cows; HLA: human lymphocyte antigen; HLA-DRA: HLA class II histocompatibility antigen, DR alpha chain; HP: Haptoglobin; IL-10: Interleukin-10; IL1B: Cytokine-interleukin-1β; IL-2: Interleukin-2; IL2R: Interleukin-2 receptor; IL-6: interleukin-6; IL-8: Interleukin 8; ILB: Interleukin beta; JUN/AP-1: JUN/AP-1 trans-activating complex; KEGG: Kyoto Encyclopedia of Genes and Genomes; LPS: Lipopolysaccharide; MHC: Proteins of major histocompatibility complex; MMP7: Matrix Metallopeptidase 7; MSCs: Milk somatic cells; PLAU: Plasminogen activator, urokinase; PTGS2: Prostaglandin endoperoxide synthase-2; qPCR: Real-time quantitative PCR; RYR3: Ryanodine receptor type 3; SAA1: Serum amyloid A1; SAA3: Serum amyloid A3; SaS: Staphylococcal culture; SCD: Stearoyl-CoA desaturase; SOD2: Superoxide dismutase 2; TGFB3: Transforming growth factor beta 3; TGF-β: Transforming growth factor beta; Th: T helper cells; TIMP1: TIMP metallopeptidase inhibitor 1; TLR-2: Toll-like receptor 2; TLR-4: Toll-like receptor 4; TNF: Tumor Necrosis Factor; UBC: Ubiquitin; ULBP3: UL16 binding protein 3

Acknowledgments
Not applicable.

Funding
Research was realized within the project "BIOFOOD – innovative, functional products of animal origin" no. POIG.01.01.02-014-090/09, co-financed by the European Union from the European Regional Development Fund within the Innovative Economy Operational Programme 2007 – 2013" and the National Science Centre of Poland No. NN311075339.
The publication was supported by KNOW Leading National Research Centre – Scientific Consortium „Healthy Animal – Safe Food".

Authors' contributions
EMK conceived the study and participated in its design, sample collection, data acquisition, molecular genetics studies including microarray analysis, analysis and interpretation of data, and drafting of the manuscript. PL participated in the study design and data analysis and interpretation. JJ participated in sample collection, data acquisition, molecular genetics studies, and drafting of the manuscript. AM performed microarray analysis. MR performed microbiological examination. DS participated in the laboratory work and data collection. LZ participated in data interpretation and critically revised the final approval of the manuscript version to be published. EB conceived the study and participated in its design, sample collection, data acquisition, analysis and interpretation of data, drafting of the manuscript and study coordination. All authors have read and approved the final manuscript.

Competing interests
The authors declare that they have no competing interests.

Consent for publication
Not applicable.

Author details
[1]Department of Animal Improvement, Institute of Genetics and Animal Breeding Polish Academy of Sciences, 36a Postepu str., Jastrzebiec 05-552, Poland. [2]Department of Physiological Sciences, Faculty of Veterinary Medicine, Warsaw University of Life Sciences, 02-776 Warsaw, Poland. [3]Department of Pre-Clinical Sciences, Faculty of Veterinary Medicine, Warsaw University of Life Sciences, 02-776 Warsaw, Poland. [4]Present address: Robert H. Lurie Comprehensive Cancer Center, Northwestern University, Chicago, IL, USA.

References

1. Petzl W, Zerbe H, Gunther J, Yang W, Seyfert H-M, Nurnberg G, et al. *Escherichia coli*, but not *Staphylococcus aureus* triggers an early increased expression of factors contributing to the innate immune defense in the udder of the cow. Vet Res. 2008;39:18.
2. Bradley A. Bovine mastitis: an evolving disease. Vet J. 2002;164(2):116–28.
3. Sender G, Korwin-Kossakowska A, Pawlik A, Galal Abdel Hameed K, Oprządek J. Genetic basis of mastitis resistance in dairy cattle – a review. Ann Anim Sci. 2013;13:663–73.
4. Sordillo LM. Factors affecting mammary gland immunity and mastitis susceptibility. Livest Prod Sci. 2005;98:89–99.
5. Oviedo-Boyso J, Valdez-Alarcón JJ, Cajero-Juárez M, Ochoa-Zarzosa A, López-Meza JE, Bravo-Patiño A, et al. Innate immune response of bovine mammary gland to pathogenic bacteria responsible for mastitis. J Inf Secur. 2007;54:399–409.
6. Bagnicka E, Strzałkowska N, Jóźwik A, Krzyżewski J, Horbańczuk J, Zwierzchowski L. Expression and polymorphism of defensins in farm animals. Acta Biochim Pol. 2010;57:487–97.
7. Kościuczuk EM, Lisowski P, Jarczak J, Strzałkowska N, Jóźwik A, Horbańczuk J, et al. Cathelicidins: family of antimicrobial peptides. A review Mol Biol Rep. 2012;39:10957–70.
8. Wilson HL, Aich P, Roche FM, Jalal S, Hodgson PD, Brinkman FSL, et al. Molecular analyses of disease pathogenesis: Application of bovine microarrays. Vet Immunol Immunopathol. 2005;105:277–87.
9. Whelehan CJ, Meade KG, Eckersall PD, Young FJ, O'Farrelly C. Experimental *Staphylococcus aureus* infection of the mammary gland induces region-specific changes in innate immune gene expression. Vet Immunol Immunopathol. 2011;140:181–9.
10. Swanson KM, Stelwagen K, Dobson J, Henderson HV, Davis SR, Farr VC, et al. Transcriptome profiling of Streptococcus uberis-induced mastitis reveals fundamental differences between immune gene expression in the mammary gland and in a primary cell culture model. J Dairy Sci. 2009;92:117–29.
11. Mitterhuemer S, Petzl W, Krebs S, Mehne D, Klanner A, Wolf E, et al. *Escherichia coli* infection induces distinct local and systemic transcriptome responses in the mammary gland. BMC Genomics. 2010;11:138.
12. Lützow YCS, Donaldson L, Gray CP, Vuocolo T, Pearson RD, Reverter A, et al. Identification of immune genes and proteins involved in the response of bovine mammary tissue to *Staphylococcus aureus* infection. BMC Vet Res. 2008;4:18.
13. Gilbert FB, Cunha P, Jensen K, Glass EJ, Foucras G, Robert-Granié C, et al. Differential response of bovine mammary epithelial cells to *Staphylococcus aureus* or *Escherichia coli* agonists of the innate immune system. Vet Res. 2013;44:40.
14. Pareek R, Wellnitz O, Van Dorp R, Burton J, Kerr D. Immunorelevant gene expression in LPS-challenged bovine mammary epithelial cells. J Appl Genet. 2005;46(2):171–7.
15. Tao W, Mallard B. Differentially expressed genes associated with *Staphylococcus aureus* mastitis of Canadian Holstein cows. Vet Immunol Immunopathol. 2007;120:201–11.
16. Krappmann K, Weikard R, Kühn C. Evaluation of a replacement method for mammary gland biopsies by comparing gene expression in udder tissue and mammary epithelial cells isolated from milk. Res Vet Sci. 2012;93:970–4.
17. Liu M-G, Li H, Xu X, Barnstable CJ, Zhang SS-M. Comparison of gene expression during in vivo and in vitro postnatal retina development. J Ocul Biol Dis Infor. 2008;1:59–72.
18. Liu XS, Zhang ZG, Zhang RL, Gregg SR, Meng H, Chopp M. Comparison of in vivo and in vitro gene expression profiles in subventricular zone neural progenitor cells from the adult mouse after middle cerebral artery occlusion. Neuroscience. 2007;146:1053–61.
19. Martignoni M, de Kanter R, Grossi P, Saturno G, Barbaria E, Monshouwer M. An in vivo and in vitro comparison of CYP gene induction in mice using liver slices and quantitative RT-PCR. Toxicol in Vitro. 2006;20:125–31.
20. Kościuczuk E, Lisowski P, Jarczak J, Krzyżewski J, Zwierzchowski L, Bagnicka E. Expression patterns of β-defensin and cathelicidin genes in parenchyma of bovine mammary gland infected with coagulase-positive or coagulase-negative Staphylococci. BMC Vet Res. 2014;10:246.
21. Jaeger A, Bardehle D, Oster M, Günther J, Muráni E, Ponsuksili S, et al. Gene expression profiling of porcine mammary epithelial cells after challenge with *Escherichia coli* and *Staphylococcus aureus* in vitro. Vet Res. 2015;46:50.
22. Ogorevc J, Mihevc SP, Hedegaard J, Benčina D, Dovč P. Transcriptomic response of goat mammary epithelial cells to Mycoplasma agalactiae challenge – a preliminary study. Anim Sci Pap Rep. 2015;33:155–63.
23. Bradley DT, Zipfel PF, Hughes AE. Complement in age-related macular degeneration: a focus on function. Eye. 2011;25:683–93.
24. Rinaldi M, Li RW, Bannerman DD, Daniels KM, Evock-Clover C, Silva MV, et al. A sentinel function for teat tissues in dairy cows: dominant innate immune response elements define early response to *E. coli* mastitis. Funct Integr Genomics. 2010;10:21–38.
25. Kołoch BF, Płoskońska GB. Efektywność bakteriobójczego działania surowicy wynikająca z obecności układu dopełniacza i lizozymu wobec bakterii, które unikają odpowiedzi immunologicznej organizmu. [The efficiency of the bactericidal action of serum raised by complement and lysozyme against

bacteria which avoid the immunological response of higher organisms, Abstrakt in English]. Post. Hig Med Dośw. 2009;63:471–84.
26. Jongerius I, Köhl J, Pandey MK, Ruyken M, van Kessel KP, van Strijp JA, et al. Staphylococcal complement evasion by various convertase-blocking molecules. J Exp Med. 2007;204:2461–71.
27. Rainard P. The complement in milk and defense of the bovine mammary gland against infections. Vet Res. 2003;34:647–70.
28. Mangalam AK, Taneja V, David CS. HLA class II molecules influence susceptibility versus protection in inflammatory diseases by determining the cytokine profile. J Immunol. 2013;190:513–8.
29. Trowsdale J, Knight JC. Major histocompatibility complex genomics and human disease. Annu Rev Genomics Hum Genet. 2013;14:301–23.
30. Brand B, Hartmann A, Repsilber D, Griesbeck-Zilch B, Wellnitz O, Kühn C, et al. Comparative expression profiling of *E. coli* and *S. aureus* inoculated primary mammary gland cells sampled from cows with different genetic predispositions for somatic cell score. Genet Select Evol. 2011;43:24.
31. Genini S, Badaoui B, Sclep G, Bishop SC,Waddington D, Pinard van der Laan MH, et al. Strengthening insights into host responses to mastitis infection in ruminants by combining heterogeneous microarray data sources BMC Genomics 2011;12:225.
32. Pisoni G, Moroni P, Genini S, Stella A, Boettcher PJ, Cremonesi P, et al. Differentially expressed genes associated with *Staphylococcus aureus* mastitis in dairy goats. Vet Immunol Immunopathol. 2010;135:208–17.
33. Fitzpatrick JL, Cripps PJ, Hill AW, Bland PW, Stokes CR. MHC class II expression in the bovine mammary gland. Vet Immunol Immunopathol. 1992;32:13–23.
34. Bonnefont CMD, Toufeer M, Caubet C, Foulon E, Tasca C, Aure M-R, et al. Transcriptomic analysis of milk somatic cells in mastitis resistant and susceptible sheep upon challenge with *Staphylococcus epidermidis* and *Staphylococcus aureus*. BMC Genomics. 2011;12:208.
35. Schukken YH, Günther J, Fitzpatrick J, Fontaine MC, Goetze L, Holst O, et al. Host-response patterns of intramammary infections in dairy cows. Vet Immunol Immunopathol. 2011;144:270–89.
36. Majewska M, Szczepaniak M. Rola receptorów toll-podobnych (TLR) w odporności wrodzonej i nabytej oraz ich funkcja w regulacji odpowiedzi immunologicznej. [The role of toll-like receptors (TLR) in innate and adaptive immune responses and their function in immune response regulation, Abstract in English]. Post Hig Med Dosw. 2006;60:52–63.
37. Buitenhuis B, Røntved CM, Edwards SM, Ingvartsen KL, Sørensen P. In depth analysis of genes and pathways of the mammary gland involved in the pathogenesis of bovine *Escherichia coli*-mastitis. BMC Genomics. 2011;12:130.
38. Günther J, Koczan D, Yang W, Nürnberg G, Repsilber D, Schuberth H-J, et al. Assessment of the immune capacity of mammary epithelial cells: comparison with mammary tissue after challenge with *Escherichia coli*. Vet Res. 2009;40:31.
39. Pure E, Cuff CA. A crucial role for CD44 in inflammation. Trends Mol Med. 2001;7:213–21.
40. DeGrendele HC, Estess P, Siegelman MH. Requirement for CD44 in activated T cell extravasation into an inflammatory site. Science. 1997;278:672–5.
41. Sladek Z, Rysanek D. Expression of macrophage CD44 receptor in the course of experimental inflammatory response of bovine mammary gland induced by lipopolysaccharide and muramyl dipeptide. Res Vet Sci. 2009;86:235–40.
42. Zhao X, Lacasse P. Mammary tissue damage during bovine mastitis: causes and control. J Anim Sci. 2008;86(Suppl):57–65.
43. Lincoln RA, Leigh JA. Characterization of the interaction of bovine plasmin with Streptococcus uberis. J Appl Microbiol. 1998;84:1104–10.
44. Moyes KM, Drackley JK, Morin DE, Bionaz M, Rodriguez-Zas SL, Everts RE, et al. Gene network and pathway analysis of bovine mammary tissue challenged with Streptococcus uberis reveals induction of cell proliferation and inhibition of PPAR gamma signaling as potential mechanism for the negative relationships between immune response and lipid metabolism. BMC Genomics. 2009;10:542.
45. Egebland M, Werb Z. New functions for the matrix metalloproteinases in cancer progression. Nat Rev Cancer. 2002;2:161–74.
46. Wang L, Sun Y, Jiang M, Zhang S, Wolfl S. FOS proliferating network construction in early colorectal cancer (CRC) based on integrative significant function cluster and inferring analysis. Cancer Investig. 2009;27:816–24.
47. Newton K, Dixit VM. Signaling in innate immunity and inflammation. Cold Spring Harb Perspect Biol. 2012;4:a006049. doi:10.1101/cshperspect.a006049.
48. Imamura F, Takaki S, Akagi K, Ando M, Yamamura K, Takatsu K, et al. The murine interleukin-5 receptor alpha-subunit gene: characterization of the gene structure and chromosome mapping. DNA Cell Biol. 1994;13:283–92.
49. Shen F, Hu Z, Goswami J, Gaffen SL. Identification of common transcriptional regulatory elements in interleukin-17 target genes. J Biol Chem. 2006;281:24138–48.
50. Ealy AD, Yang QE. Control of interferon-tau expression during early pregnancy in ruminants. Am J Reprod Immunol. 2009;61:95–106.
51. Das M, Sabio G, Jiang F, Rincón M, Flavell RA, Davis RJ. Induction of hepatitis by JNK-mediated expression of TNF-alpha. Cell. 2009;136:249–60. Ślebodzinski AB, Malinowski E, Lipczak W. Concentrations of triiodothyronine (T 3), tumor necrosis factor-a (TNF-a) and interleukin-6 (IL-6) in milk from healthy and naturally infected quarters of cows. Res Vet Sci. 2002;72:17–21.
53. Kushibiki S. Tumor necrosis factor-α-induced inflammatory responses in
52. cattle. Anim Sci J. 2011;82:504–11.
54. Riollet C, Rainard P, Poutrel B. Cells and cytokines in inflammatory secretions of bovine mammary gland. Adv Exp Med Biol. 2000;480:247–58.
55. Riollet C, Rainard P, Poutrel B. Cell subpopulations and cytokine expression in cow milk in response to chronic *Staphylococcus aureus* infection. J Dairy Sci. 2001;84:1077–84.
56. Xiu L, Fu YB, Deng Y, Shi XJ, Bian ZY, Ruhan A, et al. Deep sequencing-based analysis of gene expression in bovine mammary epithelial cells after *Staphylococcus aureus, Escherichia coli*, and *Klebsiella pneumoniae* infection. Genet Mol Res. 2015;14:16948–65.
57. Jensen K, Günther J, Talbot R, Petzl W, Zerbe H, Schuberth H-J, et al. *Escherichia coli*- and *Staphylococcus aureus*-induced mastitis differentially modulate transcriptional responses in neighbouring uninfected bovine mammary gland quarters. BMC Genomics. 2013;14:36.

A novel real-time PCR assay for quantitative detection of *Campylobacter fetus* based on ribosomal sequences

Gregorio Iraola[1,2], Ruben Pérez[1], Laura Betancor[4], Ana Marandino[1], Claudia Morsella[3], Alejandra Méndez[3], Fernando Paolicchi[3], Alessandra Piccirillo[5], Gonzalo Tomás[1], Alejandra Velilla[3] and Lucía Calleros[1*]

Abstract

Background: *Campylobacter fetus* is a pathogen of major concern for animal and human health. The species shows a great intraspecific variation, with three subspecies: *C. fetus* subsp. *fetus*, *C. fetus* subsp. *venerealis*, and *C. fetus* subsp. *testudinum*. *Campylobacter fetus fetus* affects a broad range of hosts and induces abortion in sheep and cows. *Campylobacter fetus venerealis* is restricted to cattle and causes the endemic disease bovine genital campylobacteriosis, which triggers reproductive problems and is responsible for major economic losses. *Campylobacter fetus testudinum* has been proposed recently based on genetically divergent strains isolated from reptiles and humans. Both *C. fetus fetus* and *C. fetus testudinum* are opportunistic pathogens for immune-compromised humans. Biochemical tests remain as the gold standard for identifying *C. fetus* but the fastidious growing requirements and the lack of reliability and reproducibility of some biochemical tests motivated the development of molecular diagnostic tools. These methods have been successfully tested on bovine isolates but fail to detect some genetically divergent strains isolated from other hosts. The aim of the present study was to develop a highly specific molecular assay to identify and quantify *C. fetus* strains.

Results: We developed a highly sensitive real-time PCR assay that targets a unique region of the *16S* rRNA gene. This assay successfully detected all *C. fetus* strains, including those that were negative for the *cstA* gene-based assay used as a standard for molecular *C. fetus* identification. The assay showed high specificity and absence of cross-reactivity with other bacterial species. The analytical testing of the assay was determined using a standard curve. The assay demonstrated a wide dynamic range between 10^2 and 107 genome copies per reaction, and a good reproducibility with small intra- and inter-assay variability.

Conclusions: The possibility to characterize samples in a rapid, sensitive and reproducible way makes this assay a good option to establish a new standard in molecular identification and quantification of *C. fetus* species.

Keywords: *Campylobacter fetus*, Molecular detection, Real-time PCR

Background

Members of the genus *Campylobacter* are gram-negative epsilon-proteobacteria highly adapted to vertebrate hosts. Most species are pathogens of a wide range of livestock species and have extensive reservoirs in wildlife [1–3].

The species *Campylobacter fetus* shows a remarkable level of intraspecific variation, with three subspecies: *C. fetus* subsp. *fetus*, *C. fetus* subsp. *venerealis*, and *C. fetus* subsp. *testudinum*. *Campylobacter fetus fetus* and *C. fetus venerealis* are classified on the basis of their mechanisms of transmission, clinical presentations and two key biochemical tests (tolerance to glycine and H_2S production) [4, 5]. *Campylobacter fetus fetus* infects the intestinal tract of several mammalian species and induces abortion in cattle and sheep [2, 5, 6]. In humans, it is an opportunistic pathogen that mainly infects immune-compromised patients [7, 8]. *Campylobacter fetus venerealis* is a cattle-restricted pathogen with tropism for

* Correspondence: calleros@fcien.edu.uy
[1]Sección Genética Evolutiva, Facultad de Ciencias, Iguá 4225, Montevideo 11400, Uruguay
Full list of author information is available at the end of the article

genital tissues and is the etiological agent of bovine genital campylobacteriosis (BGC), a serious reproductive disease that causes infertility and abortion [9]. *C. fetus venerealis* includes a variant, namely *C. fetus venerealis* biovar intermedius that reacts differently to the H_2S test and also causes BGC [5]. *Campylobacter fetus testudinum* has been proposed recently to cluster some reptilian and human strains of putative reptilian origin on the basis of notorious genetic divergence from *C. fetus fetus* and *C. fetus venerealis* [10].

Biochemical tests remain as the gold standard for identifying *C. fetus* and differentiating between *C. fetus fetus* and *C. fetus venerealis*, but the fastidious growth requirements and the lack of reliability and reproducibility of some assays [11], due in part to the genetic heterogeneity of some strains, motivated the development of alternative diagnostic methods.

Several studies have endeavored in determining the suitability of different genetic methods for identifying the species *C. fetus* using end-point PCRs. In particular, the multiplex-PCR assay designed by Hum et al. [12] has been vastly used for species identification. Detection of *C. fetus* in this assay is achieved using PCR primers that target signature regions of the *cstA* gene, and *C. fetus venerealis* identification is based on the *parA* gene. However, genetic divergence in the *cstA* gene could prevent their detection by this assay, as occur in reptilian strains, and thus fails as a general diagnostic tool to identify the species [10].

Other assays for *C. fetus* identification were later designed to target additional genes, like *cpn60*, which encodes the universal 60-kDa chaperonin, and *nahE*, which encodes a sodium/hydrogen exchanger protein [13, 14]. The *cpn60* and *nahE* gene-based methods have been updated to real-time PCR assays using different technologies [14–17]. Both real-time assays have been designed to detect *C. fetus* on bovine isolates, and successfully tested on this kind of samples, but may fail to detect some genetically divergent strains, particularly of reptilian origin, which have distinctive nucleotide variants in many genes. Therefore, detection of *C. fetus* can be improved by developing new real-time PCR assays able to detect strains from all subspecies and hosts. These assays should be designed to target highly stable genomic regions that are characteristic for the species. Ribosomal genes are one of the most common DNA regions used to design PCR assays for the identification and detection of microorganisms. The *16S* rRNA gene-targeted molecular tools are widely used as its variability has been thoroughly described in all *Campylobacter* species [18–23]. The sequence of the *16S* rRNA gene is species-specific within the genus and *C. fetus* has several unique nucleotide markers [24, 25]. Moreover, ribosomal genes are homogeneous for *C. fetus* subspecies and have three identical copies per genome allowing a better detection. Despite the obvious advantages of these genes, so far, there is not a real-time PCR assay targeting ribosomal sequences for the specific detection of *C. fetus*.

The aim of the present study was to develop a highly sensitive real-time PCR assay, to detect and quantify *C. fetus* strains.

Results

Strains were assigned to *C. fetus* and its subspecies using standard bacteriological methods (Table 1). Additionally, we performed the molecular characterization in the same collection of strains (Table 1). The results of bacteriological and molecular classification do not always match, particularly at the subspecies level One bovine (INTA 89/222) and the reptilian isolate (RA8/Italy/2011) were phenotypically identified as *C. fetus* but were negative for the *cstA* gene amplicon that is currently used as a marker for *C. fetus*. The bovine isolate was positive for the subspecies (*C. fetus venerealis*) markers of both tests and the reptilian isolate was negative. The assignment of these isolates to the species *C. fetus* was confirmed by sequencing a fragment of the *16S* rRNA gene, which unequivocally discriminates between *Campylobacter* species and from other bacterial species [21, 24].

The 16SPb probe is species specific and has a minimum of one mismatch with a single sequence from *C. hyointestinalis*, and a maximum of nine differences with other *Campylobacter* species (e.g. *C. rectus* and *C. showae*). The forward primer's sequence is species specific and has a minimum of one and a maximum of four mismatches with other *Campylobacter* species (Figs. 1 and 2, Additional file 1). The reverse primer's sequence is identical in some *Campylobacter* species but has one or two differences with others. The combination of primers and probe only matches perfectly with the *16S* rRNA gene of *C. fetus*.

All PCR reactions using template DNA from *C. fetus fetus*, *C. fetus venerealis*, *C. fetus venerealis* bv. intermedius, and *C. fetus testudinum* yielded a VIC signal corresponding to the *C. fetus*-specific probe. This result indicates a 100% clinical sensitivity and 95% confidence interval of 94–100% (Clopper-Pearson interval).

The analytical performance of the assay was determined using a standard curve (Fig. 3). The linear dynamic range of the assay was established between 10^2 and 10^7 genome copies per reaction. The amplification efficiency and the coefficient of determination (R^2) were 93% and 0.9973, respectively. Intra- and inter-assay reproducibility was calculated using the coefficient of variation (CV), which showed considerable low values, being the highest 2.19% (Table 2).

No fluorescent signal was observed using template DNA from non-*C. fetus* bacterial species used as negative controls (i.e. *C. geochelonis*, *C. hyointestinalis*, *C. jejuni*, *C. coli* and *C. sputorum*). This result corresponds to a clinical

Table 1 Isolates analyzed, discriminated by host, source, country and year of isolation

Isolate	Host	Source	Country	Year	Phenotypic typing[a]	Multiplex PCR A[b]	Multiplex PCR B[c]	Real-time PCR
A28	Bovine	U	Australia	1978	Cff	Cff	Cff	+
063	Bovine	Prepuce	Uruguay	1980	Cff	Cff	Cff	+
0835	Bovine	U	Uruguay	U	Cff	Cfv	Cff	+
F106	Bovine	U	Uruguay	U	Cff	Cff	Cff	+
71098	Bovine	Fetal abomasal content	Uruguay	1998	Cff	Cff	Cff	+
INTA 97/C1N3[d]	Bovine	Vaginal mucus	Argentina	1997	Cff	Cff	Cff	+
INTA 04/554	Bovine	Fetal abomasal content	Argentina	2004	Cff	Cff	Cff	+
INTA 90/189	Bovine	Fetal lung	Argentina	1990	Cff	Cfv	Cfv	+
INTA 89/222	Bovine	Prepuce	Argentina	1989	Cff	No Cf/Cfv	No Cf/Cfv	+
INTA 01/165	Bovine	Vaginal mucus	Argentina	2001	Cff	Cff	Cff	+
INTA 12/218	Bovine	Fetal abomasal content	Argentina	2012	Cff	Cfv	Cfv	+
INTA 99/801	Bovine	Prepuce	Argentina	1999	Cff	Cff	Cff	+
INTA 01/064	Bovine	Vaginal mucus	Argentina	2001	Cff	Cff	Cff	+
INTA 04/875	Bovine	Vaginal mucus	Argentina	2004	Cff	Cff	Cff	+
INTA 08/328	Bovine	Fetal lung	Argentina	2008	Cff	Cff	Cff	+
INTA 05/622	Bovine	Fetal abomasal content	Argentina	2005	Cff	Cff	Cfv	+
INTA 11/262	Bovine	Fetal abomasal content	Argentina	2011	Cff	Cfv	Cfv	+
INTA 11/295	Bovine	Fetal abomasal content	Argentina	2011	Cff	Cfv	Cfv	+
INTA 11/685A	Bovine	Vaginal mucus	Argentina	2011	Cff	Cfv	Cff	+
INTA 11/685B	Bovine	Fetal abomasal content	Argentina	2011	Cff	Cfv	Cff	+
INTA 11/677	Bovine	Fetal abomasal content	Argentina	2011	Cff	Cff	Cff	+
INTA 11/501	Bovine	Vaginal mucus	Argentina	2011	Cff	Cff	Cff	+
INTA 11/408	Bovine	Fetal abomasal content	Argentina	2011	Cff	Cff	Cff	+
INTA 11/356	Bovine	Fetal abomasal content	Argentina	2011	Cff	Cff	Cfv	+
INTA 11/360	Bovine	Fetal lung	Argentina	2011	Cff	Cfv	Cfv	+
NCTC10354[T]	Bovine	U	England	1962	Cfv	Cff	Cfv	+
D78	Bovine	U	Australia	1978	Cfv	Cfv	Cfv	+
660	Bovine	Fetal abomasal content	Uruguay	2010	Cfv	Cfv	Cfv	+
3726	Bovine	Fetal abomasal content	Uruguay	2010	Cfv	Cfv	Cfv	+
2733	Bovine	Fetal abomasal content	Uruguay	2006	Cfv	Cfv	Cfv	+
2740	Bovine	Fetal abomasal content	Uruguay	2006	Cfv	Cfv	Cfv	+
MCR03	Bovine	Prepuce	Uruguay	2009	Cfv	Cfv	Cfv	+
3837	Bovine	Fetal abomasal content	Uruguay	2010	Cfv	Cfv	Cfv	+
1198	Bovine	U	Uruguay	U	Cfv	Cff	Cfv	+
3598	Bovine	U	Uruguay	U	Cfv	Cff	Cfv	+
2432	Bovine	U	Uruguay	2010	Cfv	Cfv	Cfv	+
2370P	Bovine	Fetal abomasal content	Uruguay	2011	Cfv	Cfv	Cfv	+
2374C	Bovine	Fetal abomasal content	Uruguay	2011	Cfv	Cfv	Cfv	+
27460P	Bovine	Fetal abomasal content	Uruguay	2011	Cfv	Cfv	Cfv	+
INTA 97/608[d]	Bovine	Placenta	Argentina	1997	Cfv	Cfv	Cfv	+
INTA 83/371	Bovine	Vaginal mucus	Argentina	1983	Cfv	Cfv	Cfv	+
INTA 90/264	Bovine	Fetal abomasal content	Argentina	1990	Cfv	Cff	Cfv	+
INTA 05/355	Bovine	Fetal abomasal content	Argentina	2005	Cfv	Cfv	Cfv	+
INTA 95/258	Bovine	Vaginal mucus	Argentina	1995	Cfv	Cff	Cfv	+

Table 1 Isolates analyzed, discriminated by host, source, country and year of isolation *(Continued)*

INTA 08/382	Bovine	Fetal abomasal content	Argentina	2008	Cfv	Cff	Cfv	+
021	Bovine	U	Australia	1978	Cfvi	Cfv	Cfv	+
INTA 98/BL472	Bovine	Fetal abomasal content	Argentina	1998	Cfvi	Cfv	Cfv	+
INTA 99/541	Bovine	Prepuce	Argentina	1999	Cfvi	Cff	Cfv	+
INTA 97/384	Bovine	Fetal abomasal content	Argentina	1997	Cfvi	Cff	Cfv	+
INTA 98/472	Bovine	Fetal abomasal content	Argentina	1998	Cfvi	Cfv	Cfv	+
INTA 00/305	Bovine	Fetal abomasal content	Argentina	2000	Cfvi	Cff	Cfv	+
INTA 02/146	Bovine	Vaginal mucus	Argentina	2002	Cfvi	Cfv	Cfv	+
INTA 03/596	Bovine	Fetal abomasal content	Argentina	2003	Cfvi	Cff	Cff	+
INTA 07/379	Bovine	Fetal abomasal content	Argentina	2007	Cfvi	Cff	Cfv	+
INTA 06/341	Bovine	Fetal lung	Argentina	2006	Cfvi	Cfv	Cfv	+
H1-UY	Human	Blood	Uruguay	2013	Cf	Cff	Cff	+
HC	Human	Blood	Uruguay	2014	Cf	Cff	Cff	+
70 L	Human	Cerebrospinal fluid	Uruguay	2014	Cf	Cff	Cff	+
70H	Human	Blood	Uruguay	2014	Cf	Cff	Cff	+
RA8/Italy/2011	Turtle	Cloaca	Italy	2011	Cft	No Cf	No Cf	+
RC7	Turtle	Cloaca	Italy	2011	*C. geochelonis*	No Cf	No Cf	-
RC11	Turtle	Cloaca	Italy	2011	*C. geochelonis*	No Cf	No Cf	-
RC20	Turtle	Cloaca	Italy	2011	*C. geochelonis*	No Cf	No Cf	-
INTA 08/209	Bovine	Prepuce	Argentina	2008	*C. sputorum*	No Cf	No Cf	-
CcHB41	Human	Feces	Uruguay	2010	*C. coli*	No Cf	No Cf	-
CjHB32	Human	Feces	Uruguay	2010	*C. jejuni*	No Cf	No Cf	-
CjCP3	Chicken	Cecal content	Uruguay	2010	*C. jejuni*	No Cf	No Cf	-
CcCP60	Chicken	Cecal content	Uruguay	2009	*C. coli*	No Cf	No Cf	-
INTA 99/243	U	Vaginal mucus	Argentina	1999	*C. hyointestinalis*	No Cf	No Cf	-
NCTC 11562	Pork	U	England	1983	*C. hyointestinalis*	No Cf	No Cf	-

Cft Campylobacter fetus subsp. *testudinum*, *Cff Campylobacter fetus* subsp. *fetus*, *Cfv Campylobacter fetus* subsp. *venerealis*, *Cfvi Campylobacter fetus* subsp. *venerealis* biovar intermedius, *Cf Campylobacter fetus*, *U* unknown, *ND* not determined
[a]in *C. fetus*, glycine tolerance and H2S production, see text for details
[b]As described in Hum et al. [12]
[c]As described in Iraola et al. [41]
[d]These strains were assayed both starting from a resuspended culture and directly from bovine samples of placenta or vaginal mucus, without a previous isolation step

specificity of 100 and a 95% confidence interval of 59–100% (Clopper-Pearson interval).

Discussion

Campylobacter fetus is a pathogen of great relevance for the cattle industry and public health. It is mandatory to report the presence *C. fetus venerealis* to the World Organization for Animal Health (OIE). In humans it is necessary to detect this opportunistic pathogen to achieve a better treatment and for epidemiological surveys. Detection of *C. fetus* in humans is difficult because both *C. fetus fetus* and *C. fetus testudinum* are potential pathogens and well-established methods would fail to detect strains of reptilian origin [10]. Therefore, cost-effective, automated and straightforward tools for the unambiguous identification of *C. fetus* are of paramount importance.

Bacteriological analysis, like culture isolation and biochemical tests, are well standardized and extensively used but challenging by the slow growing and few differential phenotypic properties of *C. fetus* [26]. These methods are also laborious and time-consuming, a disadvantage when processing samples at large-scale or delivering a fast diagnosis. To improve the quality and complement the gold-standard bacteriological methods for *C. fetus* detection, some end-point PCR methods have been designed based on the presence of species-specific amplicons [12, 27–29]; these assays fulfill various criteria such as accuracy, high detection probability and well-standardized protocols for its application and interpretation. Real-time PCR methods have been also designed with the same purpose [14–17] and have provided additional technical improvements to *C. fetus*

NR115081	*C. subantarcticus*	GCACCTGTCTCTAAGTTCTAGCAAGCTAGCACCCTCATATCTCTATAAGGTTCTTAGGATATCAAGCCCAGGTAAGG
NR116923	*C. volucris*	GCACCTGTCTCTAAGTTCTAGCAAGCTAGCACCCTCATATCTCTATAAGGTTCTTAGGATATCAAGCCCAGGTAAGG
NZJFAP	*C. corcagiensis*	GCACCTGTCTTAACATTTCTGCAAGCAGACACTCTTCCATCTCTGGATGATTTGTTAGATATCAAGTCCGGGTAAGG
NZJFJK	*C. ureolyticus*	GCACCTGTCACTAAATTCTAGTAAACTAGCACTTTCTAATCTCTTAGATGTTTTAGGATGTCAAGTCCAGGTAAGG
EF621902	*C. Canadensis*	GCACCTGTCTTATGGTTCTAGCAAGCTAGCACCCTCTTATCTCTAAAAGGTTCCATAGATATCAAGCCTAGGTAAGG
AF550620	*C. coli*	GCACCTGTCTCTAAGTTCTAGCAAGCTAGCACCCTCTTATCTCTAAGAGGTTCTTAGGATATCAAGCCCAGGTAAGG
DQ174136	*C. coli*	GCACCTGTCTCTAAGTTCTAGCAAGCTAGCACCCTCTTATCTCTAAAAGGTTCTTAGGATATCAAGCCCAGGTAAGG
DQ174137	*C. coli*	GCACCTGTCTCTAAGTTCTAGCAAGCTAGCACCCTCATATCTCTATAAGGTTCTTAGGATATCAAGCCCAGGTAAGG
GQ167664	*C. concisus*	GCACCTGTCTTAACATTTCTGCAAGCAGACACTCTTCTATCTCTAGATGATTTGTTAGATATCAAGTCCGGGTAAGG
EU636820	*C. cuniculorum*	GCACCTGTCTCTAAGTTCTAGCAAGCTAGCACCCCCATATCTCTATAGGGTTCTTAGGATATCAAGCCCAGGTAAGG
DQ174165	*C. curvus*	GCACCTGTCTTAACATTTCTGCAAGCAGACACTCTTCTATCTCTAGATGATTTGTTAGATATCAAGTCCGGGTAAGG
CP012196	*C. gracilis*	GCACCTGTCTTAACATTTCTGCAAGCAGACACTCTTCCATCTCTGGATGATTTGTTAGATATCAAGTCCGGGTAAGG
DQ174163	*C. helveticus*	GCACCTGTCTCAACATTCTAGCAAGCTAGCACTTCCGTATCTCTACAGAATTTGTTGGATATCAAGCCTAGGTAAGG
DQ174182	*C. hominis*	GCACCTGTCTTAACATTTCTGCAAGCAGACACTCTTCCATCTCTGGATGATTTGTTAGATATCAAGTCCGGGTAAGG
AJ620504	*C. insulaenigrae*	GCACCTGTCTCTAAGTTCTAGCAAGCTAGCACCCTCATATCTCTATAAGGTTCTTAGGATATCAAGCCCAGGTAAGG
AY621112	*C. jejuni*	GCACCTGTCTCTAAGTTCTAGCAAGCTAGCACCCTCATATCTCTATAAGGTTCTTAGGATATCAAGCCCAGGTAAGG
DQ174142	*C. jejuni*	GCACCTGTCTCTAAGTTCTAGCAAGCTAGCACCCTCTTATCTCTAAAAGGTTCTTAGGATATCAAGCCCAGGTAAGG
DQ174201	*C. jejuni*	GCACCTGTCTCTAAGTTCTAGCAAGCTAGCACCCTCATATCTCTATAAGGTTCTTAGGATATCAAGCCCAGGTAAGG
DQ174181	*C. lanienae*	GCACCTGTCACTAAGTTCTAGCAAGCTAGCACCCTCTTATCTCTAAGAGGTTCTTAGGATATCAAGCCCAGGTAAGG
AF550664	*C. lanienae*	GCACCTGTCACTAAGTTCTAGCAAGCTAGCACCCTCGTATCTCTACAAGGTTCTTAGGATATCAAGCCCAGGTAAGG
AF550633	*C. lari*	GCACCTGTCTCTAAGTTCTAGCAAGCTAGCACCCTCTTATCTCTAAAAGGTTCTTAGGATATCAAGCCCAGGTAAGG
DQ174145	*C. lari*	GCACCTGTCTCTAAGTTCTAGCAAGCTAGCACCCTCATATCTCTATAAGGTTCTTAGGATATCAAGCCCAGGTAAGG
AF550660	*C. mucosalis*	GCACCTGTCTCAACATTCTAGCAAGCTAGCACTTCCGTATCTCTACAGAATTCGTTGGATATCAAGTCCGGGTAAGG
AF550632	*C. peloridis*	GCACCTGTCTCTAAGTTCTAGCAAGCTAGCACCCTCATATCTCTATAAGGTTCTTAGGATATCAAGCCCAGGTAAGG
DQ174170	*C. rectus*	GCACCTGTCTTAACATTTCTGCAAGCAGACACTCTTCCATCTCTGGATGATTTGTTAGATATCAAGTCCGGGTAAGG
DQ174156	*C. showae*	GCACCTGTCTTAACATTTCTGCAAGCAGACACTCTTCCATCTCTGGATGATTTGTTAGATATCAAGTCCGGGTAAGG
DQ174151	*C. sputorum*	GCACCTGTCTTAACATTTCTGCAAGCAGACACTCTTCTATCTCTAGATGATTTGTTAGATATCAAGTCCGGGTAAGG
AY621113	*C. upsaliensis*	GCACCTGTCTCAACATTCTAGCAAGCTAGCACTTCCGTATCTCTACAGAATTTGTTGGATATCAAGCCTAGGTAAGG
NR118518	*C. hyointestinalis*	GCACCTGTCACTAATTTCTTGTAAACAAGCACTATCTTATCTCTAAGATGTTATT-GGATATCAAGCCCAGGTAAGG
AB301962	*C. hyointestinalis*	GCACCTGTCTCAACATTCTAGCAAGCTAGCACTCTCTTATCTCTAAGAGATTTGTTGGATATCAAGCCTAGGTAAGG
DQ195237	*C. hyointestinalis*	GCACCTGTCTCTAAGTTCTAGCAAGCTAGCACCCTCTTATCTCTAAGAGGTTCTTAGGATATCAAGCCCAGGTAAGG
KF425532	*C. iguaniorum*	GCACCTGTCTCTAAGTTCTAGCAAGCTAGCACCCTCATATCTCTACAAGGTTCTTAGGATATCAAGCCCAGGTAAGG
DQ174127	*C. fetus fetus* ATCC 27374	GCACCTGTCTCAACTTTCTAGCAAGCTAGCACTCTCTTATCTCTAAGAGATTAGTTGGATATCAAGCCCAGGTAAGG
GQ167674	*C. fetus fetus* ATCC 33246	GCACCTGTCTCAACTTTCTAGCAAGCTAGCACTCTCTTATCTCTAAGAGATTAGTTGGATATCAAGCCCAGGTAAGG
AY621110	*C. fetus fetus* ATCC 25936	GCACCTGTCTCAACTTTCTAGCAAGCTAGCACTCTCTTATCTCTAAGAGATTAGTTGGATATCAAGCCCAGGTAAGG
NC008599	*C. fetus fetus* 8240	GCACCTGTCTCAACTTTCTAGCAAGCTAGCACTCTCTTATCTCTAAGAGATTAGTTGGATATCAAGCCCAGGTAAGG
AB301967	*C. fetus fetus* 8013-c	GCACCTGTCTCAACTTTCTAGCAAGCTAGCACTCTCTTATCTCTAAGAGATTAGTTGGATATCAAGCCCAGGTAAGG
AB301966	*C. fetus fetus* 05-338	GCACCTGTCTCAACTTTCTAGCAAGCTAGCACTCTCTTATCTCTAAGAGATTAGTTGGATATCAAGCCCAGGTAAGG
AJ306568	*C. fetus fetus* 002\82	GCACCTGTCTCAACTTTCTAGCAAGCTAGCACTCTCTTATCTCTAAGAGATTAGTTGGATATCAAGCCCAGGTAAGG
AJ306569	*C. fetus fetus* 102\80	GCACCTGTCTCAACTTTCTAGCAAGCTAGCACTCTCTTATCTCTAAGAGATTAGTTGGATATCAAGCCCAGGTAAGG
AF550618	*C. fetus fetus* F-107/4132	GCACCTGTCTCAACTTTCTAGCAAGCTAGCACTCTCTTATCTCTAAGAGATTAGTTGGATATCAAGCCCAGGTAAGG
AF550619	*C. fetus fetus* H00/415	GCACCTGTCTCAACTTTCTAGCAAGCTAGCACTCTCTTATCTCTAAGAGATTAGTTGGATATCAAGCCCAGGTAAGG
AF482990	*C. fetus fetus*	GCACCTGTCTCAACTTTCTAGCAAGCTAGCACTCTCTTATCTCTAAGAGATTAGTTGGATATCAAGCCCAGGTAAGG
M65011	*C. fetus venerealis* ATCC 19438	GCACCTGTCTCAACTTTCTAGCAAGCTAGCACTCTCTTATCTCTAAGAGATTAGTTGGATATCAAGCCCAGGTAAGG
CM001228	*C. fetus venerealis* NCTC 10354	GCACCTGTCTCAACTTTCTAGCAAGCTAGCACTCTCTTATCTCTAAGAGATTAGTTGGATATCAAGCCCAGGTAAGG
NZHG004426	*C. fetus venerealis* 84-112	GCACCTGTCTCAACTTTCTAGCAAGCTAGCACTCTCTTATCTCTAAGAGATTAGTTGGATATCAAGCCCAGGTAAGG
CP006833	*C. fetus testudinum* 03427	GCACCTGTCTCAACTTTCTAGCAAGCTAGCACTCTCTTATCTCTAAGAGATTAGTTGGATATCAAGCCCAGGTAAGG
JQ743020	*C. fetus testudinum* campy-2	GCACCTGTCTCAACTTTCTAGCAAGCTAGCACTCTCTTATCTCTAAGAGATTAGTTGGATATCAAGCCCAGGTAAGG
JQ743022	*C. fetus testudinum* campy-10	GCACCTGTCTCAACTTTCTAGCAAGCTAGCACTCTCTTATCTCTAAGAGATTAGTTGGATATCAAGCCCAGGTAAGG
JQ743023	*C. fetus testudinum* campy-11	GCACCTGTCTCAACTTTCTAGCAAGCTAGCACTCTCTTATCTCTAAGAGATTAGTTGGATATCAAGCCCAGGTAAGG
JQ743021	*C. fetus testudinum* campy-7	GCACCTGTCTCAACTTTCTAGCAAGCTAGCACTCTCTTATCTCTAAGAGATTAGTTGGATATCAAGCCCAGGTAAGG
JQ743026	*C. fetus testudinum* campy-pet2	GCACCTGTCTCAACTTTCTAGCAAGCTAGCACTCTCTTATCTCTAAGAGATTAGTTGGATATCAAGCCCAGGTAAGG
JQ743027	*C. fetus testudinum* campy-pet3	GCACCTGTCTCAACTTTCTAGCAAGCTAGCACTCTCTTATCTCTAAGAGATTAGTTGGATATCAAGCCCAGGTAAGG
JQ743028	*C. fetus testudinum* campy-pet6	GCACCTGTCTCAACTTTCTAGCAAGCTAGCACTCTCTTATCTCTAAGAGATTAGTTGGATATCAAGCCCAGGTAAGG
JQ743030	*C. fetus testudinum* campy-pet20	GCACCTGTCTCAACTTTCTAGCAAGCTAGCACTCTCTTATCTCTAAGAGATTAGTTGGATATCAAGCCCAGGTAAGG
JQ743024	*C. fetus testudinum* campy-a20	GCACCTGTCTCAACTTTCTAGCAAGCTAGCACTCTCTTATCTCTAAGAGATTAGTTGGATATCAAGCCCAGGTAAGG
JQ743031	*C. fetus testudinum* campy-Red	GCACCTGTCTCAACTTTCTAGCAAGCTAGCACTCTCTTATCTCTAAGAGATTAGTTGGATATCAAGCCCAGGTAAGG
JQ743029	*C. fetus testudinum* campy-pet21	GCACCTGTCTCAACTTTCTAGCAAGCTAGCACTCTCTTATCTCTAAGAGATTAGTTGGATATCAAGCCCAGGTAAGG
JX912510	*C. fetus testudinum* D4355	GCACCTGTCTCAACTTTCTAGCAAGCTAGCACTCTCTTATCTCTAAGAGATTAGTTGGATATCAAGCCCAGGTAAGG
JX912511	*C. fetus testudinum* D6659	GCACCTGTCTCAACTTTCTAGCAAGCTAGCACTCTCTTATCTCTAAGAGATTAGTTGGATATCAAGCCCAGGTAAGG
JX912512	*C. fetus testudinum* D6856	GCACCTGTCTCAACTTTCTAGCAAGCTAGCACTCTCTTATCTCTAAGAGATTAGTTGGATATCAAGCCCAGGTAAGG
JX912513	*C. fetus testudinum* D6683	GCACCTGTCTCAACTTTCTAGCAAGCTAGCACTCTCTTATCTCTAAGAGATTAGTTGGATATCAAGCCCAGGTAAGG
DQ997044	*C. fetus* CTA703	GCACCTGTCTCAACTTTCTAGCAAGCTAGCACTCTCTTATCTCTAAGAGATTAGTTGGATATCAAGCCCAGGTAAGG
JN585921	*C. fetus* B1-04	GCACCTGTCTCAACTTTCTAGCAAGCTAGCACTCTCTTATCTCTAAGAGATTAGTTGGATATCAAGCCCAGGTAAGG
JN585922	*C. fetus* B1-01	GCACCTGTCTCAACTTTCTAGCAAGCTAGCACTCTCTTATCTCTAAGAGATTAGTTGGATATCAAGCCCAGGTAAGG
HQ681195	*C. fetus* WCH525	GCACCTGTCTCAACTTTCTAGCAAGCTAGCACTCTCTTATCTCTAAGAGATTAGTTGGATATCAAGCCCAGGTAAGG
JX912509	*C. fetus* 2012D-9240	GCACCTGTCTCAACTTTCTAGCAAGCTAGCACTCTCTTATCTCTAAGAGATTAGTTGGATATCAAGCCCAGGTAAGG
AY621301	*C. fetus* 23D	GCACCTGTCTCAACTTTCTAGCAAGCTAGCACTCTCTTATCTCTAAGAGATTAGTTGGATATCAAGCCCAGGTAAGG
AY621302	*C. fetus* 85-388	GCACCTGTCTCAACTTTCTAGCAAGCTAGCACTCTCTTATCTCTAAGAGATTAGTTGGATATCAAGCCCAGGTAAGG
KF372434	*C. fetus* NF17692	GCACCTGTCTCAACTTTCTAGCAAGCTAGCACTCTCTTATCTCTAAGAGATTAGTTGGATATCAAGCCCAGGTAAGG
KJ081203	*C. fetus* 12S01208-4	GCACCTGTCTCAACTTTCTAGCAAGCTAGCACTCTCTTATCTCTAAGAGATTAGTTGGATATCAAGCCCAGGTAAGG
AF219233	*C. fetus* MGH_97-2126	GCACCTGTCTCAACTTTCTAGCAAGCTAGCACTCTCTTATCTCTAAGAGATTAGTTGGATATCAAGCCCAGGTAAGG
AF219234	*C. fetus* MGH_97-3574	GCACCTGTCTCAACTTTCTAGCAAGCTAGCACTCTCTTATCTCTAAGAGATTAGTTGGATATCAAGCCCAGGTAAGG
	C. fetus fetus INTA 89/222	GCACCTGTCTCAACTTTCTAGCAAGCTAGCACTCTCTTATCTCTAAGAGATTAGTTGGATATCAAGCCCAGGTAAGG
	C. fetus venerealis MCR03	GCACCTGTCTCAACTTTCTAGCAAGCTAGCACTCTCTTATCTCTAAGAGATTAGTTGGATATCAAGCCCAGGTAAGG
	C. fetus testudinum RA8/Italy/2011	GCACCTGTCTCAACTTTCTAGCAAGCTAGCACTCTCTTATCTCTAAGAGATTAGTTGGATATCAAGCCCAGGTAAGG

Fig. 1 Multiple alignment of partial sequences of *16S* gene obtained from databases. Sequences of all species of the genus from which information is available are shown. The sequences of the primers and probe are shaded

detection protocols, like the prevention of cross contamination and the minimization of manipulation and running times. However, both end-point and real-time PCR methods described to date are designed to identify *C. fetus* in bovine samples and do not deal with the intra-specific genetic variability of the bacteria that is found in diverse hosts. In comparison to conventional PCR methods, real-time PCR assays provide increased sensitivity and an accurate quantification of target DNA to study the dynamics of the bacteria in different hosts and tissues. To the best of our knowledge, there is not a real-time PCR method that uses ribosomal sequences for the identification and quantification of *C. fetus*. Here, we have improved the current molecular methods for *C. fetus* detection by designing a new real-time PCR assay that targets the multi-copy *16S* rRNA gene. The variability of these sequences within *Campylobacter* species supports its suitability as a target for amplification-based methods using fluorescent probes. The inclusion in the assay of a TaqMan-MGB probe provides higher specificity, sensitivity and accuracy than traditional TaqMan probes and discriminates between sequences that differ in just one nucleotide [30–32].

Our assay was compared to the *cstA* gene end-point PCR proposed by Hum et al. [12] and currently used as standard for molecular diagnosis of *C. fetus*. The bovine

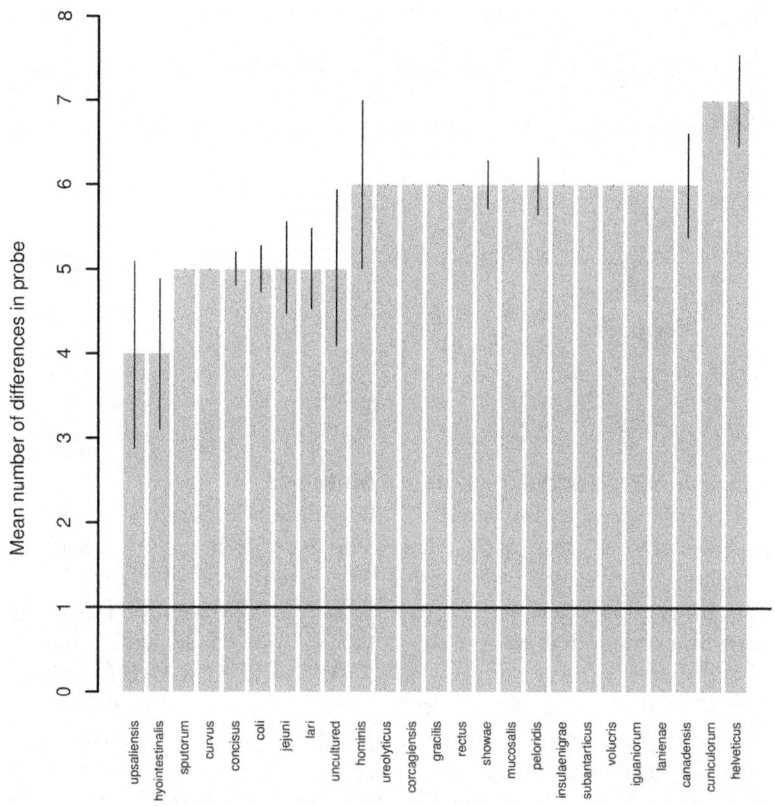

Fig. 2 Mean number of differences in probe sequence of non-*C. fetus* species *16S* gene

sample INTA 89/222 and the reptilian RA8/Italy/2011 could not be detected by Hum's PCR (Table 1), revealing that the sensitivity of this method for bovine isolates is not complete as previously reported [12, 17, 33–36]. These isolates were confirmed as belonging to *C. fetus*

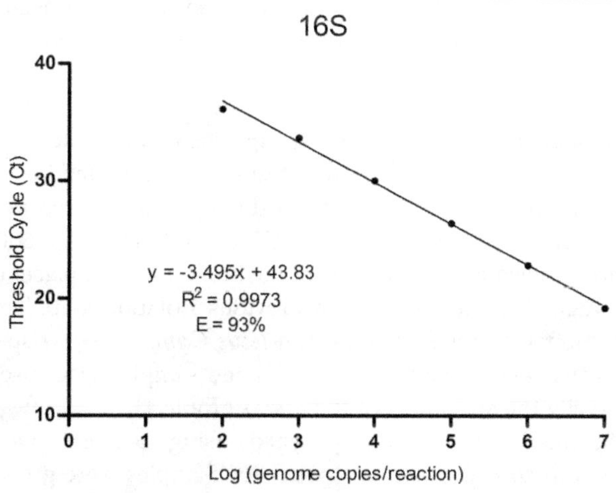

Fig. 3 Standard curve of developed TaqMan-MGB real-time PCR for *C. fetus* detection. Each point represents the mean Ct of nine different measures (three independent reactions, three replicates each). The curve equation (y), coefficient of determination (R^2) and amplification efficiency (E) are indicated

by sequencing a fragment of the *16S*rRNA gene; therefore the lack of amplification of the *cstA* gene could be due to the absence of the target *cstA* gene in these strains, or the presence of sequence variations that prevent the correct annealing of primers. Our attempt to amplify a larger region including Hum's PCR target region also failed, indicating the absence of this gene in these strains or an even greater sequence divergence within the *cstA* gene (data not shown). To test this hypothesis, it would be necessary to conduct the whole genome analysis of these strains. This notion is supported by the presence of several differences in Hum's primers binding sites in the complete genome of the reptilian strain *C. fetus* subsp. *testudinum* 03-427 (GenBank Acc. number NC_022759). This explains why the 13 isolates used for the description of this subspecies, and the RA8/Italy/2011 strain analyzed here, were negative for Hum's method based on the *cstA* gene [10]. Given the importance of this gene in the metabolism of nitrogen, and in the interaction with the host in *C. jejuni* [37], it is necessary to continue investigating its variations and possible roles in *C. fetus*.

Our novel real-time PCR assay detected all *C. fetus* tested in this study, but was negative for other *Campylobacter* species. The complete identity of primer and probe targets in all *C. fetus* strains deposited in the GenBank database (including reptilian isolates) supports that our

Table 2 Intra- and inter-assay reproducibility for the detection of *C. fetus*

Genome copies/reaction	Intra-assay variations		Inter-assay variations	
	Mean Ct (from – to)	CV (from – to)	Mean Ct	CV
1×10^1	-[a]	-	-	-
1×10^2	36.57–37.69	0.97–2.1	37.13	2.19
1×10^3	33.68–34.11	0.48–1.15	33.89	1.05
1×10^4	30–30.07	0.25–0.16	30.03	0.23
1×10^5	26.37–26.46	0.14–0.27	26.41	0.26
1×10^6	22.62–22.86	0.18–0.7	22.74	0.73
1×10^7	19.02–19.23	0.5–0.83	19.12	0.86

CV coefficient of variation of Ct values [%]
[a]Ct value out of dynamic range

assay is expected to detect the currently described subspecies from diverse hosts (Fig. 1). These results indicate the excellent sensitivity and specificity of the assay. In addition, the primers and probe sequences are conserved in the *16S*rRNA gene of the three subspecies (Fig. 1), in contrast with what happens with primers that amplify the *cstA* gene.

The assay here described has some advantages over other real-time PCR methods described in the literature. The *nahE* assay reported by Van der Graaf-van Bloois et al. [17] uses a TaqMan probe that provides high sensitivity and detection capability, but its quantification capability has not been ascertained using a standard curve. It is also uncertain whether this assay would detect reptilian *C. fetus testudinum* isolates, for which it was not designed, as the probe and the forward PCR primers have two mismatches each with respect to the *C. fetus testudinum* reference strain 03-427. The hybridization of primers and probes to the *nahE* gene could be also affected because it is embedded in a region that shows genomic rearrangements in most of the complete genome sequences available in the databases (not shown). The methodology to detect the *cpn60* gene described by Chaban et al. [14] uses specific primers and SYBR green chemistry to identify *C. fetus* species, but its performance is sub-optimal in samples with low bacterial concentrations [15], such as the uncultured samples that were successfully tested in the present assay (Table 1).

Conclusions

The *16S* rRNA gene-targeted assay here developed is excellent for the accurate detection and quantification of *C. fetus* in clinical samples and pure cultures. The possibility to characterize a large number of samples in a rapid, sensitive and reproducible way makes this assays a suitable tool for routine testing and research. For these reasons, this method has the potential to become a new standard in molecular identification of *C. fetus* species.

Methods

Real-time PCR design

The assay is based on a set of primers that amplifies a 78-bp sequence of the *16S* rRNA gene (16SFw: 5′-GCACCTGTCTCAACTTTC-3′and 16SRv: 5′-CCTTACCTGGGCTTGAT-3′) and a TaqMan-MGB probe (16SPb: 5′-VIC-ATCTCTAAGAGATTAGTTG-MGB/NFQ-3′), which targets a 19-bp polymorphic region that discriminates strains of *C. fetus* from the remaining *Campylobacter* species and other bacteria. This polymorphic region (Fig. 1) was detected by visual inspection of over 3859 partial and complete *16S* rRNA gene sequences aligned with T-Coffee [38]. The constructed alignment comprised sequences from all recognized *Campylobacter* species and from unassigned strains belonging to the genus, which were obtained from the SILVA database [39]. An alignment of 1907 representative sequences (removing identical sequences) is shown in Additional file 1. BLAST algorithm [40] was used to check *in silico* the specificity of primers and probe sequences, and to evaluate the occurrence of non-specific matches within the genomes of *C. fetus* and other bacterial species.

Bacterial strains: species and subspecies identification

The real-time PCR assay was tested with a collection of *C. fetus* strains isolated from cattle, humans and reptiles. Two of the strains (INTA 97/C1N3 and INTA 97/608) were assayed also directly from bovine samples of placenta or vaginal mucus, without a previous isolation step. Ten additional strains from four non-*fetus Campylobacter* species that occasionally occur in bovine samples were used to verify the specificity of the assays (Table 1).

Strains were previously typed using bacteriological methods to test the assay specificity. Samples were grown in Brucella semi-solid Broth and *Campylobacter* selective medium under microaerophillic conditions (85% H_2, 5% O_2, 10% CO_2) for 48 h at 37 °C. The presumptive *Campylobacter* colonies were tested by catalase and oxidase tests, and grown in Brucella broth (Sigma-Aldrich, St.

Louis, USA) with 1, 1.3, 1.5 and 1.9% glycine (Sigma-Aldrich), without glycine and in Brucella broth with NaCl and cysteine (Sigma-Aldrich) to detect H_2S production with a lead acetate paper (Sigma-Aldrich). Sodium selenite reduction test was also performed. Colonies that grew in 1% glycine were classified as *C. fetus fetus* or *C. fetus testudinum* by their positive or negative H_2S production, respectively. Glycine-sensitive colonies were assigned to the subspecies *C. fetus venerealis* (H_2S negative) or *C. fetus venerealis* bv intermedius (H_2S positive) (Table 1). Out of a total of 60 strains, 25 were *C. fetus fetus*, 20 *C. fetus venerealis*, 10 *C. fetus venerealis* bv intermedius, one was *C. fetus testudinum*, and four were not analyzed.

Strains were further characterized using the multiplex-PCR assays designed by Hum et al. [12] and Iraola et al. [41]. Both assays use the same species-specific primers to detect the *cstA* gene and different genes to identify the subspecies. The first method includes a fragment of the *parA* gene as a *C. fetus venerealis* marker, and the second uses a fragment of the *virB11* gene (Table 1) [42].

In cases where multiplex-PCR based methods failed to identify the isolates, molecular identification of species was confirmed by sequencing a fragment of the *16S* rRNA gene, which was amplified using the C412F and C1288R primers described by Linton et al [21].

Real-time PCR assays

DNA was extracted from 500 μL of a suspension of live bacteria in a phosphate-buffered saline pH 7.4 solution (1×10^8 CFU/mL), or from 1 mL of preputial washing or vaginal mucus. The QIAamp DNA Mini Kit (Qiagen, Hilden, Germany) was used for all DNA extractions and the DNA purity was measured as the ratio of absorbance at 260 and 280 nm (A260/280) using a Nanodrop 2000 (Thermo Scientific, Waltham, USA).

Real-time PCR was carried out in a 25-μL reaction containing 1 × TaqMan Genotyping Master Mix (Applied Biosystems, Foster City, USA), 1 × Custom TaqMan SNP Genotyping Assay (0.9 μM each primer and 0.2 μM probe), and 1 μL genomic DNA. Thermocycling was performed on an ABIPrism 7500 (Applied Biosystems) and consisted of a 5 min incubation step at 50 °C, denaturation for 10 min at 95 °C, followed by 40 cycles of 15 s at 95 °C and 1 min at 60 °C, and a final step of 5 min at 70 °C. Fluorescence measurements from VIC fluorophore was collected at the 5 min initial incubation stage, at the 60 °C step of each cycle, and at the end of the run.

Standard curve generation for analytical testing

To construct the standard curve for the ribosomal probe we generated 10-fold serial dilutions containing 10^0–10^7 genome copies/μL. Number of genome copies was determined by the following formula: Y (genome copies/μL) = [X (g/μL) DNA/ (nt genome length × 660)] × (6.022×10^{23}) using the DNA concentration of the dilution (X) and the genome size of the strain Cff 82-40 (1.77 Mb; GenBank accession number NC008599). The log dilution series of *C. fetus* genomes and negative controls containing nuclease-free water were tested with real-time PCR in triplicate and in three independent runs.

Standard curve was generated by plotting threshold cycle (Ct) values per three replicates per standard dilution versus the logarithm of the bacterial genome copies to determine analytical sensitivity and efficiency of the assay. The amplification efficiency was calculated with the equation $E = (10^{(-1/k)}) - 1$, where (k) is the slope of the linear regression line [43, 44]. A value of 1 corresponds to 100% amplification efficiency. The coefficient of determination (R^2) was also assessed and was considered to be suitable when it was higher than 0.980 in a single run [45, 46]. The coefficients of variation (CVs) of Ct values were assessed separately for each standard bacterial dilution by analyzing the replicates of the same analytical run (intra-assay) and the repeated analyses from different analytical runs (inter-assay).

Acknowledgments

LC and GI acknowledge support from the "Comisión Sectorial de Investigación Científica" (CSIC), and "Agencia Nacional de Investigación e Innovación" (ANII) fellowship programs from Uruguay. This work was partially financed by ANII-FSSA-2014-1-105252 Project Grant from the ANII agency.

Funding

This work was partially funded by ANII-FSSA-2014-1-105252 Project Grant from the ANII agency.

Authors' contributions

GI, LC and RP conceived and designed the experiments; GI, LC, LB, AMa, AMé, CM, GT and AV performed the experiments; GI, LC, AMa, RP and GT analyzed the data; GI, LB, LC, FP, AP and RP contributed reagents/materials/analysis tools; GI, LC and RP wrote the paper. All authors revised and approved the final version of the manuscript.

Competing interests

The authors declare that they have no competing interests.

Consent for publication

Not applicable.

Author details

[1]Sección Genética Evolutiva, Facultad de Ciencias, Iguá 4225, Montevideo 11400, Uruguay. [2]Unidad de Bioinformática, Institut Pasteur Montevideo, Montevideo, Uruguay. [3]Laboratorio de Bacteriología, Unidad Integrada INTA-Universidad Nacional de Mar del Plata, Balcarce, Argentina. [4]Departamento de Bacteriología y Virología, Instituto de Higiene, Facultad de Medicina, Universidad de la República, Montevideo, Uruguay. [5]Dipartimento di Biomedicina Comparata e Alimentazione, Università degli Studi di Padova, Padova, Italy.

References

1. Man SM. The clinical importance of emerging *Campylobacter* species. Nat Rev Gastroenterol Hepatol. 2011;8:669–85.
2. On SLW. Isolation, identification and subtyping of *Campylobacter*: where to from here? J Microbiol Methods. 2013;95:3–7.
3. On SLW. Taxonomy of *Campylobacter, Arcobacter, Helicobacter* and related bacteria: current status, future prospects and immediate concerns. J Appl Microbiol. 2001;90:1S–15S.

4. OIE. Código sanitario para los animales terrestres. CA PÍTULO 11. 3. Campilobacteriosis genital bovina. 2014. p. 10–1. Spanish version.
5. Veron M, Chatelain R. Taxonomic Study of the Genus *Campylobacter* Sebald and Veron and Designation of the Neotype Strain for the Type Species, *Campylobacter fetus* (Smith and Taylor) Sebald and Veron. Int J Syst Bacteriol. 1973;23:122–34.
6. Garcia MM, Ruckerbauer GM, Eaglesome MD, Boisclair WE. Detection of *Campylobacter fetus* in artificial insemination bulls with a transport enrichment medium. Can J Comp Med. 1983;47:336–40.
7. Wagenaar JA, van Bergen MAP, Blaser MJ, Tauxe RV, Newell DG, van Putten JPM, Van Bergen MAP, Robert V, Van Putten JPM, Diseases M, Consultancy FZ, Birches S. *Campylobacter fetus* infections in humans: exposure and disease. Clin Infect Dis. 2014;58:1–26.
8. Iraola G, Betancor L, Calleros L, Gadea P, Algorta G, Galeano S, Muxi P, Greif G, Pérez R. A rural worker infected with a bovine-prevalent genotype of *Campylobacter fetus* subsp. *fetus* supports zoonotic transmission and inconsistency of MLST and whole-genome typing. Eur J Clin Microbiol Infect Dis. 2015;34:1593–6.
9. Mshelia GD, Amin JD, Woldehiwet Z, Murray RD, Egwu GO. Epidemiology of bovine venereal campylobacteriosis: geographic distribution and recent advances in molecular diagnostic techniques. Reprod Domest Anim. 2010;45:e221–30.
10. Fitzgerald C, Tu ZC, Patrick M, Stiles T, Lawson AJ, Santovenia M, Gilbert MJ, van Bergen M, Joyce K, Pruckler J, Stroika S, Duim B, Miller WG, Loparev V, Sinnige JC, Fields PI, Tauxe RV, Blaser MJ, Wagenaar JA. *Campylobacter fetus* subsp. *testudinum* subsp. nov., isolated from humans and reptiles. Int J Syst Evol Microbiol. 2014;64(Pt 9):2944–8.
11. Alves TM, Stynen APR, Miranda KL. Campilobacteriose genital bovina e tricomonose genital bovina : epidemiologia, diagnóstico e controle. Pesqui Veterinária Bras. 2011;31:336–44.
12. Hum S, Quinn K, Brunner J, On SL. Evaluation of a PCR assay for identification and differentiation of *Campylobacter fetus* subspecies. Aust Vet J. 1997;75:827–31.
13. Abril C, Vilei EM, Brodard I, Burnens A, Frey J, Miserez R. Discovery of insertion element ISCfe1: a new tool for *Campylobacter fetus* subspecies differentiation. Clin Microbiol Infect. 2007;13:993–1000.
14. Chaban B, Musil KM, Himsworth CG, Hill JE. Development of cpn60-based real-time quantitative PCR assays for the detection of 14 *Campylobacter* species and application to screening of canine fecal samples. Appl Environ Microbiol. 2009;75:3055–61.
15. Chaban B, Chu S, Hendrick S, Waldner C, Hill JE. Evaluation of a *Campylobacter fetus* subspecies venerealis real-time quantitative polymerase chain reaction for direct analysis of bovine preputial samples. Can J Vet Res. 2012;76:166–73.
16. Selim AM, Elhaig MM, Gaede W. Development of multiplex real-time PCR assay for the detection of *Brucella* spp., *Leptospira* spp. and *Campylobacter foetus*. Vet Ital. 2014;50:269–75.
17. van der Graaf-van Bloois L, van Bergen MAP, van der Wal FJ, de Boer AG, Duim B, Schmidt T, Wagenaar JA, van Bloois LVDG. Evaluation of molecular assays for identification *Campylobacter* fetus species and subspecies and development of a *C. fetus* specific real-time PCR assay. J Microbiol Methods. 2013;95:93–7.
18. Blom K, Patton CM, Nicholson MA, Swaminathan B. Identification of *Campylobacter fetus* by PCR-DNA probe method. J Clin Microbiol. 1995;33:1360–2.
19. Cardarelli-Leite P, Blom K, Patton CM, Nicholson MA, Steigerwalt AG, Hunter SB, Brenner DJ, Barrett TJ, Swaminathan B. Rapid identification of *Campylobacter* species by restriction fragment length polymorphism analysis of a PCR-amplified fragment of the gene coding for 16S rRNA. J Clin Microbiol. 1996;34:62–7.
20. Kolbert CP, Persing DH. Ribosomal DNA sequencing as a tool for identification of bacterial pathogens. Curr Opin Microbiol. 1999;2:299–305.
21. Linton D, Owen RJ, Stanley J. Rapid identification by PCR of the genus *Campylobacter* and of five *Campylobacter* species enteropathogenic for man and animals. Res Microbiol. 1996;147:707–18.
22. Weisburg WG, Barns SM, Pelletier DA, Lane DJ. 16S ribosomal DNA amplification for phylogenetic study. J Bacteriol. 1991;173:697–703.
23. Wesley IV, Wesley RD, Cardella M, Dewhirst FE, Paster BJ. Oligodeoxynucleotide probes for *Campylobacter fetus* and *Campylobacter hyointestinalis* based on 16S rRNA sequences. J Clin Microbiol. 1991;29:1812–7.
24. Gorkiewicz G, Feierl G, Schober C, Dieber F, Köfer J, Zechner R, Zechner EL. Species-specific identification of campylobacters by partial 16S rRNA gene sequencing. J Clin Microbiol. 2003;41:2537–46.
25. Oyarzabal OA, Wesley TV, Harmon KM, Barbaree JM, Lauerman LH, Backert S, Conner DE. *Campylobacter fetus* by PCR targeting variable regions of the 16s rDNA, vol. 58. 1997. p. 61–71.
26. On SLW. Identification methods for campylobacters, helicobacters, and related organisms. Clin Microbiol Rev. 1996;9:405–22.
27. Tramuta C, Lacerenza D, Zoppi S, Goria M, Dondo A, Ferroglio E, Nebbia P, Rosati S. Development of a set of multiplex standard polymerase chain reaction assays for the identification of infectious agents from aborted bovine clinical samples. J Vet Diagn Invest. 2011;23:657–64.
28. van Bergen MA, Simons G, van der Graaf-van Bloois L, van Putten JP, Rombout J, Wesley I, Wagenaar JA. Amplified fragment length polymorphism based identification of genetic markers and novel PCR assay for differentiation of *Campylobacter fetus* subspecies. J Med Microbiol. 2005;54(Pt 12):1217–24.
29. Wang G, Clark CG, Taylor TM, Pucknell C, Barton C, Price L, Woodward DL, Rodgers FG. Colony multiplex PCR assay for identification and differentiation of *Campylobacter jejuni, C. coli, C. lari, C. upsaliensis,* and *C. fetus* subsp. *fetus*. J Clin Microbiol. 2002;40:4744–7.
30. Alonso R, Mateo E, Cisterna R. Detection of parC mutations in *Streptococcus pneumoniae* by Real-time PCR and Taqman-MGB probes. J Microbiol Methods. 2007;69:214–7.
31. Kutyavin IV, Afonina IA, Mills A, Gorn VV, Lukhtanov EA, Belousov ES, Singer MJ, Walburger DK, Lokhov SG, Gall AA, Dempcy R, Reed MW, Meyer RB, Hedgpeth J. 3'-minor groove binder-DNA probes increase sequence specificity at PCR extension temperatures. Nucleic Acids Res. 2000;28:655–61.
32. Rousselon N, Delgenès JP, Godon JJ. A new real time PCR (TaqMan® PCR) system for detection of the16S rDNA gene associated with fecal bacteria. J Microbiol Methods. 2004;59:15–22.
33. Schmidt T, Venter EH, Picard JA. Evaluation of PCR assays for the detection of *Campylobacter fetus* in bovine preputial scrapings and the identification of subspecies in South African field isolates. J S Afr Vet Assoc. 2010;81:87–92.
34. Schulze F, Bagon A, Müller W, Hotzel H. Identification of *Campylobacter fetus* subspecies by phenotypic differentiation and PCR. J Clin Microbiol. 2006;44:2019–24.
35. van der Graaf-van Bloois L, Miller WG, Yee E, Rijnsburger M, Wagenaar JA, Duim B. Inconsistency of phenotypic and genomic characteristics of *Campylobacter fetus* subspecies requires reevaluation of current diagnostics. J Clin Microbiol. 2014;52:4183–8.
36. Willoughby K, Nettleton PF, Quirie M, Maley MA, Foster G, Toszeghy M, Newell DG. A multiplex polymerase chain reaction to detect and differentiate *Campylobacter fetus* subspecies *fetus* and *Campylobacter fetus* subspecies *venerealis*: use on UK isolates of *C. fetus* and other *Campylobacter* spp. J Appl Microbiol. 2005;99:758–66.
37. Rasmussen JJ, Vegge CS, Frøkiær H, Howlett RM, Krogfelt KA, Kelly DJ, Ingmer H. *Campylobacter jejuni* carbon starvation protein A (CstA) is involved in peptide utilization, motility and agglutination, and has a role in stimulation of dendritic cells. J Med Microbiol. 2013;62:1135–43.
38. Notredame C, Higgins DG, Heringa J. T-coffee: a novel method for fast and accurate multiple sequence alignment. J Mol Biol. 2000;302:205–17.
39. Quast C, Pruesse E, Yilmaz P, Gerken J, Schweer T, Yarza P, Peplies J, Glockner FO. The SILVA ribosomal RNA gene database project: improved data processing and web-based tools. Nucleic Acids Res. 2013;41:D590–6.
40. Altschul SF, Gish W, Miller W, Myers EW, Lipman DJ. Basic local alignment search tool. J Mol Biol. 1990;215:403–10.
41. Iraola G, Hernández M, Calleros L, Paolicchi F, Silveyra S, Velilla A, Carretto L, Rodríguez E, Pérez R. Application of a multiplex PCR assay for *Campylobacter fetus* detection and subspecies differentiation in uncultured samples of aborted bovine fetuses. J Vet Sci. 2012;13:371–6.
42. Moolhuijzen PM, Lew-Tabor AE, Wlodek BM, Agüero FG, Comerci DJ, Ugalde RA, Sanchez DO, Appels R, Bellgard M. Genomic analysis of *Campylobacter fetus* subspecies: identification of candidate virulence determinants and diagnostic assay targets. BMC Microbiol. 2009;9:86–97.
43. Ginzinger DG. Gene quantification using real-time quantitative PCR: an emerging technology hits the mainstream. Exp Hematol. 2002;30:503–12.
44. Pfaffl MW. A new mathematical model for relative quantification in real-time RT-PCR. Nucleic Acids Res. 2001;29:e45.
45. Buh Gasparic M, Cankar K, Zel J, Gruden K. Comparison of different real-time PCR chemistries and their suitability for detection and quantification of genetically modified organisms. BMC Biotechnol. 2008;8:26.
46. Bustin SA, Nolan T. Pitfalls of quantitative real-time reverse-transcription polymerase chain reaction. J Biomol Tech. 2004;15:155–66.

Asymptomatic infections with highly polymorphic *Chlamydia suis* are ubiquitous in pigs

Min Li[1], Martina Jelocnik[2], Feng Yang[1], Jianseng Gong[3], Bernhard Kaltenboeck[4], Adam Polkinghorne[2], Zhixin Feng[5], Yvonne Pannekoek[6], Nicole Borel[7], Chunlian Song[8], Ping Jiang[9], Jing Li[1], Jilei Zhang[1], Yaoyao Wang[1], Jiawei Wang[1], Xin Zhou[1] and Chengming Wang[1,4*]

Abstract

Background: *Chlamydia suis* is an important, globally distributed, highly prevalent and diverse obligate intracellular pathogen infecting pigs. To investigate the prevalence and genetic diversity of *C. suis* in China, 2,137 nasal, conjunctival, and rectal swabs as well as whole blood and lung samples of pigs were collected in 19 regions from ten provinces of China in this study.

Results: We report an overall positivity of 62.4% (1,334/2,137) of *C. suis* following screening by *Chlamydia* spp. 23S rRNA-based FRET-PCR and high-resolution melting curve analysis and confirmatory sequencing. For *C. suis*-positive samples, 33.3 % of whole blood and 62.5% of rectal swabs were found to be positive for the *C. suis tetR*(C) gene, while 13.3% of whole blood and 87.0% of rectal swabs were positive for the *C. suis tet*(C) gene. Phylogenetic comparison of partial *C. suis ompA* gene sequences revealed significant genetic diversity in the *C. suis* strains. This genetic diversity was confirmed by *C. suis*-specific multilocus sequence typing (MLST), which identified 26 novel sequence types among 27 examined strains. Tanglegrams based on MLST and *ompA* sequences provided evidence of *C. suis* recombination amongst the strains analyzed.

Conclusions: Genetically highly diverse *C. suis* strains are exceedingly prevalent in pigs. As it stands, the potential pathogenic effect of *C. suis* on pig health and production of *C. suis* remains unclear and will be the subject of further investigations. Further study is also required to address the transmission of *C. suis* between pigs and the risk of 'spill-over' and 'spill-back' of infections to wild animals and humans.

Keywords: *Chlamydia suis*, Pig, FRET-PCR, *ompA*; MLST, Tanglegram

Background

Obligate intracellular bacteria of the genus *Chlamydia* are the etiological agents of chlamydiosis in wild and domestic birds, mammals and humans [1–4]. Eleven recognized *Chlamydia* spp. (*C. trachomatis, C. suis, C. muridarum, C. pneumoniae, C. abortus, C. caviae, C. felis, C. pecorum, C. psittaci, C. avium* and *C. gallinacea*) are included in the single genus *Chlamydia* under the family *Chlamydiaceae* currently contains [5].

* Correspondence: wangche@auburn.edu
[1]Yangzhou University College of Veterinary Medicine, Yangzhou, Jiangsu, People's Republic of China
[4]College of Veterinary Medicine, Auburn University, Auburn, Alabama, USA
Full list of author information is available at the end of the article

In pigs, four chlamydial species (*C. pecorum, C. abortus, C. psittaci* and *C. suis*) are regularly detected [6]. Of these, *C. abortus* and especially *C. suis* are the main species and most common involved in porcine chlamydial infections, with mixed infections occurring regularly [7–10] and only a limited number of reports finding a single species (*C. suis*) infecting cohorts of pig [10, 11].

In pigs, *C. suis* is mainly associated with subclinical infections, however it has also been found in association with respiratory disease, diarrhea, conjunctivitis and reproductive failure [3, 6]. Beyond pigs, DNA from this organism has also been detected in sheep, cattle, horses, cats, kestrels, and frogs [12–14]. Whether this PCR-based evidence represents the detection of an active infection versus exposure is, however. unknown [12–14].

Zoonotic potential of *C. suis* was suggested in the previous study, showing a single or mixed infection with *C. trachomatis* [15]. In addition, conjunctival swabs of employees in a Belgian pig slaughterhouse was identified to carry *C. suis* DNA [3] which was also found in the and pharyngeal and rectal swabs of Belgian pig farmers [10].

Consequently, pig pathogens may not only affect the pig production, but also potentially play a role in public health.

For decades, tetracyclines, as broad-spectrum antibiotics, have been extensively used in the pig industry for both prophylactic and therapeutic treatment. Interestingly, *C. suis* is the only chlamydial species to have naturally acquired genes encoding for antibiotic resistance. Over the past years, there have been accumulating reports on the occurrence of tetracycline-resistant *C. suis* strains in America, Europe and Asia [16–20]. This resistance pattern is associated with *tet*(C) islands. No standard antibiotic treatment of pigs (amoxicillin, chlortetracycline, chlortetracycline plus sulfadimidine, tylosin, trimethoprime plus sulfadimidin plus sulfathiazole) appear to be able to clear chlamydial infections at the herd level, despite individual pigs becoming negative [21]. Moreover, clear evidence of selective pressure was obvious as tetracycline treatment resulted in a higher number of tetracycline-resistant *C. suis* isolates [22]. Highlighting the additional concerns over the presence of this antibiotic-resistance genes in *C. suis*, transfer of tetracycline resistance from *C. suis* to *C. trachomatis* and *C. muridarum*, and between *C. suis* and *C. trachomatis* strains has been demonstrated *in vitro* [23].

Currently, there is no standardized typing scheme to evaluate the genetic diversity of *C. suis*. However, molecular typing schemes for other *Chlamydiaceae* are primarily based on characterizing epitopes in the major chlamydial outer membrane protein. For the closely related *C. trachomatis*, variants of this protein are subjected to selection and isolates of the same serovar may not be closely related [24, 25]. A recent study has revealed that *C. suis* had the highest whole genome recombination rate of *Chlamydia* species studied to date by whole genome sequencing [26] with *ompA*, as one of 77 *C. suis* core genes, showing significant evidence for intragenic recombination. As an alternative to *ompA*-based typing schemes, multilocus sequence typing (MLST) schemes that typically target fragments of five to seven housekeeping (HK) genes under neutral selection are widely used for determining bacterial population structures and barcoding isolates [27].

We have recently shown that, in China, a range of important livestock species, including poultry [28] and cattle [29], are infected with different endemic and epidemic strains of *Chlamydia*. Pig production is a major agricultural industry in China, however, little is known about the diversity of chlamydial infections that might impact on the health of pigs in this country. Therefore, the present study was undertaken to investigate the prevalence of *Chlamydia* spp. in pigs from China, with a particular emphasis on *C. suis* infections. Given the potential importance of tetracycline resistance for the latter species, we also investigated the presence of tetracycline resistance genes in these strains. To analyze diversity, phylogenetic and cluster analyses of *C. suis* was performed using both *ompA* and a *C. suis*-specific MLST typing scheme designed for the purpose of this study.

Methods

Ethics statement

Protocols for the collection of samples in this study were reviewed and approved by the Institutional Animal Care and Use Committee of Yangzhou University College of Veterinary Medicine (YZU-CVM#2015-057). The written permission was obtained from the owners of the pigs used in this study.

Sample collection

Nasal, rectal swabs, whole blood and lung samples

In this study, a total of 2,137 clinical samples (lung, whole blood, rectal swabs, nasal swabs, conjunctival swabs) were collected from pigs in the farms of 19 regions of 10 provinces of China between 2015 and 2016 (Table 1). A part of samples were collected from pigs in 9 regions of Jiangsu province: whole blood samples (n=308) and rectal swabs (n=55) were collected in Yangzhou City, whole blood samples (n=33) were from Nantong city, nasal swabs were from Nanjing city (n=180), Huaian city (n=70), Suqian city (n=41), Taizhou city (n=49), Wuxi city (n=36), Yancheng city (n=37), Changzhou city (n=23). In addition, nasal swabs (n=68) and rectal swabs (n=68) were collected from swine farms in Kunming city in Yunnan province; nasal swabs were from Shanghai municipality (n=52), Xihua City in Henan province (n=63), Changchun City in Jilin province (n=63), Jiangmen City in Guangdong province (n=40), Haerbin City in Heilongjiang province (n=60) and Jining City in Shandong province (n=60), respectively. Nasal swabs were also collected from Specific Pathogen Free (SPF) pigs (n=108) in two experimental animal companies in Nanjing City in Jiangsu province. Lung tissue samples (n=23) from an abattoir in Nanping city in Fujian province were also collected.

Table 1 Prevalence and copy numbers of *C. suis* of pigs from provinces of China

Province	City	Sample type	Age	Positivity	Copy /ml or swab, log10
Fujian	Nanping	Lung	NA	26.1% (6/23)	3.72 (40mg)
Jiangsu	Yangzhou	Whole blood	Finisher pig	33.4 % (103/308)	2.79
		Rectal swab	Finisher pig	98.2%(54/55)	4.50
	Nantong	Whole blood	Suckling pig	0.0% (0/11)	0.00
			Weaned pig	20.0% (2/10)	3.17
			Sow	8.3% (1/12)	2.85
	Nanjing	Nasal swab	Weaned pig*	86.1% (93/108)	3.65
			35d	95.0%(57/60)	2.61
			49d	76.7%(46/60)	1.85
			63d	91.7%(55/60)	4.19
	Huaian	Nasal swab	Suckling pig	40.9% (9/22)	2.16
			Weaned pig	18.8% (3/16)	1.99
			Finisher pig	58.3% (7/12)	2.11
			Sow	15.0% (3/20)	1.99
	Suqian	Nasal swab	Suckling pig	40.0% (6/15)	2.68
			Weaned pig	38.9% (7/17)	3.07
			Sow	12.5% (1/9)	2.20
	Taizhou	Nasal swab	Suckling pig	69.2% (18/26)	2.25
			Weaned pig	69.2 (9/13)	2.91
			Finisher pig	100.0% (5/5)	3.67
			Sow	0.0% (0/5)	0.00
	Wuxi	Nasal swab	Suckling pig	17.6% (3/17)	1.99
			Weaned pig	100.0% (5/5)	3.16
			Finisher pig	100.0% (5/5)	3.13
			Sow	0.0% (0/9)	0.00
	Yancheng	Nasal swab	Suckling pig	43.8% (7/16)	2.13
			Weaned pig	87.5% (7/8)	2.95
			Finisher pig	100.0% (3/3)	2.89
			Sow	30.0% (3/10)	2.31
	Changzhou	Nasal swab	Suckling pig	100% (7/7)	3.48
			Weaned pig	100.0% (16/16)	3.81
Shanghai	Shanghai	Nasal swab	Suckling pig	66.7% (12/18)	2.60
			Weaned pig	57.1% (8/14)	2.12
			Finisher pig	100.0% (10/10)	3.89
			Sow	20.0% (2/10)	3.00
Yunnan	Kunming	Nasal swab	Suckling pig	92.3% (12/13)	2.91
			Weaned pig	100.0% (9/9)	3.80
			Finisher pig	86.7% (13/15)	2.25
			NA	90.3% (28/31)	3.12
		Rectal swab	Suckling pig	84.6% (11/13)	3.03
			Weaned pig	100.0% (9/9)	4.14
			Finisher pig	66.7% (10/15)	2.58
			NA	93.6% (29/31)	4.54

Table 1 Prevalence and copy numbers of *C. suis* of pigs from provinces of China *(Continued)*

Province	City	Sample type	Age	Positivity	Copy /ml or swab, log10
Zhejiang	Shaoxing	Nasal swab	Suckling pig	89.0% (89/100)	3.55
			Weaned pig	95.0% (95/100)	4.26
			Finisher pig	82.0% (41/50)	3.27
			Sow	46.0% (23/50)	2.97
	Shaoxing	Nasal swab	Sow	32.0%(16/50)	2.74
		Conjunctival swab	Sow	26.0% (13/50)	2.56
		Rectal swab	Sow	20.0% (10/50)	2.89
		Whole blood	Sow	0.0% (0/50)	0.00
	Ningbo	Nasal swab	Weaned pig	100.0% (50/50)	4.86
		Conjunctival swab		100.0% (50/50)	4.87
		Rectal swab		100.0% (50/50)	5.83
		Whole blood		16.0% (8/50)	3.50
Henan	Xihua	Nasal swab	Sow	28.1%(9/32)	3.13
			Weaned pig	96.8%(30/31)	3.42
Jilin	Changchun	Nasal swab	Weaned pig	81.1%(53/63)	3.94
Guangdong	Jiangmen	Nasal swab	Weaned pig	100.0%(20/20)	4.86
			Sow	90.0%(18/20)	3.68
Heilongjiang	Haerbin	Nasal swab	Suckling pig	71.7%(43/60)	2.07
Shandong	Jining	Nasal swab	Suckling pig	53.3%(16/30)	3.68
			Sow	6.7%(2/30)	2.84

*represents SPF weaned pig from two experimental animal companies. NA: not applicable.

Nasal swabs, conjunctival and rectal swabs were collected into sterile Eppendorf tubes (Eppendorf, Shanghai, China) containing 400 µl DNA/RNA stabilization buffer (Roche Molecular Biochemicals, Indianapolis, IN, USA). Blood samples were collected into EDTA tubes (Becton, Dickinson and Company, Franklin Lakes, NJ, USA) and transported and stored at room temperature.

Nasal swabs from pigs of different ages

To compare and analyze differences in positivity and infectious load of *C. suis* among suckling pigs (age before 25 days old), weaned pigs (age after 25 d), finisher pigs (age after 100 d) and sows (age after 210 d), nasal swabs were collected from animals in each age group from Shaoxing city in Zhejiang Province: suckling pigs (n=100), weaned pigs (n=100), finisher pigs (n=50) and sows (n=50).

Nasal, conjunctival, rectal swabs and whole blood samples from pigs on two pig farms in Zhejiang province

To compare and analyze differences in the shedding of *C. suis* from different anatomical sites of animals, multiple samples (nasal, conjunctival, rectal swabs and whole blood) were collected randomly from 50 sows in a pig farm in Shaoxing of Zhejiang province and 50 weaned pigs in Ningbo of Zhejiang province. For the former, 50 sows in two blocks were randomly chosen out of 160 sows on pig farms in Shaoxing. For the latter, 50 weaned pigs in 10 blocks were chosen out of 200 weaned pigs on pig farms in Ningbo for this study. Whole blood samples (around 2 ml) were collected in EDTA tubes, nasal, conjunctival, rectal swabs were collected as above mentioned.

DNA extraction from swabs, whole blood and lung samples

The High-Pure PCR Template Preparation Kit (Roche Molecular Biochemicals, Indianapolis, IN, USA) was used to extract total nucleic acids from nasal, conjunctival, rectal swabs and whole blood and lungs from pigs, according to the manufacturer's instructions and described before [30]. The extracted DNA was eluted in 200 µl elution buffer. In this study, swabs obtained weekly from research laboratory were processed for *Chlamydia* qPCR to verify free of carry-over contamination occurred. Furthermore, diethylpyrocarbonate (DEPC)-treated ddH_2O served as a negative control to confirm that contamination between samples did not occur during the DNA extraction.

Chlamydia FRET-PCR

The FRET-PCR was performed in a LightCycler 480-II real-time PCR platform., and the protocol of the PCR in this study followed what described [28, 31]. This 23S rRNA-based FRET-PCR was able to detect all 11 *Chlamydia* species and had a detection limit of single copies/reaction. The PCR products were further verified by electrophoresis followed by DNA sequencing (BGI, Shanghai, China).

Tet(C) and *tetR*(C) PCR

Whole blood samples of both *C. suis*-positive (n=45) and *C. suis*-negative (n=40) from Yangzhou in Jiangsu province and rectal swabs of both *C. suis*-positive (n=54, 45 from Kunming in Yunnan province and 9 from Shaoxing in Zhejiang province) and *C. suis*-negative (n=53, 38 from Kunming in Yunnan province and 15 from Shaoxing in Zhejiang province) were examined for presence of the tetracycline resistance gene, *tet*(C), and the tetracycline repressor gene, *tetR*(C), by PCR as previously described [17].

C. suis-specific *ompA*-PCRs

To investigate the polymorphisms in the *C. suis ompA* gene, a set of primers were designed using Vector NTI to amplify the *ompA* VD 1-2 (amplicon size: 491bp) to interrogate 108 *C. suis* -positive samples (44 whole blood, 3 lungs samples, 12 rectal swabs, 1 conjunctival swabs, 48 nasal swabs). Twenty μl PCRs were prepared containing 10.0 μl DNA template, 0.2μl forward primer (100 μM), 0.2μl reverse primer (100 μM,), 4.0 μl 5 x PCR buffer, 0.4 μl 10 μM dNTP, 0.3 μl 5 U/μl *Taq* DNA polymerase and 4.9 μl Ultrapure H_2O. In addition, two sets of primers were designed to specifically amplify the *ompA* gene of *C. abortus* and *C. pecorum* (Table 2). Along with a set of specific primers for *C. psittaci* [29], these assays were used to confirm the detection of each species' DNA from the *Chlamydia* FRET-qPCR. PCR amplification was performed in a LightCycler 480-II real-time PCR platform using a high-stringency 18-cycle step-down temperature protocol: 6 x 1 sec @ 95°C, 12 sec @64°C, 8 sec @ 72°C; 9 x 1 sec @ 95°C, 12 sec @ 62°C, 8 sec @ 72°C; 3 x 1 sec @ 95°C, 12 sec @ 60°C, 8 sec @ 72°C; followed by 30 low-stringency cycles: 30 x 1 sec @ 95°C, 12 sec @ 55°C, 30 sec @ 67°C, and 10 sec @ 72°C. The PCR products were further verified, purified and sequenced as mentioned above.

C. suis-specific MLST analysis

In this study, a *C. suis*-specific MLST typing scheme based on a previously published *Chlamydiales* MLST scheme [32, 33] was developed. The scheme was designed to target the partial fragments of seven *C. suis* HK genes. The selected genes are not adjacent to putative outer membrane, secreted, or hypothetical and are separated widely on the chromosome. In addition, each locus for the selected genes demonstrated a

Table 2 *ompA* and MLST primers used in this study

Chlamydia	Target	Primer/probe	Sequence (5'-3')	Amplicon Size (bp)	MLST fragment (bp)
C. suis	*Cs_ompA* VD 1-2	UP	TTGAACATTTGGGATCGTTTTGA	491	_
		DN	CCAATGTAAGGAGTGAACATATTTAATCTG		
	gatA	UP	TAAAAGTGCTTTAGAATTAAGAGATGCTGT	539	425
		DN	AGATGCTGGCTGACGAATCGA		
	oppA_3	UP	AGATATCAGTGGGAATCTGCTTGC	674	468
		DN	TAAGGATTTTTTTCCAATTTAAGCCAT		
	hflX	UP	CTCTCCCTCTCAACAACGGAACTT	616	435
		DN	TTCAATAACATGCAGCAAAATATCCTC		
	gidA	UP	TTTGGGAGTTTCTACGAAGGAAGG	570	474
		DN	ATAATTTCATATTGTACATCGAAAGGCAT		
	enoA	UP	TCTCGGGGTCTCTTTAGCATTAGC	590	381
		DN	CTCCAACGAGTTGAATACGATCTCC		
	hemN	UP	GAAGAGCTTGCTATTGAATTTGATCC	608	432
		DN	CGTTTTGTAGATAGATTCCTCGAATGA		
	fumC	UP	CTCTTATGGGAAAGAATTGATGCCT	641	465
		DN	TACTTTCTCTACAAAACCTTCAGGAACATT		
C. abortus	Cab_*ompA*	UP	TACAAGCCTTGCCTGTAGGGAAC	360	_
		DN	CAGAAAATATCAAAGCGATCCCAG		
C. pecorum	Cpe_*ompA*	UP	ATGAAAAAACTCTTAAAATCGGCGT	420	_
		DN	CAGAAAATATCAAAGCGATCCCAG		

similar degree of nucleotide substitutions to provide consistency [27].

Amplification primers were designed based on the genome sequence of *C. suis* MD56 to amplify fragments of the genes encoding aspartyl/glutamyl-tRNA amidotransferase subunit A (*gatA*) (amplicon length: 539 bp), oligobinding protein (*oppA*) (674 bp), GTP-binding protein (*hflX*) (616bp), tRNA uracil-5-methyl transferase (*gidA*) (570 bp), enolase (*enoA*) (590 bp), Coproporphyrinogen III oxidase (*hemN*) (608bp), and fumarate hydratase class II (*fumC*) (641bp) (Table 2). PCR amplification of the seven HK genes was performed in a LightCycler 480-II real-time PCR platform following the above-mentioned protocol. Each sequence run was performed from a different PCR amplicon and sequence traces were obtained with automated DNA sequencing. Briefly, forward and reverse chromatograms for each sequenced HK gene fragment were aligned and trimmed, and the fragment sequence for that allele was obtained. Sequences for each gene were then aligned in MEGA 6.0 using the ClustalW multiple alignment algorithm and trimmed to appropriate lengths for *Chlamydiales* MLST fragments [32].

After the optimization and development, the *C. suis*-MLST was successfully applied to *C. suis* positive samples from nasal (n=12) and rectal (n=7) swabs, 6 whole blood (n=6) and 1 lung samples (n=1) from 26 pigs. Phylogenetic analyses were performed using DNASp 5.0 [34] and Geneious 9 [35]. DnaSP 5.0 was used to analyze the sequence polymorphisms: by determining the number of synonymous (dS) and non-synonymous (dN) substitutions per site, Jukes-Cantor corrected, the number of polymorphic sites, haplotypes and haplotypesper allele. Allele and sequence type (ST) assignation for 26 *C. suis* strains described in this study and one Italian strain-MD56 were determined and deposited at http://pubmlst.org/chlamydiales/ [36].

Phylogenetic analysis

Phylogenetic analyses were performed using the 489 bp variable region of the *ompA* gene and the concatenated *C. suis* MLST sequences. For *ompA*, a total of 127 sequences consisting of 50 publicly available sequences obtained from GenBank and 77 sequences from this study were aligned using the ClustalX 1.83. Based on these alignments, the NJ phylogenetic trees were constructed using the Kimura 2-parameter model. The MEGA 6.0. Bootstrap values were calculated by the use of 500 replicates.

A Bayesian phylogenetic tree using an alignment of a total of 40 concatenated MLST sequences from the 26 *C. suis* strains from this study, and 14 additional strains from Switzerland, USA, Italy and Austria. *C. suis* isolates was constructed with MRBAYES [37] with the GTR+G model, as implemented in Geneious 9. Run parameters included four Markov Chain Monte Carlo (MCMC) chains with a million generations, sampled every 1000 generations and with the first 10000 trees were discarded as burn-in. *C. trachomatis* MLST sequences were used as an outgroup to determine the mid-point root of the *C. suis* phylogeny. MLST gene fragments were extracted from publicly available genomes of the strains SWA-2 (GenBank acc. No. NZ_LT 821323), 14-23b (NZ_FSSG01000023), 1-28b (NZ_FTQD 01000002), 3-25a (NZ_FTQO01000003), 10-26b (NZ_FTQ J01000001), 5-22b (NZ_FTQB01000001), 8-29b (NZ_FTQ U01000001), 3-29b (NZ_FTPY01000001- NZ_FTPY010 00002), S45 (SRA accession: SRX1868493), R19 (SRX186 8490), Rogers130 (SRX1868491), R1 (SRX1868495), R16 (SRX1868494), MD56 (NZ_AYKJ00000000).

Minimum spanning tree and identification of clonal complexes (CCs) using the goeBURST algorithm [38] on the *C. suis* MLST data from this study was performed using the https://online.phyloviz.net [39]. The MLST profiles were clustered into CCs under a user-defined threshold level of identity. In this study, we used relaxed triple locus variant (TLV) level where CCs were defined as groups of sequencing types (STs) which share four out of seven alleles with at least one other ST in the group, while the satellite STs were defined as STs that differ by at least three alleles from all other STs. A 'putative progenitor' in CCs is a ST that has the most single locus variant (SLV) links to other STs.

In order to compare phylogenetic inferences based on MLST and *ompA* alignments, we have constructed a tanglegram from cladograms of Bayesian *C. suis* MLST and *ompA* phylogenetic trees, and a strict consensus tree, computed with Dendroscope 3 [40]. For this analysis, we have also constructed a mid-point rooted Bayesian phylogenetic tree using the 489 bp *ompA* fragment alignment from the same 40 (26 Chinese and 14 global) *C. suis* strains used for MLST-derived phylogeny. The tree parameters included GTR+I model and four Markov Chain Monte Carlo (MCMC) chains with a million generations, sampled every 1000 generations and with the first 10000 trees were discarded as burn-in.

In order to infer recombination break points within each alignment, we used Dual-Brothers recombination detection with default setting (as implemented in Geneious 9). DualBrothers detects recombination based on the dual Multiple Change-Point (MCP) model which finds changes in topology and evolutionary rates across sites in a multiple sequence alignment [41].

Statistical analysis

The Chi-squared Test was used to compare the positivity of *C. suis* infection in different samples of pigs. The two-tailed Tukey honest significant difference (HSD) test in one-way ANOVA was used to analyze the differences of *C. suis* copy numbers in different samples. Differences at P≤0.05 were considered significant.

Results

Prevalence of *Chlamydia* spp. in pigs

C. suis was found to be the only chlamydial species in all samples in this study with an overall positivity of 62.4% (1,334/2,137). In addition, 26.1% (6/23) of lung samples from Fujian province tested positive for *C. suis* (Table 1). Notably, a cohort of SPF pigs had 80.0% (52/65) of *C. suis* positivity in pigs less than two months old and 95.4% positivity (41/43) in pigs older than two months (Table 1).

Prevalence and copy numbers of *C. suis* affected by samples types

Nasal swabs, conjunctival swabs, rectal swabs and whole blood samples were collected from 100 pigs in Zhejiang province for *C. suis* detection. The prevalence and average bacterial genome numbers of whole blood samples was significantly lower than in other sample types (P<0.05). The *C. suis* positivity was 8.0% (8/100) in whole blood, 66.0% (66/100) in nasal swabs, 63.0% in conjunctival swabs (66/100), and 60.0% in rectal swabs (60/100). In addition, the average bacterial genome numbers of *C. suis* were $10^{3.50\pm0.20\ [SEM]}$ per ml whole blood), $10^{5.34\pm0.16}$ per rectal swab; $10^{4.39\pm0.14}$ per conjunctival swab, and $10^{4.37\pm0.14}$ per nasal swab (Fig. 1).

C. suis in pigs of different ages

C. suis positivity in nasal swabs was found to be similar in finisher pigs (84.0%; 84/100) and weaned pigs (84.0%; 262/312), which were significantly higher than in suckling pigs (69.4%, 225/324; P<0.01) and sows (31.3%, 61/195; P<0.01). Interestingly, the average copy number of *C. suis* was significantly higher in weaned pigs (P<0.01, $10^{3.88\pm0.06\ [SEM]}$ per swab) than in sows ($10^{3.11\pm0.09}$ per swab), finisher pigs ($10^{3.09\pm0.07}$ per swab) and suckling pigs ($10^{2.94\pm0.05}$ per swab) (Fig. 2).

Tet(C) and *tetR*(C) genes

For *C. suis*-positive samples, 6/45 (13.3%) of whole blood samples from Yangzhou in Jiangsu, 39/45 (86.7%) of rectal swabs from Kunming in Yunnan and 8/9 (88.9%) of rectal swabs from Shaoxing in Zhejiang province contained the *tet*(C) gene while 15/45 (33.3%) of whole blood samples and 5/8 (62.5%) of rectal swabs samples were found to be positive for the *tetR*(C) gene while 6 of 45 (13.3%) whole blood samples and 47 of 54 (87.0%) rectal swabs samples contained the *tet*(C) gene. We also tested the presence of *tet*(C) genes in *C. suis*-negative samples in this study. For *C. suis*-negative samples, no (0/40; 0.0%) whole blood samples from Yangzhou in Jiangsu and 19/38 (50%) of 53 (54.7%) rectal swabs from Kunming in Yunnan and 10/15 (66.7%) of rectal swabs from Shaoxing in Zhejiang province contained

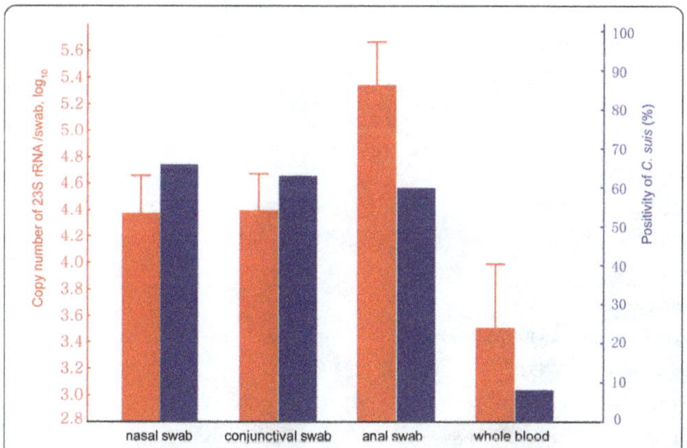

Fig. 1. Prevalence and copy numbers of *C. suis* affected by samples type of pigs. Copy number (± SEM) is shown in the left ordinate (in red). Positivity is shown in the right ordinate (in blue). FRET-qPCR were performed to determine the positivity and copy number of *C. suis* from nasal, conjunctival, rectal swabs and whole blood samples of 50 sows and 50 weaned pigs in this study. The positivity of *C. suis* in nasal swabs (66%), conjunctival swabs (63%) and rectal swabs (60%) was significantly higher than whole blood (P<0.01, 8%). The average copy number of *C. suis* was highest in rectal swab (P<0.01, $10^{5.34\pm0.16\ [SEM]}$ per swab), followed by conjunctival swab ($10^{4.39\pm0.14}$ per swab) and nasal swab ($10^{4.37\pm0.14}$ per swab), and whole blood (P<0.05, $10^{3.50\pm0.20}$ per ml).

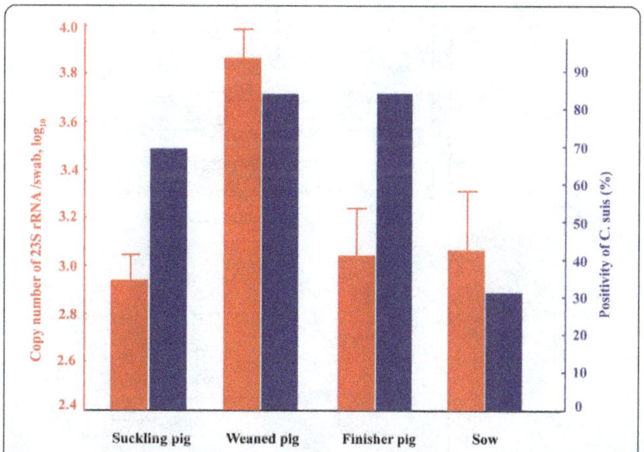

Fig. 2. Prevalence and copy numbers of *C. suis* affected by ages of pigs. Copy number (± SEM) is shown in the left ordinate (in red). Positive rate is shown in the right ordinate (in blue). FRET-qPCR were performed to determine the positivity and copy number of *C. suis* from nasal swabs of suckling pigs (n=324), weaned pigs (n=312), finisher pigs (n=100) and sows (n=195) in this study. The positivity of *C. suis* was the lowest in sow (P<0.01, 31.3%), followed by finisher pigs (84.0%) and weaned pigs (84.0%), and suckling pigs (P<0.05, 69.4%). The average copy number of *C. suis* was significantly higher in weaned pigs (P<0.01, $10^{3.88\pm0.06\ [SEM]}$ per swab) than sows ($10^{3.11\pm0.09}$ per swab), finisher pigs ($10^{3.09\pm0.07}$ per swab) and suckling pigs ($10^{2.94\pm0.05}$ per swab).

the *tet*(C) gene. Both *C. suis tet*(C) and *tetR*(C) were detected in samples from pigs in 3 provinces sampled in this study. In a word, the *tet*(C) positivity in *C. suis*-positive samples was significantly higher than in *C. suis*-negative ones for whole blood from Jiangsu (13.3%, 6/45 vs. 0.0%, 0/40; P<0.01) and rectal swabs from Yunnan and Zhejiang (87.0%, 47/54 vs. 54.7%, 29/53; P<0.01).

C. suis ompA molecular typing

We obtained 77 distinct partial *ompA* sequences encompassing the variable domain 1 and 2 (VD1-2) from 108 pig *C. suis* strains (Fig. 3, Additional file 1). Phylogenetic analyses showed that the partial *ompA* VD1-2 sequences from *C. suis* strains from China identified in this study are highly polymorphic when compared with the existing *ompA* sequences deposited in GenBank. Percent

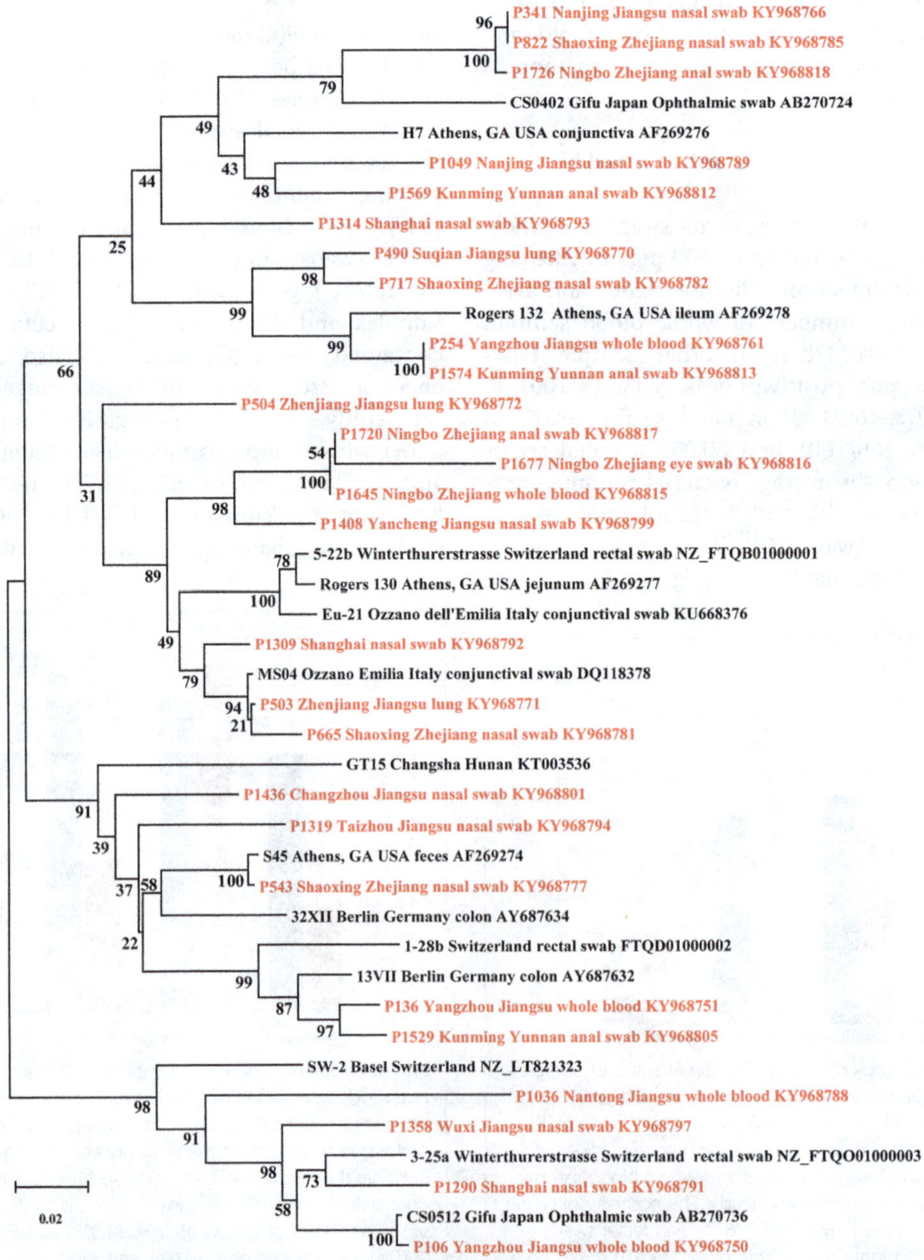

Fig. 3. Mid-point rooted NJ phylogenetic tree of the *ompA* variable domains 1-2. A 489-bp fragment encompassing *C. suis ompA* VD1-2 of 27 porcine *C. suis* strains identified in this study (in red font; name of strain, countries, sample type and accession number) are compared with 15 other *C. suis* sequences deposited in GenBank from six countries (Germany, Switzerland, Italy, USA, Japan and China). Branch lengths are measured in nucleotide substitutions and numbers show branching percentages in bootstrap replicates. Scale bar represents the percent sequence diversity.

sequence similarity observed within the Chinese cohort was 76.0%-100%, while between the Chinese cohort and the GenBank sequences, only 64.0%-100% sequence similarity could be observed. When compared with global *ompA* sequences, the Chinese *C. suis ompA* VD1-2 sequences could be resolved into four major clades of the global *ompA* VD1-2 phylogram, suggesting that the global diversity in *C. suis* strains is captured in the Chinese pig population (Figure 3). While considerable sequence variation was observed, some identical strains were also detected including the detection of at least one sequence (Ya/ChPP854/Nasal) in Zhejiang that was identical to the sequence from a *C. suis* strain (AB270743) deposited from Japan. Fine-detailed epidemiological analysis of these sequences further revealed that the same *ompA* sequences could be found in different cities and provinces, suggesting that some strains were more widely distributed than other strains.

C. suis MLST analyses

In this study, we also assessed the genetic diversity of the *C. suis* strains detected using a *C. suis*-specific MLST scheme. The MLST of the 27 global *C. suis* strains confirmed high genetic diversity for this pathogen, identifying 26 novel STs among 27 strains (0.96 ST/strain). Sequence analysis of individual as well as concatenated *C. suis* MLST gene fragments from this study confirmed that the *C. suis* HK genes are conserved and under purifying selection with dN/dS ratios < 1, yet with high haplotype diversity. The number of mutations was comparable between the *C. suis* HK alleles, ranging from 29 SNPs in *gidA* to 12 SNPs in *gatA*, with most resulting mainly in synonymous substitutions (Table 3). Each MLST allele had 3 to 8 predicted putative recombination events.

Due to its congruency with whole or core genome phylogeny, the concatenated MLST sequences have been previously used to infer phylogenetic relationships between the strains of other chlamydial species [42]. To assess the phylogenetic relationships between the Chinese and other global *C. suis* strains, a mid-point rooted Bayesian phylogenetic tree was constructed from an alignment of a total of 40 strains (Fig. 4a). Using *C. trachomatis* as an out-group, the Chinese isolates resolved into seven diverse larger clades, clustering on their own or with European and US isolates. In their own well-supported clades, Chinese *C. suis* strains formed many distinct lineages. When clustered with European and the USA isolates within a larger clade, Chinese isolates also grouped in separate but diverse sub-clades. Similarly, US and European strains also formed distinct well-supported clades (Fig. 4a).

The phylogenetic analyses further resolved the on-farm epidemiology of Chinese *C. suis* infections including evidence of sub-clades consisting of: a) related STs obtained from various anatomical sites of different hosts (as observed in the sub-clade consisting of nasal STs 190 and 177, rectal ST 192 and lung ST 189; and b) closely related STs obtained from the same anatomical site from different hosts (such as all nasal STs 172, 173, 174 and 180 sub-clade and blood STs 185 and 184, and 170 and 187 sub-clades).

The *C. suis* STs cluster analyses and minimum spanning tree also confirmed high ST diversity (Fig. 4b). Using a relaxed fit where STs must share at least 4/7 alleles, the 26 STs clustered into five clonal complexes (CCs, and 15 satellite STs (Figure 4b). Only two CCs

Table 3 Sequence analyses of the 27 *C. suis* MLST alleles and concatenated sequences

Allele	Total number of polymorphisms (Δnt)	No. of non-synonymous substitutions	No. of synonymous substitutions	dN/dS ratio	Number of haplotypes
*gat*A (425 bp)	12	1	11	0.010	11
*opp*A_3 (468 bp)	17	3	14	0.061	12
*hfl*X (435 bp)	24	2	22	0.022	18
*gid*A (474 bp)	29	4	25	0.074	18
*eno*A (381 bp)	23	1	22	0.007	23
*hem*N (432 bp)	17	2	15	0.113	14
*fum*C (465 bp)	14	2	12	0.024	14
Concatenated (3080 bp)	136	15	121	-	26

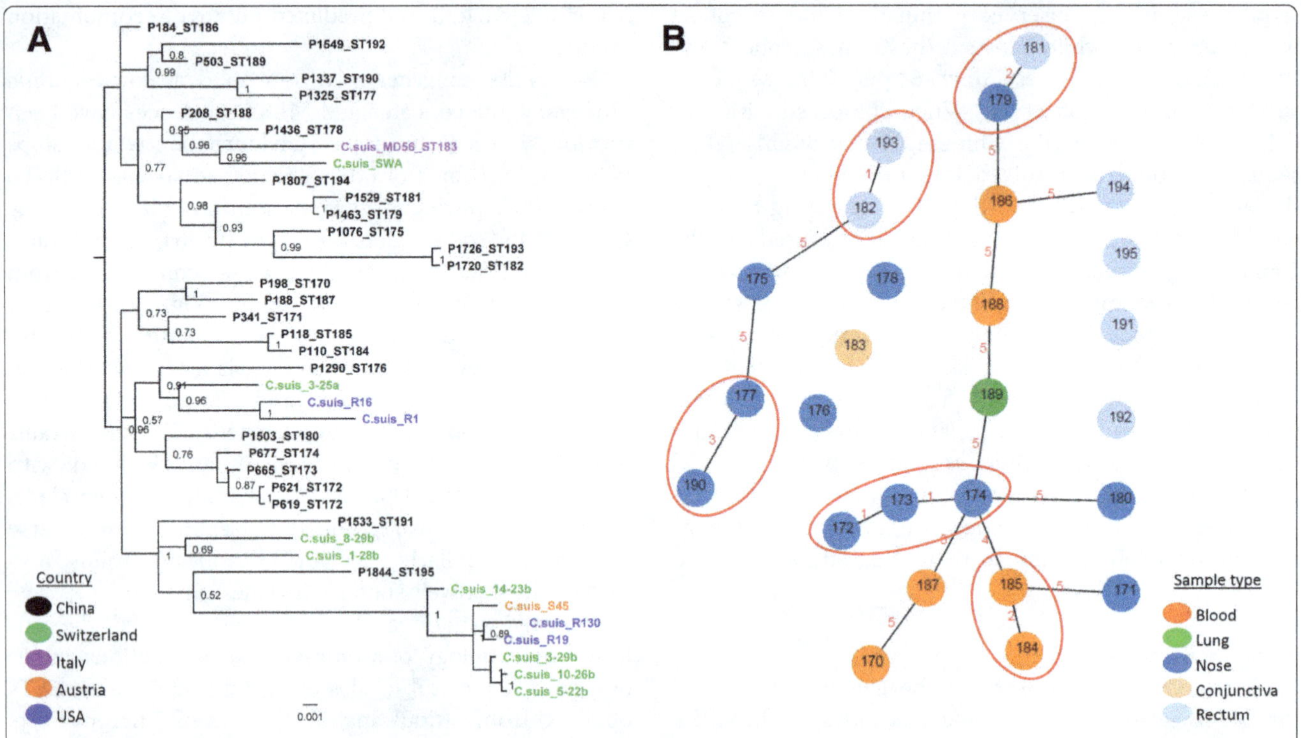

Fig. 4. Phylogenetic and cluster analyses of *C. suis* STs. **a**: Bayesian phylogenetic analysis of the concatenated sequences of seven MLST fragments of 40 *C. suis* strains. Posterior probabilities are displayed on tree nodes, while the geographical origin of the strain is indicated by different colors as outlined in the legend; **b**: Cluster analyses of *C. suis* STs, N locus difference is indicated on the link between the nodes. Clonal complexes are circled in red. Sample types from which the *C. suis* STs were derived are indicated by the colors, as outlined in the legend.

resolved based on a stringent fit differing by a single locus. CC 1 consisted of nasal only isolates denoted STs 172, 173 and 174, with ST 172 as a predicted progenitor, while CC 2 consisted of rectal STs 182 and 193, with ST 182 predicted as a putative progenitor.

Comparison of *C. suis* MLST and *ompA* phylogenies

In order to further compare phylogenetic relationships of *C. suis* strains, we produced a tanglegram of both MLST and *ompA* trees to estimate phylogenetic positioning for each taxa (strain) (Fig. 5). As observed in Fig. 5, only six taxa, including the USA R1 and R16, Chinese P619 and P621; and Swiss 5-22b and 10-26b strains, maintained the same phylogenetic clustering in both trees, whereas all other taxa clustered differently in each tree.

We additionally tested for the recombination break points and changes in topology in the MLST and *ompA* alignments using DualBrothers. Based on observed breakpoints (Additional files 2, 3 and 4), we can infer at least one putative recombination event in the *C. suis* MLST alignment, and at least four in the *ompA* alignment.

Discussion

The present study investigated the prevalence of *C. suis* in five different sample types from 2,137 pigs from 19 regions of 10 provinces in China. The present PCR methodology represents a reliable diagnostic tool for rapid, highly sensitive and specific detection of *C. suis*, bypassing the need for *C. suis* cell culture [29, 31, 43]. We reported an overall prevalence of 62.4% (1,334/2,137) positive animals in the genus-specific FRET-PCR with our results confirming a high prevalence of *C. suis* in all pig herds. We failed to detect any evidence of *C. abortus*, *C. pecorum* and *C. psittaci* DNA. This study provides the first evidence for *C. suis* infection in commercially raised pigs in China. Furthermore, this is also the first report to find that 86.1% (93/108) SPF pigs were *C. suis*-positive.

Our study was the first to show the presence of *C. suis* in blood samples. For paired samples from the same host, nasal, conjunctival and rectal swabs were *C. suis*-positive when the whole blood samples were also *C. suis*-positive. Furthermore, 6/23 lung samples were *C. suis*-positive, suggesting that systemic infection is a common outcome of the haemtogenous spread of the bacteria.

In this study, generally, the infection rate of sows was significantly lower when compared with suckling, weaned and finisher pigs (Fig. 2). These observations might be attributed to antibiotic treatment and good housing conditions for sows or protective immunity in the adult animals. Housing conditions and management systems might contribute to controlling the transmission

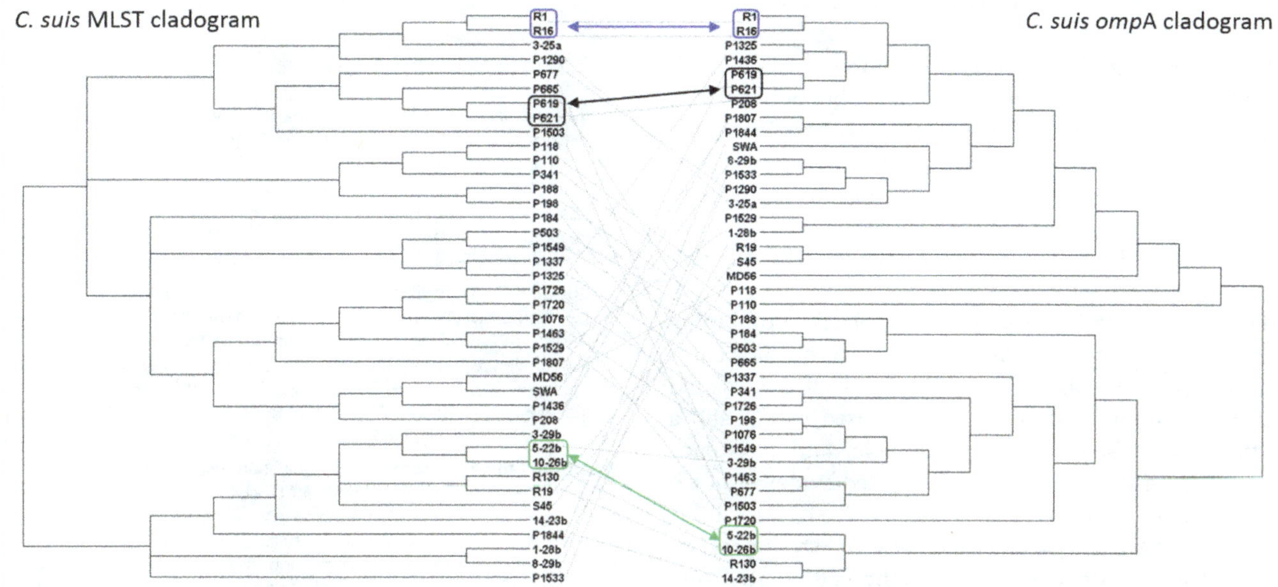

Fig. 5. Tanglegram of *C. suis* MLST and *ompA* Bayesian trees, transformed as a cladograms, from this study. Same positioning of the taxa is indicated by colored squares and arrows, where blue indicates the USA *C. suis* isolates, black Chinese and green Swiss isolates.

of chlamydial infections in pigs [10]. However, these results show that despite these practices, *C. suis* was prevalent in pigs at all stages of their production cycle.

While *C. suis* was found to be the most common species in pigs [44], this organism was mostly often found in the intestine [45–47] and conjunctiva [48, 49], and in other sites, including the genital tract [50], nasal specimens [51], lung [52] and the aborted fetuses [53].

In terms of transmission, in this study, the prevalence of *C. suis* DNA in rectal swabs was significantly higher when compared to those taken from nose and eyes, with whole blood samples having the lowest *C. suis* DNA incidence. This result is most likely due to the gastrointestinal tract being the primary site infection and chlamydial replication. Alternatively, it is also possible that pigs can swallow *C. suis* eliminated from the respiratory tract by mucociliary clearance [51]. Furthermore, the incidence of *C. suis* DNA in rectal, nasal, conjunctival swab samples and whole blood samples was significantly higher for weaned pigs when compared with sows. Data of the present study may suggest the potential *C. suis* transmission via a fecal-oral route. Besides the fecal-oral route as a potential route of transmission, the transmission may presumably also occur via exchange of body fluids, particularly secretions from the conjunctiva and nose, which may also lead to aerosol formation [10]. Hamonic et al. [54] recommended that it is possible that viable *C suis* shed in boar semen could cross current biosecurity barriers, meaning vertical transmission may also need to be considered a route of transmission.

Since 1998, the number of reports of TcR *C. suis* infections in pigs are growing in the USA, Italy, Cyprus, Germany, Israel, Switzerland and Belgium [18–20, 22, 55]. In the present study, the *tet*(C) gene was detected in clinical samples from 3 provinces, which suggests that the presence of the *tet*(C) gene in *C. suis* is common in the Chinese domestic pig population. Selective pressure from tetracycline as drug may be responsible for recent bottlenecks in *C. suis* populations [26]. In this study, we were able to test only clinical samples instead of *C. suis* isolates. However, we cannot exclude that the *tet*(C) gene of other bacteria was detected, and 54.7% *C. suis*-negative rectal swab samples was found to be *tet*(C) positive in this study. For both whole blood and rectal swabs samples in this study, the *tet*(C) positivity of *C. suis*-positive samples were significantly higher than *C. suis*-negative samples, suggesting these *C. suis* strains contained *tet*(C) gene. This may be associated with the inclusion of 10-50 gram oxytetracycline in every 1,000 kilogram pig feed in the farms examined and in the Chinese pig industry. Given the apparently prevalence of this *tet*(C) positivity in *C. suis*, it is concerning to note that, Suchland et al. [23] previously demonstrated the *in vitro* horizontal transfer of tetracycline resistance from *C. suis* to clinical strains of *C. trachomatis*, an important human pathogen. As such, *C. suis* may transfer tetracycline resistance to other chlamydial species, through mixed infections of livestock or farmers. Therefore, for the Chinese pig industry and public health, effective preventive action, such as probiotics or vaccines, should be promoted to counteract it. Targeted surveillance of tetracycline-resistant *C. suis* strains may also be warranted to curb the spread of these unusual chlamydial strains.

Phylogenetic analyses showed that the *ompA* VD1-2 gene fragment of the *C. suis* strains is highly polymorphic (Fig. 3). *C. suis* MLST confirmed these observations, possibly suggesting a shared ancestry of some Chinese strains with those described in the USA and Europe. Combining phylogenetic and cluster analyses findings, and in absence of typing paired samples from a single host, *C. suis* epidemiology nevertheless appears complex.

The genome of *C. suis* is very plastic combining unprecedented diversity with significant levels of recombination predicted between strains as well as plasmid exchange [26, 56]. Although we only used MLST and a partial *ompA* sequence, phylogenetic and sequence analyses from the present study provided evidence of recombination in Chinese *C. suis* strains. We observed differing phylogenetic positioning of the strains when constructing phylogenies using different genes, and identified of putative change points in tree topology and sequence, all indicative of recombination in the Chinese strains as well. In combination with the extreme prevalence in swine herds, the well-known fusion of chlamydial inclusion in closely related *C. trachomatis* [23], but not other chlamydial lineages, may be the pre-requisite for the unprecedented genome-wide recombination frequency of *C. suis*. If so, these mechanisms would continuously create, even within single farms, new strains that explore the full evolutionary bandwidth and enable *C. suis* escape immune protection of the host. Systematic genome sequencing may reveal if *C. suis* strains of different geographic origin that are identical at, e.g., the *ompA* locus, such as Chinese strain P854 and Japanese strain AB270743, are truly identical or are the result of convergent evolution at this locus, but are otherwise divergent across the rest of the *C. suis* chromosome.

Conclusions

The epidemiological surveys in this study indicate that *C. suis* infection in Chinese pigs is common. Molecular typing of detected strains suggest that, like elsewhere, *C. suis* are genetically diverse and that the global diversity of this pathogen is reflected in the diversity of strains detected in Chinese pigs. Further research should be performed to study the route of transmission for *C. suis*, and the potential impacts of *C. suis* on pig production.

Additional files

Additional file 1: Mid-point rooted NJ phylogeny of ompA variable domains 1-2. A 489 bp region encompassing ompA VD1-2 sequences of 77 porcine *C. suis* strains identified in this study (in red font; name of strain, countries, sample type and accession number) are compared with 50 other *C. suis* sequences deposited in GenBank from six countries: Germany, Switzerland, Italy, USA, Japan and China (in black font). Branch lengths are measured in nucleotide substitutions and numbers show branching percentages in bootstrap replicates. Scale bar represents the percent sequence diversity.

Additional file 2: DualBrother recombination detection using the 489bp *ompA* fragment alignment of 26 Chinese *C. suis* strains. The top plot shows marginal posterior probabilities of the four most probable tree topologies, where break and change points of topologies are indicative of recombination. The last two plots show 95% Bayesian confidence interval (shaded in green) of the Kappa transition/transversion ratio, and average divergence Mu.

Additional file 3: DualBrother recombination detection using the 489bp ompA fragment alignment of all 40 C. suis strains used in this study. The top plot shows marginal posterior probabilities of the four most probable tree topologies, where break and change points of topologies are indicative of recombination. The last two plots show 95% Bayesian confidence interval (shaded in green) of the Kappa transition/transversion ratio, and average divergence Mu.

Additional file 4: DualBrother recombination detection using the concatenated 3,080 bp MLST alignment of all 40 *C. suis* strains used in this study. The top plot shows marginal posterior probabilities of the four most probable tree topologies, where break and change points of topologies are indicative of recombination. The last two plots show 95% Bayesian confidence interval (shaded in green) of the Kappa transition/transversion ratio, and average divergence Mu.

Abbreviations

FRET: fluorescence resonance energy transfer; MCMC: Markov Chain Monte Carlo; *ompA*: out major protein A

Acknowledgment

This publication made use of the PubMLST website (http://pubmlst.org/) developed by Keith Jolley (16) and hosted at the University of Oxford. The development of that website was funded by the Wellcome Trust.

Funding

This work was supported by a grant from the National Key R & D Program of China (2016YFD0500804) and a grant from the National Natural Science Foundation of China (NO: 31272575), and by the Priority Academic Program Development of Jiangsu Higher Education Institutions, Yangzhou, Jiangsu, P. R. China.

Authors' contributions

Experimental design by ML and CW. Project funding secured by CW. Sample collection by ML, FY, JG, ZF, CS, PJ, JL, JZ, YW, JW and XZ. Sample processing by ML, FY, JG, ZF, CS, PJ, JL, JZ, YW, JW and XZ. Data analysis by ML, MJ, BK, AP, YP, NB and CW. Manuscript by ML, MJ, BK, AP and CW. All authors have read and approved this manuscript.

Consent for publication

Not applicable.

Competing interests

The authors declare that they have no competing interests.

Author details

[1]Yangzhou University College of Veterinary Medicine, Yangzhou, Jiangsu, People's Republic of China. [2]Centre for Animal Health Innovation, Faculty of Science, Health, Education & Engineering, University of the Sunshine Coast, QLD, Maroochydore, Australia. [3]Poultry Institute, Chinese Academy of Agricultural Sciences, Yangzhou, Jiangsu, China. [4]College of Veterinary Medicine, Auburn University, Auburn, Alabama, USA. [5]Institute of Veterinary Medicine, Jiangsu Academy of Agricultural Sciences; Key Laboratory of

Veterinary Biological Engineering and Technology, Ministry of Agriculture, National Center for Engineering Research of Veterinary Bio-Products, Nanjing, China. [6]Academic Medical Center, University of Amsterdam, Amsterdam, The Netherlands. [7]Institute for Veterinary Pathology, Vetsuisse Faculty, University of Zurich, Zurich, Switzerland. [8]Yunnan Agricultural University College of Animal Science & Technology, Kunming, Yunnan, China. [9]Key Laboratory of Animal Diseases Diagnostic and Immunology, Ministry of Agriculture, College of Veterinary Medicine, Nanjing Agricultural University, Nanjing, China.

References

1. Rohde G, Straube E, Essig A, Reinhold P, Sachse K. Chlamydial zoonoses. Dtsch Arztebl Int. 2010;107(10):174–80.
2. Reinhold P, Hartmann H, Constable PD. Characterisation of acid-base abnormalities in pigs experimentally infected with *Chlamydia suis*. Vet J. 2010;184(2):212–8.
3. De Puysseleyr K, De Puysseleyr L, Geldhof J, Cox E, Vanrompay D. Development and validation of a real-time PCR for *Chlamydia suis* diagnosis in swine and humans. PLoS One. 2014;9(5):e96704.
4. Hulin V, Oger S, Vorimore F, Aaziz R, de Barbeyrac B, Berruchon J, et al. Host preference and zoonotic potential of *Chlamydia psittaci* and *C. suis* in poultry. Pathog Dis. 2015;73(1):1–11.
5. Sachse K, Bavoil PM, Kaltenboeck B, Stephens RS, Kuo CC, Rosselló-Móra R, et al. Emendation of the family *Chlamydiaceae*: proposal of a single genus, *Chlamydia*, to include all currently recognized species. Syst Appl Microbiol. 2015;38(2):99–103.
6. Schautteet K, Vanrompay D. *Chlamydiaceae* infections in pig. Vet Res. 2011;42:29.
7. Vanrompay D, Geens T, Desplanques A, Hoang TQ, De Vos L, Van Loock M, et al. Immunoblotting, ELISA and culture evidence for *Chlamydiaceae* in sows on 258 Belgian farms. Vet Microbiol. 2004;99(1):59–66.
8. Szeredi L, Schiller I, Sydler T, Guscetti F, Heinen E, Corboz L, et al. Intestinal Chlamydia in finishing pigs. Vet Pathol. 1996;33(4):369–74.
9. Hoelzle LE, Steinhausen G, Wittenbrink MM. PCR-based detection of chlamydial infection in swine and subsequent PCR-coupled genotyping of chlamydial omp1-gene amplicons by DNA-hybridization, RFLP-analysis, and nucleotide sequence analysis. Epidemiol Infect. 2000;125(2):427–39.
10. De Puysseleyr L, De Puysseleyr K, Braeckman L, Morré SA, Cox E, Vanrompay D. Assessment of *Chlamydia suis* infection in pig farmers. Transbound Emerg Dis. 2017;64(3):826–33.
11. Chahota R, Ogawa H, Ohya K, Yamaguchi T, Everett KD, Fukushi H. Involvement of multiple *Chlamydia suis* genotypes in porcine conjunctivitis. Transbound Emerg Dis. 2017; https://doi.org/10.1111/tbed.12645.
12. Polkinghorne A, Borel N, Becker A, ZH L, Zimmermann DR, Brugnera E, et al. Molecular evidence for chlamydial infections in the eyes of sheep. Vet Microbiol. 2009;135(1-2):142–6.
13. Pantchev A, Sting R, Bauerfeind R, Tyczka J, Sachse K. Detection of all *Chlamydophila* and *Chlamydia* spp. of veterinary interest using species-specific real-time PCR assays. Comp Immunol Microbiol. 2010;33(6):473–84.
14. Lemus JA, Fargallo JA, Vergara P, Parejo D, Banda E. Natural cross chlamydial infection between livestock and free-living bird species. PLoS One. 2010; 5(10):e13512.
15. Dean D, Rothschild J, Ruettger A, Kandel RP, Sachse K. Zoonotic Chlamydiaceae Species Associated with Trachoma, Nepal. Emerg Infect Dis. 2013;19(12):1948–55.
16. Lenart J, Andersen AA, Rockey DD. Growth and development of tetracycline-resistant *Chlamydia suis*. Antimicrob. Agents Chemother. 2001; 45(8):2198–203.
17. Dugan J, Rockey DD, Jones L, Andersen AA. Tetracycline resistance in *Chlamydia suis* mediated by genomic islands inserted into the chlamydial inv-like gene. Antimicrob Agents Chemother. 2004;48(10):3989–95.
18. Di Francesco A, Donati M, Rossi M, Pignanelli S, Shurdhi A, Baldelli R, et al. Tetracycline-resistant *Chlamydia suis* isolates in Italy. Vet Rec. 2008; 163(8):251–2.
19. Borel N, Regenscheit N, Di Francesco A, Donati M, Markov J, Masserey Y, et al. Selection for tetracycline-resistant *Chlamydia suis* in treated pigs. Vet Microbiol. 2012;156(1-2):143–6.
20. Schautteet K, De Clercq E, Miry C, Van Groenweghe F, Delava P, Kalmar I, et al. Tetracycline-resistant *Chlamydia suis* in cases of reproductive failure on Belgian, Cypriote and Israeli pig production farms. J Med Microbiol. 2013; 62(Pt 2):331–4.
21. Hoffmann K, Schott F, Donati M, Di Francesco A, Hässig M, Wanninger S, et al. Prevalence of chlamydial infections in fattening pigs and their influencing factors. PLoS One. 2015;10(11):e0143576.
22. Wanninger S, Donati M, Di Francesco A, Hässig M, Hoffmann K, Seth-Smith HM, et al. Selective Pressure Promotes Tetracycline Resistance of *Chlamydia suis* in Fattening Pigs. PLoS One. 2016;11(11):e0166917.
23. Suchland RJ, Sandoz KM, Jeffrey BM, Stamm WE, Rockey DD. Horizontal transfer of tetracycline resistance among Chlamydia spp. in vitro. Antimicrob Agents Chemother. 2009;53(11):4604–11.
24. Gomes JP, Bruno WJ, Nunes A, Santos N, Florindo C, Borrego MJ, et al. Evolution of *Chlamydia trachomatis* diversity occurs by widespread interstrain recombination involving hotspots. Genome Res. 2007;17(1):50–60.
25. Brunelle BW, Sensabaugh GF. The *ompA* gene in *Chlamydia trachomatis* differs in phylogeny and rate of evolution from other regions of the genome. Infect Immun. 2006;74(1):578–85.
26. Joseph SJ, Marti H, Didelot X, Read TD, Dean D. Tetracycline Selective Pressure and Homologous Recombination Shape the Evolution of *Chlamydia suis*: A Recently Identified Zoonotic Pathogen. Genome Biol Evol. 2016;8(8):2613–23.
27. Maiden MC. Multilocus sequence typing of bacteria. Annu Rev Microbiol. 2006;60:561–88.
28. Guo W, Li J, Kaltenboeck B, Gong J, Fan W, Wang C. *Chlamydia suis*, not *C. psittaci*, is the endemic chlamydial species in chicken (Gallus gallus). Sci Rep. 2016;6:19638.
29. Li J, Guo W, Kaltenboeck B, Sachse K, Yang Y, Lu G, et al. *Chlamydia pecorum* is the endemic intestinal species in cattle while *C. gallinacea*, *C. psittaci* and *C. pneumoniae* associate with sporadic systemic infection. Vet Microbiol. 2016;193:93–9.
30. Wei L, Kelly P, Zhang J, Yang Y, Zheng X, Tao J, et al. Use of a universal hydroxymethylbilane synthase (HMBS)-based PCR as an endogenous internal control and to enable typing of mammalian DNAs. Appl Microbiol Biotechnol. 2014;98(12):5579–87.
31. De Graves FJ, Gao D, Hehnen HR, Schlapp T, Kaltenboeck B. Quantitative detection of *Chlamydia psittaci* and *C. pecorum* by high-sensitivity real-time PCR reveals high prevalence of vaginal infection in cattle. J Clin Microbiol. 2003;41(4):1726–9.
32. Pannekoek Y, Morelli G, Kusecek B, Morré SA, Ossewaarde JM, Langerak AA, et al. Multi locus sequence typing of Chlamydiales: clonal groupings within the obligate intracellular bacteria *Chlamydia trachomatis*. BMC Microbiol. 2008;8:42.
33. Pannekoek Y, Dickx V, Beeckman DS, Jolley KA, Keijzers WC, Vretou E, et al. Multi Locus Sequence Typing of Chlamydia Reveals an Association between *Chlamydia psittaci* Genotypes and Host Species. PLoS One. 2010;5(12):e14179.
34. Librado P, Rozas J. DnaSP v5: a software for comprehensive analysis of DNA polymorphism data. Bioinformatics. 2009;25(11):1451–2.
35. Kearse M, Moir R, Wilson A, Stones-Havas S, Cheung M, Sturrock S, et al. Geneious Basic: an integrated and extendable desktop software platform for the organization and analysis of sequence data. Bioinformatics. 2012;28(12):1647–9.
36. Jolley KA, Maiden MC. BIGSdb: Scalable analysis of bacterial genome variation at the population level. BMC Bioinformatics. 2010;11:595.
37. Huelsenbeck JP, Ronquist FMRBAYES. Bayesian inference of phylogenetic trees. Bioinformatics. 2001;17(8):754–5.
38. Francisco AP, Bugalho M, Ramirez M, Carriço JA. Global optimal eBURST analysis of multilocus typing data using a graphic matroid approach. BMC Bioinformatics. 2009;10:152.
39. Ribeiro-Gonçalves B, Francisco AP, Vaz C, Ramirez M, Carriço JA. PHYLOViZ Online: web-based tool for visualization, phylogenetic inference, analysis and sharing of minimum spanning trees. Nucleic Acids Res. 2016;44(W1): W246–51.
40. Huson DH, Scornavacca C. Dendroscope 3: an interactive tool for rooted phylogenetic trees and networks. Syst Biol. 2012;61(6):1061–7.
41. Minin VN, Dorman KS, Fang F, Suchard MA. Dual multiple change-point model leads to more accurate recombination detection. Bioinformatics. 2005;21(13):3034–42.
42. Jelocnik M, Walker E, Pannekoek Y, Ellem J, Timms P, Polkinghorne A. Evaluation of the relationship between *Chlamydia pecorum* sequence types

and disease using a species-specific multi-locus sequence typing scheme (MLST). Vet Microbiol. 2014;174(1-2):214–22.

43. Sachse K, Grossmann E, Jäger C, Diller R, Hotzel H. Detection of *Chlamydia suis* from clinical specimens: comparison of PCR, antigen ELISA, and culture. J Microbiol Methods. 2003;54(2):233–8.
44. Longbottom D. Chlamydial infections of domestic ruminants and swine: new nomenclature and new knowledge. Vet J. 2004;168(1):9–11.
45. Zahn I, Szeredi L, Schiller I, Straumann Kunz U, Bürgi E, Guscetti F, et al. Immunohistochemical determination of *Chlamydia psittaci/pecorum* and *C. trachomatis* in the piglet gut. Zentralbl Veterinarmed B. 1995;42(5):266–76.
46. Schiller I, Koesters R, Weilenmann R, Kaltenboeck B, Pospischil A. PCR detection of porcine *Chlamydia trachomatis* and ruminant *Chlamydia psittaci* serovar 1 DNA in formalin-fixed intestinal specimens from swine. Zentralbl Veterinarmed B. 1997;44(3):185–91.
47. Pollmann M, Nordhoff M, Pospischil A, Tedin K, Wieler LH. Effects of a probiotic strain of *Enterococcus faecium* on the rate of natural *Chlamydia* infection in swine. Infect Immun. 2005;73(7):4346–53.
48. Becker A, Lutz-Wohlgroth L, Brugnera E, ZH L, Zimmermann DR, Grimm F, et al. Intensively kept pigs predisposed to chlamydial associated conjunctivitis. J Vet Med A Physiol Pathol Clin Med. 2007;54(6):307–13.
49. Davidson HJ, Rogers DP, Yeary TJ, Stone GG, Schoneweis DA, Chengappa MM. Conjunctival microbial flora of clinically normal pigs. Am J Vet Res. 1994;55(7):949–51.
50. Kauffold J, Melzer F, Berndt A, Hoffmann G, Hotzel H, Sachse K. Chlamydiae in oviducts and uteri of repeat breeder pigs. Theriogenology. 2006;66(8): 1816–23.
51. Reinhold P, Liebler-Tenorio E, Sattler S, Sachse K. Recurrence of *Chlamydia suis* infection in pigs after short-term antimicrobial treatment. Vet J. 2011; 187(3):405–7.
52. Sachse K, Hotzel H, Slickers P, Ellinger T, Ehricht RDNA. microarray-based detection and identification of *Chlamydia* and *Chlamydophila* spp. Mol Cell Probes. 2005;19(1):41–50.
53. Schiller I, Koesters R, Weilenmann R, Thoma R, Kaltenboeck B, Heitz P, et al. Mixed infections with porcine *Chlamydia trachomatis/pecorum* and infections with ruminant Chlamydia psittaci serovar 1 associated with abortion in swine. Vet Microbiol. 1997b;58(2-4):251–60.
54. Hamonic G, Pasternak JA, Käser T, Meurens F, Wilson HL. Extended semen for artificial insemination in swine as a potential transmission mechanism for infectious *Chlamydia suis*. Theriogenology. 2016;86(4):949–56.
55. Andersen A, Rogers D. Resistance to tetracycline and sulfadiazine in swine C. trachomatis isolates. Editors: Stephens, R. S. *In*: Ninth International Symposium on Human Chlamydial Infection. San Fransico: Conference Proceedings. 1998; pp. 313-316
56. Seth-Smith HM, Wanninger S, Bachmann N, Marti H, Qi W, Donati M, et al. The *Chlamydia suis* genome exhibits high levels of diversity, plasticity and mobile antibiotic resistance: comparative genomics of a recent livestock cohort shows influence of treatment regimes. Genome Biol Evol. 2017;9(3): 750–60.

18

Otitis in a cat associated with *Corynebacterium provencense*

Sonja Kittl[1], Isabelle Brodard[1], Lorenz Rychener[1], Jörg Jores[1], Petra Roosje[2,3] and Stefanie Gobeli Brawand[1*]

Abstract

Background: The role of corynebacteria in canine and feline otitis has not been investigated in detail; however, members of this genus are increasingly recognized as pathogens of otitis in both human and veterinary medicine.

Case presentation: Here we report the first case of feline otitis associated with the recently described species *Corynebacterium provencense*. A seven-month old cat presented with a head tilt and ataxia was diagnosed with peripheral vestibular syndrome associated with an otitis media/interna. This took place 6 weeks after resection of a polyp, having initially shown a full recovery with topical ofloxacin and glucocorticoid treatment. Bacteriology of an ear swab yielded a pure culture of corynebacteria, which could not be identified at the species level using routine methods. However, the 16S rRNA gene sequence was 100% identical to the recently published novel corynebacterium species, *Corynebacterium provencense*. Whole genome sequencing of the cat isolate and calculation of average nucleotide identity (99.1%) confirmed this finding. The cat isolate was found to contain additional presumptive iron acquisition genes that are likely to encode virulence factors. Furthermore, the strain tested resistant to clindamycin, penicillin and ciprofloxacin. The cat was subsequently treated with chloramphenicol, which lead to clinical improvement.

Conclusion: Corynebacteria from otitis cases are not routinely identified at the species level and not tested for antimicrobial susceptibility in veterinary laboratories, as they are not considered major pathogens. This may lead to underreporting of this genus or animals being treated with inappropriate antimicrobials since corynebacteria are often resistant to multiple drugs.

Keywords: Feline otitis, *Corynebacterium*, Neglected pathogen

Background

The genus *Corynebacterium* consists of 128 species [1], with a large number pathogenic to humans and animals [2]. The main animal pathogens include *C. pseudotuberculosis*, *C. kutscheri*, the *C. renale* group, *C. bovis* and *C. ulcerans* while *C. diphtheriae* is considered the main human pathogen [3]. Many other *Corynebacterium* spp. have been isolated from opportunistic infection sites in humans and animals, sometimes also with a zoonotic origin [2]. Besides the diphtheria toxin, which is the major virulence factor in *C. diphtheriae* (also found in other species like *C. ulcerans*) [4], and phospholipase D, a virulence factor of *C. pseudotuberculosis* and *C. ulcerans* [5], relatively little is known about virulence traits in the genus *Corynebacterium*.

Recently human and veterinary diagnostic laboratories have begun to investigate the role of *Corynebacterium* spp. as causative agents for otitis with a study [6] finding *Corynebacterium* spp. to be present in 33% of human patients with otologic infections. These cases were often resistant to fluoroquinolones, an antibiotic frequently used as a first-line in treatment [6]. In dogs, *Corynebacterium* spp. are also increasingly recognized as otitis-associated pathogens, however, in most cases they are isolated together with other pathogens [7, 8]. There are even fewer publications describing corynebacteria-associated otitis in cats than in dogs. Henneveld et al. described four cats with otitis externa/media from which corynebacteria were

* Correspondence: stefanie.gobeli@vetsuisse.unibe.ch
[1]Institute of Veterinary Bacteriology, Vetsuisse Faculty, University of Bern, Laenggassstrasse 122, CH-3001 Bern, Switzerland
Full list of author information is available at the end of the article

isolated, albeit in association with other bacterial species [7]. Two of these cats also suffered from an aural polyp.

In addition to scant information linking corynebacteria and otitis, knowledge is also limited concerning the microbiome of the healthy feline ear canal. Kose et al. investigated the flora of the normal tympanic bulla in cats but did not detect any corynebacteria, although the sample size was very small (five animals) [9].

Thus, further research is needed to elucidate the role of pathogenic bacteria in feline otitis. In this study, we present a case of feline otitis media and interna from which the recently described species *Corynebacterium provencense* was isolated in pure culture.

Case presentation

A 7-month-old male, neutered Maine Coon cat was presented to the Small Animal Teaching Hospital at the University of Bern with acute neurological signs consistent with unilateral otitis media/interna. Six weeks earlier an inflammatory aural polyp had been removed by traction and flushing of the ear canal. The cat had fully recovered after three weeks of treatment with oral and topical glucocorticoids and topical ofloxacin (Floxal, Bausch & Lomb Swiss AG). Otoscopic and cytologic examinations revealed brown-colored fluid in the external canal with numerous extra- and intracellular rod-shaped bacteria and neutrophils. A deep ear swab was submitted for culture and subsequent antimicrobial susceptibility testing.

The ear swab was cultured on sheep blood agar at 37 °C for 2 days, yielding a pure culture of small white colonies (strain number 17KM38). Gram staining showed Gram-positive, polymorphic rods and the bacteria were catalase positive. Thus, the bacteria were classified as belonging to the genus *Corynebacterium*, however species identification was not possible with either Maldi-Tof MS (MALDI Biotyper, Bruker using the in-house database and MBT 6903 MSP Library, Bruker) or VITEK® 2 Compact (Biomérieux) (cards GP and CBC). Therefore, the 16S rRNA gene was amplified and Sanger sequenced using universal primers [10]. Sequence analysis and sequence comparison using the BLAST program (NCBI, 'rRNA_typestrains/prokaryotic_16S_ribosomal_RNA' database) revealed 98.6% identity to *Corynebacterium variabile* (NR_025314.1), 98.0% to *Corynebacterium terpenotabidum* (NR_121699.1) and 97.8% to *Corynebacterium glyciniphilum* (NR_121782.1), thus the strain 17KM38 could not be assigned to any species present in the database. However, the 16S rRNA sequence showed a 100% identity with the whole genome shotgun sequence of the recently described *Corynebacterium provencense* SN15 (GenBank accession no.: NZ_LT160593.1) isolated from faeces of an obesity patient [11].

In order to select the appropriate antimicrobial therapy, the isolate was tested for antimicrobial resistance using broth microdilution (Sensititre EUST, Thermo Fisher Scientific) initially following in-house guidelines. Minimum inhibitory concentration (MIC) testing was however repeated according to the most recent EUCAST (European Committee on Antimicrobial Susceptibility Testing) guidelines [12] using *Streptococcus pneumoniae* ATCC 49619 as a quality control. Briefly, the bacteria were grown on sheep blood agar at 37 °C for 24 h. They were then suspended in Mueller-Hinton broth with 5% lysed horse blood (Thermo Fisher Scientific) and 20 mg/l β-NAD to a concentration of 5×10^5 CFU/ml and used for plate inoculation. Our strain tested resistant to clindamycin, penicillin and ciprofloxacin but susceptible to tetracycline, gentamicin and vancomycin. In addition, high MIC values were found for cefoxitin (8 mg/l), mupirocin (≥256 mg/l) and trimethoprim (≥32 mg/l) while the MIC for chloramphenicol was low (≤4 mg/l) (Table 1).

To better characterize the strain, whole genome sequencing was performed using the PacBio method. The strain was grown on sheep blood agar at 37 °C for 24 h and the harvested cells were used to extract gDNA according to a protocol published earlier [13]. Sequencing was performed by the Lausanne Genomic Technologies Facility (University

Table 1 Minimal inhibitory concentrations for 17KM38, interpretation according to EUCAST clinical breakpoints where available

Antimicrobial	MIC (mg/l)	Interpretation
Clindamycin	2	R
Tetracycline	1	S
Rifampin	0.25	I
Streptomycin	≤4	–
Fusidate	1	–
Penicillin	1	R
Chloramphanicol	≤4	–
Kanamycin	≤4	–
Tiamulin	≥4	–
Quinupristin/dalfopristin	1	–
Vancomycin	≤1	S
Gentamicin	≤1	S
Trimethoprim	≥32	–
Erythromycin	≤0.25	–
Ciprofloxacin	≥8	R
Cefoxitin	8	–
Linezolid	≤1	–
Mupirocin	≥256	–
Sulfamethoxazole	≤64	–

of Lausanne, Switzerland). The genome was assembled from PacBio reads using Canu 1.4 [14]. A single contig was built after assembly of the obtained reads, and circularized using amos 3.1.0 [15]. Subsequently the genome was annotated using Prokka 1.12 [16] and submitted to GenBank (Accession No. CP024988). The genome of 17KM38 has a size of 3.11 Mb and 2682 coding sequences were detected. Of these, 862 out of 2682 were annotated as hypothetical proteins. In order to confirm that 17KM38 belongs to the same species as SN15 and is indeed distinct from its closest relatives, average nucleotide identity (ANI) was calculated according to Goris et al. [17] using an online tool (ANI calculator) developed by Rodriguez-R and Konstantinidis [18] with default settings. The ANI of 17KM38 was found to be 81.5% with *C. variabile* (NC_015859.1), 81.0% with *C. terpenotabidum* (NC_021663.1), 79.1% with *C. glyciniphilum* (CP006842.1) and 99.1% with SN15 (FIZC01). Since the recommended cutoff point for species delineation is 95% ANI [17], these results confirm that SN15 [11] and 17KM38 indeed belong to the same species which is distinct from related species. Furthermore, a phylogenetic tree was constructed from the theoretical proteome according to Qi et al. [19] applying the online tool CVTree [20] (Fig. 1).

The genome of 17KM38 was compared to the genome of the strain SN15 using mauve [21]. Gap regions were extracted and annotated resulting in 280 coding sequences (CDS), 113 of which could be assigned a putative function (Additional file 1). Interestingly, 12 CDS unique to 17KM38 are related to iron acquisition (Fig. 2), which is important for bacterial survival in the host and thus for virulence [22]. Most interesting is an approximately 17kbp region containing nine genes for siderophore synthesis and transport organized in two presumptive operons (Fig. 3) [23]. Genes *dhbBCEF* are related to the corresponding genes in *Bacillus subtilis* (between 36 and 52% identity in blastx) where they form the biosynthetic pathway for the catecholic siderophore bacillibactin [24]. The whole gene cluster has similarity to the enterobactin gene cluster in *E. coli* which also includes *fep* genes and the *fes* gene [25]. A gene corresponding to *dhbA*/*entA* is missing from this cluster in 17KM38, but is located elsewhere on the genome (1,026,704 - > 1,027,528). *C. variabile*, the closest relative to *C. provencense*, also possesses a repertoire of iron acquisition genes, since its habitat is the iron-restricted environment found in cheese [26]. Interestingly the genome of *C. variabile* also encodes a pathway similar to that for bacillibactin. However, the *dhbBCEF* genes in 17KM38 are no closer related to those in *C. variabile* than those in *B. subtilis*.

In terms of virulence factors 17KM38 encodes a candidate adhesin (Csp1_16740) related to (82% query cover, 51% identity in blastx) a cell wall-associated hydrolase of *C. resistens* (encoded by *cwlH*) [27]. The exact function

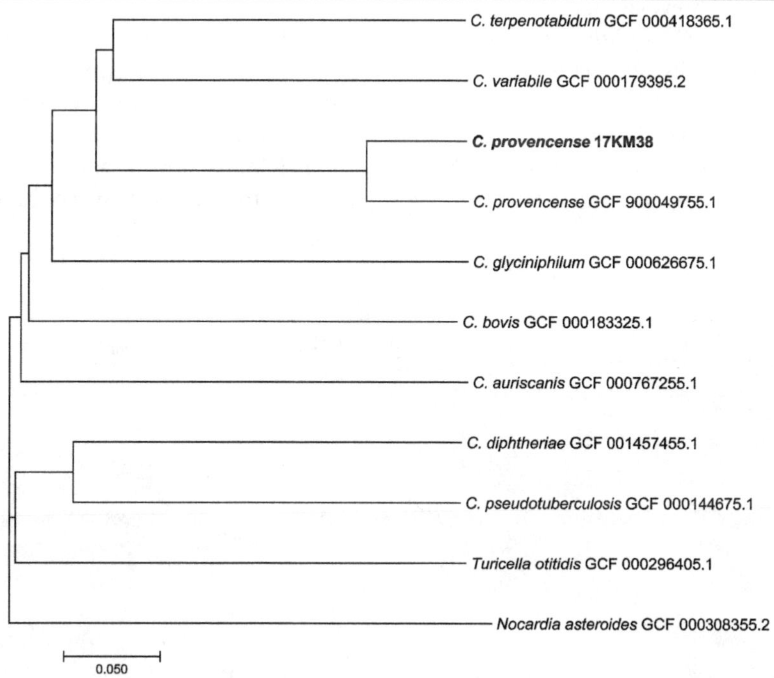

Fig. 1 Phylogenetic tree based on the proteome, showing 17KM38 in relation to other corynebacteria. The tree was constructed using CVTree with K = 6. *Nocardia asteroides* was used as outgroup. The scale bar indicates normalized distance between composition vectors

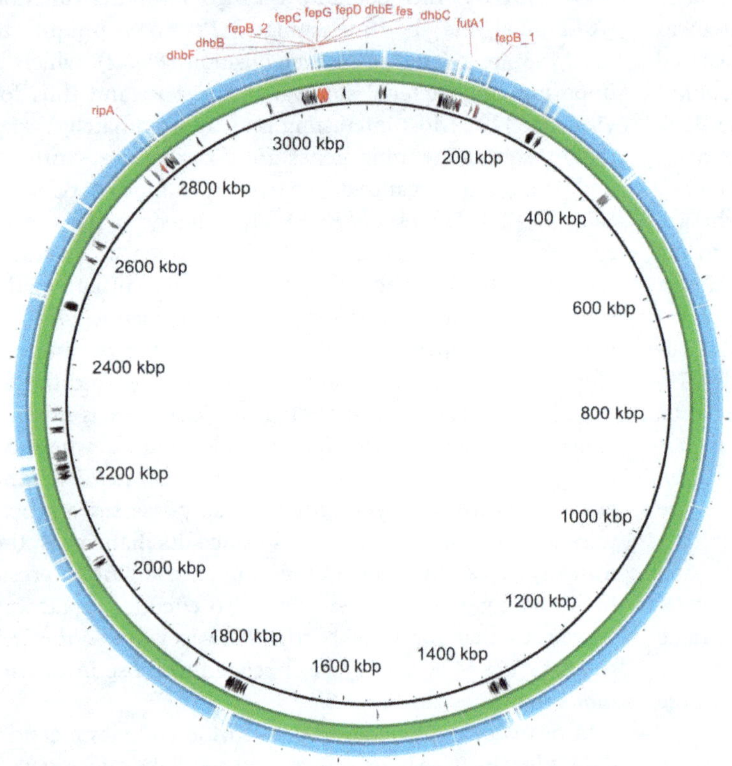

name	product
futA1	Iron uptake protein A1
fepB_1	Ferrienterobactin-binding periplasmic protein
ripA	HTH-type transcriptional regulator RipA
dhbF	Dimodular nonribosomal peptide synthase
dhbB	Isochorismatase
fepB_2	Ferrienterobactin-binding periplasmic protein
fepC	Ferric enterobactin transport ATP-binding protein FepC
fepG	Ferric enterobactin transport system permease protein FepG
fepD	Ferric enterobactin transport system permease protein FepD
dhbE	2,3-dihydroxybenzoate-AMP ligase
fes	Enterochelin esterase
dhbC	Isochorismate synthase DhbC

Fig. 2 Comparison of 17KM38 (green) with SN15 *Corynebacterium provencense* (blue). CDS in gap regions are shown. Hypothetical proteins are shown in grey, proteins presumptively related to iron acquisition are shown in red. The image was constructed with BRIG (BLAST Ring Image Generator v0.95)

of this protein is unknown, however knockout of the homologous gene DIP1621 in *C. diphtheriae* led to reduced adherence to epithelial cells [28]. This gene is also present in strain SN15.

As mentioned above, 17KM38 showed resistance to several antibiotics. Quinolone resistance in corynebacteria has been described to rely on mutations in the quinolone resistance determining region (QRDR) of *gyrA* leading to changes in the SAIYD (aa 87–91 in *C. glutamicum*) motif of susceptible strains [29]. Mutations of Ser-87 to Arg in *C. amycolatum* and to Val in *C. striatum* have been shown to confer quinolone resistance [29]. 17KM38 showed a mutation in this region changing Ser to Ala, which could explain the quinolone

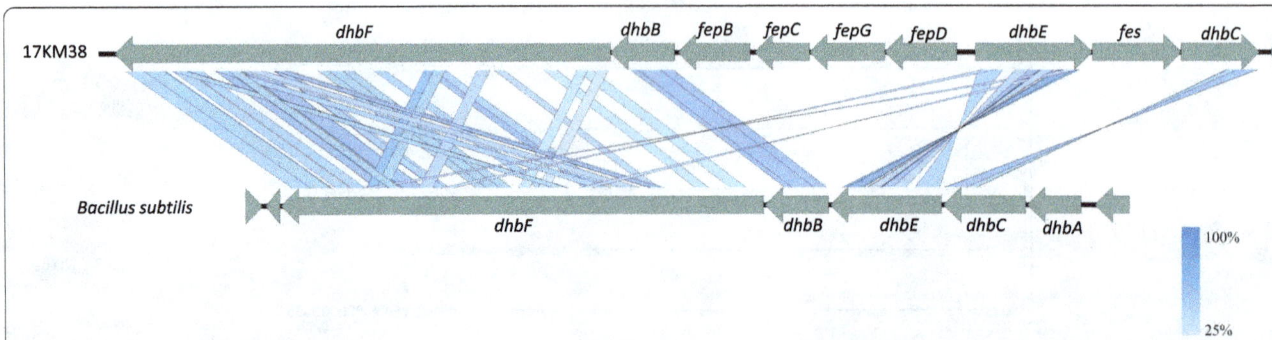

Fig. 3 Comparison of the presumptive siderophore synthesis genomic region in 17KM38 and the *dhb* genes containing region in Bacillus subtilis (NC_000964 region: 3280000–3,293,000). The graph was generated using Easyfig 2.2.2 [23]. Comparisons were performed using tblastx, min. Length 50, max. e value 0.001

resistance. A mechanism for resistance to ß-lactams in corynebacteria has been demonstrated for *C. jeikeium* where acquisition of the gene *pbp2C* encoding the low-affinity class B penicillin binding protein 2C was shown to confer resistance [30]. 17KM38 has four genes encoding penicillin binding proteins one of which is related to *pbp2C* (Csp1_14570, 96% query cover, 44% identity), however, if this gene is actually related to penicillin resistance remains to be shown.

Following sensitivity testing results, the cat was treated with oral chloramphenicol *palmitate solution (Cloropal,* Dr. E. Gräub AG) 20 mg/kg twice daily for three weeks and an ear cleaner containing chlorhexidine digluconate (Otodine®, Ufamed AG) twice daily for two weeks. Re-examination after three weeks of therapy revealed that the head tilt was much improved and the cat was no longer ataxic and cytology of the ear canal did not show any bacteria or neutrophils.

Discussion and conclusion

Ear infections with corynebacteria in dogs and cats are rather rare; however, they are of concern to clinicians as they can be difficult to treat due to antibiotic resistance. This has also been described in human medicine where fluoroquinolones are normally used as a first-line therapy for otitis media [6]. A retrospective study by Crowson et al. found 58% of *Corynebacterium sp.* isolates from otitis patients were resistant to ciprofloxacin, compared to only 32% of non-*Corynebacterium* isolates [6]. In dogs and cats, quinolones are also frequently used to treat otitis. Aalbaek et al. found US *Corynebacterium* isolates from canine otitis to show a high percentage of enrofloxacin resistance when compared to Danish isolates [8]. In the case described here, the animal had also initially received topical quinolone therapy from the referring veterinarian before removal of the ear polyp. As cultures were not performed prior to this treatment, the nature of the initial infectious agent is unknown. Possibly a different bacterium caused the first infection, and the *Corynebacterium provencense* was able to proliferate under therapy. Alternatively, as quinolone resistance is presumably caused by a point mutation, the bacteria may have developed resistance under therapy as has been described for other species [31].

As mentioned before, not much is known about virulence factors of corynebacteria, however, iron acquisition systems are known to contribute to virulence in many pathogens [22]. Interestingly, the strain in this study contained a genomic region coding for a siderophore synthesis pathway that was not present in the human *C. provencense* strain and therefore might contribute to its virulence. As corynebacteria from ear infections are not routinely identified to species level in many laboratories, cases with this species may have been previously underreported. It is therefore desirable to pay more attention to corynebacterial ear infections in dogs and cats with importance placed on resistance testing as is increasingly done in human medicine. Consequently, this will improve the treatment success rate for otitis in veterinary medicine.

Abbreviations

ANI: Average Nucleotide Identity; CDS: Coding Sequence; EUCAST: European Committee on Antimicrobial Susceptibility Testing; MIC: Minimum Inhibitory Concentration

Acknowledgements

We thank Valentine Jaquier for performing phenotypic analyses of the isolate. Calculations were performed on UBELIX (http://www.id.unibe.ch/hpc), the HPC cluster at the University of Bern. Additional financial support was received from the University of Bern and the Swiss Federal Food Safety and Veterinary Office.

Authors' contributions

SK performed wet lab and bioinformatics analyses and wrote the manuscript, IB performed wet lab analyses, LR contributed to bioinformatics analysis, PR provided clinical data and contributed to the manuscript, JJ and SG helped writing the manuscript. All authors read and approved the final manuscript.

Consent for publication

Not applicable.

Competing interests

The authors declare that they have no competing interests.

Author details

[1]Institute of Veterinary Bacteriology, Vetsuisse Faculty, University of Bern, Laenggassstrasse 122, CH-3001 Bern, Switzerland. [2]Division of Clinical Dermatology, Department of Clinical Veterinary Medicine, Vetsuisse Faculty, University of Bern, Bremgartenstrasse 109a, CH-3001 Bern, Switzerland. [3]DermFocus, Vetsuisse Faculty, University of Bern, Bern, Switzerland.

References

1. LPSN List of prokaryotic names with standing in nomenclature http://www.bacterio.net/corynebacterium.html Accessed 19 June 2017.
2. Bernard K. The genus corynebacterium and other medically relevant coryneform-like bacteria. J Clin Microbiol. 2012;50(10):3152–8.
3. Markey BK. Clinical veterinary microbiology. 2nd ed. Edinburgh: Elsevier; 2013.
4. Meinel DM, Margos G, Konrad R, Krebs S, Blum H, Sing A. Next generation sequencing analysis of nine Corynebacterium ulcerans isolates reveals zoonotic transmission and a novel putative diphtheria toxin-encoding pathogenicity island. Genome Med. 2014;6(11):113.
5. Tauch A, Burkovski A. Molecular armory or niche factors: virulence determinants of Corynebacterium species. FEMS Microbiol Lett. 2015; 362(23):fnv185.
6. Crowson MG, Callahan K, Saunders JE. Review of otorrhea microbiology: is there a pathogenic role of corynebacter? Otol Neurotol. 2015;36(2):244–9.
7. Henneveld K, Rosychuk RA, Olea-Popelka FJ, Hyatt DR, Zabel S. Corynebacterium spp. in dogs and cats with otitis externa and/or media: a retrospective study. J Am Anim Hosp Assoc. 2012;48(5):320–6.
8. Aalbaek B, Bemis DA, Schjaerff M, Kania SA, Frank LA, Guardabassi L. Coryneform bacteria associated with canine otitis externa. Vet Microbiol. 2010;145(3–4):292–8.
9. Klose TC, MacPhail CM, Schultheiss PC, Rosychuk RA, Hawley JR, Lappin MR. Prevalence of select infectious agents in inflammatory aural and nasopharyngeal polyps from client-owned cats. J Feline Med Surg. 2010; 12(10):769–74.

10. Kuhnert P, Frey J, Lang NP, Mayfield L. Phylogenetic analysis of Prevotella nigrescens, Prevotella intermedia and Porphyromonas gingivalis clinical strains reveals a clear species clustering. Int J Syst Evol Microbiol. 2002;52(Pt 4):1391–5.
11. Ndongo S, Andrieu C, Fournier PE, Lagier JC, Raoult D. Actinomyces provencensis' sp. nov., 'Corynebacterium bouchesdurhonense' sp. nov., 'Corynebacterium provencense' sp. nov. and 'Xanthomonas massiliensis' sp. nov., 4 new species isolated from fresh stools of obese French patients. New Microbes New Infect. 2017;18:24–7.
12. Breakpoint tables for interpretation of MICs and zone diameters. Version 8.1, 2018. http://www.eucast.org
13. Pitcher DG, Saunders NA, Owen RJ. Rapid extraction of bacterial genomic DNA with guanidium thiocyanate. LettApplMicrobiol. 1989;8:151–6.
14. Koren S, Walenz BP, Berlin K, Miller JR, Bergman NH, Phillippy AM. Canu: scalable and accurate long-read assembly via adaptive k-mer weighting and repeat separation. Genome Res. 2017;27(5):722–36.
15. AMOS http://amos.sourceforge.net/wiki/index.php/AMOS Accessed 03 July 2017.
16. Seemann T. Prokka: rapid prokaryotic genome annotation. Bioinformatics. 2014;30(14):2068–9.
17. Goris J, Konstantinidis KT, Klappenbach JA, Coenye T, Vandamme P, Tiedje JM. DNA-DNA hybridization values and their relationship to whole-genome sequence similarities. Int J Syst Evol Microbiol. 2007;57(Pt 1):81–91.
18. Online tools Environmental Microbial Genomics Laboratory http://enve-omics.ce.gatech.edu/ Accessed 07 June 2017.
19. Qi J, Wang B, Hao BI. Whole proteome prokaryote phylogeny without sequence alignment: a K-string composition approach. *J Mol Evol*. 2004; 58(1):1–11.
20. Composition Vector Tree Version 2 http://tlife.fudan.edu.cn/cvtree Accessed 17 July 2017.
21. Darling AC, Mau B, Blattner FR, Perna NT. Mauve: multiple alignment of conserved genomic sequence with rearrangements. Genome Res. 2004; 14(7):1394–403.
22. Chu BC, Garcia-Herrero A, Johanson TH, Krewulak KD, Lau CK, Peacock RS, Slavinskaya Z, Vogel HJ. Siderophore uptake in bacteria and the battle for iron with the host; a bird's eye view. Biometals. 2010;23(4):601–11.
23. Sullivan MJ, Petty NK, Beatson SA. Easyfig: a genome comparison visualizer. Bioinformatics. 2011;27(7):1009–10.
24. May JJ, Wendrich TM, Marahiel MA. The dhb operon of Bacillus subtilis encodes the biosynthetic template for the catecholic siderophore 2,3-dihydroxybenzoate-glycine-threonine trimeric ester bacillibactin. J Biol Chem. 2001;276(10):7209–17.
25. Crosa JH, Walsh CT. Genetics and assembly line enzymology of siderophore biosynthesis in bacteria. Microbiol Mol Biol Rev. 2002;66(2):223–49.
26. Schroder J, Maus I, Trost E, Tauch A. Complete genome sequence of Corynebacterium variabile DSM 44702 isolated from the surface of smear-ripened cheeses and insights into cheese ripening and flavor generation. BMC Genomics. 2011;12:545.
27. Schroder J, Maus I, Meyer K, Wordemann S, Blom J, Jaenicke S, Schneider J, Trost E, Tauch A. Complete genome sequence, lifestyle, and multi-drug resistance of the human pathogen Corynebacterium resistens DSM 45100 isolated from blood samples of a leukemia patient. BMC Genomics. 2012;13:141.
28. Kolodkina V, Denisevich T, Titov L. Identification of Corynebacterium diphtheriae gene involved in adherence to epithelial cells. Infect Genet Evol. 2011;11(2):518–21.
29. Sierra JM, Martinez-Martinez L, Vazquez F, Giralt E, Vila J. Relationship between mutations in the gyrA gene and quinolone resistance in clinical isolates of Corynebacterium striatum and Corynebacterium amycolatum. Antimicrob Agents Chemother. 2005;49(5):1714–9.
30. Lavollay M, Arthur M, Fourgeaud M, Dubost L, Marie A, Riegel P, Gutmann L, Mainardi JL. The beta-lactam-sensitive D,D-carboxypeptidase activity of Pbp4 controls the L, D and D, D transpeptidation pathways in Corynebacterium jeikeium. Mol Microbiol. 2009;74(3):650–61.
31. Luo N, Sahin O, Lin J, Michel LO, Zhang Q. In vivo selection of campylobacter isolates with high levels of fluoroquinolone resistance associated with gyrA mutations and the function of the CmeABC efflux pump. Antimicrob Agents Chemother. 2003;47(1):390–4.

Antibiotic resistance pattern and virulence genes content in avian pathogenic *Escherichia coli* (APEC) from broiler chickens in Chitwan, Nepal

Manita Subedi[1], Himal Luitel[2], Bhuminanda Devkota[2], Rebanta Kumar Bhattarai[3], Sarita Phuyal[4], Prabhat Panthi[5], Anil Shrestha[6] and Dhiraj Kumar Chaudhary[7*]

Abstract

Background: Avian pathogenic *Escherichia coli* (APEC) are causative agent of extraintestinal infections, collectively known as colibacillosis, which results significant losses in poultry industries. The extraintestinal survival of *E. coli* is facilitated by numerous virulence factors which are coded by virulence genes. This study was conducted to find out the pattern of antibiotic resistance and virulence genes content in the APEC strains isolated from broiler chickens at National Avian Disease Investigation Laboratory and Veterinary Teaching Hospital, Rampur, Chitwan, Nepal.

Results: A total of 50 *E. coli* strains were isolated from 50 colibacillosis suspected broiler chickens. Out of 50 isolates of *E. coli*, 47 (94%) showed resistant to three or more antimicrobials. The highest levels (22%) of multidrug-resistant *E. coli* were observed for five different types of antimicrobials. Antibiogram profiles of 50 *E. coli* strains showed the maximum resistance to ampicillin (98%), followed by co-trimoxazole (90%), and doxycycline (62%). The highest intermediate resistance was shown by colistin (50%) and the highest sensitivity was against amikacin (84%), followed by nitrofurantoin (55%). Based on the genetic criteria, 45 (90%) *E. coli* isolates were considered as pathogenic (APEC) which contained more than five virulence genes. Out of total APEC genes detected, we found the combination of *iss, iucD, hlyF, ompT, iroN,* and *iutA* genes were mostly associated with the APEC and additionally, to some lesser extent *irp2, papC, Cva/cvi,* and *tsh* genes showed the critical role for virulent traits of APEC strains.

Conclusion: In this study, high prevalent of antimicrobial resistant pattern was found with avian pathogenic *E. coli* strains isolated from broiler chickens. To our knowledge, this is the first molecular analysis which confirmed the prevalence of APEC strains in poultry sector in Nepal. These finding suggest the need of surveillance and intervention system to control misuse of antibiotics and APEC outbreak in the poultry farm.

Keywords: Avian pathogenic *Escherichia coli* (APEC), Antimicrobial resistance, Virulence gene, Broiler chicken, PCR

Background

Escherichia coli are considered as normal inhabitant of gastrointestinal tract of man and animals. It is also a part of normal intestinal microflora in bird [1]. But, certain pathogenic strains of *E. coli* invade different organs of bird and causes pericarditis, air sacculitis, perihepatitis, peritonitis, and other extraintestinal diseases, collectively termed as colibacillosis [1, 2]. Colibacillosis may be localized or systemic and caused by avian pathogenic *Escherichia coli* (APEC) [3]. The pathogenic ability of *E. coli* strain is facilitated by broad range of virulence factors which are coded by virulence-associated genes (*iutA, iss, papC, iucD, tsh, irp-2, ompT, hlyF, iron, cva/cvi,* and *astA*). According to the genetic criteria, the pathogenicity of APEC strain is determined by presence of at least five virulence genes [1]. Some human and avian extraintestinal pathogenic *E.coli* (ExPEC) has similar phylogenic backgrounds and shares similar virulence

* Correspondence: dhirajchaudhary2042@gmail.com
[7]Department of Microbiology, Prithu Technical College, Institute of Agriculture and Animal Science, Tribhuvan University, Lamahi, Dang, Nepal
Full list of author information is available at the end of the article

genes possessing zoonotic risk [4]. The sequencing of the genome of the APEC strain O1:K1:H7 revealed a high similarity to the genome of human uropathogenic *E. coli* (UPEC) and neonatal meningitis *E. coli* (NMEC) [5].

Antibiotics are commonly used in the poultry farm to circumvent the challenges arise due to APEC strains. In many countries including Nepal, there is excessive use of antibiotics in poultry industries. Studies have reported that antibiotics have been used in chicken broilers as growth promoter and disease preventive measures [6, 7]. However, utilization of antimicrobials in food producing animals have created several adverse effects, such as changes in intestinal micro flora, presence of residual antibiotics in food products, impact on public environment, and emergence of antimicrobial resistance in microorganisms [8, 9]. Multiple antibiotic resistant microbes have challenged in the treatment of zoonotic diseases and its transmission from animal to human have led to the threatening situation in health sectors [10].

Poultry industries are emerging rapidly in the developing countries like Nepal. Chitwan, Kathmandu, and Kaski districts are the major areas of poultry farms in Nepal [6]. Chitwan district solely produces 68% and 10% of total eggs and chicken meats, respectively in the country [11]. But, outbreaks of different types of diseases in the poultry farms cause significant economic losses. Among the diseases reported, the outbreak of colibacillosis is one of the major problems of poultry industries [12]. Colibacillosis among broiler chicken is endemic in Nepal. Studies have reported that the prevalence of colibacillosis ranges from 10 to 60% in Chitwan district. The frequent incidence of avian diseases has been increased tremendously [11, 13]. In the context of Nepal, only few literatures are available regarding assessment and investigation of APEC disease. In addition, the trend of pathological investigations of colibacillosis in Nepal is based on clinical symptoms and isolation of *E. coli* from fecal samples [11]. These conventional approaches of investigations always pose the risk of reporting non-pathogenic *E. coli*. Furthermore, studies on virulence genes and molecular detection of APEC strains from broiler chicken of Nepal have not been reported yet. Therefore, this study was conducted to find the pattern of antibiotic resistance and virulence genes content among APEC strains isolated from broiler chickens.

Methods

Sample collections, bacterial isolation and identification

Fifty liver samples were collected from 50 colibacillosis suspected broiler chickens which were attended from May 2016 to March 2017 for routine diagnosis at National Avian Disease Investigation Laboratory (NADIL) and Veterinary Teaching Hospital, Rampur, Nepal. For isolation of *E. coli* strains, swab from the liver sample was aseptically streaked directly on the MacConkey agar (HiMedia, M081) and incubated aerobically at 37 °C for 24 h. The pure colonies were further streaked in the eosine methylene blue (EMB) agar (HiMedia, M317) and incubated overnight at 37 °C. Colonies with the green metallic sheen on EMB agar were suspected as *E. coli* strains and the further confirmation was done by following the standard microbiological techniques which include studies of colony morphology, Gram staining, and biochemical tests (indole, methyl red, Voges-Proskauer, citrate, catalase, oxidase, and motility indole ornithinase test) [14, 15].

Antibiotic susceptibility testing

Antibiotic susceptibility test of the isolates was performed following modified Kirby-bauer disk diffusion method as recommended by Clinical and Laboratory Standards Institute (CLSI) [16]. The antibiotics used in this study were amikacin (AK), nitrofurantoin (NIT), ciprofloxacin (CIP), levofloxacin (LE), gentamicin (GEN), ampicillin (AMP), co-trimoxazole (COT), doxycycline hydrochloride (DO), and colisitin (CL). These antibiotics were selected due to their extensive consumption in the poultry feed and treatment of colibacillosis and other avian diseases [7, 11, 13]. All the antibiotic discs used in this study were purchased from Himedia, India. For quality control, *E coli* ATCC 25922 and *Pseudomonas aeruginosa* ATCC 27853 were used as reference strains.

Detection of virulence genes

Isolated *E. coli* strains were investigated for the presence of eleven virulence genes (*iutA, iss, papC, iucD, tsh, irp-2, ompT, hlyF, iron, cva/cvi,* and *astA*) which are associated with colibacillosis. For the detection of virulence genes, genomic DNA was extracted from pure cultures of *E. coli* grown overnight in the MacConkey agar at 37 °C by using the DNeasy Blood and Tissue Kit (Qiagen, catalogue no. 69506). The quality of genomic DNA was checked by gel electrophoresis and measuring absorbance at A_{260}/A_{280} and A_{260}/A_{230} ratios using the MaestroNano spectrophotometer (MaestroGen; Model name: MN-913). The conventional PCR was used to amplify the virulence genes. The primers used for amplification were those described previously (Table 1) [17, 18]. The PCR was performed in 25 μL volume containing 12.5 μL Hot start Taq 2X master mix (BioLab Inc., New England), 1 μL each primer, 2 μL DNA template, and 8.5 μL nuclease free water. The PCR amplifications were conducted in MultiGene OptiMax Thermal Cycler (Labnet International, Inc., North America) and the cycling conditions were identical for all the samples as follows: 94 °C for 4 min; 35 cycles of 30 s at 94 °C, 1 min at 60 °C, and 2 min at 68 °C; and 72 °C for 7 min. The amplicons were analyzed by agarose gel electrophoresis with 1.5% agarose gel (Sigma-Aldrich, A4718)

Table 1 Primer sets for detection of target virulence genes from avian pathogenic *Escherichia coli* (APEC) isolates

Genes	Primer Sequence (5′–3′)	Amplicon size (bp)
iutA	F: GGCTGGACATCATGGGAACTGG R: CGTCGGGAACGGGTAGAATCG	302
iss	F: CAGCAACCCGAACCACTTGATG R: AGCATTGCCAGAGCGGCAGAA	323
papC	F: TGATATCACGCAGTCAGTAGC R: CCGGCCATATTCACATAA	501
iucD	F: ACAAAAAGTTCTATCGCTTCC R: CCTGATCCAGATGATGCTC	714
tsh	F: ACTATTCTCTGCAGGAAGTC R: CTTCCGATGTTCTGAACGT	824
irp-2	F: AAGGATTCGCTGTTACCGGAC R: AACTCCTGATACAGGTGGC	413
ompT	F: TCATCCCGGAAGCCTCCCTCACTACTAT R: TAGCGTTTGCTGCACTGGCTTCTGATAC	496
hlyF	F: GGCCACAGTCGTTTAGGGTGCTTACC R: GGCGGTTTAGGCATTCCGATACTCAG	450
iroN	F: AATCCGGCAAAGAGACGAACCGCCT R:GTTCGGGCAACCCCTGCTTTGACTTT	553
cva/cvi	F: TGGTAGAATGTGCCAGAGCAAG R: GAGCTGTTTGTAGCGAAGCC	1181
astA	F: TGCCATCAACACAGTATATCC R: TCAGGTCGCGAGTGACGGC	116

prepared in 1× TBE buffer (ThermoFisher Scientific, B52). All the PCR products were stained with ethidium bromide. After electrophoresis, the bands were visualized and photographed under UV light. The amplified product was considered to contain virulence gene if it produced band of the expected size.

Statistical analysis

Data entry and analysis were done using the program Microsoft Office Excel 2010 and *Chi*-square test was performed. The *p*-value was calculated and considered significant only when it was less than 0.05. The Multiple Antibiotic Resistance (MAR) index was calculated as a/b [19], where 'a' is the number of resistance antibiotics and 'b' is the number of antibiotics used.

Results

A total of 50 *E. coli* strains were isolated from 50 liver swab samples of colibacillosis suspected broiler chickens. The antibiogram profile of *E. coli* isolates showed highest resistance to ampicillin (98%) and least resistance to amikacin (16%) (Fig. 1). Out of 50 *E. coli* isolates, 47 (94%) isolates were resistant to three or more antibiotics. The MAR index analysis showed 94% of *E. coli* isolates had MAR index value of > 0.2 and 6% had MAR index value of ≤0.2. The proportions of isolates with the MAR index values of 0.3, 0.4, 0.5, and 0.6 were 31%, 21%, 22%, and 20%, respectively. There was no significant association of prevalence of antibiotic resistant strains with the type of *E. coli* strains ($P > 0.05$).

Based on the genetic criteria for the pathogenicity, isolates containing at least five virulence genes were considered as the APEC strains and isolates containing less than five virulence genes were considered as the avian non-pathogenic *Escherichia coli* (non-APEC) strains. Out of 50 *E. coli* isolates, 45 (90%) isolates were found to be APEC strains and 5 (10%) isolates were found to be non-APEC strains (Table 2). Among 50 *E. coli* strains, 7 strains contained all the eleven virulence genes, 14 strains contained ten virulence genes, 15 strains contained nine virulence genes, 5 strains contained eight virulence genes, 2 strains contained seven virulence genes, 2 strains contained five virulence genes, 4 strains contained 4 virulence genes, and 1 strain contained 3 virulence genes. The virulence genes *iss, ompT, hlyF,* and *iroN* were detected from all the 45 APEC strains. The frequencies of *iucD, astA, iutA, irp-2,* and *tsh* genes in the APEC strains were 97.8%, 95.6%, 82.2%, 73.3%, and 62.2%, respectively. The presence of virulence genes *cva/cvi* and *papC* showed the lowest

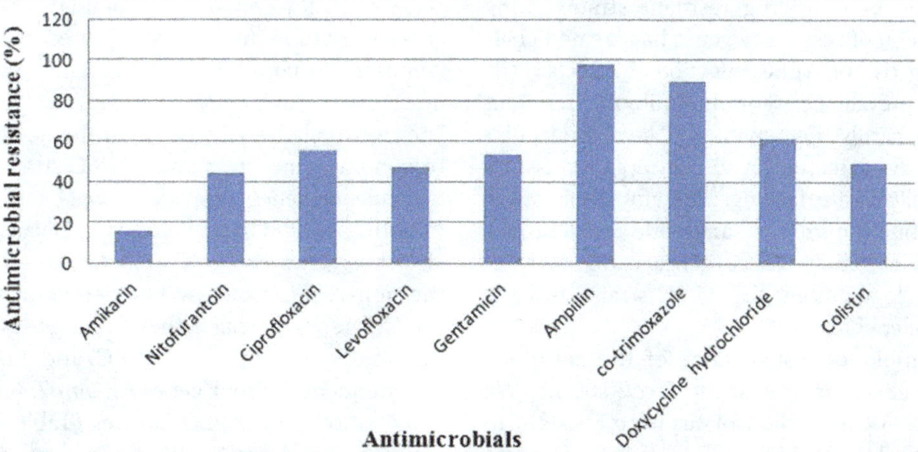

Fig. 1 Antimicrobial resistance pattern of tested antibiotics among *E. coli* strains isolated from colibacillosis suspected broiler chickens

Table 2 Virulence gene frequency in avian pathogenic *Escherichia coli* (APEC) and avian non-pathogenic *Escherichia coli* (Non-APEC) isolates

Genes	APEC isolates ($n = 45$) n(%)	Non-APEC isolates ($n = 5$) n(%)	Total ($n = 50$) n(%)
iutA	37(82.2)	1 (20)	38 (76)
iss	45 (100)	0 (0)	45 (90)
papC	25 (55.6)	0 (0)	25 (50
iucD	44 (97.8)	3 (60)	47 (94)
tsh	28 (62.2)	0 (0)	28 (56)
irp-2	33 (73.3)	3 (60)	36 (72)
ompT	45 (100)	4 (80)	49 (98)
hlyF	45 (100)	3 (60)	48 (96)
iroN	45 (100)	1 (20)	46 (92)
cva/cvi	26 (57.8)	2 (40)	28 (56)
astA	43 (95.6)	2 (40)	45 (90)

frequency among APEC strains (Table 2; Additional file 1: Figure S1). High frequency of the five virulence genes (*iss, ompT, hlyF, iroN,* and *iucD*) was observed among the APEC isolates compared to the non-APEC. Statistical analysis showed that the distribution of virulence genes was significantly associated with the APEC and the non-APEC strains of *E. coli* ($P < 0.05$).

Discussion

Commercialized poultry industries consume wide range of antibiotics for disease prevention and growth promotion [20]. Globally, the consumption of antimicrobials in food animal production is projected to rise by 67%, by 2030. The antimicrobial use in the chicken is expected to rise by 129%, by 2030 in the Asia-Pacific region [21]. Avian colibacillosis is the major disease in chicken which has been reported by several previous studies [3, 12, 22]. The therapeutic use of antimicrobials in poultry industries is considered as efficient control measure for colibacillosis. However, evolution of multidrug resistant strains along with the transmission of resistance genes has created challenges in reducing risk of APEC infections. In Nepal, the accurate data of prevalence of multi-antibiotic resistant APEC strains is hardly documented. Next, molecular based studies for the detection of virulence genes associated with colibacillosis are lacking. Therefore, this study has attempted to find the multiple antibiotic resistant patterns and detects eleven virulence genes using conventional PCR technology among the APEC strains isolated from diseased broiler chicken.

Out of nine antibiotics tested, none of the antibiotic showed 100% effectiveness against the *E coli* strains. We found the highest 98% of *E. coli* isolates were resistant to ampicillin and the lowest 16% of *E. coli* isolates were resistant to amikacin. Cotrimoxazole, doxycycline hydrochloride, and ciprofloxacin account more than 60% resistivity among the tested *E. coli* isolates. These antibiotic resistivity patterns of *E. coli* strains are comparable with the previous studies [3, 7, 13, 23]. Conversely, aminoglycoside amikacin was the most effective against 84% of *E. coli* strains, which is close to the study published by Bist et al. [24]. Inappropriate utilization of different types of antibiotics in the poultry feed and for disease prevention is the common practice in Chitwan districts and other regions of Nepal. Previous data have showed the marked increase in veterinary antibiotic sales in Nepal [13, 25]. Indiscriminate use of the antibiotics exerts a selection pressure leading to the development of drugs resistance strain of bacteria. The antibiotic resistant patterns found in this study suggest a threatening situation of prevalence of the antibiotic resistant *E. coli* strains among broiler chickens in Chitwan district. Multiple antibiotic resistant patterns showed 94% of the isolates were resistant to the three or more antimicrobials. The high prevalent of multidrug resistance in *E. coli* have been reported in Bangladesh [3], China [26], and Korea [27]. The proportion of the isolates with MAR index greater than 0.2 is 94%, and less than or equal to 0.2 is 6%. MAR index value greater than 0.2 indicates high-risk sources of contamination, where several antibiotics may often use for the control of diseases [28]. This suggests the strong indication about an indiscriminative and abusive administration of multiple antibiotics for prophylaxis or infection. Such multi-drug resistances ultimately replace the drug sensitive microorganisms from the antibiotic saturated environment [29].

In this study, the frequency of eleven virulence genes and their role in the pathogenicity was evaluated among APEC and non-APEC strains. APEC strains are characterized by the possession of at least five virulence genes, which enable them to survive an extraintestinal life [1]. To the best of our knowledge, this is the first report in Nepal regarding the study of APEC virulence associated genes by PCR technique. We found the virulence associated genes were more frequently appeared among APEC strains compared to non-APEC strains. The detection rates of *iss, iucD, ompT, hlyF, iroN, astA,* and *iutA* among APEC isolates were relatively higher than the detection rates of corresponding genes in the non-APEC strains. High frequency of virulence genes *ompT, hlyF, iucD,* and *irp-2* were found in both the APEC and non-APEC isolates. In contrast, the virulence genes *iss, papC,* and *tsh* were not detected from the non-APEC isolates. The detection rate of *irp-2* and *cva/cvi* genes revealed that these genes were frequently distributed in both the APEC and non-APEC strains. The frequency of four genes *iss, ompT, hlyF,* and *iroN* were 100% among the APEC isolates (Table 2). The virulence genes *irp2* and *iucD,* both are related to iron acquisition system which demonstrated different detection frequency between the APEC and non-APEC isolates. Among the 45 APEC isolates, 97.8% showed presence of *iucD* genes, whereas, presence of *irp-2* gene was lower (73.3%). Due to the comparable detection rate, this study indicates the possession of *iucD* gene is important characteristics of both APEC and non-APEC isolates. The frequency of virulence genes detected in this study is comparable with other studies. Kwon et al. studied the presence of eight genes among 18 APEC strains and found the frequency of virulence genes as: *iss* (100%), *tsh* (94%), *vat* (89%), *iucD* (83%), *irp-2* (67%), *astA* (56%), *cva/cvi* (16%), and *papC* (11%) [30]. In another study, De Carli et al. has reported high frequency of virulence genes (*hlyF,* 100%; *iroN,* 98. 8%; *ompT,* 100%; *iss,* 96.3%; and *iutA,* 81.5%) among the APEC strains [1]. The detection rate of *papC* is low (55.6%) among the APEC isolates and not detected among the non-APEC isolates. Due to the higher detection rates (80–90%), virulence genes *astA, iucD,* and *iutA* are considered as essential genes for pathogenicity. This study also revealed that there was no uniform and absolute combination of the virulence genes which can differentiate APEC and non-APEC strains of *E. coli.* Additionally, the detection of *iss, papC,* and *tsh* genes exclusively only among the APEC strains could be considered as important virulent factors for colibacillosis. The high prevalence of APEC strains of *E. coli* found in this study based on molecular investigation is the first report to reveal the severity of APEC strains in Chitwan district.

Conclusions

This study showed high prevalence of multiple antimicrobials resistant *E. coli* and high frequency of virulence genes in APEC strains isolated from the colibacillosis suspected broiler chickens in Chitwan, Nepal. Regular screening and monitoring of the virulence genes associated with the antibiotic resistant APEC strains is essential for implementing intervention program to reduce risk of colibacillosis. A holistic approach is required for the prevention and the control of avian colibacillosis in Nepal and other regions of the country. This can be achieved with the active involvement and cooperation of farmers, hatchery operators, drug importers and marketers, veterinary and allied professionals, and government regulatory agencies.

Abbreviations

APEC: Avian pathogenic *Escherichia coli*; ATCC: American Type Culture Collection; CLSI: Clinical and Laboratory Standards Institute; EMB: Eosine methylene blue; ExPEC: Avian extraintestinal pathogenic *E.coli*; MAR: Multiple Antibiotic Resistance; NADIL: National Avian Disease Investigation Laboratory; NMEC: Neonatal meningitis *E. coli*; UPEC: Human uropathogenic *E. coli*

Acknowledgements

We express sincere gratitude to all the members of the advisory committee, National Avian Disease Investigation Laboratory (NADIL) and faculty members of Agriculture and Forestry University.

Funding

This work was supported financially by the National Avian Disease Investigation Laboratory (NADIL) and National Agricultural Research Development Fund (NARDEF), Nepal.

Authors' contributions

HL, BD and RKB conceived the concept, design, and supervised this study. MS and SP performed experimental work. MS, SP, AS, PP, and DKC analyzed data and prepared the final draft of the manuscript. All authors read and approved the final manuscript.

Consent for publication

Not applicable.

Competing interests

The authors declare that they have no competing interests.

Author details

[1]Department of Drug Administration, Government of Nepal, Bijulibazar, Kathmandu, Nepal. [2]Center for Biotechnology, Agriculture and Forestry University, Rampur, Chitwan, Nepal. [3]Department of Veterinary Microbiology and Parasitology, Agriculture and Forestry University, Rampur, Chitwan, Nepal. [4]Department of Veterinary Science & Animal Husbandry, Himalayan College of Agriculture Sciences and Technology, Kathmandu, Nepal. [5]Department of Microbiology, National College, Kathmandu, Nepal. [6]Department of Microbiology, Balkumari College, Bharatpur, Chitwan, Nepal. [7]Department of Microbiology, Prithu Technical College, Institute of Agriculture and Animal Science, Tribhuvan University, Lamahi, Dang, Nepal.

References

1. De Carli S, Ikuta N, Lehmann FK, da Silveira VP, de Melo Predebon G, Fonseca AS, et al. Virulence gene content in *Escherichia coli* isolates from poultry flocks with clinical signs of colibacillosis in Brazil. Poult Sci. 2015;94:2635–40.
2. Matter LB, Barbieri NL, Nordhoff M, Ewers C, Horn F. Avian pathogenic *Escherichia coli* MT78 invades chicken fibroblasts. Vet Microbiol. 2011;148:51–9.
3. Matin MA, Islam MA, Khatun MM. Prevalence of colibacillosis in chickens in greater Mymensingh district of Bangladesh. Vet World. 2017;10:29–33.
4. Manges AR, Johnson JR. Food-borne origins of *Escherichia coli* causing extraintestinal infections. Clin Infect Dis. 2012;55:712–9.
5. Johnson TJ, Kariyawasam S, Wannemuehler Y, Mangiamele P, Johnson SJ, Doetkott C, et al. The genome sequence of avian pathogenic *Escherichia coli* strain O1:K1:H7 shares strong similarities with human extraintestinal pathogenic *E. coli* genomes. J Bacteriol. 2007:3228–36.
6. Osti R, Bhattarai D, Chaudhary H, Singh V. Poultry production in Nepal: characteristics, productivity and constraints. Int J Appl Sci Biotechnol. 2017;5:222–6.
7. Shrestha A, Bajracharya AM, Subedi H, Turha RS, Kafle S, Sharma S, et al. Multi-drug resistance and extended spectrum beta lactamase producing gram negative bacteria from chicken meat in Bharatpur metropolitan, Nepal. BMC Res Notes. 2017;10:574.
8. Miles TD, McLaughlin W, Brown PD. Antimicrobial resistance of *Escherichia coli* isolates from broiler chickens and humans. BMC Vet Res. 2006;2:7.
9. Umolu PI, Ohenhen ER, Okwu IG, Ogiehor IS. Multiple antibiotic resistant index and plasmid of *Escherichia coli* in beef in Ekpoma. J Am Sci. 2006;2:16–8.
10. Centers for Disease Control and Prevention (CDC). Antibiotic resistance threats in the United States. U. S. CDC: Department of Health and Human Services; 2013. p. 2013.
11. Gautam G, Devkota B, Thapaliya S. Recent case flow pattern in veterinary teaching Hospital of Agriculture and Forestry University, Chitwan, Nepal. Journal of Agriculture and Forestry University. 2017;1:119–28.
12. Mellata M. Human and avian extraintestinal pathogenic *Escherichia coli*: infections, zoonotic risks, and antibiotic resistance trends. Foodborne Pathog Dis. 2013;10:916–32.

13. Shrestha EK, Dhakal IP, Sapkota M, Manandhar P, Rijal TB. Antimicrobial resistance pattern of *Eshcerichia coli* isolates from chicken and human samples in Chitwan. Nepalese. Vet J. 2011;30:38–44.
14. da Silva N, Taniwaki MH, Junqueira VC, Silveira N, do Nascimento MS, RAR G. Microbiological examination methods of food and water: a laboratory manual. London, UK: Taylor & Francis Group; 2013.
15. Overdevest I, Willemsen I, Rijnsburger M, Eustace A, Xu L, Hawkey P, et al. Extended-spectrum β-lactamase genes of *Escherichia coli* in chicken meat and humans, the Netherlands. Emerg Infect Dis. 2011;17:1216–22.
16. Clinical Laboratory Standards Institute (CLSI). Performance standards for antimicrobial susceptibility testing; 24th informational supplement (M100-S23). Wayne PA, USA: CLSI; 2014.
17. Ewers C, Janssen T, Kiessling S, Philipp HC, Wieler LH. Rapid detection of virulence-associated genes in avian pathogenic *Escherichia coli* by multiplex polymerase chain reaction. Avian Dis. 2005;49:269–73.
18. Radwan IAE, Salam HSH, Abd-Alwanis AA, Al-Sayed MAY. Frequency of some virulence associated genes among multidrug-resistant *Escherischia coli* isolated from septicemic broiler chicken. Int. J Adv Res. 2014;2:867–74.
19. Krumperman PH. Multiple antibiotic resistance indexing of *Escherichia coli* to identify high-risk sources of fecal contamination of foods. Appl Environ Microbiol. 1983;46:165–70.
20. Bhandari S, Singh S. Annual consumption of veterinary medicines and feed supplement in Nepal. Nepalese Vet J. 2004;28:25–32.
21. Van Boeckel TP, Brower C, Gilbert M, Grenfell BT, Levin SA, Robinson TP, et al. Global trends in antimicrobial use in foods animals. Proc Natl Acad Sci U S A. 2015;112:5649–54.
22. Tonu NS, Sufian MA, Sarkar S, Kamal MM, Rahman MH, Hossain MM. Pathological study on colibacillosis in chickens and detection of *Escherichia coli* by PCR. Bangladesh. J Vet Med. 2001;9:17–25.
23. Bakhshi M, Bafghi MF, Astani A, Ranjbar VR, Zandi H, Vakili M. Antimicrobial resistence pattern of *Escherichia coli* isolated from chickens with colibacillosis in Yazd, Iran. J Food Qual Hazards Control. 2017;4:74–78.
24. Bist B, Sharma B, Jain U. Virulence associated factors and antibiotic sensitivity pattern of *Escherichia coli* isolated from cattle and soil. Vet World. 2014;3:69–72.
25. Basnyat B, Pokharel P, Dixit S, Giri S. Antibiotic use, its resistance in Nepal and recommendations for action: a situation analysis. J Nepal Health Res Counc. 2015;13:102–11.
26. Yang H, Chen S, White DG, Zhao S, Mc Dermott P, Walker R, et al. Characterization of multiple-antimicrobial-resistant *Eshcerichia coli* isolates from diseased chickens and swine in China. J Clin Microbiol. 2004;42:3483–9.
27. Kim TE, Jeong YW, Cho SH, Kim SJ, Kwon HJ. Chronological study of antibiotic resistances and their relevant genes in Korean avian pathogenic *Eshcerichia coli* isolates. J Clin Microbiol. 2007;45:3309–15.
28. Chitanand MP, Kadam TA, Gyananath G, Totewad ND, Balhal DK. Multiple antibiotic resistance indexing of coliforms to identify high risk contamination sites in aquatic environment. Indian J Microbiol. 2010;50:216–20.
29. Van den Bogaard AE, London N, Driessen C, Stobberingh EE. Antibiotic resistance of faecal *Escherichia coli* in poultry, poultry farmers and poultry slaughterers. J Antimicrob Chemother. 2001;47:763–71.
30. Kwon SG, Cha SY, Choi EJ, Kim B, Song HJ, Jang HK. Epidemiological prevalence of avian pathogenic *Escherichia coli* differentiated multiplex PCR from commercial chickens and hatchery in Korea. J Bacteriol Virol. 2008;38:179–88.

20

The value of necropsy reports for animal health surveillance

Susanne Küker[1*], Celine Faverjon[1], Lenz Furrer[2], John Berezowski[1], Horst Posthaus[3], Fabio Rinaldi[2] and Flavie Vial[1,4]

Abstract

Background: Animal health data recorded in free text, such as in necropsy reports, can have valuable information for national surveillance systems. However, these data are rarely utilized because the text format requires labor-intensive classification of records before they can be analyzed with using statistical or other software. In a previous study, we designed a text-mining tool to extract data from text in necropsy reports. In the current study, we used the tool to extract data from the reports from pig and cattle necropsies performed between 2000 and 2011 at the Institute of Animal Pathology (ITPA), University of Bern, Switzerland. We evaluated data quality in terms of credibility, completeness and representativeness of the Swiss pig and cattle populations.

Results: Data was easily extracted from necropsy reports. Data quality in terms of completeness and validity varied a lot depending on the type of data reported. Diseases of the gastrointestinal system were reported most frequently (54.6% of pig submissions and 40.8% of cattle submissions). Diseases affecting serous membranes were reported in 16.0% of necropsied pigs and 27.6% of cattle. Respiratory diseases were reported in 18.3% of pigs and 21.6% of cattle submissions.

Conclusions: This study suggests that extracting data from necropsy reports can provide information of value for animal health surveillance. This data has potential value for monitoring endemic disease syndromes in different age and production groups, or for early detection of emerging or re-emerging diseases. The study identified data entry and other errors that could be corrected to improve the quality and validity of the data. Submissions to veterinary diagnostic laboratories have selection biases and these should be considered when designing surveillance systems that include necropsy reports.

Keywords: Electronic necropsy records, Veterinary, Informatics, Surveillance, Text-mining

Background

In veterinary public health, active and passive surveillance most often relies on the definitive diagnosis of specific diseases using laboratory tests for known pathogens. However, when a previously unknown or unexpected pathogen emerges in a population, this approach can take additional time and many result in a delay in pathogen identification and detection [1–3]. The same may apply to multifactorial diseases such as production diseases where detection of a single pathogen is often insufficient to unravel the underlying causal factors contributing to the disease problem.

Syndromic surveillance systems (SYS) were developed to enhance traditional passive surveillance systems and for this reason they are currently increasing in importance in veterinary medicine [4–6]. Through the analysis and interpretation of pre-diagnostic health-related data, veterinary SYS supports the early identification of disease threats that may require veterinary public health action [7]. Various sources of data have been evaluated for use in veterinary SYS worldwide [6]. These include clinical observations collected from veterinary practitioners [8], diagnostic laboratory test requests [9], post-mortem meat inspection information [10–14] and examinations of fallen stock [15–18]. Data quality in terms of completeness, validity, representativeness, usefulness and timeliness are important characteristics for determining the effectiveness of a SYS for detecting changes in animal health [19].

* Correspondence: susanne.kueker@vetsuisse.unibe.ch
[1]Veterinary Public Health Institute, Vetsuisse Faculty, University of Bern, Schwarzenburgstrasse 155, 3097, Liebefeld, Switzerland
Full list of author information is available at the end of the article

Necropsies performed by diagnostic laboratories on fallen stock or diseased animals could provide additional information about animal health that could have value for SYS [4]. Necropsies are a common diagnostic tool in veterinary medicine and play an important role in the investigation of disease outbreaks [20–22]. Veterinarians may be called by farmers to investigate a sudden increase in morbidity or mortality of an unknown or unrecognized disease. If animals died suspiciously or were euthanized, veterinarians may perform a field necropsy or arrange for the transport of the carcasses to a diagnostic laboratory, where a more detailed post-mortem examination and diagnostic workup can take place [23, 24]. In most disease investigations involving food-producing animals, the main purpose of a post-mortem examination is to provide additional information about the cause of death. The information present in necropsy reports is in the form of patho-morphological diagnoses, which are very specific descriptions of the gross and microscopic lesions, and the results of diagnostic tests. They also contain information about the geographic location of the farm, the affected animal(s), species, breed, sex, age, production group, clinical presentation of affected animal(s), and other farm-level characteristics, which are valuable for disease surveillance [4].

Necropsy reports could potentially have value for identifying unexpected health events that occur in a population. Syndromes representing a broad range of diseases could be defined and monitored in a SYS based on pathological findings from necropsies. Recent examples of the use of syndromes from pathology data for disease surveillance include abortion and fetal anomalies that occurred in the Schmallenberg virus epidemic in Europe [25] and central nervous system lesions in cattle infected with Astroviruses [26]. These examples suggest that monitoring of necropsy data from food production animals can be of value for early detection of new diseases or detection of changing endemic disease patterns in a population [21]. However, necropsy data from food production animals are rarely used for SYS. One challenge for using necropsy reports in routine surveillance is that these reports are commonly created and stored in natural language (free text format). This makes it difficult to extract the structured data required for the computer based data manipulation and analysis needed for surveillance. Furthermore, no internationally accepted unifying clinical terminology or coding system, such as the International Classification of Diseases (ICD) developed for human medicine, exists in animal health, although there have been attempts to create such systems [27, 28]. This makes automated classification and integration of multiple datasets difficult [4, 27].

Natural language processing (NLP) methods such as text mining are becoming increasingly important for dealing with natural language records [29]. Text mining is used to extract data from text found in electronic documents such as medical records, by automatically classifying text data into a defined set of categories which are monitored over time [30]. This approach has been used in human [31, 32] and in animal health surveillance [33–35]. However, text mining has not yet been systematically applied to livestock necropsy reports.

The objective of our study was to evaluate the quality of the data extracted from necropsy reports from food animals in order to estimate their value for SYS. A text-mining tool that classifies necropsy reports based on topographical organ systems was developed in a previous study [36] and used in the current study to classify necropsy reports into syndromes that could be used for SYS. We used these results to estimate the distribution of syndromes in the population and make inferences about the applicability of the tool and necropsy reports for veterinary SYS.

Methods

Necropsy data

We analyzed 12 years of pig and cattle necropsy data recorded at the Institute of Animal Pathology (ITPA), Vetsuisse Faculty, University of Bern, Switzerland. Post-mortem findings were entered manually as free text by veterinary pathologists, using a record keeping and reporting software application and database (Qualicare, Qualidoc AG). Final necropsy reports contained several separate sections, such as macroscopic findings, histologic findings and morphological diagnoses, as well as results from additional diagnostic tests such as microbiological investigations.

Necropsy reports were extracted from the Qualicare software as a Microsoft Excel file. The dataset ($n = 6031$ pig records and $n = 2911$ cattle records) included necropsies performed on whole carcasses. Reports from examinations of partial carcasses, entries without text and double entries were excluded.

Necropsy reports included the following additional variables: a unique necropsy submission number, species, breed, sex, weight, date, animal age (in days), how the animal died (e.g., euthanized) and address of the owner. For cattle, the breed and the unique animal identification number registered in the Swiss central animal movement database (Tierverkehrsdatenbank, TVD) were also recorded. Information about the clinical history of necropsied animals was not available in 99% of the reports and for this reason clinical history was excluded from study.

Data quality

Data quality was assessed by evaluating the completeness, validity, and representativeness of the data [19]. Data quality was assessed for the following fields: Submission number, Sex, Age (in days), Weight (in Kg), How the animal died, Owner name, Owner address, (postal code) Breed, TVD number. Complete records were records that had an entry in the record for the field that was valid. Entries were valid if they were logically or biologically plausible.

Age and weight validity were assessed by checking for biologically unlikely entries (e.g., > 250 kg weight for pigs were classified as invalid). For cattle reports, the unique animal identification number (TVD number) was classified as invalid if it was not exactly 8 digits long or contained punctuation or letters.

The number of dead cattle and pigs was not available for the full period of the study. Therefore, to assess the representativeness of the submissions, the distributions of sex, age, breed and geographical origin of necropsied animals were compared to those of the overall Swiss pig and cattle living populations using data provided by the Swiss Federal Veterinary Office.

Syndrome categories & text-mining classification tool

We defined 12 syndrome categories based primarily on affected organ systems. This classification included the following systems: gastrointestinal (GI), respiratory (RESP), heart (HEART), lymphatic (LYMPH), nervous (NEURO), musculoskeletal (MUSCO), urinary (URI), reproductive (REPRO) and serous membrane systems (SERO). Three additional non-organ system syndrome categories were defined, one for congenital malformations (MAL), one for neoplasia (NEO) and one named OTHER for diagnoses or terms that referred to pathologic patterns that could not be assigned to one of the previous syndrome categories. Examples of reports classified as OTHER included intoxications, macroscopic findings of the skin and septicemia (details can be found in Additional file 1). We constructed a German veterinary terminology resource to classify necropsy reports into at least one of the above syndrome categories. Each report could be classified into more than one category. The construction of the ontology is thoroughly described in [36] but is summarized below. We started with a frequency-ranked list of the words found in all of the reports and implemented methods for dealing with spelling mistakes, inflections, negations and abbreviations. We selected "key terms" that were likely to indicate diagnoses in the reports. These key terms ($n = 484$) were mostly morphological diagnoses (e.g., bronchopneumonia or enteritis), macroscopic findings (e.g., "bladder stone", which relates to urolithiasis), diagnosis synonyms (e.g., "Sohlengeschwür-pododermatitis") or sub terms (e.g., "jejunitis", which can be stated as enteritis). The key terms were then assigned to the syndrome categories listed above (Table 1 and Additional file 1). A further selection criterion was the proportion of correctly classified reports: if a key term resulted in many incorrect classifications, it was excluded. The evaluation of classification is reported in [36].

Table 1 List of the 12 syndrome categories used for classification of necropsy records by a text-mining tool, with examples of key terms that resulted in classification into the categories

Syndromic category	Examples of diagnoses
Gastrointestinal system	enteritis, colon perforation, mesenteric torsion, typhlocolitis, abomasitis
Respiratory system	pneumonia, bronchitis, laryngitis, sinusitis, tracheitis
Heart	endocarditis, cardiomyopathy, heart infarct, myocarditis
Lymphatic system	lymphadenitis, splenitis, lymphomegaly, tonsillitis, splenic torsion
Reproductive system	abortion, ovarian cyst, metritis, uterus torsion, vaginitis
Urinary system	cystitis, kidney cyst, tubular necrosis, nephritis, bladder rupture
Neurologic system	encephalitis, meningitis, brain edema, paralysis, brain abscess
Musculoskeletal system	arthrosis, callus, fracture, muscle degeneration, osteochondrosis
Other	hydrothorax, intoxication, otitis, skin perforation, dermatitis
Congenital malformation	atresia, ectopy, heart malformation, septal defect, malformation
Neoplasia	osteosarcoma, tumor, neoplasia, carcinoma, metastases
Serous membranes	peritonitis, pleuritis, pericarditis, polyserositis, serositis

After classification by the text-mining tool, we analyzed the most common syndrome categories for each species, sex and age. Special attention was paid to records that were not classified. Unclassified records either did not contain any pathological information or they contained words that were not used for classification because they would have increased the number of misclassifications.

Statistical analysis

Descriptive analyses were performed using R version 3.2.4 [37] with the packages: ggplot2 [38], rgdal [39], rgeos [40] and RColorBrewer [41]. The shape file used to plot the maps of Switzerland was obtained from the Swiss cadastral system (https://www.swisstopo.admin.ch/en/knowledge-facts/swiss-cadastral-surveying.html).

Time series analysis was conducted on the total number of submissions for each species and on the three most frequent syndromes per species. Three temporal patterns were investigated: long-term trend, monthly effect and day-of-the-week effect. Trend was defined as a continuous time variable. Months and days of the week were included using categorical variables for each month and day. A zero-inflated negative binomial model was fitted to the daily time-series to evaluate the effect of day of the week using the R package *pscl* [42]. A negative binomial model was used to evaluate the trend and the monthly effect with the *MASS* R package [43]. Models including temporal patterns were compared with the null model using likelihood ratio tests with a statistical significance level of 0.05.

The pig age classification of our dataset was linked to that of the Swiss pig industry, in which the age is classified based on the production status of the pig, as follows: piglets (1 to 4 weeks), weaner pigs (> 4 to 10 weeks), fattening pigs (> 10 to 22 weeks) and adults (> 22 weeks). Cattle were grouped into the following age classes: 0 to 1 month, > 1 to 6 months, > 6 months to 1 year, > 1 to 2 years and > 2 years.

Results

Data quality

The variables date, owner name and submission number were the most complete with 0 to 0.3% incomplete or invalid entries (Table 2). The variables: age, breed and production type (the latter two being cattle-specific) had 20 to 35% missing or invalid entries. The TVD number was missing or improperly transcribed in 80% of the cattle reports. A small number of zip codes of owner addresses were missing in the dataset, and 4.5% for pigs and 3.5% for cattle were invalid. Only a small proportion of necropsied animals had no geographical information associated with them (1.2% of pigs and 2% of cattle).

Descriptive analysis of necropsied animals

Necropsied animals submitted to the ITPA originated mostly from west and central parts of Switzerland (Fig. 1.a1 for pigs and Fig. 2.a1 for cattle; "count" = number of animals). Cattle submissions came from a larger area of Switzerland than swine submissions. Registered pig and cattle farms were more widely distributed throughout Switzerland (Fig. 1.a2 for pigs and Fig. 2.a2 for cattle, "count" = number of animals); indicating that submissions to the ITPA did not provide complete coverage of the Swiss cattle or and swine populations.

The proportion of males to female pigs was slightly higher (2258 males to 1834 females). The majority of pigs were piglets (1–4 weeks of age) or weaner (> 4–10 weeks of age), (Fig. 1.b1). This contrasts with the age distribution of the pig population in Switzerland, where the majority of pigs are fattening pigs (11–22 weeks of age; Fig. 1.b2).

The greatest proportion of necropsied cattle (26%) were in the age class "2 years and above" (Fig. 2.b1). These animals were almost exclusively (702/715) females. However, when the < 1 month and 1–6 month categories were combined, we found that 53% of necropsied cattle (586/1040 females) were 6 months of age or younger. This age distribution is in contrast to the Swiss cattle population, which consists predominately of female cattle over 2 years old (Fig. 2.b2).

The most common breeds of necropsied cattle were Holstein Friesian ($n = 573$), Simmental Fleckvieh ($n = 371$), Red Holstein ($n = 365$), and crosses of Simmental Fleckvieh and Red Holstein ($n = 250$), which aligns with the main breeds reported to be present in the Swiss cattle population [44]. However, data on the breed distribution of cattle in Switzerland were not available to make direct comparisons.

Syndrome classification

The four most frequent syndrome categories were the same for both species: GI (pigs 54.6%, cattle 40.8%), SERO (pigs 16.0%, cattle 27.6%), RESP (pigs 18.3%, cattle 21.6%) and OTHER (pigs 14.7%, cattle 13.8%). In cattle, REPRO also represented a large proportion of necropsies (19.1%), but this syndrome was less frequently encountered in pigs (4.4%). Thirty-six percent of pig necropsy reports and 45% of cattle necropsy reports were classified into more than one syndrome. The most frequent combinations of syndromes were GI and/or RESP and/or SERO and/or OTHER for both species. The majority (90.2%) of post-mortem records were classified into at

Table 2 Data quality (completeness and validity) for the 13 descriptive variables extracted from the post-mortem reports for pigs and cattle between 2000 and 2011. The TVD number is the unique Swiss cattle identification number

	Cattle			Pig			Cattle	Pig
	Complete	Missing	Invalid	Complete	Missing	Invalid	% unusable entries	% unusable entries
Submission number	2862	0	0	5997	0	0	0	0
Sex	2753	109	0	5823	174	0	4	3
Age (days)	2114	549	199	4361	1471	165	27	27
Weight (kg)	2742	1	119	5888	1	108	4	2
How animal died	2786	76	0	5901	96	0	3	2
Owner name	2862	0	0	5996	1	0	0	< 1
Owner address	2611	251	0	5809	188	0	9	3
Owner address (zip code)	2847	15	0	5983	14	0	< 1	< 1
Breed	2279	583	0	NA	NA	NA	21	NA
TVD number	1604	9	1284	NA	NA	NA	80	NA

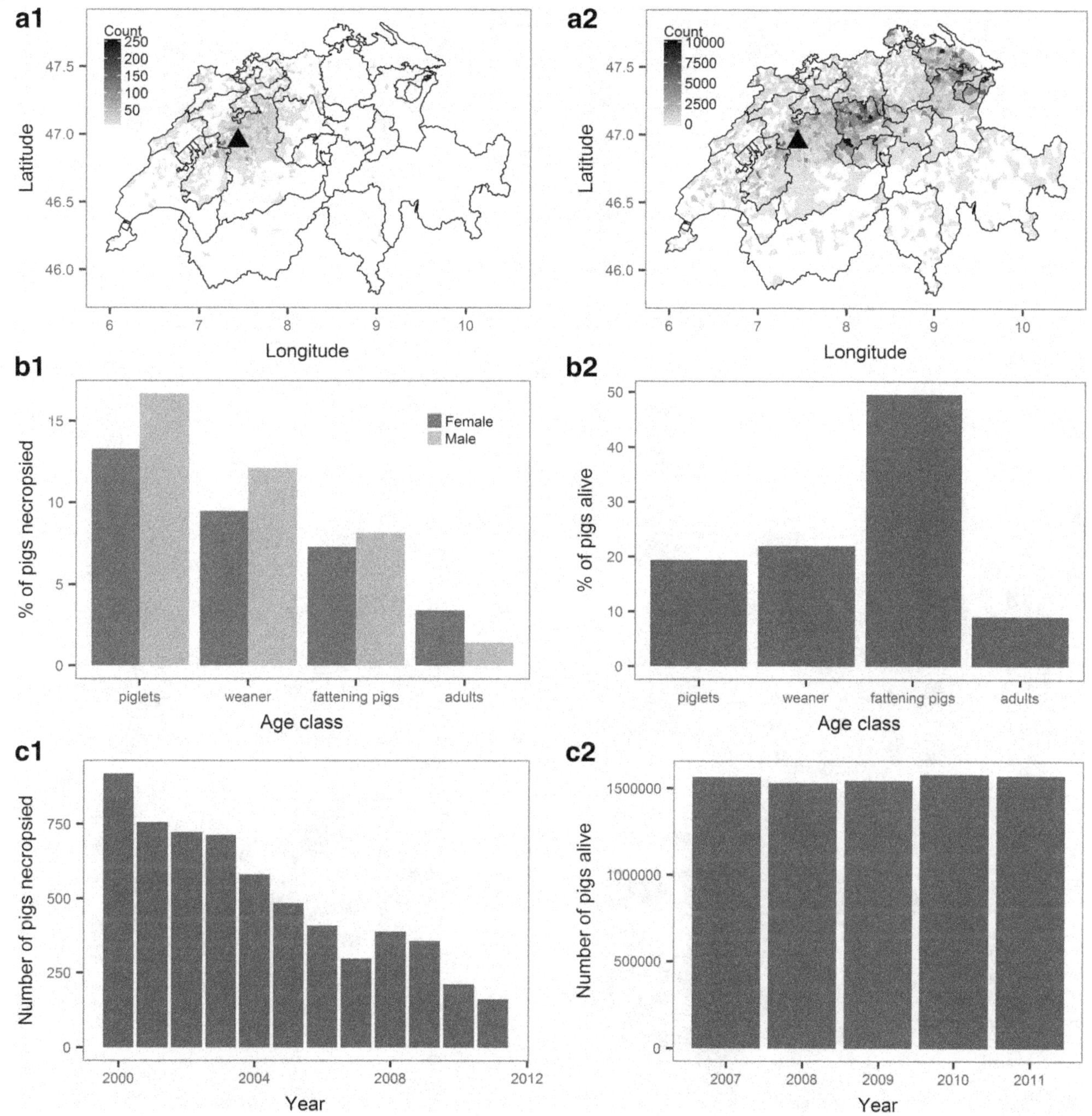

Fig. 1 Results for pigs. The left row (1) presents results of data collected at the Animal Pathology Institute (ITPA) of the University of Bern, Switzerland in 2000–2012. The right row (2) presents data for the pig population in 2007–2011 in Switzerland, provided by the farm census database (Agrarpolitisches Information system AGIS, Federal Office for Agriculture FOAG). Data were only available for the period 2007–2011; the sex ratio could not be determined. Column A represents the geographical distribution of pigs ("count" = number of pigs); column B the age groups and their ex ratio and column C the number of animals per year

least one category. The main reason reports were not classified was the absence of any key term in the text. Records without any categories represented between 6.3 and 15.0%, depending on the species and age class.

The proportion of each syndrome varied between species and age categories (Fig. 3). In pigs, respiratory syndromes (69%) were most common in animals greater than 2 years old. Heart (19.8%) and urinary (20.7%) syndromes were especially frequent in pigs between 6 months and 1 year of age. Musculoskeletal syndromes were found in 35.4% of pigs between 1 and 2 years of age, but the number of pigs in this age group was very small.

The most common syndrome in calves less than 1 month of age was GI (54.0%). Gastrointestinal syndromes were

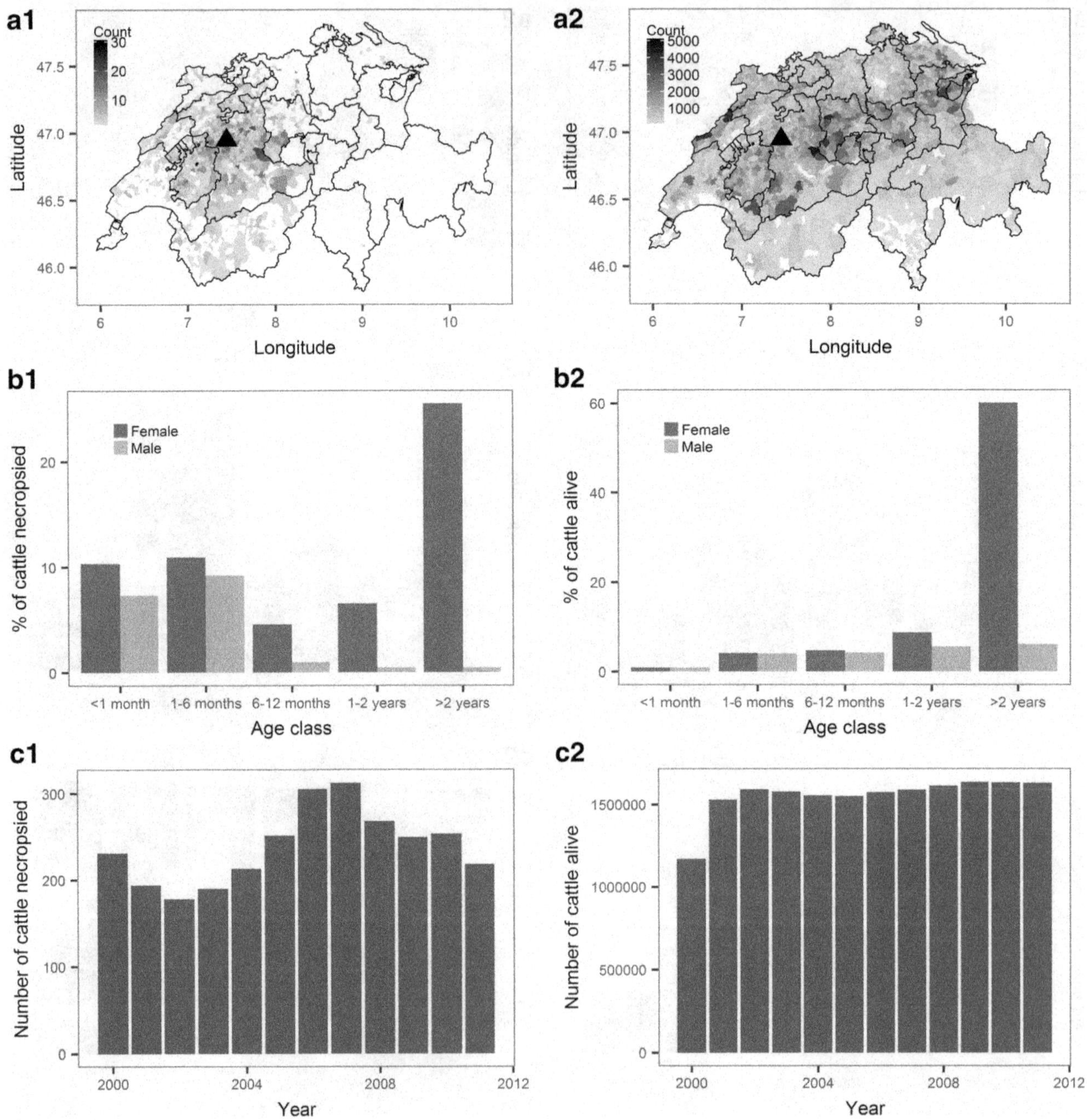

Fig. 2 Results for cattle. The left row (1) presents results of data collected at the Animal Pathology Institute (ITPA) of the University of Bern, Switzerland in 2000–2012. The right row (2) presents data for the cattle population in 2000–2011 in Switzerland, provided by the Swiss central animal movement database (TVD database 2014; http://www.tierverkehr.ch). Column A represents the geographical distribution of cattle ("count" = number of cattle), column B the age groups and their ex ratio and column C the number of animals per year

important across all age groups of cattle, but to a lesser extent in older age groups. In calves between 1 and 12 months, gastrointestinal (43.0%) and respiratory (34.0%) syndromes were the most common. In cattle between 1 and 2 years of age, the proportion of cattle classified as having a respiratory syndrome decreased to less than 20.0%. Reproductive syndromes were most important in cattle 2 years old or older, where they represented 33.5% of the submissions.

Time series analysis

There was a decreasing trend in the number of pigs necropsied per year at the ITPA between the years 2000 and 2011. The number of cattle necropsied at the ITPA per year remained stable over the same period (Fig. 1.c1 for pigs and 2.c1 for cattle).

The number of submissions for both species was lower during summer (June and July) than winter months

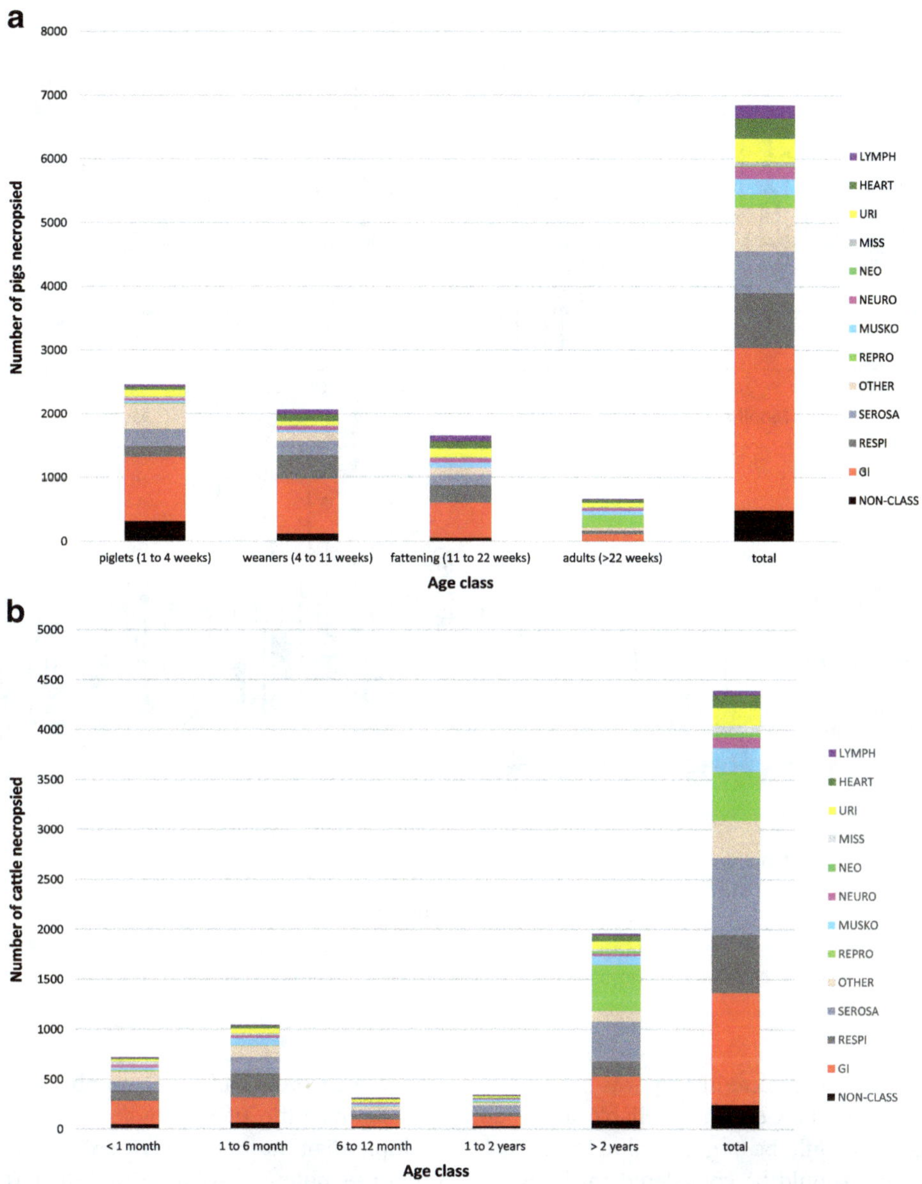

Fig. 3 Total number of animals classified into each syndrome by their age classes (the classification numbers are higher than the total number of necropsies because more than one syndrome class per report was possible), based on the automatic categorization of necropsy reports using a text-mining tool with data collected at the Animal Pathology Institute (ITPA) of the University of Bern, Switzerland in 2000–2011. Panel A presents pigs, panel B presents cattle

(January and February; Fig. 4). The number of submissions for both species was also affected by the day of the week. Fewer animals were necropsied during the weekend and more on Mondays (data not shown). For both species, the three main syndromes showed a seasonal trend that mirrored the seasonal trend in the total number of submissions.

Discussion

In this study, we evaluated the quality of data extracted post-mortem reports from a veterinary diagnostic pathology laboratory and assessed their potential value for animal health surveillance. Extracting data from the text records was relatively easy. Data completeness and validity varied a lot depending on the type of data. Geographical information and personal information such as name and address were present and considered to be valid in most of the reports (i.e., less than 9% of owner addresses and less than 1% of zip codes were unusable), making the data suitable for spatio-temporal analyses and traceability [45]. This information represents an added value that is not often found in other animal health data

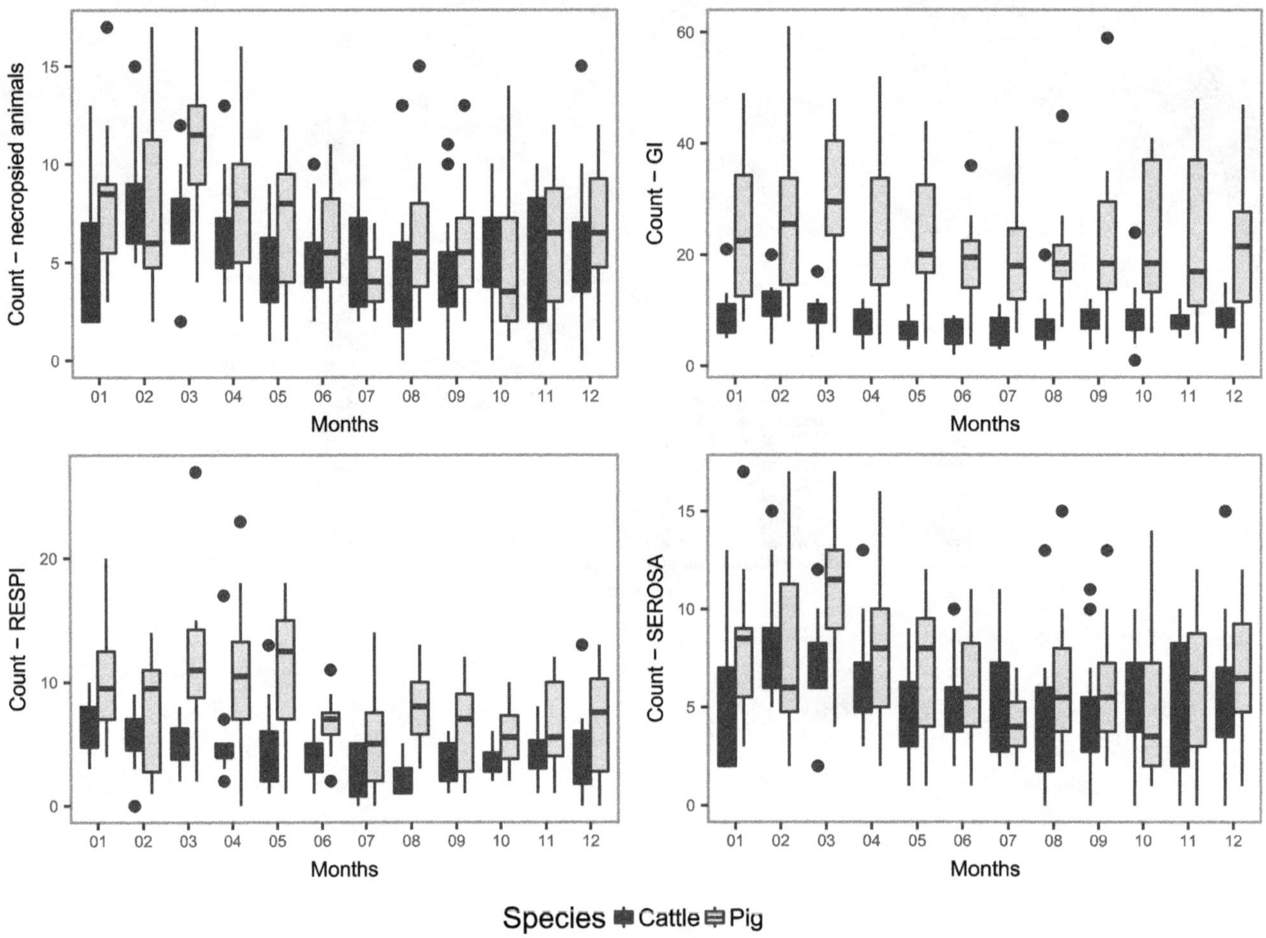

Fig. 4 Temporal pattern of the three main syndromes (GI-Gastrointestinal system; RESPI-respiratory system; SEROSA-serous membrane system) of pigs and cattle submissions to the Animal Pathology Institute (ITPA) of the University of Bern, Switzerland in 2000–2012. The count scale is differs among the panels

sources [4]. In contrast, the clinical history was missing in 99% of the necropsy reports. Collecting reliable information on clinical histories could be of great value for animal health surveillance and should be considered for improving the overall value of diagnostic laboratory data. Processes to ensure the quality and reliability of the clinical history reported would also be helpful because clinical histories ranged from owner observations without veterinary consultation to detailed clinical diagnoses made by veterinary specialists (data not shown). Twenty-seven percent of the ages (for pigs and cattle) and 80% of the TVD numbers (for cattle) were also unusable because of missing or invalid values. Poor recording of animal age may limit the use of these data for individual monitoring of different age groups. The TVD number could be used to link necropsy reports to the nationwide animal movement database and track the origin of cases necropsied at ITPA [46]. Improving the recording of these two parameters may thus offer additional opportunities for using the necropsy reports. The most commonly reported problems with the recording of TVD numbers were missing numbers at the time of submission and typing errors when multiple-digit numbers were entered into the computer system. A potential solution to reduce these errors would be to implement an automatic voice recognition system, as already shown to be effective in other fields [47, 48]. In addition, barcode scanners could be used to record the TVD number present on Swiss cattle ear tags and to store it directly in the database [49]. Another potential method to reduce errors would be to implement completeness and correctness checks in the electronic forms that are used for data entry.

The profile of animals necropsied at ITPA was compared to the overall Swiss population to assess the representativeness of these data. In cattle, the balanced sex ratio in young age classes and the preponderance of females in adults was consistent with the Swiss cattle population. Over half (53%) of the cattle necropsied in the study period were less than 6 months of age, which differs from much the smaller proportion of young cattle in the Swiss cattle population [50]. Explanations for this could be a generally higher risk of morbidity and mortality in young animals, or there could be greater difficulty in reaching an on farm clinical diagnosis in young animals. An additional explanation could be that the predominant health problems in adult cattle, such as mastitis, reproductive failure, dystocia and hoof problems typically do not require post-mortem diagnoses. Finally, farmers frequently opt to slaughter an older diseased animal to retain the value of its meat, rather than submitting it for necropsy and further diagnostics. It is not surprising to have differences between the living population and the necropsied population. For a better assessment of the data representativeness, it would be necessary to compare information from necropsy reports to all-cause-mortality data. This data does not exist for pigs in Switzerland, and for cows, the data is only available since 2010. Even though these data have deficiencies, they may still have value for animal health surveillance. There are many factors that might influence the submission (or not) of dead livestock for necropsy. These include factors that affect the behavior of farmers and veterinarians including the economic or sentimental value of the animal, cost of the post mortem examination, postmortem skills of the veterinarian, confidence of the veterinarian in the diagnostic laboratory and others. However, the characteristics of the disease also can influence the submission of dead animal for necropsy. We expect that important diseases that are clinically unusual and the cause significant morbidity and mortality would be submitted to a diagnostic laboratory, and that these rather important diseases should be contained within the data. Monitoring these over time could help to identify new disease emergences.

The seasonality of cattle submitted for necropsy was similar to the seasonality of reported on-farm deaths in Switzerland [17]. We were unable to make the same comparisons for pigs because information to make the comparison was not available.

The ITPA reports did not cover the whole of Switzerland, and the catchment areas for cattle and pigs were clearly centered on the geographic location of the ITPA. This finding is likely due to there being other diagnostic services available to the farmers and the travel distance, as farmers have to transport their animals to the ITPA for necropsy. As expected, as the distance from the farm to Bern increased, the number of necropsied animals decreased. For production animals, there are four additional laboratories, offering necropsy diagnostics in Switzerland. Furthermore, in Switzerland veterinarians commonly perform on farm necropsies especially in the case of small piglets, which can be easily disposed of by the farmer following the necropsy. Additional studies from other laboratories in Switzerland could be performed to see if similar biases are present in other laboratories.

The number of cattle submitted per year remained stable over the 12 years of the study period (200 to 2011), however the number of pigs submitted to the ITPA continuously declined. The reason for the decline in pig submissions could not be determined in this study. Submissions to diagnostic laboratories have been reported to be influenced not only by disease trends, but also by the economic situation in the meat market and other factors [51, 52]. If the reduction in submissions could be determined to be caused by non-disease related factors, it would be a cause of concern if the diagnostic pathology data were used in a national animal health surveillance system. Additional work is needed to determine whether the reduction in swine submissions observed in this study was due to a decline in disease or to other factors. However, these variations could also be of value for animal health surveillance, as investigating them may help improve the understanding of farmer and veterinarian practices, which is essential for building efficient surveillance programs.

The text-mining tool used in this study allowed us to identify pathological patterns in the study population of ITPA necropsy reports. Respiratory and gastrointestinal syndromes were the most common categories identified in both species, which is consistent with previous studies reporting morbidity, mortality and affected organ systems of pigs and cattle in Switzerland, Germany and the USA [53–58]. As expected, reproductive syndromes were most common in animals of reproductive age for both species. Ten percent of the submissions were not classified into a specific syndrome category. There were two types of non-classified animals: animals with an unclear cause of death, and animals that were misclassified (i.e., they should have been classified into at least one syndrome category but the text-mining tool failed to correctly classify them due to misinterpretation). The proportion of misclassified reports (906/8859) was estimated to be low in this dataset, and these cases were mainly caused by undetected negations in the text [36]. However, the number of misclassified reports should be reduced as much as possible to ensure that data is a valid representation of the pathologists' reports. More standardized procedures for data collection (e.g., avoiding negated diagnoses in the reports) could help to improve the classification performance of the text-mining tool and reduce bias in the data. Monitoring truly unclassified reports might be of value for animal health surveillance, as deaths caused by unknown pathogens might cause an increase in the number of reports in this category [25, 26].

The syndrome categories used in this study were primarily based on the topography of organ systems. The categories chosen are suitable for a wide range of situations and especially for non-specific health monitoring.

However, monitoring more specific disease conditions can have advantages. For example, abortions could be identified as a separate syndrome category instead of grouping them into the category reproductive disorders [59], or combining respiratory syndromes and reproductive disorders in pigs might help to monitor Porcine Reproductive & Respiratory Syndrome (PRRS). On the other hand, the more key terms that are grouped into one category, the fewer specific changes that can be detected within that category. For example, the category "other" covers a considerable number of key terms related to a broad range of topographical regions. An increase in a specific pathology, such as conjunctivitis or mastitis, might therefore be masked by the background noise in this category. Thus, further classifications could be necessary, depending on the surveillance objective and its required sensitivity. The text classifying tool used in this study was designed to be highly flexible [36] which means that it is possible to easily modify the syndrome categories in any way that fits with the data and the surveillance objectives. The syndromes that should be used and their characteristics should be determined by the specific goals of the surveillance system. So for example a surveillance system that has the goal of early detection of unusual, previously unseen disease could be based upon a syndrome or set of syndromes that include cases that were classified into the "other" category. These would include cases for which pathologists could not establish a pathological diagnosis [60].

Conclusion

In this study we have demonstrated that data can be extracted from free text necropsy reports, and that it could potentially be of value for animal health surveillance. The most frequent syndrome categories per species, sex and age, and their respective temporal patterns could serve as a basis for implementing a syndromic surveillance system. This information would not have been obtained without the use of text classification tool. While these methods and necropsy data have potential, the data does have biases and there are improvements that should be made to improve the validity of the data if their value is to be fully realized.

Abbreviations

AGIS: Agrarpolitical Information System; AI: Artificial insemination; FSVO: Federal Food Safety Authority; ICD: International Classification of Diseases; ITPA: Animal Pathology Institute University of Bern, Switzerland; NLP: Natural language processing; TVD: Swiss animal movement database (Tierverkehrsdatenbank)

Acknowledgments

We would like to thank Corinne Gurtner of the ITPA for helping to develop the terminology, Sara Schaerrer (FSVO) for extracting data from the TVD and Michael Binggeli (FSVO) for extracting data from the AGIS.

Funding

This study was funded by the FSVO.

Authors' contributions

FV and JB were responsible for the conception and design of the study. LF, SK and FR designed the text-mining system and created the terminological resource, which was approved and adapted by HP. SK, FV and CF actively participated in the analysis and data interpretation. All authors participated in organizing and drafting the manuscript and including updated information in it. Once completed, all authors read and approved the final manuscript.

Competing interests

The authors declare that they have no competing interests.

Author details

[1]Veterinary Public Health Institute, Vetsuisse Faculty, University of Bern, Schwarzenburgstrasse 155, 3097, Liebefeld, Switzerland. [2]Institute of Computational Linguistics, University of Zürich, Andreasstrasse 15, 8050 Zürich, Switzerland. [3]Institute of Animal Pathology, University of Bern, Länggassstrasse 122, 3012 Bern, Switzerland. [4]Present Address: Epi-Connect, Skogås, Sweden.

References

1. Henning KJ. What is syndromic surveillance? 2004. https://www.cdc.gov/mmwr/preview/mmwrhtml/su5301a3.htm. Accessed 20 Jan 2016.
2. Wendt A, Kreienbrock L, Campe A. Zoonotic disease surveillance - inventory of systems integrating human and animal disease information. Zoonoses Public Health. 2015;62:61–74.
3. Morse SS. Public health surveillance and infectious disease detection. Biosecur Bioterror. 2012;10:6–16.
4. Dórea FC, Sanchez J, Revie CW. Veterinary syndromic surveillance: current initiatives and potential for development. Prev Vet Med. 2011:1:1–17.
5. Dupuy C, Morignat E, Maugey X, Vinard J-L, Hendrikx P, Ducrot C, et al. Defining syndromes using cattle meat inspection data for syndromic surveillance purposes: a statistical approach with the 2005–2010 data from ten French slaughterhouses. BMC Vet Res. 2013;9:88.
6. Dórea FC, Vial F. Animal health syndromic surveillance: a systematic literature review of the progress in the last 5 years (2011–2016). Vet Med Res Reports. 2016;7:157–70.
7. Hulth A. First European guidelines on syndromic surveillance in human and animal health published. Euro Surveill. 2014;19:9806.
8. Vourc'h G, Bridges VE, Gibbens JC, De Groot BD, McIntyre L, Poland R, et al. Detecting emerging diseases in farm animals through clinical observations. Emerg Infect Dis. 2006;12:204–10.
9. Dórea FC, Revie CW, McEwen BJ, McNab WB, Kelton D, Sanchez J. Retrospective time series analysis of veterinary laboratory data: preparing a historical baseline for cluster detection in syndromic surveillance. Prev Vet Med. 2013;109:219–27.
10. Alton GD, Pearl DL, Bateman KG, McNab WB, Berke O. Factors associated with whole carcass condemnation rates in provincially-inspected abattoirs in Ontario 2001-2007: implications for food animal syndromic surveillance. BMC Vet Res. 2010;6:42.
11. Sanchez-Vazquez MJ, Strachan WD, Armstrong D, Nielen M, Gunn GJ. The British pig health schemes: integrated systems for large-scale pig abattoir lesion monitoring. Vet Rec. 2011;169:413–3.
12. Thomas-Bachli AL, Pearl DL, Friendship RM, Berke O. Suitability and limitations of portion-specific abattoir data as part of an early warning system for emerging diseases of swine in Ontario. BMC Vet Res. 2012;8:3.
13. Dupuy C, Morignat E, Dorea F, Ducrot C, Calavas D, Gay E. Pilot simulation study using meat inspection data for syndromic surveillance: use of whole carcass condemnation of adult cattle to assess the performance of several algorithms for outbreak detection. Epidemiol Infect. 2015;143:2559–69.
14. Vial F, Thommen S, Held L. A simulation study on the statistical monitoring of condemnation rates from slaughterhouses for syndromic surveillance: an evaluation based on Swiss data. Epidemiol Infect. 2015; https://doi.org/10.1017/S0950268815000989.

15. Perrin J-B, Ducrot C, Vinard J-L, Morignat E, Gauffier A, Calavas D, et al. Using the National Cattle Register to estimate the excess mortality during an epidemic: application to an outbreak of bluetongue serotype 8. Epidemics. 2010;2:207–14.
16. Alba A, Dórea F, Arinero L, Sanchez J, Cordón R, Revie C. Exploring the surveillance potential of mortality data: Nine years of bovine fallen stock data collected in Catalonia (Spain). 2015; doi:https://doi.org/10.1371/journal.pone.0122547.
17. Struchen R, Reist M, Zinsstag J, Vial F. Investigating the potential of reported cattle mortality data in Switzerland for syndromic surveillance. Prev Vet Med. 2015;121:1–7.
18. Tapprest J, Borey M, Dornier X, Morignat E, Calavas D, Hendrikx P, et al. Assessment of fallen equine data in France and their usefulness for epidemiological investigations. Res Vet Sci. 2016;104:96–9.
19. Avram C, Bosman A, Brusin S, Ciancio B, Coulombier D, Devaux I, et al. Data quality monitoring and surveillance system evaluation. Eur Cent Epidemiol. 2014; https://doi.org/10.2900/35329.
20. Mörner T, Obendorf DL, Artois M, Woodford MH. Surveillance monitoring of wildlife diseases. Rev Sci Tech. 2002;21:67–76.
21. O'Toole D. Monitoring and investigating natural disease by veterinary pathologists in diagnostic laboratories. Vet Pathol. 2010;47:40–4.
22. World Organization for Animal Health (OIE). Collection, Submission and Storage of Diagnostic Secimens. In: OIE. Manual of Diagnostic Tests and Vaccines for Terrestrial Animals Paris; 2012. p. 4.
23. Nietfeld JC. Field necropsy techniques and proper specimen submission for investigation of emerging infectious diseases of food animals. Vet Clin North Am Food Anim Pract. 2010;26:1–13.
24. Griffin D. Field necropsy of cattle and diagnostic sample submission. Vet Clin North Am Food Anim Pract. 2012;28:391–405.
25. van den Brom R, Luttikholt SJ, Lievaart-Peterson K, Peperkamp NH, Mars MH, van der Poel WH, et al. Epizootic of ovine congenital malformations associated with Schmallenberg virus infection. Tijdschr Diergeneeskd. 2012;137:106–11.
26. Seuberlich T, Wüthrich D, Selimovic-Hamza S, Drögemüller C, Oevermann A, Bruggmann R, et al. Identification of a second encephalitis-associated astrovirus in cattle. Emerg Microbes Infect. 2016; https://doi.org/10.1038/emi.2017.56.
27. McGreevy P, Thomson P, Dhand N, Raubenheimer D, Masters S, Mansfield C, et al. VetCompass Australia: a National big Data Collection System for veterinary science. Animals. 2017;7:74.
28. Palotay JL. SNOMED-SNOVET: an information system for comparative medicine. Med Inf 1983; 8:17–21+59.
29. Chen HCH, Zeng D. AI for global disease surveillance. IEEE Intell Syst. 2009; https://doi.org/10.1109/MIS.2009.126.
30. Kao A. Text mining and natural language processing: introduction for the special issue. SIGKDD Explor Newsl. 2005; https://doi.org/10.1145/1089815.1089816.
31. Lu H, Zeng D, Trujillo L, Komatsu K, Chen H. Ontology-enhanced automatic chief complaint classification for syndromic surveillance. J Biomed Inform. 2008;41:340–56.
32. Conway M, Dowling JN, Chapman WW. Using chief complaints for syndromic surveillance: a review of chief complaint based classifiers in North America. J Biomed Inform. 2013;46:734–43.
33. Zhang Y, Dang Y, Chen H, Thurmond M, Larson C. Automatic online news monitoring and classification for syndromic surveillance. Decis Support Syst. 2009;47:508–17.
34. Dórea FC, Muckle CA, Kelton D, McClure J, McEwen BJ, McNab WB, et al. Exploratory analysis of methods for automated classification of laboratory test orders into syndromic groups in veterinary medicine. PLoS One. 2013; https://doi.org/10.1371/journal.pone.0057334.
35. Arsevska E, Roche M, Hendrikx P, Chavernac D, Falala S, Lancelot R, et al. Identification of terms for detecting early signals of emerging infectious disease outbreaks on the web. Comput Electron Agric. 2016;123:104–15.
36. Furrer L, Küker S, Berezowski J, Posthaus H, Vial F, Rinaldi F. Constructing a syndromic terminology resource for veterinary text mining. Proc 11th Int Conf Terminol Artif Intell. 2015; https://doi.org/10.5167/uzh-114496.
37. R Core Team. R: A language and Enviroment for statistical Computing. Vienna: R Foundation for Statiscal Programming; 2016.
38. Wickham H. ggplot2: elegant graphics for data analysis. New York: Springer-Verlag; 2009.
39. Bivand R, Keitt T, Rowlingson B. Rgdal: bindings for the geospatial data abstraction Library 2016. https://cran.r-project.org/web/packages/rgdal/index.html. Acessed 04 June 2018.
40. Bivand R, Rundel C. rgeos: Interface to Geometry Engine - Open Source (GEOS). 2016. https://cran.r-project.org/web/packages/rgeos/index.html. Acessed 04 June 2018.
41. Neuwirth E. RColorBrewer: ColorBrewer Palettes. 2014. https://cran.r-project.org/web/packages/RColorBrewer/RColorBrewer.pdf . Acessed June 2018.
42. Zeileis A, Kleiber C, Jackman S. Regression models for count data in R. J Stat Softw. 2008;27(8):1–25.
43. Venables WN, Ripley BD. Modern applied statistics with S. 4th ed. New York: Springer; 2002.
44. Tierverkehrsdatenbank 2014. http://www.tierverkehr.ch. Accessed 20 Nov 2014.
45. Lawson AB, Kleinman K. Introduction: spatial and syndromic surveillance for public health. In: Lawson AB, Kleinman K, editors. Spatial and syndromic surveillance for public health. Chichester: John Wiley & Sons; 2005. p. 4.
46. Schärrer S, Widgren S, Schwermer H, Lindberg A, Vidondo B, Zinsstag J, et al. Evaluation of farm-level parameters derived from animal movements for use in risk-based surveillance programmes of cattle in Switzerland. BMC Vet Res. 2015;11:149.
47. Hoyt R, Yoshihashi A. Lessons learned from implementation of voice recognition for documentation in the military electronic health record system. Perspect Health Inf Manag. 2010;1e:7.
48. Ajami S. Use of speech-to-text technology for documentation by healthcare providers. Natl Med J India. 2016;29:148–52.
49. Identitas TVD App. 2012. https://play.google.com/store/apps/details?id=tvdapp.tvd&hl=de_CH. Acessed 04 June 2018.
50. Schärrer S, Presi P, Hattendorf J, Chitnis N, Reist M, Zinsstag J, et al. Demographic model of the Swiss cattle population for the years 2009-2011 stratified by gender, age and production type. PLoS One. 2014; https://doi.org/10.1371/journal.pone.0109329.
51. Stärk KDC, Nevel A. Strengths, weaknesses, opportunities and threats of the pig health monitoring systems used in England. Vet Rec. 2009;165:461–5.
52. O'Sullivan T, Friendship R, Pearl DL, McEwen B, Ker A, Dewey C. The association between submission counts to a veterinary diagnostic laboratory and the economic and disease challenges of the Ontario swine industry from 1998 to 2009. Prev Vet Med. 2012;106:275–83.
53. Tubbs RC. Preweaning morbidity and mortality in the United States swine herd. J Swine Heal Prod. 1993;1:21–8.
54. Busato A, Steiner L, Martin SW, Shoukri MM, Gaillard C. Calf health in cow-calf herds in Switzerland. Prev Vet Med. 1997;30:9–22.
55. Bähler C, Steiner A, Luginbühl A, Ewy A, Posthaus H, Strabel D, et al. Risk factors for death and unwanted early slaughter in Swiss veal calves kept at a specific animal welfare standard. 2012; 92:162–168.
56. Luginbühl A, Bähler C, Steiner A, Kaufmann T, Regula G, Ewy A. Ergebnisse der Integrierten Tierärztlichen Bestandesbetreuung in der Kälbermast. Schweiz Arch Tierheilkd. 2012;154:277–85.
57. Viviane de Vries. Erhebung von Organbefunden und Konfiskatabzügen von Schlachtschweinen an Schlachthöfen in der Schweiz und deren Korrelation mit Betriebs- und Managementdaten. 2010. http://www.zora.uzh.ch. Acessed 13 Aug 2016.
58. Katrin Pill. Untersuchungen zur Verwendung von klinischen und pathologisch/anatomischen Befunden am Schlachthof für die Einschätzung der Tiergesundheit und des Tierschutzes in Schweine- und Rinderbeständen. 2014. https://d-nb.info/1053385609/04Acessed 13 Aug 2016.
59. Bronner A, Morignat E, Fournié G, Vergne T, Vinard JL, Gay E, et al. Syndromic surveillance of abortions in beef cattle based on the prospective analysis of spatio-temporal variations of calvings. Sci Rep. 2015; https://doi.org/10.1038/srep18285.
60. Vial F, Berezowski J. A practical approach to designing syndromic surveillance systems for livestock and poultry. Prev Vet Med. 2015;120:27–38.

21

Expression kinetics of natural resistance associated macrophage protein (NRAMP) genes in *Salmonella* Typhimurium-infected chicken

Mashooq Ahmad Dar[1,2], Raashid Ahmed[1], Uneeb Urwat[1], Syed Mudasir Ahmad[1*], Pervaiz Ahmad Dar[3], Zahid Amin Kushoo[3], Tanveer Ali Dar[2], Peerzada Tajamul Mumtaz[1], Shakil Ahmad Bhat[1], Umar Amin[4], Nadeem Shabir[1], Hina Fayaz Bhat[1], Riaz Ahmad Shah[1], Nazir Ahmad Ganai[5] and Mohammad Heidari[6]

Abstract

Background: *Salmonella enterica serovar* Typhimurium (*Salmonella* Typhimurium) is a zoonotic pathogen responsible for severe intestinal pathology in young chickens. Natural resistance-associated macrophage protein (NRAMP) family has been shown to be associated with resistance to intracellular pathogens, including *Salmonella* Typhimurium. The role of NRAMP proteins in macrophage defence against microbial infection has been ascribed to changes in the metal-ion concentrations inside the bacteria-containing phagosomes. The present study was conducted to investigate tissue-specific (liver, spleen and caecum) expression kinetics of NRAMP gene family (NRAMP1 and NRAMP2) in broilers from day 0 to day 15 after *Salmonella* Typhimurium challenge concomitant to clinical, blood biochemical and immunological parameters survey.

Results: Clinical symptoms appeared 4 days post-infection (dpi) in infected birds. Symptoms like progressive weakness, anorexia, diarrhoea and lowering of the head were seen in infected birds one-week post-infection. On postmortem examination, liver showed congestion, haemorrhage and necrotic foci on the surface, while as the spleen, lungs and intestines revealed congestion and haemorrhages. Histopathological alterations were principally found in liver comprising of necrosis, reticular endothelial hyperplasia along with mononuclear cell and heterophilic infiltration. Red Blood Cell (RBC) count, Haemoglobin (Hb) and Packed Cell Volume (PCV) decreased significantly ($P < 0.05$) in blood while heterophil counts increased up to 7 days post-infection. Serum glucose, aspartate transaminase (AST) and alanine transaminase (ALT) enzymes concentrations increased significantly throughout the study. A gradual increase of specific humoral IgG response confirmed *Salmonella* infection. Meanwhile, expression of NRAMP1 and NRAMP2 genes was differentially regulated after infection in tissues such as liver, spleen and caecum known to be the target of *Salmonella* Typhimurium replication in the chicken.

Conclusion: Thus the specific roles of NRAMP1 and NRAMP2 genes in Salmonella Typhimurium induced disease may be supposed from their differential expression according to tissues and timing after per os infection. However, these roles remain to be analyzed related to the severity of the disease which can be estimated by blood biochemistry and immunological parameters.

Keywords: *Salmonella* Typhimurium, Poultry, Histopathology, Biochemistry, Real time expression, NRAMP

* Correspondence: mudasirbio@gmail.com
[1]Division of Biotechnology, Faculty of Veterinary Sciences and Animal Husbandry, Shuhama, Sher-e- Kashmir University of Agricultural Sciences and Technology – Kashmir, Srinagar, India
Full list of author information is available at the end of the article

Background

Salmonella is an intracellular pathogenic, gram negative, facultative anaerobe, non-spore forming, and usually motile bacilli that leads to salmonellosis in the host. Among the different diseases occurring in poultry, those caused by the genus *Salmonella* are the most common, causing serious economic losses to the poultry industry in terms of mortality, reduced growth and loss in egg production [1]. Salmonella infection can reach eggs either through vertical or horizontal transmission thus making it an important zoonotic disease [2]. Salmonellosis is a big socioeconomic threat worldwide that causes considerable mortality and morbidity in both humans and animals [3]. Owing to growing public health concern, prevention of foodborne transmission of *Salmonella* spp. remains one of the major foci for the poultry sector [4]. The gastrointestinal (GI) tract of newly hatched chickens is usually sterile and presents an empty ecological niche that provides easy access for the pathogen to colonize with limited restriction making them highly susceptible to enteric bacterial infections, such as *Salmonella* [5]. After ingestion, the bacteria can survive the acidic pH of the stomach and is taken via microfold (M)-cells and reach liver and spleen through the hepatic portal system where the bacteria multiply in macrophages of reticuloendothelial system [6]. Many genes such as Major Histocompatibility Complex (MHC), Caspasel, NRAMP Family, inducible nitric oxide synthase (iNOS), those encoding complement proteins and Toll-like Receptor 4 (TLR4) have been found to be associated with resistance against *Salmonella* infection in poultry [7].

The Solute Carrier Family (SLC11A), formerly known as natural resistance associated macrophage protein family functions as metal ion transporters in diverse organisms from bacteria to human [8]. Iron is essential for the survival of bacteria inside the macrophages and any impairment in iron homeostasis may promote inappropriate immune responses thereby affecting the host resistance to infectious diseases [9]. Iron transporter natural resistance-associated macrophage protein 1 (NRAMP1/SLC11A1), the member of the solute carrier (SLC11A) family of ion transporters [10] has certain genotypes that provide resistance to wide range of intracellular pathogens including *Salmonella* Typhimurium [11]. NRAMP1 is an antiporter, expressed on phagosomes and primary phagolysosomes [12] that transports iron into the phagosome [13], where it catalyzes the Haber-Weiss reaction [14]. This results in an increase in the production of highly microbicidal hydroxyl radicals that inhibit bacterial growth. SLC11A2 formerly known as NRAMP2/ DMT1 is ubiquitously expressed in all tissues including the brush border of intestinal epithelial cells and is involved in transport of divalent cations into the cytosol of cells as well as intestinal absorption of iron, while as NRAMP1 has more restricted expression but is especially associated with myeloid lineage cells and the liver, thymus and spleen [15–18]. Polymorphisms in the NRAMP1 gene have been found to be significantly associated with caecal *Salmonella* colonization, and expression of NRAMP1 gene can accelerate inflammatory responses in caecum [19]. NRAMP1 plays an important role in modulating the growth of bacteria that reach the reticuloendothelial system during early infection [20]. Association of NRAMP1 Ser^{379} polymorphism with *Salmonella* colonization of the spleen has been found in young chickens and also linkage analysis studies have shown that NRAMP1 is associated with resistance in *Salmonella* Typhimurium-infected chicken and mice [21–23]. NRAMP2 is expressed in almost all tissues in *Salmonella*-infected chicken [24]. However, detailed studies of expression kinetics of NRAMP genes in liver and spleen (that form the hepatoportal system) and caecum in chicken at different days post *Salmonella* Typhimurium infection has not been carried out. Thus, the present study was conducted to investigate the mRNA expression kinetics of NRAMP1 and NRAMP2 in liver, spleen and caecum of birds challenged with *Salmonella* Typhimurium in relation with blood physiological and immunological parameters along with the disease severity.

Methods

Experimental birds

Cobb breeding flock procured from the Hariparbat hatchery Srinagar, Department of Animal Husbandry government of Jammu and Kashmir, India, was maintained under strict hygienic conditions at the experimental housing of Faculty of Veterinary Science and Animal Husbandry, Sher-e-Kashmir University of Agricultural Sciences and Technology, Kashmir, India and the work was agreed upon by the Institutional Animal Ethics Committee on ethical standards in animal experimentation (No: AU/FVS/PS-57/4461) (IAEC/15/01).

Salmonella Typhimurium strain

For the development of infection in experimental birds, *Salmonella* Typhimurium was isolated in the field from fecal and liver samples of salmonellosis-suspected chicks at the Division of Veterinary Pathology, F.V.Sc and AH, Shuhama, Srinagar Jammu and Kashmir-India. Samples were inoculated in tetrathionate broth (TTB) and incubated at 37 °C for 48 h. The cultures were identified by a method as recommended [25]. The *Salmonella* Typhimurium was confirmed by PCR as described previously [26] and biochemical (IMViC) tests. For further confirmation serotyping was done at National Salmonella and Escherichia Centre (NSEC), Himachal Pradesh, India.

Experimental design

A total of 170 one day-old chickens were divided into two groups (control and infected) and were checked to be free of *Salmonella* infection before the challenge. After three days of acclimatization, the chicks in the infected group were challenged orally with 2×10^8 CFU of *Salmonella* Typhimurium. Chicks in the control group were given 1 ml of nutrient broth.

Confirmation of infection

Faecal swabs were taken 12 h after infection and cultured in TTB broth and incubated for 18 h at 37 °C. The growth of TTB broth was streaked on BGA and MacConkey agar. These plates were incubated for 24–48 h at 37 °C. The plates were examined for typical colonies of *Salmonella* i.e. pale colonies on MacConkey agar, pink colonies on Brilliant Green Agar (BGA).

Sampling

The birds were euthanized with CO_2 and subsequently sharp cut was made in the neck to drain blood from vessels. Blood samples were collected for blood cell enumeration and biochemical analysis, and organs (liver, spleen and caecum) were collected for histopathological and gene expression studies from 6 birds randomly selected in each group at 0, 1, 3, 5, 7, 9, 11, 13 and 15 days post infection. For real time gene expression, tissue samples were collected in Trizol (Invitrogen, USA) and stored at − 80 °C for RNA extraction. The blood samples were analyzed for haemoglobin (Hb), packed cell volume (PCV), red blood cell (RBC) count, white blood cell (WBC) count, heterophils and lymphocyte count using Sysmex (KX-21) automated haematology analyzer. Serum samples were analyzed for alanine transaminase (ALT), aspartate transaminase (AST), total protein, serum albumin and glucose using commercially available kits.

Histopathology

For histopathological studies, representative liver tissue samples from infected and control birds were collected and fixed in 10% neutral buffered formalin. These were processed for paraffin embedding using alcohol as dehydrating agent and benzene as the clearing agent. The sections were cut at 4–5 μm thickness and stained by the routine haematoxylin and eosin method [27].

Enzyme linked immunosorbent assay (ELISA)

Indirect ELISA was performed to detect the anti-Salmonella IgG antibodies in serum as per the method described [28]. Sonicated *Salmonella* Typhimurium (20 ng/100 μl) was used as antigen. One hundred μl of goat anti-chicken antibody (Sigma 1:15000) diluted in PBS-T (Phosphate buffered saline -tween) was added to each well and plate was incubated at 37 °C for 2 h. Plates were washed with PBS Tween-20 (0.05%) and incubated with 100 μl O-phenylene diamine dihydrochloride in the dark at room temperature for 15 min. The reaction was stopped by adding 2 N H_2SO_4 @ 50 μl per well. Absorbance was determined using ELISA reader (PerkinElmer) at 492 nm. Known positive ($n = 5$) and known negative ($n = 22$) controls were used in this study. The specificity was statistically calculated as.

Specificity = $T_N/T_N + F_P$.

Where T_N denotes total negatives and F_P denotes false positives.

Gene expression analysis

RNA extraction

Total RNA was extracted from the tissue samples by Trizol method (Invitrogen, USA) as per manufacturer's protocol. The quantity and quality of isolated RNA were checked at 260 and 280 nm with UV–Visible spectrophotometer. Prior to cDNA synthesis, RNA samples were run on 1% agarose gel. DNase treatment using DNase1 kit (Sigma, USA) was given to rule out any genomic DNA contamination.

cDNA synthesis

cDNA synthesis was done with an equal concentration of RNA (1.5 μg) in all the samples using Thermo Scientific RevertAid First Strand cDNA Synthesis Kit™ (Lithuania) using oligo dT primers following manufacturer protocol. In conventional PCR, all primers produce only one amplification band visualized by agarose gel electrophoresis, indicating the specificity of the amplification. The primers used for NRAMP1 and β-actin gene amplification were already reported [24]. Primers for NRAMP2 were designed using PRIMER 3 Plus. (Table 1).

Table 1 List of primers used for real time PCR

Target	Primer sequence (5′→3′)		Size of Amplicon	T_m °C	Reference
β Actin	Forward primer	TGGCATTGCTGACAGGAT	160 bp	63.1	[24]
	Reverse primer	CTGCTTGCTGATCCACAT		60.0	
NRAMP1	Forward primer	CCCCCACATCACCCCGTCC	180 bp	74.2	[24]
	Reverse primer	GGCCCCACACTGCAGGTCTGAC		74.4	
NRAMP2	Forward primer	GTACTCAGGGCAGTTCGTCA	162 bp	63.0	This study
	Reverse primer	GCACGTTGAGGAAGTCGTTC		64.8	

Quantitative PCR

For real time PCR, β-actin was used as internal control and SYBR green as fluorescent dye to quantify the mRNA level of chicken NRAMP1 and NRAMP2 genes by RT-PCR analysis. To confirm reproducibility, all determinations were performed at least two times. The reaction mixture contained 10 μL 2X Q-PCR SYBR Green Mix (Roche), 0.3 μL 10 μM of each primer, 8.9 μL ultrapure RNase-free water, and 0.5 μL cDNA to a final volume of 20 μL. Running program was performed in a Light cycler 480 II (Roche). All Aliquots were then amplified by 40 cycles of denaturation at 95 °C for 5 min, annealing at 60 °C for 15 s and extension at 72 °C for 15 s. Melting curve analysis was performed to confirm the specificity of the product. NRAMP1 and NRAMP2 mRNA relative expression was indicated by $2^{-\Delta\Delta C_T}$, where $\Delta\Delta C_T$ corresponded to the difference between the C_T measured for the mRNA level of each tissue and the C_T measured for the mRNA level of the reference tissue, $\Delta C_T = C_T$ (target gene) - C_T (β-actin).

Statistical analysis

The data obtained in the current study was analyzed using a computer-aided statistical software package SPSS 20.0. The differences between means were analyzed by unpaired Student's t-test and by one way ANOVA followed by Fisher's LSD test and significance was determined at $P < 0.05$.

Results

Clinical signs

After inoculating 2×10^8 CFU of *Salmonella* Typhimurium, clinical symptoms appeared within 4 dpi and included dullness, depression, inappetence and reluctance to move with both eyes closed. After one week of infection, birds showed progressive weakness, anorexia, increased thirst, diarrhoea, dropping of wings, ruffled feathers and lowering of the head.

Gross pathology

The birds in the control group did not exhibit any gross lesion in any of the organs examined throughout the experimental trial. However, in infected birds, liver revealed severe congestion, haemorrhages and enlargement. Congestion of liver was observed up to 15 dpi. Formation of pinpoint foci on the surface of the liver was observed at 9 dpi. Spleen and lungs of infected birds revealed congestion and haemorrhages from 1 to 15 dpi. Mild catarrhal enteritis, congestion and severe haemorrhages throughout the intestinal tract were noticed. Mostly, severe haemorrhages were observed in the second week post-infection.

Histopathology

Liver of birds infected with *Salmonella* Typhimurium revealed congestion of blood vessels at all time points. Chicks mostly showed degeneration of hepatic parenchyma along with distortion of hepatic cords and leukocytic infiltration comprising of lymphocytes and heterophils at 13 dpi (Fig. 1a, b).

Haematology

The haematological results are presented in Table-2. The mean values of Hb, RBC and PCV were significantly lower ($P < 0.05$) in the infected group as compared to control group starting day 1 post-infection. There was a significant decrease in the lymphocyte count in the infected birds as compared to their respective controls ($P < 0.05$). After an initial decrease, recovery in the number of circulating lymphocytes in infected birds was observed. Further there was a significant increase in the heterophil count in the infected birds compared to their respective controls up to day 5 post- infection, followed by a gradual increase thereafter. (Table 2).

Serum biochemical profile

The mean values of glucose levels were significantly elevated in the infected birds when compared to their respective controls starting day 1 post-infection. Serum protein contents were lower in the infected group when compared with corresponding values in the control group after day 0 post-infection, as shown in Table 3. Similarly, mean values of serum albumin were significantly lower ($P < 0.05$) in the infected group at almost all intervals except at 0 dpi where no significant changes were seen. The AST and ALT in the infected group showed a sharp and significant increase ($P < 0.05$) when compared to their respective controls from day 1 post infection till the end of the experiment (Table 3).

Elisa

Specific serum (IgG) antibody response to *Salmonella* Typhimurium as the mean OD values of the chicks challenged orally with *Salmonella* Typhimurium increased from 0.0545 to 0.2088 up to 15 dpi as shown in Fig. 2. The overall antibody (IgG) response of the infected group was found to be statistically significant ($P < 0.05$). The mean OD values of the infected group were higher as compared to their respective controls.

NRAMP gene family mRNA expression

The mRNA expression levels of NRAMP1 and NRAMP2 increased significantly at all time intervals starting day 1post-infection. Following infection with *Salmonella* Typhimurium, expression of NRAMP1 mRNA was significantly up-regulated in all the three tissues (liver, spleen, caecum) compared to control group. Peak expression of NRAMP1

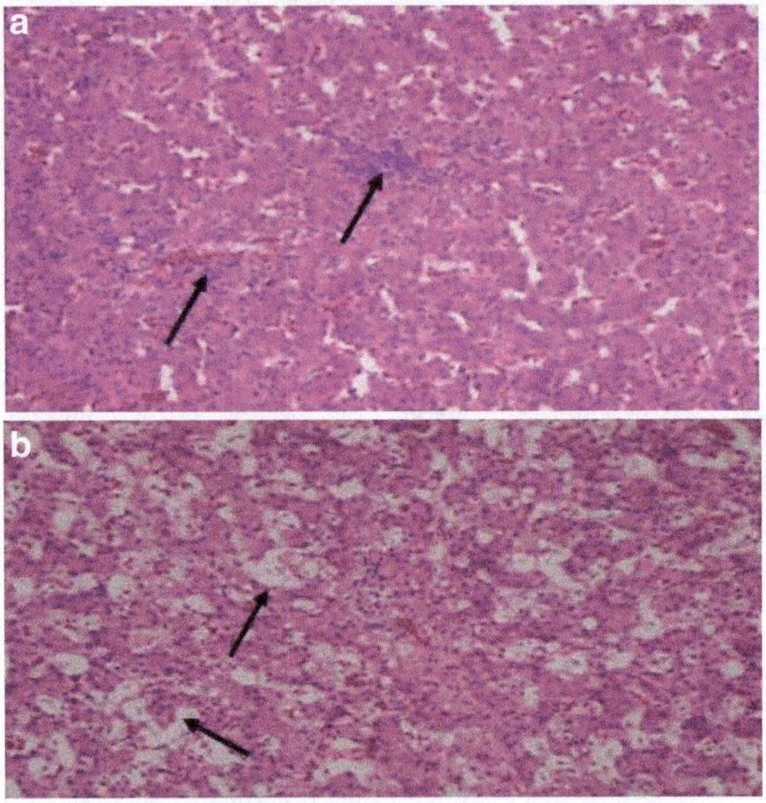

Fig. 1 a Histopathological examination of liver showing leukocytic infiltration of the infected birds at 13 dpi. H&E × 10. **b** Histopathological examination showing hepatic parenchyma degeneration in infected birds at 13 dpi. H&E × 10

was found on day 3 in liver (37 fold, $P < 0.05$) (Fig. 3a), day 5 in spleen (247 fold, $P < 0.05$) (Fig. 3b) and on day 7 in caecum (144 fold, $P < 0.05$) (Fig. 3c). Similarly, expression of NRAMP2 mRNA was significantly up-regulated in infected birds from day 1 up to day 9 (32 fold, $P < 0.05$) in liver (Fig. 3a), up to day 5 (20 fold, $P < 0.05$) in the spleen (Fig. 3b) and up to day 9 (359 fold, $P < 0.05$) in caecum (Fig. 3c). After day 9 in liver and caecum and day 5 in the spleen, NRAMP2 mRNA started returning to basal levels in the infected birds.

Discussion

Although expression pattern of disease resistance genes against *Salmonella* Typhimurium infection has been studied in mammals [8, 19, 22], information regarding tissue-specific expression of these genes is poorly available in poultry. The non-specific clinical observations that we observed in our study were similar to the earlier studies [29, 30] and clinical signs of ruffled feathers, dullness and diarrhoea were also found in Fowl typhoid outbreak [31]. It was also reported in *Salmonella* Typhimurium infection, chicken showed high mortalities, decreased body weight, lameness, inappetence, conjunctivitis, respiratory manifestation, and pasty diarrhoea [32]. In post-mortem examination of infected birds, we observed congestion and haemorrhages in spleen and lungs, whereas necrosis, congestion and haemorrhages followed by leukocytic infiltration primarily seen in liver, as also reported previously [33, 34]. Small intestines revealed mild catarrhal enteritis, congestion and severe haemorrhages mostly in the second week of infection, as that of earlier reports [35, 36].

Haematological profile in animals is an important indicator of the physiological or pathophysiological status of the body [37]. In the present study, we observed that the mean haematological values of Hb, RBC and PCV decreased markedly after *Salmonella* Typhimurium infection. Similar findings were also reported in Japanese quail infected with Salmonella enteric Serovar Gallinarum [38]. The mean values of Hb and PCV showed marked decrease from day 0 to day 9 post-infection in infected group. As with PCV, younger chicken have lower total erythrocyte count and mean corpuscular heamoglobin (MCH) than adult ones [39]. A decrease in Hb and PCV in broiler chicken infected with Fowl typhoid was also reported earlier [33]. Heterophils display high phagocytic and killing activity. Thus an increase of blood heterophil number is an indication of acute infection and tissue damages [39]. Our observations related to heterophil and lymphocyte counts coincide with earlier

Table 2 Effect of *Salmonella* Typhimurium infection on haematological parameters at different days post infection (dpi)

Parameter	Group (Control ($N = 6$) (Infected ($N = 6$)	0 (dpi)	1 (dpi)	3 (dpi)	5 (dpi)	7 (dpi)	9 (dpi)	11 (dpi)	13 (dpi)	15 (dpi)
RBC (10^6/μl)	Control	1.745^a ± 0.024	1.860^a ± 0.021	1.941^a ± 0.025	2.031^a ± 0.024	2.045^a ± 0.038	2.108^a ± 0.023	2.155^a ± 0.032	2.228^a ± 0.032	2.265^a ± 0.021
	Infected	1.723^a ± 0.008	1.700^b ± 0.020	1.671^b ± 0.014	1.655^b ± 0.024	1.623^b ± 0.100	1.585^b ± 0.009	1.615^b ± 0.023	1.633^b ± 0.013	1.658^b ± 0.027
Haemoglobin (g/dl)	Control	10.018^a ± 0.226	10.621^a ± 0.118	11.04^a ± 0.13	11.790^a ± 0.147	12.011^a ± 0.126	12.343^a ± 0.059	12.516^a ± 0.060	12.553^a ± 0.104	12.800^a ± 0.064
	Infected	10.001^a ± 0.211	9.368^b ± 0.078	9.041^b ± 0.074	8.880^b ± 0.105	8.806^b ± 0.074	8.675^b ± 0.070	8.791^b ± 0.023	8.830^b ± 0.038	8.963^b ± 0.063
PCV (%)	Control	26.656^a ± 0.055	26.855^a ± 0.076	27.29^a ± 0.070	27.590^a ± 0.123	27.805^a ± 0.143	28.080^a ± 0.061	28.258^a ± 0.057	28.628^a ± 0.109	28.990^a ± 0.170
	Infected	26.605^a ± 0.042	26.263^b ± 0.053	25.91^b ± 0.113	25.743^b ± 0.079	25.470^b ± 0.057	25.141^b ± 0.080	25.365^b ± 0.059	25.408^b ± 0.048	25.446^b ± 0.063
WBC (10^3/μl)	Control	20.125^a ± 0.390	20.828^a ± 0.385	21.48^a ± 0.325	21.675^a ± 0.276	21.730^a ± 0.599	22.038^a ± 0.720	22.396^a ± 0.324	23.010^a ± 0.474	23.160^a ± 0.426
	Infected	20.303^a ± 0.248	27.085^b ± 0.300	32.76^b ± 0.399	38.368^b ± 0.431	36.160^b ± 0.318	34.060^b ± 0.320	32.556^b ± 0.486	27.980^b ± 0.444	25.046^b ± 0.416
Heterophils (10^3/μl)	Control	10.545^a ± 0.079	10.46^a ± 0.077	10.35^a ± 0.065	10.293^a ± 0.059	10.183^a ± .037	10.030^a ± 0.047	9.676^a ± 0.100	9.393^a ± 0.064	9.180^a ± 0.036
	Infected	10.531^a ± 0.079	15.055^b ± 0.100	21.32^b ± 0.038	26.146^b ± 0.018	23.205^b ± 0.017	20.465^b ± 0.032	18.140^b ± 0.033	17.185^b ± 0.027	15.963^b ± 0.161
Lymphocytes (10^3/μl)	Control	6.888^a ± 0.010	7.170^a ± 0.020	7.330^a ± 0.012	7.518^a ± 0.009	7.796^a ± 0.014	8.170^a ± 0.017	8.340^a ± 0.020	8.513^a ± 0.014	8.930^a ± 0.050
	Infected	6.873^a ± 0.026	6.583^b ± 0.208	5.755^b ± 0.318	4.970^b ± 0.110	8.453^b ± 0.178	10.773^b ± 0.279	12.833^b ± 0.335	15.188^b ± 0.362	17.115^b ± 0.471

Values are presented as mean ± SE

Values having different superscript (a and b) differ significantly ($P < 0.05$)

Number of birds from each group that were evaluated at each time point (dpi) was 6, each sample was run in duplicates. Statistical analysis was done using unpaired Student's t-test and by one way ANOVA followed by Fisher's LSD test

Table 3 Effect of *Salmonella* Typhimurium infection on serum biochemical parameters at different days post infection (dpi)

Parameter	Group (Control ($N = 6$) (Infected ($N = 6$)	0 (dpi)	1 (dpi)	3 (dpi)	5 (dpi)	7 (dpi)	9 (dpi)	11 (dpi)	13 (dpi)	15 (dpi)
ALT (IU/L)	Control	$8.98^{a} \pm 0.097$	$9.27^{a} \pm 0.123$	$9.40^{a} \pm 0.135$	$9.63^{a} \pm 0.138$	$9.76^{a} \pm 0.097$	$10.05^{a} \pm 0.085$	$10.19^{a} \pm 0.109$	$10.43^{a} \pm 0.124$	$10.87^{a} \pm 0.175$
	Infected	$9.08^{a} \pm 0.138$	$25.62^{b} \pm 0.221$	$45.60^{b} \pm 0.380$	$63.90^{b} \pm 0.219$	$67.88^{b} \pm 0.237$	$73.96^{b} \pm 0.317$	$78.34^{b} \pm 0.218$	$82.41^{b} \pm 0.276$	$86.28^{b} \pm 0.364$
AST (IU/L)	Control	$39.20^{a} \pm 0.127$	$39.99^{a} \pm 0.282$	$41.08^{a} \pm 0.388$	$42.94^{a} \pm 0.178$	$42.94^{a} \pm 0.452$	$43.45^{a} \pm 0.405$	$44.34^{a} \pm 0.261$	$45.45^{a} \pm 0.332$	$46.06^{a} \pm 0.251$
	Infected	$39.77^{a} \pm 0.177$	$44.48^{b} \pm 0.638$	$49.73^{b} \pm 0.779$	$54.46^{b} \pm 0.910$	$67.27^{b} \pm 1.136$	$77.81^{b} \pm 0.438$	$90.26^{b} \pm 0.535$	$108.44^{b} \pm 0.763$	$120.81^{b} \pm 0.862$
Albumin (g/dl)	Control	$0.848^{a} \pm 0.006$	$0.888^{a} \pm 0.004$	$0.901^{a} \pm 0.003$	$0.927^{a} \pm 0.003$	$0.964^{a} \pm 0.002$	$0.985^{a} \pm 0.003$	$1.011^{a} \pm 0.006$	$1.063^{a} \pm 0.008$	$1.111^{a} \pm 0.013$
	Infected	$0.839^{a} \pm 0.005$	$0.837^{b} \pm 0.001$	$0.845^{b} \pm 0.001$	$0.851^{b} \pm 0.001$	$0.871^{b} \pm 0.001$	$0.891^{b} \pm 0.002$	$0.911^{b} \pm 0.004$	$0.932^{b} \pm 0.002$	$0.950^{b} \pm 0.001$
Protein (g/dl)	Control	$1.698^{a} \pm 0.004$	$1.756^{a} \pm 0.006$	$1.876^{a} \pm 0.008$	$1.990^{a} \pm 0.012$	$2.051^{a} \pm 0.013$	$2.150^{a} \pm 0.005$	$2.215^{a} \pm 0.008$	$2.365^{a} \pm 0.007$	$2.543^{a} \pm 0.014$
	Infected	$1.680^{aa} \pm 0.003$	$1.726^{b} \pm 0.004$	$1.745^{b} \pm 0.008$	$1.798^{b} \pm 0.009$	$1.816^{b} \pm 0.009$	$1.861^{b} \pm 0.003$	$1.925^{b} \pm 0.004$	$1.981^{b} \pm 0.007$	$2.021^{b} \pm 0.017$
Glucose (mg/dl)	Control	$145.31^{a} \pm 0.672$	$155.94^{a} \pm 0.407$	$162.1^{a} \pm 0.667$	$170.44^{a} \pm 0.322$	$195.60^{a} \pm 0.440$	$210.54^{a} \pm 0.211$	$235.52^{a} \pm 0.588$	$256.00^{a} \pm 0.470$	$275.84^{a} \pm 0.741$
	Infected	$148.36^{a} \pm 0.297$	$170.89^{b} \pm 0.672$	$178.7^{b} \pm 0.759$	$197.51^{b} \pm 0.634$	$211.34^{b} \pm 0.978$	$232.04^{b} \pm 0.293$	$247.13^{b} \pm 0.694$	$269.92^{b} \pm 0.297$	$290.03^{b} \pm 0.752$

Values are presented as mean ± SE

Values having different superscript (a and b) differ significantly ($P < 0.05$)

Number of birds from each group that were evaluated at each time point (dpi) was 6, each sample was run in duplicates. Statistical analysis was done using unpaired Student's t-test and by one way ANOVA followed by Fisher's LSD test

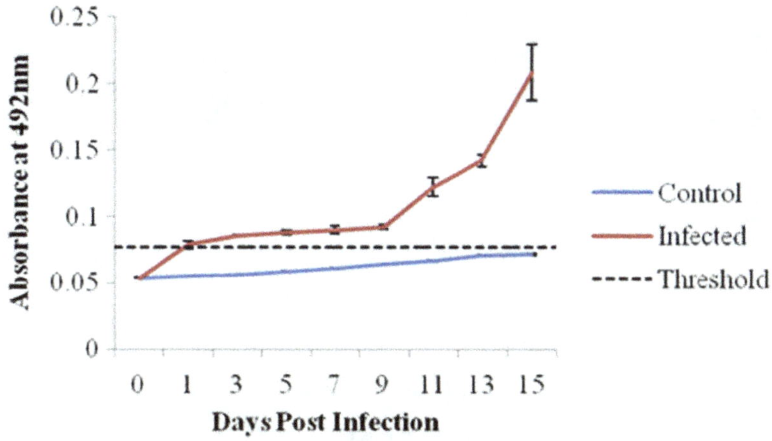

Fig. 2 Level of Salmonella Typhimurium specific IgG response (mean OD ± SEM) detected in sera of Salmonella Typhimurium infected chicks and their respective uninfected controls at 0,1,3,5,7,9,11,13 and 15 days post infection (dpi). Number of birds from each group that were evaluated at each time point (dpi) was 6, each sample was run in duplicates. Statistical analysis was done using unpaired Student's t-test and by one way ANOVA followed by Fisher's LSD test

studies for increased blood heterophils and lymphocytes counts in Fowl typhoid infection [33].

Serum biochemistry profiling is a major tool to identify the occurrence of acute infection in birds and mammals to predict the severity of disease [40]. The increase in serum glucose of infected chickens is possibly due to increased expression of glucose transporters in intestinal tract plus more glucose consumption for bacterial replication within macrophages [41, 42]. A decrease in serum protein and albumin levels has also been reported in chicken infected with acute fowl typhoid [33, 43]. The significant decrease in protein and albumin could be due to severe liver and kidney damage of infected birds that resulted in the failure of synthesis of plasma proteins and protein loss or decreased appetite [44]. Elevation in AST and ALT in infected birds is possibly due to hepatocellular damage with alteration in cell membrane permeability and leakage of cytoplasmic ALT into the blood [45]. Elevation in AST levels has also been reported in fowl typhoid infection of chicken [33].

Strong antigen-specific cell and humoral immune responses have both been temporally linked to clearance of *Salmonella* Typhimurium infection in chicks [46]. Oral infection of chickens with *Salmonella* Typhimurium stimulates systemic immunity and a significant increase of specific humoral response after 10 days post *Salmonella* Typhimurium infection was found in the present study. These results are in conformity with other studies showing a steady increase in specific IgG and/or IgA starting one week after infection in chickens with *Salmonella* Enteritidis [47] and *Salmonella* Typhimurium [48].

In the present study, during the early stages of *Salmonella* Typhimurium infection, mRNA expression of NRAMP1 upregulated significantly in all the three tissues under study which dropped to the basal expression levels thereafter. NRAMP1 has a major effect on survival of chicken during the first phase of *Salmonella* Typhimurium infection [22]. Previous studies using mouse models have shown that NRAMP1 is involved in the control of exponential growth of bacteria in reticuloendothelial organs and has also been found to be involved in *Salmonella* clearance [20, 49]. Our findings were in accordance with the earlier studies that showed that there occurs a rapid increase in NRAMP1 expression in the lamina propia of caecum following infection with *Salmonella* Typhimurium and further suggesting a role of NRAMP1 in the early inflammatory response [50]. NRAMP genes often show tissue-specific expression [51]. In the present study, the NRAMP2 mRNA expression showed an initial upregulation in all the tissues of infected birds under study. In agreement with our results, an increased mRNA expression of both NRAMP2 and NRAMP1 following infection of macrophages with the intracellular bacterium *Mycobacterium avium* has been found [22]. Also, lipopolysaccharide (LPS) stimulation resulted in increased NRAMP2 mRNA expression in mice macrophages [52]. NRAMP2 is expressed in the intestinal tract where it plays an important role in iron uptake and in liver NRAMP2 is responsible for iron transport from endosomes into the intracellular space [53, 54]. Unlike earlier studies on Partridge chicken, where the expression of NRAMP genes was found predominantly in liver and spleen compared to caecum [24], we found mRNA expression of NRAMP1 and NRAMP2 in salmonella-infected birds was predominant in caecum which was followed by liver and spleen. The differences of expression levels in various tissues could

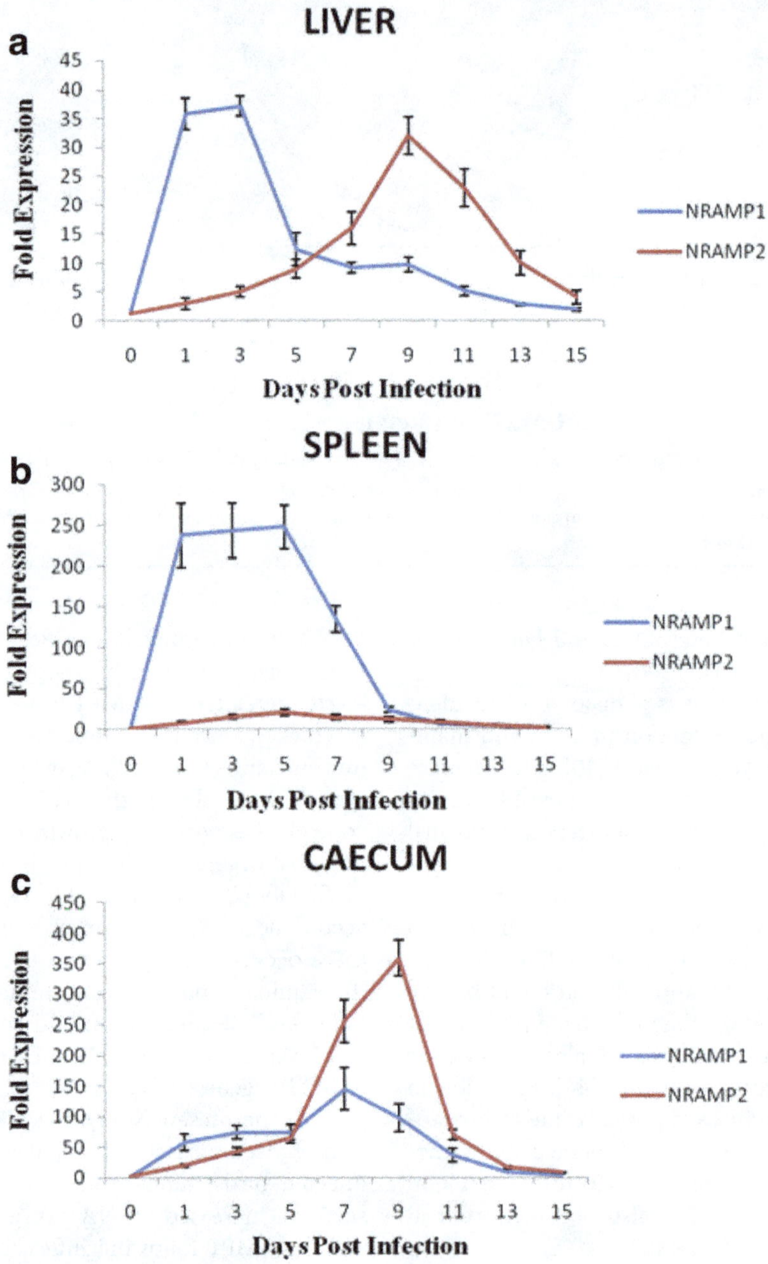

Fig. 3 a mRNA expression of NRAMP1 and NRAMP2 at 0,1,3,5,7,9,11,13 and 15 days post infection (dpi) in liver of birds infected with *Salmonella* Typhimurium. The values are expressed as mean fold expression±standard error of mean. Number of birds from each group that were evaluated at each time point (dpi) was 6, each sample was run in duplicates. Statistical analysis was done using unpaired Student's t-test and by one way ANOVA followed by Fisher's LSD test. **b** mRNA expression of NRAMP1 and NRAMP2 at 0,1,3,5,7,9,11,13 and 15 days post infection (dpi) in spleen of birds infected with *Salmonella* Typhimurium. The values are expressed as mean fold expression±standard error of mean. Number of birds from each group that were evaluated at each time point (dpi) was 6, each sample was run in duplicates. Statistical analysis was done using unpaired Student's t-test and by one way ANOVA followed by Fisher's LSD test. **c** mRNA expression of NRAMP1 and NRAMP2 at 0,1,3,5,7,9,11,13 and 15 days post infection (dpi) in caecum of birds infected with *Salmonella* Typhimurium. The values are expressed as mean fold expression±standard error of mean. Number of birds from each group that were evaluated at each time point (dpi) was 6, each sample was run in duplicates. Statistical analysis was done using unpaired Student's t-test and by one way ANOVA followed by Fisher's LSD test

be due to the higher colonization of *Salmonella* Typhimurium in lower GIT followed by dispersion to peripheral organs and response to defence signals in various tissues. NRAMP genes have an important role in iron homeostasis as discussed in the background of the manuscript, so evaluating the role of NRAMP family in the regulation of serum and cellular iron in a state of bacterial infection can open new avenues to investigate the role of iron metabolism in bacterial infection in the chicken model.

Conclusion

In conclusion, the significant increase in mRNA expression of NRAMP genes in caecum, liver and spleen of the infected chicken could enhance our understanding the importance of NRAMP genes in salmonellosis. With further well designed studies and thorough validation, the present study may serve as a base in development of blood markers for genetic selection of *Salmonella* resistant chicken with respect to NRAMP polymorphisms and iron metabolism. Additionally, blood investigations for biochemical and haematological parameters may aid in monitoring the physiological and pathological changes in *Salmonella* infection in poultry.

Abbreviations

ALT: Alanine transaminase; ANOVA: Analysis of variance; AST: Aspartate transaminase; cDNA: Complementary deoxyribonucleic acid; CFU: Colony forming unit; CO_2: Carbon dioxide; C_T: Threshold value; DMT: Divalent metal ion transporter; dpi: Days post infection; FP: False positives; GIT: Gastrointestinal tract; Hb: Haemoglobin; Ig: Immunoglobulin; LPS: Lipopolysaccharide; LSD: Least square difference; MCH: Mean corpuscular heamoglobin; mRNA: Messenger ribonucleic acid; NRAMP: Natural resistance-associated macrophage protein; NSEC: National Salmonella and Escherichia Centre; OD: Optical density; PBS-T: Phosphate buffered saline; PCV: Packed cell volume; RBC: Red blood cells; RNA: Ribonucleic acid; SLC: Solute carrier; SLC: Solute carrier; SPSS: Statistical package for social sciences; TN: Total negatives; WBC: White blood cell

Acknowledgements

We are highly thankful to Prof. Shakil Ahmad Wani, Faculty of Veterinary science and AH, SKUAST-Kashmir for his suggestions and providing microbiology laboratory facilities. We appreciate the help and support provided by Dean Faculty of Veterinary science and AH, SKUAST-Kashmir.

Authors' contributions

MAD, RA and UU helped in expression studies, acquisition, analysis and interpretation of data. SMA designed the experiment and overall coordinated the project. PAD, ZAK and UA helped in microbiological, infectious dose preparation, and histopathological studies. NS, TAD, PTM and SAB helped in drafting of manuscript and manuscript revision. HF, RAS, NAG and MH helped in statistical analysis and proofreading of the manuscript. All authors read and approved the final manuscript.

Competing interests

The authors declare that they have no competing interests.

Author details

[1]Division of Biotechnology, Faculty of Veterinary Sciences and Animal Husbandry, Shuhama, Sher-e- Kashmir University of Agricultural Sciences and Technology – Kashmir, Srinagar, India. [2]Depatment of Biochemistry, University of Kashmir, Srinagar, India. [3]Division of Veterinary Microbiology, Faculty of Veterinary Sciences and Animal Husbandry, Shuhama, SKUAST-K, Srinagar, India. [4]Division of Veterinary Pathology, Faculty of Veterinary Sciences and Animal Husbandry, Shuhama, SKUAST-K, Srinagar, India. [5]Division of Animal Breeding and Genetics, Faculty of Veterinary Sciences and Animal Husbandry, Shuhama, SKUAST-K, Srinagar, India. [6]USDA, Agricultural Research Service, Avian Disease and Oncology Laboratory, 4279 E. Mount Hope Rd., East Lansing, MI 48823, USA.

References

1. Dar MA, Ahmad SM, Bhat SA, Ahmad R, Urwat U, Mumtaz PT, Bhat SA, Dar TA, Shah RA, Ganai NA. *Salmonella* typhimurium in poultry: a review. Worlds Poult Sci J. 2017;73:345–54.
2. Vivek VP, Rebecca LD, Pardeep S, Andrea RM, Kapil KC. Study of Salmonella typhimurium infection in laying hens. Front Microbiol. 2016;7:203.
3. Smith SI, Seriki A, Ajayi A. Typhoidal and non-typhoidal *Salmonella* infections in Africa. Eur J Clin Microbiol Infect Dis. 2016;35:1913–22.
4. Oliveira DD, Silva EN. Salmonella in table eggs: occurrence in retails, storage conditions and eggshell disinfections. Arq Bras Med Vet Zootec. 2000;52:6.
5. Crhanova M, Hradecka H, Faldynova M, Matulova M, Havlickova H, Sisak F, Rychlik I. Immune response of chicken gut to natural colonization by gut microflora and to Salmonella enterica serovar enteritidis infection. Infect Immun. 2011;79:2755–63.
6. Niedergang F, Sirard JC, Blanc CT, Kraehenbuhl JP. Entry and survival of Salmonella typhimurium in dendritic cells and presentation of recombinant antigens do not require macrophage-specific virulence factors. Proc Natl Acad Sci. 2000:14650–5.
7. R T, Idris IB, Malar PJ, Hair BM. The effects of polymorphisms in 7 candidate genes on resistance to Salmonella Enteritidis in native chickens. Poult Sci. 2013;92:900–9.
8. Nevo Y, Nelson N. The NRAMP family of metal-ion transporters. Biochimica et Biophysica Acta (BBA)-Mol Cell Res. 2006;(7):609–20.
9. Wessling RM. Nramp1 and other transporters involved in metal withholding during infection. J Biol Chem. 2015;290:18984–90.
10. Horin P, Matiasovic J. Two polymorphic markers for the horse SLC11A1 (NRAMP1) gene. Anim Genet. 2000;31:152.
11. G F, Nairz M, Libby SJ, Fang FC, Weiss G. Slc11a1 (Nramp1) impairs growth of Salmonella enterica serovar typhimurium in macrophages via stimulation of lipocalin-2 expression. J Leukoc Biol. 2012;92:353–9.
12. Gruenheid S, Pinner E, Desjardins M, Gros P. Natural resistance to infection with intracellular pathogens: the Nramp1 protein is recruited to the membrane of the phagosome. The J Exp Med. 1997;185:717–30.
13. Kuhn DE, Baker BD, Lafuse WP, Zwilling BS. Differential iron transport into phagosomes isolated from the RAW264. 7 macrophage cell lines transfected with Nramp1Gly169 or Nramp1Asp169. J Leukoc Biol 1999;66:113–119.
14. Zwilling BS, Kuhn DE, Wikoff L, Brown D, Lafuse W. Role of iron in Nramp1-mediated inhibition of mycobacterial growth. Infect Immun. 1999;67:1386–92.
15. Blackwell JM, Goswami T, Carlton AW, Sibthorpe D, Papo N, Jacqueline K, Susan SE, Miller N, Christopher SP, Mohammed H, Ibrahim M. SLC11A1 (formerly NRAMP1) and disease resistance. Cell Microbiol. 2001;3:773–84.
16. Canonne-Hergaux F, Gruenheid S, Ponka P, Gros P. Cellular and subcellular localization of the Nramp2 iron transporter in the intestinal brush border and regulation by dietary iron. Blood. 1999;93:4406–17.
17. Fleet JC. Identification of Nramp2 as an iron transport protein: another piece of the intestinal iron absorption puzzle. Nutr Rev. 1998;56:88–9.
18. Wood RJ, Han O. Recently identified molecular aspects of intestinal iron absorption. J Nutr. 1998;128:1841–4.
19. Paul W. Genetic resistance to Salmonella infection in domestic animals. Res Vet Sci. 2004;76:165–9.
20. Vidal SM, Malo D, Vogan K, Skamene E, Gros P. Natural resistance to infection with intracellular parasites: isolation of a candidate for Bcg. Cell. 1993;73:469–85.
21. W L, Kaiser MG, Lamont SJ. Natural resistance-associated macrophage protein 1 gene polymorphisms and response to vaccine against or challenge with Salmonella enteritidis in young chicks. Poult Sci. 2003;82:259–66.
22. Hu J, Bumstead N, Barrow P, Sebastiani G, Olien L, Morgan K, Malo D. Resistance to salmonellosis in the chicken is linked to NRAMP1 and TNC. Genome Res. 1997;7:693–704.
23. Vidal SM, Gros P, Skamene E. Natural resistance to infection with intracellular parasites: molecular genetics identifies Nramp1 as the Bcg/Ity/Lsh locus. J Leukoc Biol. 1995;58:382–90.
24. He XM, Fang MX, Zhang ZT, Hu YS, Jia XZ, He DL, Liang SD, Nie QH, Zhang XQ. Characterization of chicken natural resistance-associated macrophage

protein encoding genes (Nramp1 and Nramp2) and association with salmonellosis resistance. Genet Mol Res. 2013;12:618–30.
25. Edwards PR, Ewing WH. Identification of Enterobacteriaceae, Burgess Publication Company, Minneapolis, Minnesota. 3rd ed; 1972.
26. Wani SA, Hussain I, Beg SA, Rather MA, Kabli ZA, Mir MA, Nishikawa Y. Diarrhoeagenic Escherichia coli and salmonellae in calves and lambs in Kashmir: absence, prevalence and antibiogram. Rev sci tech Off int Epiz. 2013;32:1–7.
27. Luna LG. Manual of histologic staining methods of the armed forces institute of pathology. 3rd ed. New York, NY: McGraw-Hill; 1968.
28. Holt PS, Gast RK, Porter RE, Stone HD. Hyporesponsiveness of the systemic and mucosal humoral immune systems in chickens infected with Salmonella enterica serovar enteritidis at one day of age. Poult Sci. 1999;78:1510–7.
29. Shivprasad HL. Fowl typhoid and pullorum disease. Review Science Technology. 2000;19:405–24.
30. Chacana PA, Terzolo HR. New light on old views of avian Pullorosis: avian Typhosis. Rev Inst Med Trop. 2003;84:14–20.
31. Bhattacharya A, Majumder P, Isolation DMK. Characterization and antibiotic spectra of S. Gallinarum from an outbreak of fowl typhoid in adult broiler parent flock in Tripura. Indian j. Comp. Microbiol. Immunol Infect Dis. 2001;22:56–8.
32. Sharkawy H, Tahoun A, Gohary AE, Abasy M, Khayat F, Gillespie T, Kitade Y, Hafez HM, Neubauer H, Adawy H. Epidemiological, molecular characterization and antibiotic resistance of Salmonella enterica serovars isolated from chicken farms in Egypt. Gut Pathog. 2017;10:8.
33. Shah SN, Kamil SA, Darzi MM, Mir MS, Bhat SA. Haematological and some biochemical changes in experimental fowl typhoid infection in broiler chickens. Comp Clin Path. 2013;22:83–91.
34. Chishti MA, Khan MZ, Irean M. Pathology of liver and spleen in avian salmonellosis. Pak Vet J. 1985:5157–60.
35. Parsons BN, Humphrey S, Salisbury AM, Mikoleit J, Hinton JC, Gordon MA, Wigley P. Invasive non-typhoidal Salmonella typhimurium ST313 are not host-restricted and have an invasive phenotype in experimentally infected chickens. PLoS Negl Trop Dis. 2013;77:10.
36. Withanage GS, Kaiser P, Wigley P, Powers C, Mastroeni P, Brooks H, Barrow P, Smith A, Maskell D, McConnell I. Rapid expression of chemokines and proinflammatory cytokines in newly hatched chickens infected with Salmonella enterica serovar typhimurium. Infect Immun. 2004;72:2152–9.
37. Khan AT, Zafar F. Hematological study in response of varying doses of estrogen in broiler chicken. Int J Poult Sci. 2005;4:748–51.
38. Barde JO, Bale O, Oladele SB, Fatihu MY, Kumbish PR, Rimfa AG, Teki IS, Moses GD, Ahmed JS, Okewole PA. Study of some Haematological parameters of Japanese quail (Coturnix coturnix japonica) experimentally infected with Salmonella enterica Serovar Gallinarum. Annu res rev biol. 2015;7:222–8.
39. Greenacre CB, Morishita Y, editors. Backyard poultry medicine and surgery, a guide for veterinary practitioners. Ames: John Wiley and Sons Inc; 2015.
40. Smith CM, Reynard A. Text Book of Pharmacology, W. B. Saunders, London, 1992.
41. Feng Y, Yang XJ, Wang YB, Li WL, Liu Y, Yin RQ, Yao JH. Effects of immune stress on performance parameters, intestinal enzyme activity and mRNA expression of intestinal transporters in broiler chickens. ASIAN AUSTRAL J ANIM. 2012;25:701.
42. Bowden SD, Rowley G, Hinton JC, Thompson A. Glucose and glycolysis are required for the successful infection of macrophages and mice by Salmonella enterica serovar typhimurium. Infect and immunity. 2009;77:3117–26.
43. Kokosharov T. Bacterial colonization and endotoxin activity during experimental acute fowl typhoid in chickens. Onder J Vety Res. 2000;67:297.
44. Coles EH. Vet Clin Pathol, 4th edn. Saunders WB Company, Philadelphia, 1986: 486.
45. Benjamin MN. Outline of veterinary clinical pathology, University, Iowa; 1978. p. 229–32.
46. Saif YM, Barnes HJ, Glisson Glisson RJ, Fadly MA, RL MD, Swayne ED. Diseases of Poultry. 11th ed.
47. Olabisi IO, Peter HS. Salmonella Enteritidis experimental infection in chickens; effects of challenge dose on serum immunoglobulin G antibody response. Afr J Biotechnol. 2008;20:3783–7.
48. Hassan JO, Barrow PA, Mockett APA, McLeod S. Antibody response to experimental *Salmonella* typhimurium infection in chickens measured by ELISA. Vet Rec. 1990;12:519–22.
49. Caron J, Loredo-Osti JC, Laroche L, Skamene E, Morgan K, Malo D. Identification of genetic loci controlling bacterial clearance in experimental Salmonella enteritidis infection: an unexpected role of Nramp1 (Slc11a1) in the persistence of infection in mice. Genes Immun. 2002;(4):196–204.
50. Yanet V, Guntram AG, Julian AG, Bryan C, Phillipe G, Bruce AV, Brett F. Nramp1 drives an accelerated inflammatory response during Salmonella-induced colitis in mice. Cell Microbiol. 2009;11:351–62.
51. Xiangjun Z, Yang Y. Differential expression of rice Nramp genes in response to pathogen infection, defense signal molecules and metal ions. Physiol Mol Plant Pathol. 2004;65:235–43.
52. Wardrop SL, Richardson DR. Interferon-g and lipopolysaccharide regulate the expression of Nramp2 and increase the uptake of iron from low relative molecular mass complexes by macrophages. Eur J Biochem. 2000;267:6586–93.
53. Simovich MJ, Conrad ME, Umbreit JN, Moore EG, Hainsworth LN, Smith HK. Cellular location of proteins related to iron absorption and transport. Am J Hematol. 2002;69:164–70.
54. Foot NJ, Gembus KM, Mackenzie K, Kumar S. Ndfip2 is a potential regulator of the iron transporter DMT1 in the liver. Sci Rep. 2016;6:24045.

Computer simulation of syringomyelia in dogs

Srdjan Cirovic[1*], Robert Lloyd[1,5], Jelena Jovanovik[3], Holger A. Volk[4] and Clare Rusbridge[2,3]

Abstract

Background: Syringomyelia is a pathological condition in which fluid-filled cavities (syringes) form and expand in the spinal cord. Syringomyelia is often linked with obstruction of the craniocervical junction and a Chiari malformation, which is similar in both humans and animals. Some brachycephalic toy breed dogs such as Cavalier King Charles Spaniels (CKCS) are particularly predisposed. The exact mechanism of the formation of syringomyelia is undetermined and consequently with the lack of clinical explanation, engineers and mathematicians have resorted to computer models to identify possible physical mechanisms that can lead to syringes. We developed a computer model of the spinal cavity of a CKCS suffering from a large syrinx. The model was excited at the cranial end to simulate the movement of the cerebrospinal fluid (CSF) and the spinal cord due to the shift of blood volume in the cranium related to the cardiac cycle. To simulate the normal condition, the movement was prescribed to the CSF. To simulate the pathological condition, the movement of CSF was blocked.

Results: For normal conditions the pressure in the SAS was approximately 400 Pa and the same applied to all stress components in the spinal cord. The stress was uniformly distributed along the length of the spinal cord. When the blockage between the cranial and spinal CSF spaces forced the cord to move with the cardiac cycle, shear and axial normal stresses in the cord increased significantly. The sites where the elevated stress was most pronounced coincided with the axial locations where the syringes typically form, but they were at the perimeter rather than in the central portion of the cord. This elevated stress originated from the bending of the cord at the locations where its curvature was high.

Conclusions: The results suggest that it is possible that repetitive stressing of the spinal cord caused by its exaggerated movement could be a cause for the formation of initial syringes. Further consideration of factors such as cord tethering and the difference in mechanical properties of white and grey matter is needed to fully explore this possibility.

Keywords: Cavalier king Charles spaniels, Mathematical modelling, Chiari malformation, Pathophysiology, Syrinx

Background

Syringomyelia is a severe progressive pathological condition characterised by the presence of abnormal fluid-filled cavities (singular syrinx and plural syringes) within the spinal cord [1–8]. Clinical signs of syringomyelia include pain, loss of sensation, and motor dysfunction [2]. Syringomyelia affects both humans and animals (mainly dogs and cats) [9–11]. In humans, syringomyelia has a low prevalence of about one in 10,000 [3, 4]. In contrast, in some toy breed of dogs such as Cavalier King Charles Spaniels (CKCS), King Charles spaniels, Griffon Bruxellois, Maltese, Chihuahuas, and Pomeranians the prevalence is high. In the CKCS up to 70% of the total population is affected by the condition although in many dogs it may be asymptomatic [12]; in the Griffon Bruxellois, 50% of the American population was affected with again many dogs being asymptomatic [11].

Syringomyelia is associated with the obstruction of CSF channels and the subarachnoid space (SAS), particularly if the obstruction is at the foramen magnum [4]. The most common cause of foramen magnum obstruction in humans is Chiari malformation and in animals the analogous condition, Chiari-like malformation, to which brachycephalic toy breed dogs such as Cavalier King Charles Spaniels (CKCS) are particularly predisposed [13]. A common feature of Chiari-like malformation in several toy breeds is occipital

* Correspondence: s.cirovic@surrey.ac.uk
[1]The Centre for Biomedical Engineering, University of Surrey, Guildford GU2 7XH, UK
Full list of author information is available at the end of the article

bone hypoplasia and reduced caudal fossa volume associated with a compensatory increase in height of the cranial fossa [14]. Traits that increase the risk of syringomyelia in CKCS include brachycephaly with rostral displacement of the atlas and axis, acute angulation between the sphenoid and basioccipital bone, reduced occipital crest and increased cervical flexure and odontoid (dens) angulation [14–17]. Chiari-like malformation is analogous to Chiari type 1 and 0 malformation in humans which is also associated with syringomyelia [18].

The pathogenesis of syringomyelia is still unknown and this ultimately compromises the effectiveness of clinical (surgical) management of syringomyelia [2, 4, 8, 19]. It is widely believed that variation to the normal flow pathways of the cerebrospinal fluid (CSF) plays the main role in the formation and expansion of syringes [20]. CSF constantly moves in a pulsatile manner between the cranial and spinal SAS via the foramen magnum to compensate for transient shifts in the cranial blood volume associated with the arterial pulse [21, 22]. In Chiari malformation, the obstruction of the foramen magnum compromises the normal communication between the cranial and spinal CSF compartments [3, 23]. Similarly, stenoses in the SAS due to traumatic injury obstruct the flow of CSF [4]. In-vivo and in-vitro experiments [24–27] indicate that such blockages can result in pressure dissociation in the SAS and in excessive motion of the spinal cord [28]. Typically, syringes form caudally from a blockage. In dogs most affected with syringomyelia, the emergence and progression of cavities has a breed-related pattern. Thus, for example in Cavalier King Charles Spaniels the initial cavities usually first emerge in the cranial-cervical and thoracic-spinal cord segments (C1-C4 and T1-T4, respectively) [29]. The twelfth thoracic-second lumbar (T12-L2) segment is also a common site where syringes may form [29]. By comparison, in some breeds such as Griffon Bruxellois the cavities are often widest in the cervicothoracic junction and cranial thoracic region (unpublished data). In humans the analogous condition Chiari-I malformation is more likely to be associated with a cervical syringe [30].

Early theories on the origins of syringomyelia speculated that syringes form because bulk CSF flow is redirected to the central canal of the spinal cord which is connected with the ventricular system of the brain [1, 25]. However, these theories were abandoned since they could not account for non-caninular syringes (not continuous with the central canal) or syringes emerging in the absence of a patent central canal [20]. Current theories focus mainly on the accumulation of fluid into the spinal cord parenchyma [31–37] and on excessive stressing of the spinal cord tissue [38–40]. Most of the current theories are derived from in-vitro and computer models that can simulate propagation of CSF pulse waves in the spine under various scenarios [31–35, 38–50]. These models can capture the interaction between elastic structures (spinal cord and dura) and the CSF as well as predict spatial and temporal variation of parameters such as CSF pressure, CSF velocity, and stress in the spinal cord. Cirovic et al. [41, 49], and Bertram et al. [39, 51] used mathematical/computer models to identify four pulse modes in the spinal cord. Three of the four modes are involved in the movement of the CSF and have speeds of the order of several metres per second. More recently Støverud et al. predicted pulse speeds between 2 and 5 m/s using an anatomically realistic computer model of poroelastic spinal cord [52]. The findings from the computer modelling studies are consistent with the pulse speed data obtained from in-vivo human and animal experiments [24, 53, 54]. Elliot [40] further examined the pulse modes and concluded that stenoses in the SAS lead to elevated stress in the cord which is released with the emergence of a syrinx (branding this "a homeostatic mechanism for syringomyelia"). Bertram developed a fluid-structure interaction computer model of the human spinal cavity that included the cord with a syrinx, the SAS fluid compartment, and the elastic dura [38, 39, 45]. The model geometry was idealised to be axisymmetric neglecting the spinal curvature. He concluded that arachnoiditis can lead to excessive stressing of the cord, and that the sloshing of the fluid in an existing syrinx can induce stresses at the caudal end of the syrinx. Recently, Bertram and Heil [32, 35] extended Bertram's original model to examine the case of a stenosis overlaying a large syrinx for a poro-elastic spinal cord. They concluded that this situation results in a "diastolic valve" that may pump small amounts of fluid from the SAS to the syrinx with each cardiac cycle. While these results are promising, they mainly apply to the enlargement of an existing syrinx or a "presyrinx" (an initial state of increased fluid in the spinal cord [55]) rather than with its emergence. None of the models convincingly explain why syringes emerge at specific anatomical locations even in the absence of arachnoiditis or an initial small "pre-syrinx".

We hypothesize that preferential locations for the emergence of syringes may be related to the curvature of the spine. This cannot be examined with existing computer models of syringomyelia since they all approximate the spinal cord as a straight cylindrical structure. In order to investigate this possibility, we constructed a three-dimensional computer model of the canine spine. The CKCS spine was chosen for the study due to a high prevalence of syringomyelia in this breed and because of a highly regular pattern in the development of cavities in the spinal cord.

Methods

The dynamics of the canine spinal cord was investigated using a finite element model of a canine spinal cavity.

The finite element method is an approximate method for solving engineering problems involving complex geometries and material properties that cannot be solved analytically. In this method, the domain of interest is "discretized" by breaking it into a large number of small geometric components called "elements". For each element in the model, simplifying approximations are applied to the equations governing the mechanical behaviour of the system examined. The resulting set of equations involving all the elements is solved using computers to yield quantities such as displacement, speed, strain and stress in each element.

The model

The computational model was developed from a CKCS with a Chiari-like malformation and fully developed syrinx (C2-L3; Fig. 1a). The geometry of the spinal canal was extracted from T2-weighted transverse anatomical magnetic resonance imaging (MRI) scans. The imaging was obtained as part of the necessary diagnostic work and consent was obtained from the owner. Due to the size of the subject, two series of transverse scans were compiled to cover the full length of the spine (C1 – S1) at 5 mm intervals with a 10% interslice gap. During the MRI scan the dog was placed in dorsal recumbency with its pelvic limbs extended caudally on the scanning couch, with the spine being as straight as possible to avoid any external distortions of the images. The following T2-weighted imaging parameters were applied: Time to Repetition (TR) 3200, Echo Time (TE) 102, Field of View (FOV) 150, matrix resolution 384 × 320, and averages 5, using combination of spine table integrated coil and torso array coil for maximum signal collection.

In order to reduce the complexity of the model and create a high quality mesh, the components of the spinal canal were assumed to be circular and concentric. Previous studies have demonstrated that the CSF pressures are relatively unaffected by the concentricity and shape of the anatomic layers [56, 57]. The geometry of the spinal canal (C2 - S1) was manually segmented using the Simpleware software package (Simpleware Ltd., Exeter, UK) generating two-dimensional (2D) transverse masks for the following components of the spinal canal; the epidural space (EDS), the subarachnoid space, the spinal cord and the syrinx cavity (Fig. 1b). The 2D masks were exported into ImageJ, an open source image processing platform [58], to calculate the cross-sectional areas and the corresponding radii of each component. The centroids of the spinal cord masks were assumed to be the centres for all components. The reconstructed geometric data is summarised in Table 1 and in the Additional file 1.xlsx. A volumetric model was generated in ANSYS (ANSYS Inc., Pittsburgh USA) by connecting the transverse sections with splines. It was found that it is sufficient to use only 13 sections to construct a smooth three-dimensional geometry that conforms well with the reconstructed 68 transverse sections (see Table 1). The spine was assumed to be symmetric about the mid-sagittal plane and mediolateral motion was neglected. The cranial end of the model was extended by 15 mm (transparent section in

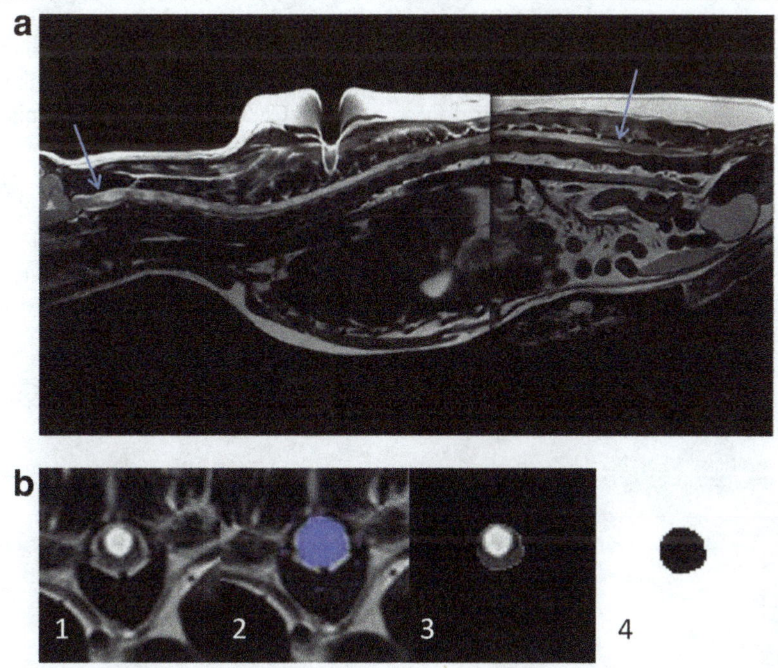

Fig. 1 **a** T2-weighted mid-sagittal MRI of a CKCS suffering from a large syrinx (syrinx ends indicated with arrows). **b** The geometry reconstruction process. 68 transverse plane scans were obtained (1). Each anatomical layer was segmented to create a mask (2). The mask was filtered out (3) and then binarised (4) to create a pure black and white image

Table 1 Geometric parameters of the model

x [mm]	y[mm]	R_syrinx [mm]	R_cord [mm]	R_SAS [mm]	R_EDS [mm]
0	0	2.2	4.5	6.4	7.2
20	3.4	3.7	4.6	5.6	6.3
45	−7.9	4.5	5.1	6.3	7.1
75	−22.8	2.5	4.3	5.6	6.2
95	−24.2	2.6	3.8	5.1	6.0
125	−20.0	3.0	3.6	4.5	5.4
170	−9.3	3.1	3.5	4.6	5.5
205	−5.7	2.7	3.3	4.3	5.1
245	−12.0	3.0	3.7	4.9	5.5
275	−22.3	2.4	3.9	5.3	6.2
285	−25.7	1.8	4.1	5.2	6.2
325	−35.2	–	2.5	4.0	5.0
335	−34.5	–	–	3.8	4.3

Coordinates of the centroids and radii of the syrinx, cord, SAS, and EDS used in the model. The x coordinate is in the cranial-to-caudal direction. The y coordinate is in the ventral-to-dorsal direction. The raw data for syrinx, cord, and SAS radii and centroids are given in the Additional file 1

Fig. 2). This was done to remove spurious stress concentrations which would form in the cranial end of spine if the model was loaded directly at the C2 section of the model. Hexagonal "brick" elements of 0.5 mm overall size were used to discretize the model. The element size was chosen so that each layer has at least two elements across the thickness. The finite element model comprised of 903,232 elements in total. Figure 2 detail A shows all the layers in the final model, with the finite element mesh. The dura mater was modelled as a layer of shell elements with 1 mm thickness between the SAS and the EDS.

The mechanical properties for the materials of the layers comprising the model were taken from the published literature [20]; the cord, dura, and the epidural fat were represented as linear elastic solids, and the CSF was represented as an inviscid fluid with the compressibility equal to that of water (Table 2). Treating CSF as inviscid in the first approximation is justified since the pulsatile flow of the CSF in the spine is dominated by inertia rather than viscous effects [56]. From a practical point of view, inviscid approximation was useful since it allowed for the simultaneous solution of solid and fluid equations using a Lagrangian approach. The model was constrained from moving at the outer edge of the EDS to account for the constraint imposed by the vertebrae. Constraint to movement was also imposed to the caudal ends of the spinal cord and the SAS.

Simulations

An input with amplitude and frequency representative of CSF movement generated by the arterial pulse in the cranium were used to excite the model. This was done by imposing a sinusoidal volumetric flow with a period of 0.4 s (150 beats per minute as the upper limit of heart rate for CKCS [59]) and an amplitude of 0.35 cm^3/s. This resulted in a peak CSF speed of about 0.02 m/s which is within a physiologically plausible range [28, 53, 56, 60–62]. The volumetric input was applied at the cranial end of the extruded section of the model. Three extreme hypothetical situations were considered by varying the boundary conditions at the cranial end of the extruded section and by excluding or including the syrinx:

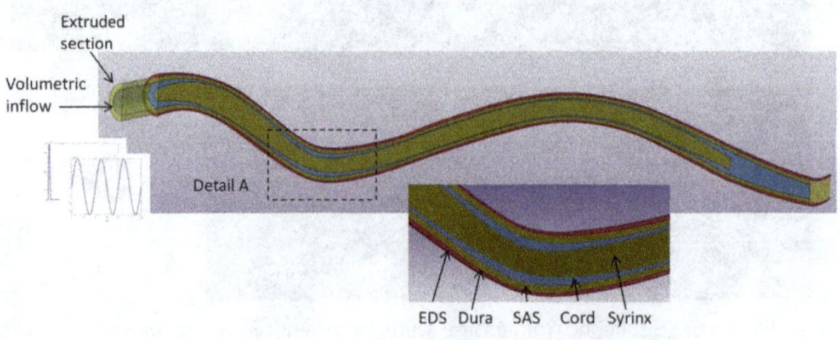

Fig. 2 The finite element model of the CKCS suffering from a large syrinx. The anatomical layers are indicated in Detail A. The transparent cranial segment was added to the original geometry and the inputs were applied at its cranial end

Table 2 Material properties

Spinal cord	E = 62.5 kPa, ν = 0.49, ρ = 1000 kg/m^3
Dura	E = 1.25 MPa, ν = 0.4, ρ = 1000 kg/m^3
EDS fat tissue	E = 1 kPa, ν = 0.25, ρ = 900 kg/m^3
CSF and the fluid in the syrinx	K = 2.2 GPa, G = 0, ρ = 1000 kg/m^3

Material properties of the anatomical layers. E = Young's modulus, ν = Poisson's ratio, K = bulk modulus, G = shear modulus, ρ = density

1) Cord without syrinx; cranial end of the cord constrained from movement and the CSF allowed to flow freely at the cranial end (representing the normal condition).
2) Cord without syrinx; cranial end of the cord allowed to move freely and the CSF blocked at the cranial end (representing Chiari with the syrinx still not formed).
3) Cord with syrinx; cranial end of the cord allowed to move freely and the CSF blocked at the cranial end (representing Chiari with the syrinx formed).

Prior to applying the above listed scenarios, a preliminary simulation was run in which the model was excited with a short transient pulse of 0.01 s duration and 0.35 cm^3/s volumetric flow amplitude. This was done to test if the model can predict the pulse modes reported in the published theoretical and computational studies. All simulations were performed using the LS-DYNA finite element package for dynamic simulations (LS-DYNA Version 971, Livermore Software Technology Corp., Livermore, CA).

Results

Figure 3 shows the distribution of the axial (cranial-to-caudal) component of speed for a short pulse excitation. Only the syrinx, cord, and SAS layers are shown since the movement in the EDS was very small. At 5 ms after the excitation, there was a single disturbance at the cranial end of the model. At 25 ms that disturbance split into three waves that moved at different speeds and covered different distances. For the fastest wave modes, all three layers moved in the same (caudal) direction. For the second fastest mode, the fluids in the syrinx and SAS moved in the opposite direction from the spinal cord. For the slowest mode, the syrinx and the spinal cord moved in the opposite direction from the CSF in the SAS. From the distance covered and the time elapsed, the speeds of the three modes can be estimated to be approximately 1.5 m/s, 7 m/s, and 11 m/s. The speed of movement of the tissues in the anatomical layers of the spine generated by the pulse modes is of the order of 10^{-2} m/s (see Fig. 3).

The "cardiac" excitation of the model generated an oscillatory motion of the SAS and/or spinal cord at the cranial end of the model. For the "normal condition" the peak speed of the CSF at the cranial end of the SAS was approximately 0.02 m/s. The amplitude of the speed in the SAS diminished in a linear way from the cranial to the caudal end. For the "Chiari" conditions, the peak speed of the cord at the cranial end was just below 0.01 m/s and the same linear tendency of amplitude decrease towards the caudal end was observed. In all three cases considered, the excitation resulted in harmonic pressure fluctuations in the SAS with a peak amplitude of approximately 400 Pa (about 3 mmHg). The pressure amplitude was approximately constant along the length of the spine; the pressure gradient between the cranial and the caudal ends did not exceed 0.5 mmHg over the cardiac cycle.

Figure 4 shows the distribution of stress in the cord along the axis of the spine for the three inputs. The displayed results were obtained in the following way: for each element comprising the discretized spinal cord, a stress-versus-time curve was obtained and the peak value of stress was determined. Next, the cord was divided into segments of one millimetre width in the cranial-to-caudal direction and the maximal value of peak stress recorded in the elements within each segment was determined. Thus, each point in a curve represents the maximal value of stress within a 1 mm thick slice of the cord over the whole simulated event. Please note that the normal stresses in the

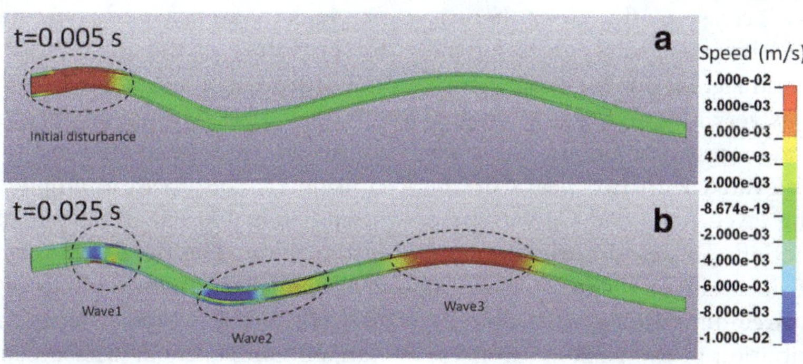

Fig. 3 Axial (cranial-to-caudal) speed of tissue movement in the spinal column due to a short transient cranial excitation. **a** At $t = 0.005$ s from the onset of excitation an initial disturbance with the amplitude of 0.01 m/s (1 cm/s) formed at the cranial end. **b** At $t = 0.025$ s the initial disturbance split into three waves which travelled at speeds of 1.5 m/s (wave 1), 7 m/s (wave 2), and 11 m/s (wave 3). The waves generated tissue movement in the range of ±0.01 m/s

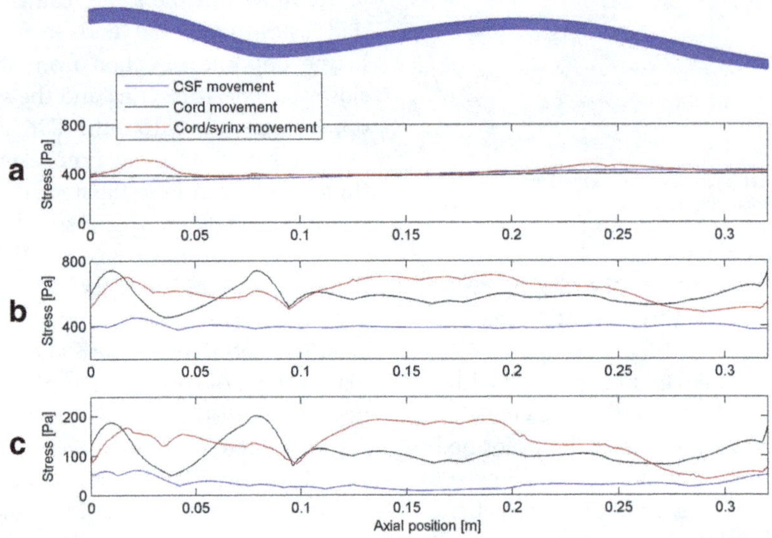

Fig. 4 The distribution of maximal stress in the axial (cranial-to-caudal) direction along the spinal cord. The axial coordinate is measured from C2; the shape of the spinal cord is shown at the top for reference. **a** Radial normal stress. **b** Axial normal stress. **c** Shear stress

cord were entirely negative (compressive) and that the values shown represent the absolute maximal values. The radial stress perpendicular to the sagittal plane is shown in Fig. 4a. The stress was fairly uniform along the length of the cord for all three cases considered and approximately equal to the pressure in the SAS (400 Pa). The same was found for the radial stress in the sagittal plane (not shown in the figure). The radial stress was thus a reflection of the pressure in the SAS. For the normal case, the axial normal stress (cranial-to-caudal direction) showed little variation along the length of the spine and had the same amplitude as the radial stress. In contrast, for the Chiari case without a syrinx, the axial normal stress had two prominent peaks of just under 800 Pa, which were located at the level of C2 and C3 vertebrae and cervico-thoracic junction. Elsewhere, the stress values were about 200 Pa higher than for the normal condition. With the syrinx introduced, the stress levels remained elevated, the peaks were less distinct and there was a further stress increase in the lower thoracic portion of the spinal cord. This was also observed for the shear stress, as can be seen in Fig. 5c. For the normal condition, the shear stress was very low, an order of magnitude lower than the normal stress. For Chiari, the shear stress was considerably elevated with two peaks of approximately 200 Pa at the level of C2 and C3 vertebrae and cervico-thoracic junction. To get a more complete understanding as to the location of maximal stresses, we must look at the three-dimensional distribution. Figure 5 shows the distribution of the peak shear stress in the cranial portion of the spinal cord for the case of Chiari without a syrinx. The results displayed were obtained by assigning to each element the peak value of the shear stress recorded in that element during the simulated event. It can be seen that regions with the highest level of stress were on the ventral side of the cranial-cervical cord and at the dorsal side of the caudal-cervical/cranial thoracic spine. The same type of result was obtained for the normal axial stress. This suggests that regions of localised high stress are due to the bending deformation of the spinal cord.

Discussion

The results for the short transient excitation show that the model can successfully predict the wave modes of the CSF pulse propagation reported in the open literature. The speeds of the three modes estimated from the results, as well as the associated movement of the anatomical layers are consistent with the theoretical models presented by Cirovic [41, 49]. They are also within the physiologically plausible range determined from in-vivo experiments on humans and animals [53, 54]. As the previous theoretical and computational studies neglected the curvature of the spine, it can be concluded that the curvature has a negligible effect on the propagation of the CSF pulse. The spinal curvature also had little effect on the pressure generated in the SAS; for all three cases considered, the pressure amplitude in the SAS was approximately 400 Pa, and it was uniform along the length of the spine. The predicted small spatial pressure gradient is consistent with findings of other published studies [63]. In other words, the spinal cavity behaved as a lumped compartment whose compliance was chiefly determined by the elasticity of the dural sac. This is because the time scales of the cardiac input are larger than the time needed for the CSF pulse to traverse the entire spinal cord. For all cases considered all the stress components in

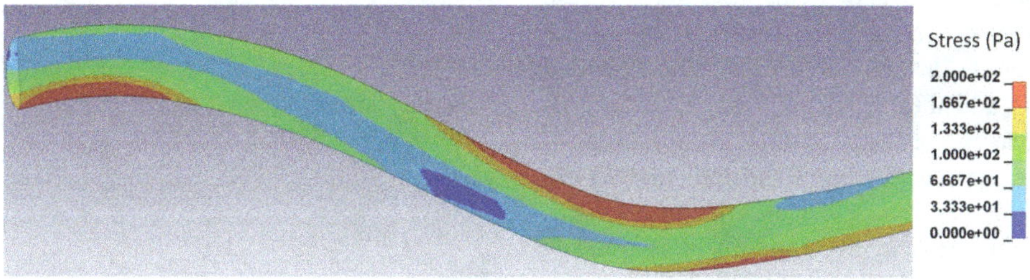

Fig. 5 The distribution of peak shear stress in the cervical and cranial thoracic part of the spinal cord (Chiari without a syrinx case). The regions in red are the locations of the highest shear stress

the cord were of the same order of magnitude as the pressure in the SAS (several hundreds of Pa). For the normal case where the cranial end of the cord was fixed, all the components of the normal stress were compressive and effectively equal to the pressure in the SAS. In other words, the pressure in the SAS generated an equal "hydrostatic pressure" (average normal stress) in the spinal cord. When the CSF was blocked and the cord was allowed to move, the radial normal stress did not change, but the axial (cranio-caudal) stress increased. We attribute this result to the fact that the axial movement of the cord resulted in bending in the sagittal plane. Bending deformation generates normal axial stresses that are largest at the perimeter of the section, and this is consistent with the predictions of the model. It should be noted that the maximal displacement of the cord in the caudal direction was small; about 1 mm in total. The axial normal stress was particularly prominent at the locations where the spinal cord had large curvature and the bending effect was pronounced. The same case was for the shear stress which is also generated by bending. Furthermore, these locations are also the locations where the cavities usually first start forming in the CKCS affected with syringomyelia. When a large syrinx was present, stress concentration moved to the lower thoracic region which is the next most likely site of syrinx formation [29]. This is an interesting result, and to our knowledge this is the first case where computer simulation predicts stress concentration at specific regions of the spinal cord in absence of stenosis and arachnoiditis. Although the stress magnitude at the most affected regions increased by as much as 100% from the normal values, the overall stress levels were generally quite low, and should not be able to cause an immediate damage to the spinal cord tissue. However, it is still feasible that exaggerated stressing repeated with each cardiac pulse does cause pathological changes to the spinal cord tissue over a long period of time. Actually, this is consistent with the fact that syringes take months or years to form [2, 8]. While the axial location of the increased cord stressing is coincident with the sites where the syringes tend to form, the model predicted that the stress was concentrated at the perimeter of the spinal cord rather than at the central portion. This is not in agreement with the fact that the cavities are usually located more centrally. Therefore, as it stands now, the results of this study cannot fully support the assumption that stressing of the cord near the maximum curvature locations may initiate the formation of syringes via direct mechanical damage. However, it should be considered that the model presented in this study does not include numerous factors that could modify the current result. Such factors include non-concentric realistic geometry of the anatomical layers, different material properties of the white and grey matter of the spinal cord, and the effect of denticulate ligaments and tethering in general. It is also possible that the syrinx initiation mechanism is less direct; it has been shown that the damage of microstructure at the surface of the cord may disrupt the blood-spinal cord barrier and affect fluid content of the spinal cord [37, 64, 65], thus leading to fluid accumulation.

Similar to other computer models, the model presented in this paper is based on a number of idealisations. Furthermore, the material properties of the spinal compartments are still not well characterised. We opted for choosing the material properties of the dura and the spinal cord that are most commonly used in the current (human) models of the spinal cavity [32, 35, 38, 39, 45]. Prior to making this choice, the model had been tested with the full range of spinal cord and dura material properties reported in the literature as summarised by Elliot et al. [20]. The tests showed that the dura properties listed in Table 2 lead to the most realistic results in terms of SAS pressure magnitude. When a lower stiffness was assigned to the spinal cord tissue, this resulted in proportionately lower stresses in the cord. However, the general trends remained the same; there was a significant increase in the axial and shear stresses at the upper cervical and thoracic spinal cord for the Chiari condition. This suggests that the conclusions for the current model are largely independent of the material constants, as long as they are within a plausible range. On the other hand, this also means that all the quantitative values of stress reported in this paper should not be taken literally, but rather in reference to the set of material properties used in the current model.

Virtually all computer models of syringomyelia end at the cranial end of the cervical spine or at best extend into the cranio-cervical junction. In this model, an ad hoc extruded cranial segment was added to avoid spurious stress concentrations at the cranial end of the cord. Effectively, this problem arises from the fact that the brain and the cranium are not included in the model. As Chiari deformation results in the brain being "crammed" in the cranium, it is possible that the lower portion of the brain and perhaps cranial section of the cervical spinal cord are under permanent stressing. Therefore, ultimately, a more complete model of syringomyelia should include both the cranial and spinal compartments.

Conclusions

A computer model was used to investigate the effect of excess movement of the spinal cord in dogs suffering from Chiari-like malformations with the goal of identifying possible factors that could promote the emergence of fluid-filled cavities in the spinal cord. It was found that small movements of the spinal cord associated with a cardiac pulse can result in a significant increase in shear and axial normal stresses and that this effect is most pronounced in the cervical and upper thoracic regions where the spinal curvature is high. The regions of high stress as predicted by the model are at the locations where syringes first form, but they are positioned near the perimeter, rather than at the central portion of the cord which is where the cavities usually are. We believe that the latter may be due to simplifying assumptions inherent to the model, and that this mechanism should be further investigated.

Acknowledgements
We are grateful to the staff at Fitzpatrick Referrals Orthopaedic and Neurology Service for facilitating the MRI imaging and ensuring good patient care and also to the owners and dogs that contributed to our understanding of this condition.

Funding
RL was supported by EPSRC Vacation Bursary in the initial stages of this project (June–August 2014). The bursary was a part of EP/L505092 DTG Training Grant and it covered RL's salary and consumables.
Fitzpatrick Referrals Ltd., provided support in the form of salaries and materials for authors JJ, and CR. The funders had no role in study design, data collection and analysis, decision to publish, or preparation of the manuscript.

Authors' contributions
SC and CR were responsible for the study concept, supervision and funding acquisition. SC and CR and RL were responsible for the methodology. The investigation was performed by RL and SC. Formal analysis was the responsibility of RL and SC. Resources were provided by JJ, CR and HV. SC prepared the original draft which was reviewed and edited by CR, JJ, HV, and RL. SC prepared the figures. All authors read and approved the final manuscript.

Consent for publication
Not applicable

Competing interests
RL was as undergraduate student at the University of Surrey where CR and SC are employed. JJ, was and CR is employed by Fitzpatrick Referrals Ltd., Surrey, GU7 Q22. HJV is employed by the Royal Veterinary College, University of London.
The Universities of Surrey and London and Fitzpatrick Referrals did not play a role in the study design, data collection and analysis, decision to publish, or preparation of the manuscript and only provided financial support in the form of authors' salaries and/or research materials. None of the authors have personal or financial relationships with other people or organizations that might inappropriately influence or bias the content of the paper. There are no patents, products in development, or marketed products to declare.

Author details
[1]The Centre for Biomedical Engineering, University of Surrey, Guildford GU2 7XH, UK. [2]The School of Veterinary Medicine, University of Surrey, Guildford GU2 7AD, UK. [3]Fitzpatrick Referrals, Eashing, Halfway Lane, Goadalming GU7 2QQ, UK. [4]Clinical Science and Services, Royal Veterinary College, Hatfield AL9 7TA, UK. [5]Neuroscience Research Australia and Prince of Wales Clinical School, University of New South Wales, Sydney, NSW 2031, Australia.

References

1. Williams B. On the pathogenesis of syringomyelia: a review. J R Soc Med. 1980;73(11):798–806.
2. Levine DN. The pathogenesis of syringomyelia associated with lesions at the foramen magnum: a critical review of existing theories and proposal of a new hypothesis. J Neurol Sci. 2004;220(1–2):3–21.
3. Heiss JD, Patronas N, DeVroom HL, Shawker T, Ennis R, Kammerer W, Eidsath A, Talbot T, Morris J, Eskioglu E, et al. Elucidating the pathophysiology of syringomyelia. J Neurosurg. 1999;91(4):553–62.
4. Brodbelt AR, Stoodley MA. Post-traumatic syringomyelia: a review. J Clin Neurosci. 2003;10(4):401–8.
5. Stoodley MA, Jones NR, Yang L, Brown CJ. Mechanisms underlying the formation and enlargement of noncommunicating syringomyelia: experimental studies. Neurosurg Focus. 2000;8(3):E2.
6. Milhorat TH, Kotzen RM, Anzil AP. Stenosis of central canal of spinal cord in man: incidence and pathological findings in 232 autopsy cases. J Neurosurg. 1994;80(4):716–22.
7. Milhorat TH, Capocelli AL Jr, Anzil AP, Kotzen RM, Milhorat RH. Pathological basis of spinal cord cavitation in syringomyelia: analysis of 105 autopsy cases. J Neurosurg. 1995;82(5):802–12.
8. Rusbridge C, Greitz D, Iskandar BJ. Syringomyelia: current concepts in pathogenesis, diagnosis, and treatment. J Vet Intern Med. 2006;20(3):469–79.
9. Rusbridge C, Knowler SP, Pieterse L, McFadyen AK. Chiari-like malformation in the griffon Bruxellois. J Small Anim Pract. 2009;50(8):386–93.
10. Chandler K, Volk H, Rusbridge C, Jeffery N. Syringomyelia in cavalier king Charles spaniels. Vet Rec. 2008;162(10):324.
11. Freeman AC, Platt SR, Kent M, Huguet E, Rusbridge C, Holmes S. Chiari-like malformation and syringomyelia in American Brussels griffon dogs. J Vet Intern Med. 2014;28(5):1551–9.
12. Parker JE, Knowler SP, Rusbridge C, Noorman E, Jeffery ND. Prevalence of asymptomatic syringomyelia in cavalier king Charles spaniels. Vet Rec. 2011; 168(25):667.
13. Marino DJ, Loughin CA, Dewey CW, Marino LJ, Sackman JJ, Lesser ML, Akerman MB. Morphometric features of the craniocervical junction region in dogs with suspected Chiari-like malformation determined by combined use of magnetic resonance imaging and computed tomography. Am J Vet Res. 2012;73(1):105–11.
14. Knowler SP, Kiviranta AM, McFadyen AK, Jokinen TS, La Ragione RM, Rusbridge C. Craniometric analysis of the hindbrain and Craniocervical

junction of Chihuahua, Affenpinscher and cavalier king Charles spaniel dogs with and without Syringomyelia secondary to Chiari-like malformation. PLoS One. 2017;12(1):e0169898.
15. Knowler SP, Cross C, Griffiths S, McFadyen AK, Jovanovik J, Tauro A, Kibar Z, Driver CJ, La Ragione RM, Rusbridge C. Use of morphometric mapping to characterise symptomatic Chiari-like malformation, secondary Syringomyelia and associated Brachycephaly in the cavalier king Charles spaniel. PLoS One. 2017;12(1):e0170315.
16. Driver CJ, Rusbridge C, McGonnell IM, Volk HA. Morphometric assessment of cranial volumes in age-matched cavalier king Charles spaniels with and without syringomyelia. Vet Rec. 2010;167(25):978–9.
17. Rusbridge C, Knowler SP. Inheritance of occipital bone hypoplasia (Chiari type I malformation) in cavalier king Charles spaniels. J Vet Intern Med. 2004;18(5):673–8.
18. Rusbridge C. Veterinary aspects. In: Flint G, Rusbridge C, editors. Syringomyelia: a disorder of CSF circulation. Heidelberg, New York, Dordecht, London: Springer; 2014. p. 209–30.
19. Rusbridge C. Chiari-like malformation with syringomyelia in the cavalier king Charles spaniel: long-term outcome after surgical management. Veterinary surgery : VS. 2007;36(5):396–405.
20. Elliott NSJ, Bertram CD, Martin BA, Brodbelt AR. Syringomyelia: a review of the biomechanics. J Fluid Struct. 2013;40:1–24.
21. Alperin N. MR-intracranial compliance and pressure: a method for noninvasive measurement of important neurophysiologic parameters. Methods Enzymol. 2004;386:323–49.
22. Alperin NJ, Lee SH, Loth F, Raksin PB, Lichtor T. MR-intracranial pressure (ICP): a method to measure intracranial elastance and pressure noninvasively by means of MR imaging: baboon and human study. Radiology. 2000;217(3):877–85.
23. Martin BA, Kalata W, Shaffer N, Fischer P, Luciano M, Loth F: Hydrodynamic and longitudinalimpedance analysis of cerebrospinal fluid dynamics at the craniovertebral junction in type I Chiari malformation. PloS one 2013;8(10):e75335.
24. Williams B. Simultaneous cerebral and spinal fluid pressure recordings. I. Technique, physiology, and normal results. Acta Neurochir. 1981;58(3–4): 167–85.
25. Williams B. Cerebrospinal fluid pressure changes in response to coughing. Brain. 1976;99(2):331–46.
26. Martin BA, Loth F. The influence of coughing on cerebrospinal fluid pressure in an in vitro syringomyelia model with spinal subarachnoid space stenosis. Cerebrospinal Fluid Res. 2009;6:17.
27. Martin BA, Labuda R, Royston TJ, Oshinski JN, Iskandar B, Loth F. Spinal subarachnoid space pressure measurements in an in vitro spinal stenosis model: implications on syringomyelia theories. J Biomech Eng. 2010;132(11):111007.
28. Vavasour IM, Meyers SM, MacMillan EL, Madler B, Li DK, Rauscher A, Vertinsky T, Venu V, MacKay AL, Curt A. Increased spinal cord movements in cervical spondylotic myelopathy. Spine J. 2014;14(10):2344–54.
29. Loderstedt S, Benigni L, Chandler K, Cardwell JM, Rusbridge C, Lamb CR, Volk HA. Distribution of syringomyelia along the entire spinal cord in clinically affected cavalier king Charles spaniels. Vet J. 2011;190(3):359–63.
30. Strahle J, Muraszko KM, Garton HJ, Smith BW, Starr J, Kapurch JR 2nd, Maher CO. Syrinx location and size according to etiology: identification of Chiari-associated syrinx. J Neurosurg Pediatr. 2015;16(1):21–9.
31. Martin BA, Reymond P, Novy J, Baledent O, Stergiopulos N. A coupled hydrodynamic model of the cardiovascular and cerebrospinal fluid system. Am J Phys Heart Circ Phys. 2012;302(7):H1492–509.
32. Heil M, Bertram CD. A poroelastic fluid-structure interaction model of syringomyelia. J Fluid Mech. 2016;809:360–89.
33. Bilston LE, Stoodley MA, Fletcher DF. The influence of the relative timing of arterial and subarachnoid space pulse waves on spinal perivascular cerebrospinal fluid flow as a possible factor in syrinx development. J Neurosurg. 2010;112(4): 808–13.
34. Bilston LE, Fletcher DF, Brodbelt AR, Stoodley MA. Arterial pulsation-driven cerebrospinal fluid flow in the perivascular space: a computational model. Comput Methods Biomech Biomed Engin. 2003;6(4):235–41.
35. Bertram CD, Heil M, Poroelastic Fluid A. Structure-interaction model of cerebrospinal fluid dynamics in the cord with Syringomyelia and adjacent subarachnoid-space stenosis. J Biomech Eng. 2017;139(1)
36. Kim M, Cirovic S. A computational model of the cerebrospinal fluid system incorporating lumped-parameter cranial compartment and one-dimensional distributed spinal compartment. J Biorheol. 2011;25(1):78–87.
37. Hemley SJ, Biotech B, Tu J, Stoodley MA. Role of the blood-spinal cord-barrier in posttraumatic syringomyelia. Laboratory investigation J Neurosurg-Spine. 2009;11(6):696–704.
38. Bertram CD, Bilston LE, Stoodley MA. Tensile radial stress in the spinal cord related to arachnoiditis or tethering: a numerical model. Med Biol Eng Comput. 2008;46(7):701–7.
39. Bertram CD. A numerical investigation of waves propagating in the spinal cord and subarachnoid space in the presence of a syrinx. J Fluid Struct. 2009;25:1189–205.
40. Elliott NSJ, Lucey AD, Lockerby DA, Brodbelt AR. Fluid-structure interactions in a cylindrical layered wave guide with application in the spinal column to syringomyelia. J Fluid Struct. 2017;70:464–99.
41. Cirovic S. A coaxial tube model of the cerebrospinal fluid pulse propagation in the spinal column. J Biomech Eng. 2009;131(2):021008.
42. Chang HS, Nakagawa H. Hypothesis on the pathophysiology of syringomyelia based on simulation of cerebrospinal fluid dynamics. J Neurol Neurosurg Psychiatry. 2003;74(3):344–7.
43. Carpenter PW, Berkouk K, Lucey AD. Pressure wave propagation in fluid-filled co-axial elastic tubes. Part 2: mechanisms for the pathogenesis of syringomyelia. J Biomech Eng. 2003;125(6):857–63.
44. Martin BA, Kalata W, Loth F, Royston TJ, Oshinski JN: Syringomyelia hydrodynamics: an in vitro study based on in vivo measurements. J Biomech Eng. 2005;127(7):1110–1120.
45. Bertram CD. Evaluation by fluid/structure-interaction spinal-cord simulation of the effects of subarachnoid-space stenosis on an adjacent syrinx. J Biomech Eng. 2010;132(6):061009.
46. Berkouk K, Carpenter PW, Lucey AD. Pressure wave propagation in fluid-filled co-axial elastic tubes. Part 1: basic theory. J Biomech Eng. 2003;125(6): 852–6.
47. Elliott NS, Lockerby DA, Brodbelt AR. A lumped-parameter model of the cerebrospinal system for investigating arterial-driven flow in posttraumatic syringomyelia. Med Eng Phys. 2011;33(7):874–82.
48. Elliott NS. Syrinx fluid transport: modeling pressure-wave-induced flux across the spinal pial membrane. J Biomech Eng. 2012;134(3):031006.
49. Cirovic S, Kim M. A one-dimensional model of the spinal cerebrospinal-fluid compartment. J Biomech Eng. 2012;134(2):021005.
50. Clarke EC, Fletcher DF, Stoodley MA, Bilston LE. Computational fluid dynamics modelling of cerebrospinal fluid pressure in Chiari malformation and syringomyelia. J Biomech. 2013;46(11):1801–9.
51. Bertram CD, Brodbelt AR, Stoodley MA. The origins of syringomyelia: numerical models of fluid/structure interactions in the spinal cord. J Biomech Eng-T Asme. 2005;127(7):1099–109.
52. Stoverud KH, Alnaes M, Langtangen HP, Haughton V, Mardal KA. Poro-elastic modeling of Syringomyelia - a systematic study of the effects of pia mater, central canal, median fissure, white and gray matter on pressure wave propagation and fluid movement within the cervical spinal cord. Comput Methods Biomech Biomed Engin. 2016;19(6):686–98.
53. Khani M, Xing T, Gibbs C, Oshinski JN, Stewart GR, Zeller JR, Martin BA. Nonuniform moving boundary method for computational fluid dynamics simulation of Intrathecal cerebrospinal flow distribution in a Cynomolgus monkey. J Biomech Eng. 2017;139(8)
54. Kalata W, Martin BA, Oshinski JN, Jerosch-Herold M, Royston TJ, Loth F. MR measurement of cerebrospinal fluid velocity wave speed in the spinal canal. IEEE Trans Biomed Eng. 2009;56(6):1765–8.
55. Fischbein NJ, Dillon WP, Cobbs C, Weinstein PR. The "presyrinx" state: is there a reversible myelopathic condition that may precede syringomyelia? Neurosurg Focus. 2000;8(3):E4.
56. Loth F, Yardimci MA, Alperin N. Hydrodynamic modeling of cerebrospinal fluid motion within the spinal cavity. J Biomech Eng. 2001;123(1):71–9.
57. Heidari Pahlavian S, Yiallourou T, Tubbs RS, Bunck AC, Loth F, Goodin M, Raisee M, Martin BA. The impact of spinal cord nerve roots and denticulate ligaments on cerebrospinal fluid dynamics in the cervical spine. PLoS One. 2014;9(4):e91888.
58. Schneider CA, Rasband WS, Eliceiri KW. NIH image to ImageJ: 25 years of image analysis. Nat Methods. 2012;9(7):671–5.
59. Hezzell MJ, Dennis SG, Humm K, Agee L, Boswood A. Relationships between heart rate and age, bodyweight and breed in 10,849 dogs. J Small Anim Pract. 2013;54(6):318–24.
60. Cerda-Gonzalez S, Olby NJ, Broadstone R, McCullough S, Osborne JA. Characteristics of cerebrospinal fluid flow in cavalier king Charles spaniels analyzed using phase velocity cine magnetic resonance imaging. Vet Radiol Ultrasound. 2009;50(5):467–76.

61. Yildiz S, Thyagaraj S, Jin N, Zhong X, Heidari Pahlavian S, Martin BA, Loth F, Oshinski J, Sabra KG. Quantifying the influence of respiration and cardiac pulsations on cerebrospinal fluid dynamics using real-time phase-contrast MRI. J Magn Reson Imaging. 2017;46(2):431–9.
62. Martin BA, Sass L, Khani M, Gibbs C, Freeman T, Pluid J, Elliot A, Oshinski JN, Zeller J, Stewart GR et al: Are Monkeys Like Humans? Comparison of Intrathecal CSF Dynamics across Mammalian Species. 4th International Cerebrospinal Fluid Dynamics Symposium 2017 https://csfdynamics.org/atlanta2017/scientific-program/ Accessed 24 July 2017.
63. Fric R, Lindstrom EK, Ringstad GA, Mardal KA, Eide PK. The association between the pulse pressure gradient at the cranio-cervical junction derived from phase-contrast magnetic resonance imaging and invasively measured pulsatile intracranial pressure in symptomatic patients with Chiari malformation type 1. Acta Neurochir. 2016;158(12):2295–304.
64. Perdiki M, Farooque M, Holtz A, Li GL, Olsson Y. Expression of endothelial barrier antigen immunoreactivity in blood vessels following compression trauma to rat spinal cord. Temporal evolution and relation to the degree of the impact Acta Neuropathol. 1998;96(1):8–12.
65. Whetstone WD, Hsu JY, Eisenberg M, Werb Z, Noble-Haeusslein LJ. Blood-spinal cord barrier after spinal cord injury: relation to revascularization and wound healing. J Neurosci Res. 2003;74(2):227–39.

Development and evaluation of a broadly reactive reverse transcription recombinase polymerase amplification assay for rapid detection of murine norovirus

Lei Ma[1†], Fanwen Zeng[2†], Feng Cong[1], Bihong Huang[1], Yujun Zhu[1], Miaoli Wu[1], Fengjiao Xu[1], Wen Yuan[1], Ren Huang[1] and Pengju Guo[1*]

Abstract

Background: Murine norovirus (MNV) is recognized as the most prevalent viral pathogen in captive mouse colonies. The rapid detection assay for MNV would be a useful tool for monitoring and preventing MNV infection. A recombinase polymerase amplification (RPA) assay was established in this study to provide a solution for rapid and sensitive detection of MNV.

Results: The detection limit of the RT-RPA assay for the detection of MNV was 1×10^2 copies of RNA molecules per reaction. The assay was specific since there was no cross-reaction with other common murine viruses. In addition, the broad reactivity of the RT-RPA assay was validated using the synthesized template carrying seven point mutations among several MNV strains. The MNV RT-RPA assay could detect as few as 1×10^2 copies of the mutant per reaction, suggesting the assay could be broadly reactive against a large diversity of MNV strains. Forty eight clinical samples including 16 gastric tissue specimens, 16 cecal tissue specimens and 16 fecal specimens were tested for the validation of the new developed RT-RPA assay. The detection results of RT-RPA and RT-qPCR for clinical samples were very similar, except that a gastric tissue sample which was positive by RT-qPCR, with a RNA titer of 27 copies, was negative by RT-RPA.

Conclusions: A broadly reactive RT-RPA assay was successfully established for MNV detection.

Keywords: Murine norovirus, Recombinase polymerase amplification, Genetic diversity, Detection

Background

Norovirus is a class of viral pathogens that could infect a variety of hosts [1]. Norovirus have been tentatively classified as five genogroups based on the sequences of major capsid protein (VP1) [1]. In a previous study, standard norovirus classification tree made with the alignment of 68 NoV sequences was proposed for nomenclature: 29 genetic clusters are classified in the 5 genogroups, 8 in GI, 17 in GII, 2 in GIII, and 1 each in GIV and GV [1]. GI, GII, and GIV strains, are found in humans, and GIII and GV strains are found in cows and mice, respectively. MNV, belongs to genogroup GIII, is one of the most common pathogens in laboratory mice [2, 3].

Since the prototype strain MNV-1 was firstly detected in immunocompromised mice [3], multiple strains of MNV have been discovered and/or isolated from the laboratory and wild rodents [4–6]. Although different MNV strains exhibited the considerable genetic and biological diversity, they belonged to a single serotype determined by cross-neutralization test [7]. Serological investigations in North America, Europe and Japan demonstrated the high prevalence of specific antibodies against MNV in laboratory rodents [8–10]. Currently,

* Correspondence: vetbio2016@hotmail.com
†Lei Ma and Fanwen Zeng contributed equally to this work.
[1]Guangdong Key Laboratory of Laboratory Animals, Guangdong Laboratory Animals Monitoring Institute, Guangzhou, China
Full list of author information is available at the end of the article

MNV has become the most prevalent pathogen in laboratory mice worldwide.

The mice are the most commonly used laboratory animals in biomedical research. The high prevalence of MNV in laboratory mice may interfere in the result of biomedical research. Several experiments have been performed to investigate the effects of MNV infection on scientific research. For examples, experimental infection of the mice revealed that MNV-1 lead to the persistent infection and long fecal virus shedding [2]. MNV-4 infection induced multiple inflammatory hallmarks of human Crohn's disease in Atg16L1^{HM} mice after dextran sodium sulfate administration [11]. Whereas, another study reported that transient or persistent norovirus infection didn't alter the pathology of intestinal inflammation and fibrosis induced by *Salmonella Typhimurium* infection in C57BL/6 mice [12]. As no clear conclusion can be made from the previous studies regarding to the effects of MNV infection on biomedical research in mice, the use of MNV-free mice was recommended for fundamental research and drug safety evaluation. Thus, the rapid and sensitive detection methods for MNV infection played a critical role in the quality control of the laboratory mice.

To monitor and detect MNV rapidly and specifically, several molecular methods such as reverse transcription polymerase chain reaction (RT-PCR) assays and RT-quantitative PCR (RT-qPCR) assays have been developed [8, 13–15]. Considering that the RT-PCR and RT-qPCR methods are time-consuming, the loop-mediated isothermal amplification (LAMP) method for detection of MNV was developed [16]. However four to six primers were required in the LAMP assay [16]. Recombinase polymerase amplification (RPA), another isothermal amplification method, which requires only two primers, has been recently used for pathogen detection and only takes less than 30 min to perform the amplification reaction [17–21]. RPA primers bind to DNA template by bacterial recombinase enzyme, then the extension and amplification reaction is initiated by an isothermal polymerase [22]. These enzymes are in concert with a reverse transcriptase and a fluorescent probe for real-time detection of the viruses containing RNA genomes [23].

Previous study has reported the RT-RPA assay for detection of human norovirus [24]. However, the whole genome sequence of human norovirus shared poor identity with MNV [2]. The RT-RPA assay used for human norovirus cannot be applied to the detection of MNV. Thus the aim of the present study is to establish a broadly reactive RT-RPA assay for rapid and sensitive detection of MNV which is widely present in laboratory mice across the world.

Results

Screening of the primer sets

Six primer sets were screened by the basic RT-RPA assay using the 10^4 copies RNA standard as the template. As clearly showed in Fig. 2a, the product of the primer set f5/r5 emitted the strongest light under ultraviolet light. The probe was designed based on the target sequence of the primer set f5/r5. All the sequences of primers and probe used in this study were displayed in Table 1.

Sensitivity and specificity of the real-time RT-RPA

The detection limit of the RT-RPA assay was assessed using the 10-fold serially diluted RNA standards. As illustrated in Fig. 1b, the dynamic detection range of the assay ranged from 10^6 to 10^2 copies per reaction, demonstrating that the limit of detection of the assay was 10^2 copies/μL molecular RNA. The RT-RPA assay was performed eight times on the serially diluted RNA standards, in which 8 out of 8 (8/8) runs were positive when viral load are 10^6–10^2 copies per reaction; 5/8 runs were positive when 10 copies per reaction; and 0/8 positive when 1 copy per reaction was used. To evaluate the reproducibility of the RT-RPA assay, semi-logarithmic regression analysis was performed using the data from the 8 runs (Fig. 3a). A probit regression analysis using the results of 8 runs was performed to determine the exact detection limit, and the results showed that RT-RPA could detect 70 RNA molecules in 95% of cases (Fig. 3b). The synthesized templates carrying seven point mutations were

Table 1 Primers and probe

Name	Sequence	Amplicon length
MNV-F	ATGCATGGTGAAAAGTACTAT	788 bp
MNV-R	TAGAAAGAAGGCGACCAGAGA	
f1	CAGTCTTTGTGAATGAGGATGAGTGATG	189 bp
r1	AAAATTTTGGAAGATCCAGGGGTCAATTT	
f2	CAAATCAACCAAATTGACCCCTGGATCTT	151 bp
r2	ACCTCCATGTTCCCAACCCAGCCGGTGTACAT	
f3	CAAAATTTTGTCCAGTGCCCCCTTGGTGAGTT	135 bp
r3	AGGACCAGCTGAACCTCCATGTTCCCAACCCA	
f4	CACGCCACCGGTCTGTTCTGCGCTGGGTGC	154 bp
r4	AAGGAACAAGATCCTGGCCGCTGGCTTC	
f5	TTCCAAAATTTTGTCCAGTGCCCCCTTGGT	131 bp
r5	GCTGAACCTCCATGTTCCCAACCCAGCCGGTG	
f6	TTCAGCTGGTCCTCGCCGGCAATGCCTTTA	141 bp
r6	CCAGGGTGCGCACATCACACATGACATGTG	
probe	TCGAAACACCCCAGGCGAAATATTGTTTGA (BHQ)(THF)(FAM)GGCCCTCGGGCCAGG	

BHQ1-dT dT-fluorophore, *THF* tetrahydrofuran, *FAM-dT* dT-quencher group

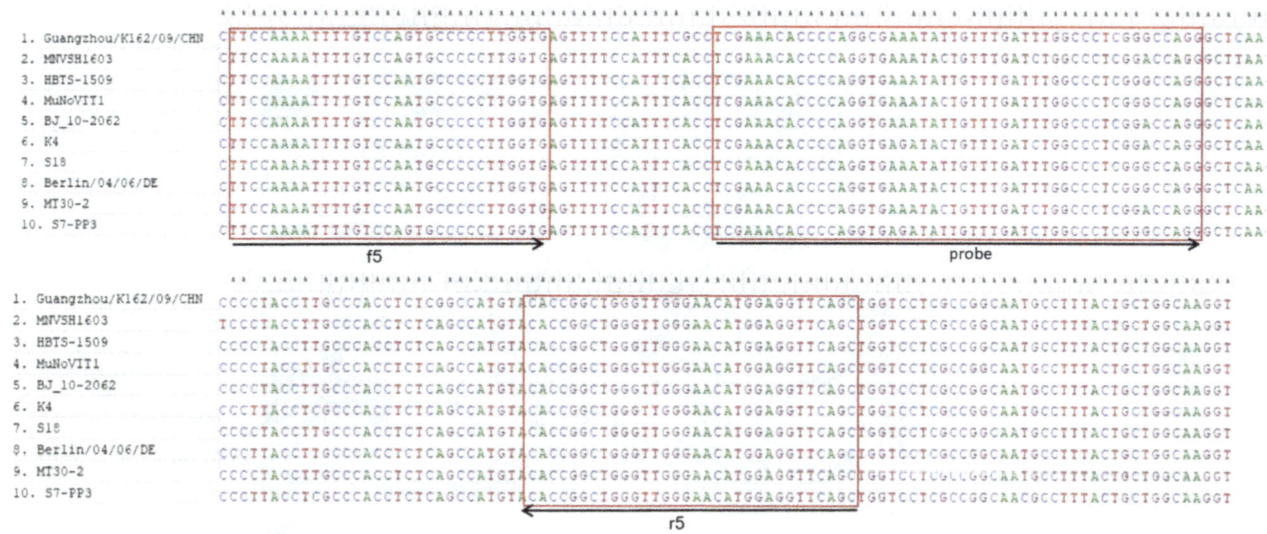

Fig. 1 Alignment of nucleotide sequences from the ORF1–ORF2 junctions of 10 MNV strains. Nucleotide sequences of 10 MNV strains are aligned from nt 5220 to nt 5420 in Guangzhou/K162/09/CHN. Asterisks indicate consensus nucleotide sequences among the 10 MNV genes. The positions with no asterisk indicate bases that are different from the nucleotide sequence of Guangzhou/K162/09/CHN. The positions of RPA primers (forward primer: nt 5221–5250, reverse primer: nt 5352–5383) and probe (nt 5268–5315) are indicated in the red box

also tested by the RT-RPA assay to evaluate the broadly reactive capacity of the assay. The result showed that the RT-RPA assay can detect the mutant template as few as 10^2 copies/μL molecular RNA (data not shown), indicating that the point mutations had no effect on the sensitivity of RT-RPA assay.

RNA genomes from other common murine viral pathogens were tested by the RT-RPA assay. Figure 2c revealed that the amplification curve was only observed for MNV; no amplification signal was detected for TMEV, SeV, MHV, PVM, Reo-3 and distilled water.

Assay performance on clinical samples

The performance of RT-RPA was compared with probe-based RT-qPCR using RNA isolated from 48 murine samples. Eight of 16 cecal samples and 9 of 16 fecal samples were positive by both assays. In contrast, 6 of 16 gastric tissue samples were by RT-RPA while 7 of 16 gastric tissue samples were positive by RT-qPCR. The viral load in the gastric tissue sample which was negative by RT-RPA, was 27 copies per reaction determined by RT-qPCR, which was lower than the detection limit of the RT-RPA assay. Linear regression analysis demonstrated a poor correlation between C_T values determined by RT-qPCR and TT values determined by RT-RPA (Fig. 3c), suggesting the RT-RPA assay could not be applied to quantitative analysis of MNV viral loads in the samples. This phenomenon was also reported in the RT-RPA assay for detection of avian influenza virus in clinical samples [25].

Discussion

In present study, a real-time RT-RPA assay was established for rapid and specific detection of MNV. The primer-probe set was designed based on the sequences of the highly conserved ORF1-ORF2 junction. This new assay could detect a broad range of genetically diverse MNV isolates with the same detection sensitivity.

MNV is considered the most prevalent viral pathogen in laboratory mice worldwide. MNV infection may affect the results of biomedical researches [16], so it is of vital importance to confirm the MNV-free status of the laboratory mice. Several real-time RT-PCR assays have been developed for detecting MNV. However, these techniques could not detect all the MNV strains due to the genetic diversity of MNV [5, 15, 26]. Thus two broadly reactive real-time RT-PCR assays were established to detect MNV infection [27, 28]. Although the real-time RT-PCR assay is sensitive and specific, it is expensive, time-consuming and labor-intensive. To overcome the shortcomings of the real-time RT-PCR, a broadly reactive LAMP assay was developed for detection of MNV. However, the LAMP assay required five primers, which increased the difficulty of primer design for MNV with genetic diversity. A portable and user-friendly method is therefore necessary for rapid detection of MNV on site. One promising solution is the RPA assay. Due to its convenience and portability, the RPA technique has been used for rapid detection of various pathogens, such as foot-and-mouth disease virus [29], Zika virus [30], human norovirus [24] and

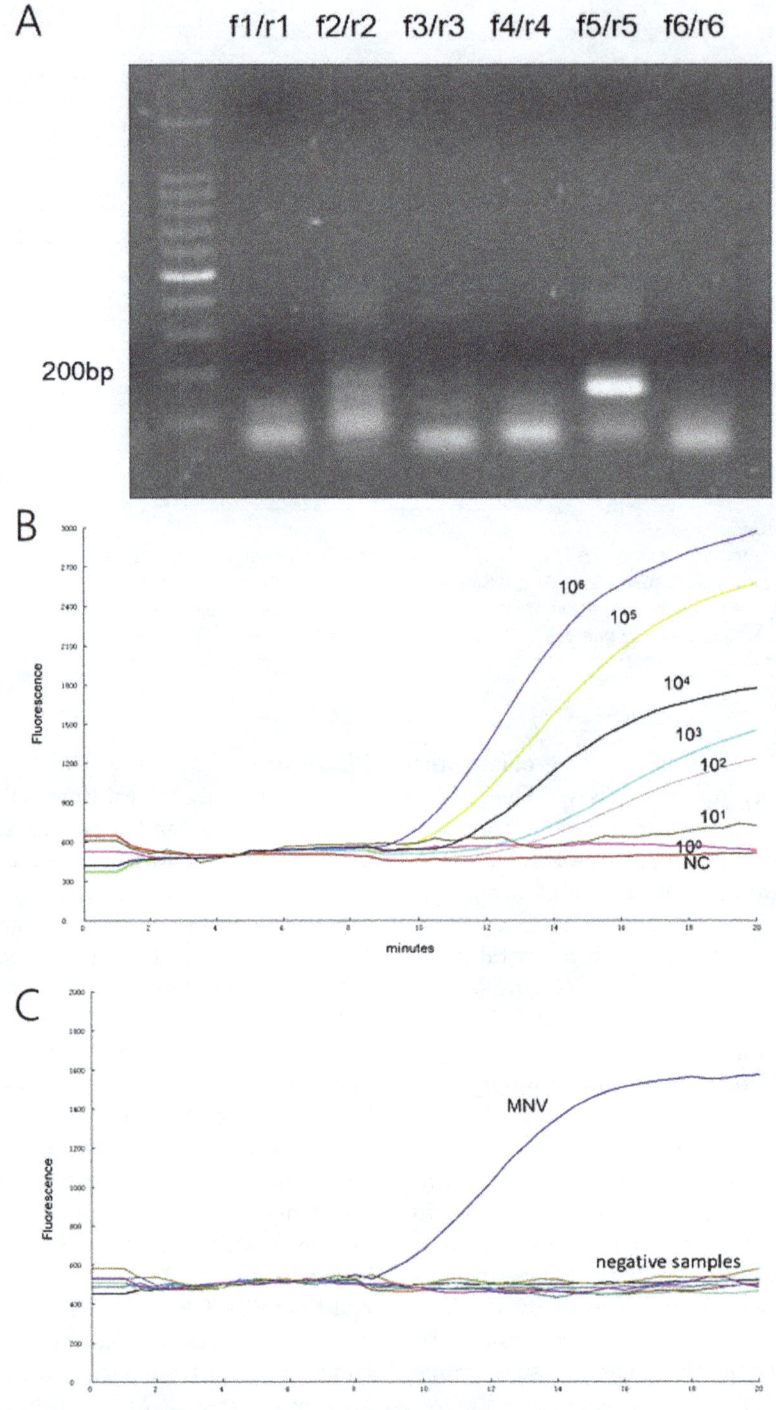

Fig. 2 Primers sets screening; sensitivity and specificity of the RT-RPA assay. **a** The products of RT-RPA using six primers pairs were separated on agarose gel electrophoresis. **b** Fluorescence signal over time using the RNA standards ranging from 10^6 to 10^0 copies. **c** Specificity of the RT-RPA assay. TMEV, SeV, MHV, MPV, Reo-3 and distilled water were the negative samples

pathogenic bacteria [31]. Up to date, there is only one report about the RPA assay for the laboratory animal health monitoring [32].

Design of the primer set plays a vital role in the performance of the RPA assay. Up to now, no software is available for RPA primer design. The primers used in

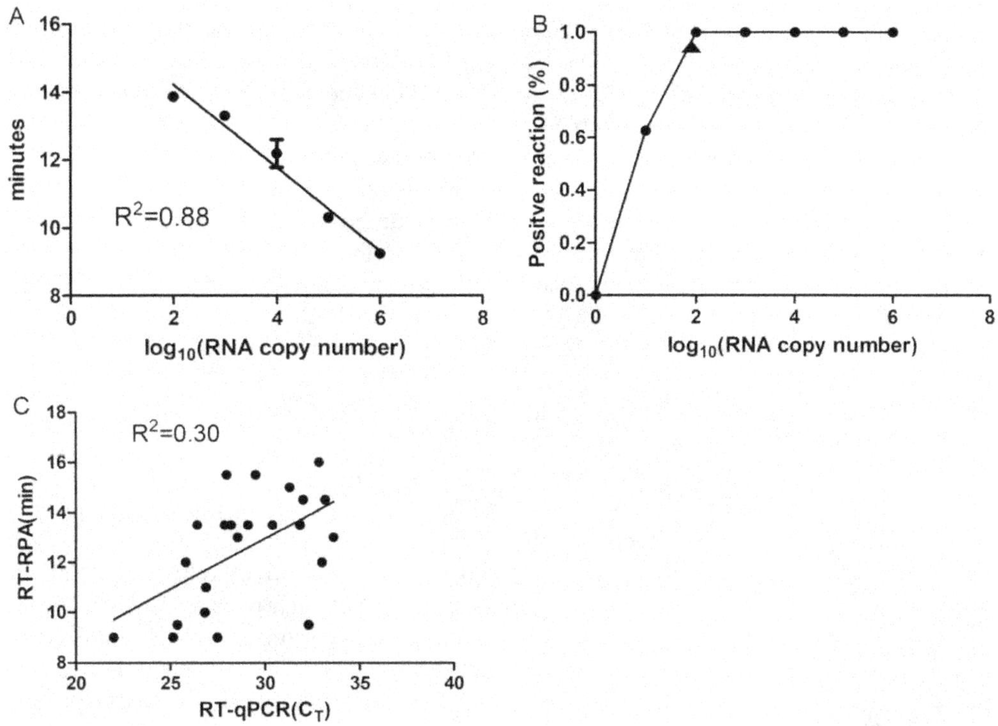

Fig. 3 Performance of the RT-RPA assay. **a** Semi-logarithmic regression of the data collected from 8 runs using the RNA standard analyzed by GraphPad Prism 5.0. **b** Probit regression analysis using the data of the 8 runs. The detection limit at 95% probability (95 molecules) is depicted by a triangle. **c** Linear regression analysis of RT-RPA threshold time (TT, y axis) and RT-qPCR cycle threshold (CT) values (x axis) were performed by Prism software. R^2 value was 0.3

this study were manually designed following the manufacturer's instruction. In this study, six primer sets were tested by the RPA assay, only one primer set (f5/r5) produced strong gene amplification signal. The probe was designed based on the target region of the primers set (f5/r5). The primer-probe set produced satisfied result (Fig. 2b). This result demonstrated that it is efficient and cost-effective to screen the primer sets through basic RPA assay, followed by gel electrophoresis.

Although the target region of the RT-RPA assay is highly conserved within the whole MNV genome sequence, it still possesses several point mutations among different strains that may affect the diagnostic sensitivity of the RPA assay. The sequences of 10 represent MNV strains in different countries were aligned. There are six different nucleotides at the binding site of the forward primer and the probe between the MNV strain Guangzhou/K162/09/CHN and strain K4. In addition, one more point mutation was present at other strains. To determine the effect of all the mutations on the performance of the RT-RPA assay, the templates containing all the seven point mutations were synthesized and tested by the RT-RPA assay. The result demonstrated that the mutations have no effect on the performance of the RT-RPA assay, which was consistent with previous studies proving that up to nine point mutations were tolerated [33, 34], suggesting that the RT-RPA assay could detect a diverse array of MNV strains.

The clinical performance of the RT-RPA assay was evaluated using 48 field samples. The MNV positive rate was 47.9% (23/48) determined by RT-RPA and 50.0% determined by RT-qPCR. The sensitivity of the RT-RPA technique for detection of MNV in clinical samples was 95.8% when compared with the RT-qPCR assay. Only one sample containing low RNA titer (27 RNA copies) was tested negative by RT-RPA. We believe that this was due to the low RNA copies (27 RNA copies) in the sample and low analytical sensitivity of the RT-RPA technique. However, the MNV RT-RPA assay was 10 times more sensitive than the RT-RPA for detection of human norovirus reported in a previous study [24]. It is worthy to note that the limit of detection of the human norovirus RT-RPA assay was performed on serially diluted RNA extract of stool. The sensitivity of present study was determined using a purified in vitro transcribed RNA rather than RNA extract of stool which may contain a lot of other RNA that interacts with recombinase proteins and thus can harm sensitivity. This may explained the difference of sensitivity between the two RPA assays. The RT-RPA assay could detect human norovirus in directly boiled stool, and displayed better resistance to inhibitors than a commonly used RT-qPCR assay [24]. It is promising to detect MNV in directly boiled animal tissue or stool samples by the RT-RPA assay in the future. This procedure would be valuable to reduce sample processing time and increase portability.

Conclusion

A rapid, sensitive and specific method for detection of MNV was successfully established based on RPA assay. The RT-RPA had several advantages over RT-qPCR, including: (i.) a cost-effective portable device is sufficient; (ii) quicker time-to-result; (iii) the use of enzyme pellet in one tube reduces the laborious work and the likelihood of contaminant; (iv.) tolerance to common PCR/qPCR inhibitors [24]; (v.) the potential of point-of-care detection of the clinical samples. Thus, the assay provides an easy-to-use platform for rapid detection and monitoring of MNV infection which circulates in laboratory mice across the world.

Methods

Virus

MNV Guangzhou/K162/09/CHN strain was isolated and preserved in our laboratory [35], Theiler's mouse encephalomyelitis virus (TMEV) BeAn8386 strain, sendai virus (SeV) Sendai/52 strain, mouse hepatitis virus A59 strain (MHV), reovirus type 3 (Reo-3) Dearing strain, pneumonia virus of mice (PVM) number 15 strain were purchased from American Type Culture Collection (ATCC). Nucleic acid for lymphocytic choriomeningitis virus (LCMV) Armstrong strain were kindly provided by Dr. Zheng Ming He, from the Laboratory Animal Institute, National Institutes for Food and Drug Control, China.

Generation of MNV RNA standard

The ORF1-ORF2 junction sequence on MNV genome was demonstrated to be highly conserved [16]. A pair of primers (MNV-F: 5'-ATGCATGGTGAAAAGTACTAT-3', MNV-R: 5'-TAGAAAGAAGGCGACCAGAGA3') were designed and used to amplify the highly conserved ORF1-ORF2 junction. RNA of MNV strain Guangzhou/K162/09/CHN (Accession No: HQ317203) was used to amplify the target region by One Step RT-PCR kit (Takara, China). The reaction condition was set up as follows: reverse transcription (RT) at 50 °C for 30 min, denaturation at 95 °C for 5 min, 30 cycles of 94 °C for 30 s, 50 °C for 30 s and 72 °C for 45 s, a final extension step at 72 °C for 5 min. The amplicon was subjected to gel electrophoresis and recovered. The purified amplicon was cloned into the pGEM-T vector (Promega, USA) and designated as pGEM-MNV. The positive plasmid was confirmed by Sanger sequencing and in vitro transcribed using RiboMAX™ Large Scale RNA Production Systems (Promega, USA) according to the manufacturer's instruction. The in vitro transcribed RNA was quantified by Nano2000 (GE, USA) and converted to copy number.

Primer and probe design

There is no software available for RPA primer and probe design up to now. The primer sets were manually designed following the manufacturer recommendation (TwistDx), based on the sequence of MNV RNA molecular standard. Basic RPA assay was performed to screen the primer set with the best amplification efficiency. Thereafter, the probe was designed based on the target sequence of the primer pair.

RT-RPA assay

Basic RT-RPA reaction was carried out in a 50 μl volume using the TwistAmp Basic RT kit (TwistDx, UK), which consisted of 30.1 μl of rehydration buffer, 1 μl of template, 2.1 μl of each primer (10 μM), 12.2 μl of water and 2.5 μl of magnesium acetate (280 mM). The microtubes were immediately placed in the heating block and incubated at 39 °C for 20 min. The RPA product was cleaned using a clean-up kit (Beyotime, China) to remove the inhibitors that might affect the agrose electrophoresis and separated on a 2% agarose gel.

Real time RT-RPA assay was performed using the TwistAmp exo RT kit. The reaction conditions for real-time RT-RPA were the same as for the basic RT-RPA, except that 0.6 μl of water was replaced by 0.6 μl of probe. The mircotubes were placed in the Deaou-308C tubescanner (DEAOU Biotechnology, China) set to 39 °C to start the reaction. After incubating for 4 min, the mircotubes were mixed, spun down, and placed back on the tubescanner for 16 min at 39 °C. A sample was considered positive when it generated an exponential amplification curve above the threshold of the negative control.

Sensitivity and specificity of the RT-RPA assay

The transcribed RNA standard was 10-fold serially diluted by distilled water and used to evaluate the detection limit of the MNV real-time RT-RPA assay. Each RNA dilution was tested in 8 replicates. A semi-log regression was performed by plotting the threshold time against the $\log_{10}$ RNA copy numbers using Prism 5.0 software (GraphPad, USA). To determine the analytical sensitivity of the RT-RPA technique, a probit regression was performed using Prism 5.0 software (GraphPad, USA).

Due to the high genetic diversity of different MNV strains, the broad reactivity of the RT-RPA technique was investigated. Multiple alignments of sequences from 10 isolates retrieved from Genebank were performed.

These 10 MNV strains were isolated from different countries and are the dominant strains in these countries, the point mutations at the primer-probe set may represent a large diversity of MNV. Six point mutations were present at the binding site of the probe and one mutation was present at the RPA forward primer (Fig. 1). The sequence containing all the seven point mutations were synthesized by Sangon Biotech (Sangon, China) and cloned in pGEM-T vector. The sensitivity of the RT-RPA assay using the mutants as the template was evaluated by the above method.

The specificity of the MNV RT-RPA assay was evaluated by testing a panel of viruses including TMEV, Reo-3, SeV, PVM and MHV.

Detection of clinical samples

Forty eight frozen clinical samples (16 gastric tissue specimens, 16 cecal tissue specimens and 16 fecal specimens) from previous experiment stored at − 80 °C at our laboratory were subjected to the RT-RPA assay [36]. Homogenates of the tissues were produced with Dulbecco's Modified Eagle Medium (DMEM). The homogenates after two freezing-thawing cycles were clarified by high-speed centrifugation and the supernatant fluids were collected for RNA extraction and RT-RPA assay. All the samples were also tested by the RT-qPCR method previously described [27]. Linear regression analysis of RT-RPA threshold time (TT) and RT-qPCR cycle threshold (C_t) values were performed by Prism 5.0 software (GraphPad, USA).

Abbreviations

MNV: Murine norovirus; RT-PCR: Reverse transcriptase polymerase chain reaction; RT-RPA: Reverse transcriptase recombinase polymerase amplification

Acknowledgments

We would like to thank LetPub (www.letpub.com) for providing linguistic assistance during the preparation of this manuscript.

Funding

This work was supported by grants from Science and Technology Program of Guangdong Province, China (2017A030303026, 2017B030314171, 2017A070702001, 2017A030303025, 2016A030303016) and Science and Technology Program of Guangzhou, China (201707010440). The funders had no role in the design of the study, collection, analysis, and interpretation of data, nor writing of the manuscript.

Authors' contributions

PJG and LM designed the study and drafted the manuscript. LM and FWZ conducted the experiments, data analysis, and participated in drafting of the manuscript. FC, BHH, YJZ, MLW, FJX, RH helped with the experiments. WY contributed to the revision of the manuscript. All the authors read and approved the final manuscript.

Consent for publication

Not applicable

Competing interests

The authors declare that they have no competing interests.

Author details

[1]Guangdong Key Laboratory of Laboratory Animals, Guangdong Laboratory Animals Monitoring Institute, Guangzhou, China. [2]College of Veterinary Medicine, South China Agricultural University, Guangzhou 510640, China.

References

1. Zheng DP, Ando T, Fankhauser RL, Beard RS, Glass RI, Monroe SS. Norovirus classification and proposed strain nomenclature. Virology. 2006;346(2):312–23.
2. Hsu CC, Riley LK, Livingston RS. Molecular characterization of three novel murine noroviruses. Virus Genes. 2007;34(2):147–55.
3. Karst SM, Wobus CE, Lay M, Davidson J, Virgin HW. STAT1-dependent innate immunity to a Norwalk-like virus. Science. 2003;299(5612):1575–8.
4. Hsu CC, Riley LK, Wills HM, Livingston RS. Persistent infection with and serologic cross-reactivity of three novel murine noroviruses. Comp Med. 2006;56(4):247–51.
5. Muller B, Klemm U, Mas Marques A, Schreier E. Genetic diversity and recombination of murine noroviruses in immunocompromised mice. Arch Virol. 2007;152(9):1709–19.
6. Smith DB, McFadden N, Blundell RJ, Meredith A, Simmonds P. Diversity of murine norovirus in wild-rodent populations: species-specific associations suggest an ancient divergence. J Gen Virol. 2012;93(Pt 2):259–66.
7. Thackray LB, Wobus CE, Chachu KA, Liu B, Alegre ER, Henderson KS, Kelley ST. Virgin HWt: murine noroviruses comprising a single genogroup exhibit biological diversity despite limited sequence divergence. J Virol. 2007;81(19):10460–73.
8. Hsu CC, Wobus CE, Steffen EK, Riley LK, Livingston RS. Development of a microsphere-based serologic multiplexed fluorescent immunoassay and a reverse transcriptase PCR assay to detect murine norovirus 1 infection in mice. Clin Diagn Lab Immunol. 2005;12(10):1145–51.
9. Pritchett-Corning KR, Cosentino J, Clifford CB. Contemporary prevalence of infectious agents in laboratory mice and rats. Lab Anim. 2009;43(2):165–73.
10. Kitagawa Y, Tohya Y, Ike F, Kajita A, Park SJ, Ishii Y, Kyuwa S, Yoshikawa Y. Indirect ELISA and indirect immunofluorescent antibody assay for detecting the antibody against murine norovirus S7 in mice. Exp Anim. 2010;59(1):47–55.
11. Cadwell K, Patel KK, Maloney NS, Liu TC, Ng AC, Storer CE, Head RD, Xavier R, Stappenbeck TS, Virgin HW. Virus-plus-susceptibility gene interaction determines Crohn's disease gene Atg16L1 phenotypes in intestine. Cell. 2010;141(7):1135–45.
12. Higgins PD, Johnson LA, Sauder K, Moons D, Blanco L, Taube S, Wobus CE. Transient or persistent norovirus infection does not alter the pathology of Salmonella typhimurium induced intestinal inflammation and fibrosis in mice. Comp Immunol Microbiol Infect Dis. 2011;34(3):247–57.
13. Compton SR. Prevention of murine norovirus infection in neonatal mice by fostering. J Am Assoc Lab Anim Sci. 2008;47(3):25–30.
14. Tajima M, Kotani Y, Kurosawa T, Miyasaka M. Pitfalls in mouse norovirus (MNV) detection in fecal samples using RT-PCR, and construction of new MNV-specific primers. Exp Anim. 2013;62(2):127–35.
15. Baert L, Wobus CE, Van Coillie E, Thackray LB, Debevere J, Uyttendaele M. Detection of murine norovirus 1 by using plaque assay, transfection assay, and real-time reverse transcription-PCR before and after heat exposure. Appl Environ Microbiol. 2008;74(2):543–6.
16. Hanaki K, Ike F, Kajita A, Yasuno W, Yanagiba M, Goto M, Sakai K, Ami Y, Kyuwa S. Detection of murine norovirus by reverse transcription loop-mediated isothermal amplification. J Virol Methods. 2014;204:17–24.
17. Lillis L, Siverson J, Lee A, Cantera J, Parker M, Piepenburg O, Lehman DA, Boyle DS. Factors influencing recombinase polymerase amplification (RPA) assay outcomes at point of care. Mol Cell Probes. 2016;30(2):74–8.
18. Yang Y, Qin X, Wang G, Zhang Y, Shang Y, Zhang Z. Development of a fluorescent probe-based recombinase polymerase amplification assay for rapid detection of Orf virus. Virol J. 2015;12:206.
19. Yang Y, Qin X, Wang G, Jin J, Shang Y, Zhang Z. Development of an isothermoal amplification-based assay for rapid visual detection of an Orf virus. Virol J. 2016;13:46.

20. Yang Y, Qin X, Zhang X, Zhao Z, Zhang W, Zhu X, Cong G, Li Y, Zhang Z. Development of real-time and lateral flow dipstick recombinase polymerase amplification assays for rapid detection of goatpox virus and sheeppox virus. Virol J. 2017;14(1):131.
21. Yang Y, Qin X, Song Y, Zhang W, Hu G, Dou Y, Li Y, Zhang Z. Development of real-time and lateral flow strip reverse transcription recombinase polymerase amplification assays for rapid detection of peste des petits ruminants virus. Virol J. 2017;14(1):24.
22. Piepenburg O, Williams CH, Stemple DL, Armes NA. DNA detection using recombination proteins. PLoS Biol. 2006;4(7):e204.
23. Amer HM, Abd El Wahed A, Shalaby MA, Almajhdi FN, Hufert FT, Weidmann M. A new approach for diagnosis of bovine coronavirus using a reverse transcription recombinase polymerase amplification assay. J Virol Methods. 2013;193(2):337–40.
24. Moore MD, Jaykus LA. Development of a recombinase polymerase amplification assay for detection of epidemic human noroviruses. Sci Rep. 2017;7:40244.
25. Yehia N, Arafa AS, Abd El Wahed A, El-Sanousi AA, Weidmann M, Shalaby MA. Development of reverse transcription recombinase polymerase amplification assay for avian influenza H5N1 HA gene detection. J Virol Methods. 2015;223:45–9.
26. Bae J, Schwab KJ. Evaluation of murine norovirus, feline calicivirus, poliovirus, and MS2 as surrogates for human norovirus in a model of viral persistence in surface water and groundwater. Appl Environ Microbiol. 2008; 74(2):477–84.
27. Kitajima M, Oka T, Takagi H, Tohya Y, Katayama H, Takeda N, Katayama K. Development and application of a broadly reactive real-time reverse transcription-PCR assay for detection of murine noroviruses. J Virol Methods. 2010;169(2):269–73.
28. Hanaki K, Ike F, Kajita A, Yasuno W, Yanagiba M, Goto M, Sakai K, Ami Y, Kyuwa S. A broadly reactive one-step SYBR green I real-time RT-PCR assay for rapid detection of murine norovirus. PLoS One. 2014;9(5):e98108.
29. Wang HM, Zhao GM, Hou PL, Yu L, He CQ, He HB. Rapid detection of foot-and-mouth disease virus using reverse transcription recombinase polymerase amplification combined with a lateral flow dipstick. J Virol Methods. 2018;261:46–50.
30. Vasileva Wand NI, Bonney LC, Watson RJ, Graham V, Hewson R. Point-of-care diagnostic assay for the detection of Zika virus using the recombinase polymerase amplification method. J Gen Virol. 2018;99(8):1012–26.
31. Chen J, Xu Y, Yan H, Zhu Y, Wang L, Zhang Y, Lu Y, Xing W. Sensitive and rapid detection of pathogenic bacteria from urine samples using multiplex recombinase polymerase amplification. Lab Chip. 2018;18(16):2441–52.
32. Ma L, Cong F, Zhu Y, Wu M, Xu F, Huang R, Moore RJ, Guo P. Development of a reverse transcription recombinase polymerase amplification assay for rapid detection of Theiler's murine encephalomyelitis virus. Mol Cell Probes. 2018;41:27–31.
33. Abd El Wahed A, El-Deeb A, El-Tholoth M, Abd El Kader H, Ahmed A, Hassan S, Hoffmann B, Haas B, Shalaby MA, Hufert FT, et al. A portable reverse transcription recombinase polymerase amplification assay for rapid detection of foot-and-mouth disease virus. PLoS One. 2013;8(8):e71642.
34. Boyle DS, Lehman DA, Lillis L, Peterson D, Singhal M, Armes N, Parker M, Piepenburg O, Overbaugh J. Rapid detection of HIV-1 proviral DNA for early infant diagnosis using recombinase polymerase amplification. mBio. 2013;4(2): e00135–13. https://doi.org/10.1128/mBio.00135-13.
35. Yuan W, Zhang Y, Wang J, Liu XM, Zhao WB, Huang R. Isolation, identification and genetic analysis of a murine norovirus strain. Bing Du Xue Bao = Chin J Virol. 2014;30(4):359–68.
36. Yuan W, Wang J, Xu F, Huang B, Lian Y, Rao D, Yin X, Wu M, Zhu Y, Zhang Y, et al. Development of a duplex real-time RT-PCR for the simultaneous detection and differentiation of Theiler's murine encephalomyelitis virus and rat theilovirus. J Virol Methods. 2016;236:139–46.

Permissions

All chapters in this book were first published in VR, by BioMed Central; hereby published with permission under the Creative Commons Attribution License or equivalent. Every chapter published in this book has been scrutinized by our experts. Their significance has been extensively debated. The topics covered herein carry significant findings which will fuel the growth of the discipline. They may even be implemented as practical applications or may be referred to as a beginning point for another development.

The contributors of this book come from diverse backgrounds, making this book a truly international effort. This book will bring forth new frontiers with its revolutionizing research information and detailed analysis of the nascent developments around the world.

We would like to thank all the contributing authors for lending their expertise to make the book truly unique. They have played a crucial role in the development of this book. Without their invaluable contributions this book wouldn't have been possible. They have made vital efforts to compile up to date information on the varied aspects of this subject to make this book a valuable addition to the collection of many professionals and students.

This book was conceptualized with the vision of imparting up-to-date information and advanced data in this field. To ensure the same, a matchless editorial board was set up. Every individual on the board went through rigorous rounds of assessment to prove their worth. After which they invested a large part of their time researching and compiling the most relevant data for our readers.

The editorial board has been involved in producing this book since its inception. They have spent rigorous hours researching and exploring the diverse topics which have resulted in the successful publishing of this book. They have passed on their knowledge of decades through this book. To expedite this challenging task, the publisher supported the team at every step. A small team of assistant editors was also appointed to further simplify the editing procedure and attain best results for the readers.

Apart from the editorial board, the designing team has also invested a significant amount of their time in understanding the subject and creating the most relevant covers. They scrutinized every image to scout for the most suitable representation of the subject and create an appropriate cover for the book.

The publishing team has been an ardent support to the editorial, designing and production team. Their endless efforts to recruit the best for this project, has resulted in the accomplishment of this book. They are a veteran in the field of academics and their pool of knowledge is as vast as their experience in printing. Their expertise and guidance has proved useful at every step. Their uncompromising quality standards have made this book an exceptional effort. Their encouragement from time to time has been an inspiration for everyone.

The publisher and the editorial board hope that this book will prove to be a valuable piece of knowledge for researchers, students, practitioners and scholars across the globe.

List of Contributors

Salvatore Catania and Elisa Baldasso
Istituto Zooprofilattico Sperimentale delle Venezie, viale dell'Universita' 10, Legnaro, 35020 Padova, Italy

Federica Gobbo and Maria Luisa Moronato
Istituto Zooprofilattico Sperimentale delle Venezie, viale dell'Universita' 10, Legnaro, 35020 Padova, Italy
Università degli Studi di Padova, Dipartimento di Medicina Animale, Produzioni e Salute (MAPS), Legnaro, Padova, Italy

Ana S. Ramirez
Unidad de Epidemiología y Medicina Preventiva, Facultad de Veterinaria, Universidad de Las Palmas de Gran Canaria, C/Trasmontala s/n, Arucas 35413Islas Canarias, Spain

Davide Guadagnini
Parco Faunistico LE CORNELLE, Valbrembo, Bergamo, Italy

Robin A. J. Nicholas
Nutshell Lane, Farnham, Surrey GU9 0HG, UK

James Wabwire Oguttu
Department of Agriculture and Animal Health, College of Agriculture and Environmental Sciences, University of South Africa, Florida Science Campus, Johannesburg, South Africa

Agricola Odoi
Department of Agriculture and Animal Health, College of Agriculture and Environmental Sciences, University of South Africa, Florida Science Campus, Johannesburg, South Africa
Biomedical and Diagnostic Sciences, College of Veterinary Medicine, University of Tennessee, Knoxville, USA

Daniel Nenene Qekwana
Section Veterinary Public Health, Department of Paraclinical Sciences, Faculty of Veterinary Sciences, University of Pretoria, Pretoria, South Africa

Tommaso Banzato and Alessandro Zotti
Department of Animal Medicine, Production and Health, Clinical Section, Radiology Unit, University of Padua, Viale dell'Università 16, Legnaro 35020, Padua, Italy

Federico Bonsembiante and Luca Aresu
Department of Comparative Biomedicine and Food Science, University of Padua, Viale dell'Università 16, Legnaro 35020, Padua, Italy

Bitsu Kiflu
Ministry of Livestock and Fisheries, Addis Ababa, Ethiopia

Haile Alemayehu, Yohannes Negash and Tadesse Eguale
Aklilu Lemma Institute of Pathobiology, Addis Ababa University, Addis Ababa, Ethiopia

Mukarim Abdurahaman
College of Agriculture and Veterinary Medicine, Jimma University

Fuchang Yu, Yayun Wu, Jianke Cao, Suhui Hu, Sumei Zhang, Rongjun Wang, Changshen Ning and Longxian Zhang
College of Animal Science and Veterinary Medicine, Henan Agricultural University, Zhengzhou 450002, People's Republic of China
International Joint Research Laboratory for Zoonotic Diseases of Henan, Zhengzhou 450002, People's Republic of China

Huili Zhu
College of Animal Science and Veterinary Medicine, Henan Agricultural University, Zhengzhou 450002, People's Republic of China
College of Animal Science, Henan Institute of Science and Technology, Xinxiang 453003, People's Republic of China

Jiantang Wang and Tongyi Li
Zhengzhou Zoo, Zhengzhou 450000, People's Republic of China

Sarah C. Roode
Department of Molecular Biomedical Sciences, College of Veterinary Medicine, North Carolina State University, CVM Research Building – Room 348, 1060 William Moore Drive, Raleigh 27607, NC, USA

Matthew Breen
Department of Molecular Biomedical Sciences, College of Veterinary Medicine, North Carolina State University, CVM Research Building - Room 348, 1060 William Moore Drive, Raleigh 27607, NC, USA
Comparative Medicine Institute, North Carolina State University, Raleigh, NC, USA
Cancer Genetics Program, Lineberger Comprehensive Cancer Center, University of North Carolina, Chapel Hill, NC, USA

Daniel Rotroff
Bioinformatics Research Center, Department of Statistics, North Carolina State University, Raleigh, NC, USA

Alison Motsinger-Reif
BioinformaticsResearch Center, Department of Statistics, North Carolina State University, Raleigh, NC, USA
Comparative Medicine Institute, North Carolina State University, Raleigh, NC, USA

Kristy L. Richards
Department of Medicine, University of North Carolina, Chapel Hill, NC, USA
Comparative Medicine Institute, North Carolina State University, Raleigh, NC, USA
Cancer Genetics Program, Lineberger Comprehensive Cancer Center, University of North Carolina, Chapel Hill, NC, USA
Department of Biomedical Sciences, Cornell University, Ithaca, NY, USA

Steven E. Suter
Comparative Medicine Institute, North Carolina State University, Raleigh, NC, USA
Cancer Genetics Program, Lineberger Comprehensive Cancer Center, University of North Carolina, Chapel Hill, NC, USA
Department of Clinical Sciences, College of Veterinary Medicine, North Carolina State University, CVM Research Building - Room 308, 1051 William Moore Drive, Raleigh, NC 27607, USA

Peter Moore
Department of Pathology, Microbiology, and Immunology, College of Veterinary Medicine, University of California, Davis, CA, USA

Yasuhiko Okamura
Veterinary Teaching Hospital, Faculty of Agriculture, Iwate University, Morioka, Japan

Takuya Mizuno
Laboratory of Veterinary Internal Medicine, Faculty of AgricultureYamaguchi University, Yamaguchi, Japan

Hajime Tsujimoto
Graduate School of Agricultural and Life Sciences, University of Tokyo, Bunkyo, Japan

Victor R. Simpson
Wildlife Veterinary Investigation Centre, Chacewater, Truro, Cornwall TR4 8PB, UK

David N. Fisher
Centre for Ecology and Conservation, University of Exeter, Penryn, Cornwall TR10 9FE, UK
Department for Integrative Biology, University of Guelph, Guelph, ON N1G 2W1, Canada

Xiaoxing Wang, Yanyan Cui, Yan Zhang, Ke Shi, Yaqun Yan, Fuchun Jian, Longxian Zhang, Rongjun Wang and Changshen Ning
College of Animal Science and Veterinary Medicine, Henan Agricultural University, Zhengzhou 450002, People's Republic of China

S. Cériac, D. Feuillet, Y. Félicité, H. Archimède and J.-C. Bambou
URZ, INRA, 97170 Petit-Bourg, Guadeloupe, France

C. Jayles and R. Arquet
PTEA, INRA, 97170 Le Moule, Guadeloupe, France

Yang Yu, Yu Feng Zhou, Jian Sun and Xiao Ping Liao
National Risk Assessment Laboratory for Antimicrobial Resistance of Animal Original Bacteria, South China Agricultural University, Guangzhou 510642, China
Guangdong Provincial Key Laboratory of Veterinary Pharmaceutics Development and Safety Evaluation, South China Agricultural University, Guangzhou 510642, China
Laboratory of Veterinary Pharmacology, College of Veterinary Medicine, South China Agricultural University, Guangzhou, Guangdong 510642, China

Wei Shi
National Risk Assessment Laboratory for Antimicrobial Resistance of Animal Original Bacteria, South China Agricultural University, Guangzhou 510642, China
Laboratory of Veterinary Pharmacology, College of Veterinary Medicine, South China Agricultural University, Guangzhou, Guangdong 510642, China

Ya Hong Liu
National Risk Assessment Laboratory for Antimicrobial Resistance of Animal Original Bacteria, South China Agricultural University, Guangzhou 510642, China
Guangdong Provincial Key Laboratory of Veterinary Pharmaceutics Development and Safety Evaluation, South China Agricultural University, Guangzhou 510642, China
Laboratory of Veterinary Pharmacology, College of Veterinary Medicine, South China Agricultural University, Guangzhou, Guangdong 510642, China
College of Veterinary Medicine, National Reference Laboratory of Veterinary Drug Residues, South China Agricultural University, Guangzhou 510642, China

Yaxin Li, Jianjun Dai, Xiangkai Zhuge, Haojin Wang, Lin Hu, Jianluan Ren, Ling Chen, Dezhi Li and Fang Tang
Key Laboratory Animal Bacteriology, Ministry of Agriculture, College of veterinary medicine, Nanjing Agricultural University, No.1 Weigang, Nanjing 210095, Jiangsu province, People's Republic of China

Kamelia M. Osman and Ahmed Orabi
Department of Microbiology, Faculty of Veterinary Medicine, Cairo University, Giza, Egypt

Khalid S. Al-Maary, Aymen S. Mubarak, Turki M. Dawoud and Ihab M. I. Moussa
Department of Botany and Microbiology, College of Science, King Saud University, Riyadh, Kingdom of Saudi Arabia

Mai D. S. Ibrahim
Department of Public Health, College of Applied Medical Science, King Khalid University, Abha, Kingdom of Saudi Arabia

Ashgan M. Hessain
Department of Health Science, College of Applied Studies and Community Service, King Saud University, Riyadh, Kingdom of Saudi Arabia

Nehal M. Fawzy
Department of Fish Diseases and Management, Animal Health Research Institute, Dokki, Giza, Egypt

Isa Serrano, José Pedro Santos, Alexandre Leitão, Luis Tavares and Manuela Oliveira
CIISA/Faculty of Veterinary Medicine, University of Lisbon, Lisbon, Portugal

Daniel De Vos, Florence Bilocq and Jean-Paul Pirnay
Laboratory for Molecular and Cellular Technology, Queen Astrid Military Hospital, Brussels, Belgium

Giancarlo Avallone
Department of Veterinary Medical Sciences (DIMEVET), University of Bologna, Ozzano dell'Emilia, Italy

Elena Riccardi and Annalisa Forlani
IDEXX Laboratories Ltd. Grange House, Sandbeck Way, Wetherby, West Yorkshire LS22 7DN, UK

Guido Grilli, Paola Roccabianca and Marco Tecilla
Department of Veterinary Medicine, University of Milan, Via Celoria 10, 20100 Milan, Italy

Sara Belluco
Equipe recherche UPSP ICE 2011-03-101: Oncology, and Laboratoire de Pathologie et Morphologie Clinique, Vetagro-sup, France

Sara Francesca Santagostino
Laboratory of Comparative Pathology, Memorial Sloan Kettering Cancer Center, 1275 York Av, New York, USA

Kiumars Khadivi
Private practicioner, Milan, Italy

Paweł Lisowski, Justyna Jarczak, Lech Zwierzchowski and Emilia Bagnicka
Department of Animal Improvement, Institute of Genetics and Animal Breeding Polish Academy of Sciences, 36a Postepu str., Jastrzebiec 05-552, Poland

Ewa M Kosciuczuk
Department of Animal Improvement, Institute of Genetics and Animal Breeding Polish Academy of Sciences, 36a Postepu str., Jastrzebiec 05-552, Poland
Robert H. Lurie Comprehensive Cancer Center, Northwestern University, Chicago, IL, USA

Alicja Majewska
Department of Physiological Sciences, Faculty of Veterinary Medicine, Warsaw University of Life Sciences, 02-776 Warsaw, Poland

Magdalena Rzewuska
Department of Pre-Clinical Sciences, Faculty of Veterinary Medicine, Warsaw University of Life Sciences, 02-776 Warsaw, Poland

Ruben Pérez, Ana Marandino, Gonzalo Tomás and Lucía Calleros
Sección Genética Evolutiva, Facultad de Ciencias, Iguá 4225, Montevideo 11400, Uruguay

Gregorio Iraola
Sección Genética Evolutiva, Facultad de Ciencias, Iguá 4225, Montevideo 11400, Uruguay
Unidad de Bioinformática, Institut Pasteur Montevideo, Montevideo, Uruguay

Claudia Morsella, Alejandra Méndez, Fernando Paolicchi and Alejandra Velilla
Laboratorio de Bacteriología, Unidad Integrada INTA-Universidad Nacional de Mar del Plata, Balcarce, Argentina

Laura Betancor
Departamento de Bacteriología y Virología, Instituto de Higiene, Facultad de Medicina, Universidad de la República, Montevideo, Uruguay

Alessandra Piccirillo
Dipartimento di Biomedicina Comparata e Alimentazione, Università degli Studi di Padova, Padova, Italy

Min Li, Feng Yang, Jing Li, Jilei Zhang, Yaoyao Wang, Jiawei Wang and Xin Zhou
Yangzhou University College of Veterinary Medicine, Yangzhou, Jiangsu, People's Republic of China

Chengming Wang
Yangzhou University College of Veterinary Medicine, Yangzhou, Jiangsu, People's Republic of China
College of Veterinary Medicine, Auburn University, Auburn, Alabama, USA

Martina Jelocnik and Adam Polkinghorne
Centre for Animal Health Innovation, Faculty of Science, Health, Education & Engineering, University of the Sunshine Coast, QLD, Maroochydore, Australia

Jianseng Gong
Poultry Institute, Chinese Academy of Agricultural Sciences, Yangzhou, Jiangsu, China

Bernhard Kaltenboeck
College of Veterinary Medicine, Auburn University, Auburn, Alabama, USA

Zhixin Feng
Institute of Veterinary Medicine, Jiangsu Academy of Agricultural Sciences; Key Laboratory of Veterinary Biological Engineering and Technology, Ministry of Agriculture, National Center for Engineering Research of Veterinary Bio-Products, Nanjing, China

Yvonne Pannekoek
Academic Medical Center, University of Amsterdam, Amsterdam, The Netherlands

Nicole Borel
Institute for Veterinary Pathology, Vetsuisse Faculty, University of Zurich, Zurich, Switzerland

Chunlian Song
Yunnan Agricultural University College of Animal Science & Technology, Kunming, Yunnan, China

Ping Jiang
Key Laboratory of Animal Diseases Diagnostic and Immunology, Ministry of Agriculture, College of Veterinary Medicine, Nanjing Agricultural University, Nanjing, China

Sonja Kittl, Isabelle Brodard, Lorenz Rychener, Jörg Jores and Stefanie Gobeli Brawand
Institute of Veterinary Bacteriology, Vetsuisse Faculty, University of Bern, Laenggassstrasse 122, CH 3001 Bern, Switzerland

Petra Roosje
Division of Clinical Dermatology, Department of Clinical Veterinary Medicine, Vetsuisse Faculty, University of Bern, Bremgartenstrasse 109a, CH-3001 Bern, Switzerland
DermFocus, Vetsuisse Faculty, University of Bern, Bern, Switzerland

Manita Subedi
Department of Drug Administration, Government of Nepal, Bijulibazar, Kathmandu, Nepal

Himal Luitel and Bhuminanda Devkota
Center for Biotechnology, Agriculture and Forestry University, Rampur, Chitwan, Nepal

Rebanta Kumar Bhattarai
Department of Veterinary Microbiology and Parasitology, Agriculture and Forestry University, Rampur, Chitwan, Nepal

Sarita Phuyal
Department of Veterinary Science & Animal Husbandry, Himalayan College of Agriculture Sciences and Technology, Kathmandu, Nepal

Prabhat Panthi
Department of Microbiology, National College, Kathmandu, Nepal

Anil Shrestha
Department of Microbiology, Balkumari College, Bharatpur, Chitwan, Nepal

Dhiraj Kumar Chaudhary
Department of Microbiology, Prithu Technical College, Institute of Agriculture and Animal Science, Tribhuvan University, Lamahi, Dang, Nepal

Susanne Küker, Celine Faverjon and John Berezowski
Veterinary Public Health Institute, Vetsuisse Faculty, University of Bern, Schwarzenburgstrasse 155, 3097, Liebefeld, Switzerland

Flavie Vial
Veterinary Public Health Institute, Vetsuisse Faculty, University of Bern, Schwarzenburgstrasse 155, 3097, Liebefeld, Switzerland
Epi-Connect, Skogås, Sweden

Lenz Furrer and Fabio Rinaldi
Institute of Computational Linguistics, University of Zürich, Andreasstrasse 15, 8050 Zürich, Switzerland

Horst Posthaus
Institute of Animal Pathology, University of Bern, Länggassstrasse 122, 3012 Bern, Switzerland

Raashid Ahmed, Uneeb Urwat, Syed Mudasir Ahmad, Peerzada Tajamul Mumtaz, Shakil Ahmad Bhat1, Nadeem Shabir, Hina Fayaz Bhat and Riaz Ahmad Shah
Division of Biotechnology, Faculty of Veterinary Sciences and Animal Husbandry, Shuhama, Sher-e Kashmir University of Agricultural Sciences and Technology – Kashmir, Srinagar, India

Mashooq Ahmad Dar
Division of Biotechnology, Faculty of Veterinary Sciences and Animal Husbandry, Shuhama, Sher-e-Kashmir University of Agricultural Sciences and Technology – Kashmir, Srinagar, India
Depatment of BiochemistryUniversity of Kashmir, Srinagar, India

Tanveer Ali Dar
Depatment of BiochemistryUniversity of Kashmir, Srinagar, India

Zahid Amin Kushoo and Pervaiz Ahmad Dar
Division of Veterinary Microbiology, Faculty of Veterinary Sciences and Animal Husbandry, Shuhama, SKUAST-K, Srinagar, India

Umar Amin
Division of Veterinary Pathology, Faculty of Veterinary Sciences and Animal Husbandry, Shuhama, SKUAST-K, Srinagar, India

Nazir Ahmad Ganai
Division of Animal Breeding and Genetics, Faculty of Veterinary Sciences and Animal Husbandry, Shuhama, SKUAST-K, Srinagar, India

Mohammad Heidari
USDA, Agricultural Research Service, Avian Disease and Oncology Laboratory, 4279 E. Mount Hope Rd., East Lansing, MI 48823, USA

Srdjan Cirovic
The Centre for Biomedical Engineering, University of Surrey, Guildford GU2 7XH, UK

Robert Lloyd
The Centre for Biomedical Engineering, University of Surrey, Guildford GU2 7XH, UK
Neuroscience Research Australia and Prince of Wales Clinical School, University of New South Wales, Sydney, NSW 2031, Australia

Clare Rusbridge
The School of Veterinary Medicine, University of Surrey, Guildford GU2 7AD, UK
Fitzpatrick Referrals, Eashing, Halfway Lane, Goadalming GU7 2QQ, UK

Jelena Jovanovik
Fitzpatrick Referrals, Eashing, Halfway Lane, Goadalming GU7 2QQ, UK

Holger A. Volk
Clinical Science and Services, Royal Veterinary College, Hatfield AL9 7TA, UK

Lei Ma, Feng Cong, Bihong Huang, Yujun Zhu, Miaoli Wu, Fengjiao Xu, Wen Yuan, Ren Huang and Pengju Guo
Guangdong Key Laboratory of Laboratory Animals, Guangdong Laboratory Animals Monitoring Institute, Guangzhou, China

Fanwen Zeng
College of Veterinary Medicine, South China Agricultural University, Guangzhou 510640, China

Index

CPSIA information can be obtained
at www.ICGtesting.com
Printed in the USA
BVHW021123170223
658734BV00006B/642

9 781639 275243